Contempo

CHRISTOPHER P. CANNON, MD

SERIES EDITOR

More information about this series at
http://www.springer.com/series/7677

M. Gabriel Khan

Cardiac Drug Therapy

8th Edition

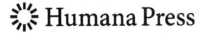 Humana Press

M. Gabriel Khan, MD, FRCPC, FRCP (London), FACC
University of Ottawa
The Ottawa Hospital
Ottawa, ON, Canada

ISSN 2196-8969   ISSN 2196-8977 (electronic)
ISBN 978-1-61779-961-7   ISBN 978-1-61779-962-4 (eBook)
DOI 10.1007/978-1-61779-962-4
Springer Totowa Heidelberg New York Dordrecht London

Library of Congress Control Number: 2014952818

Printed on acid-free paper

Humana Press is a brand of Springer
Springer is part of Springer Science+Business Media (www.springer.com)

To My wife Brigid
and to our
Children
Susan, Christine, Yasmin,
Jacqueline, Stephen,
and Natasha
And to our
Grandchildren
Sarah, Patrick, Emma,
Kathleen, Michael, Roxanna,
Fiona, Jaxson, James, Fraea,
Esmé, Jordan, and Joshua

Preface

Several foreign translations and favorable reviews of earlier editions provided the impetus to produce an eighth edition of *Cardiac Drug Therapy*. Here is a review of the fifth edition in *Clinical Cardiology*: "this is an excellent book. It succeeds in being practical while presenting the major evidence in relation to its recommendations. Of value to absolutely anyone who prescribes for cardiac patients on the day-to-day basis. From the trainee to the experienced consultant, all will find it useful. The author stamps his authority very clearly throughout the text by very clear assertions of his own recommendations even when these recommendations are at odds with those of official bodies. In such situations the 'official' recommendations are also stated but clearly are not preferred."

And for the fourth edition a cardiologist reviewer states that it is "by far the best handbook on cardiovascular therapeutics I have ever had the pleasure of reading. The information given in each chapter is up-to-date, accurate, clearly written, eminently readable and well referenced."

The entire text has been revised and, most importantly, continues to give practical clinical advice. New chapters include:

• Endocrine Heart Diseases
• Management of Cardiomyopathies
• Newer Agents

A new feature involves diagnosis.

- Because appropriate therapy requires sound diagnosis the short sections on diagnosis given in previous editions have been expanded.

Other highlights include:

- Chapter 11: "Acute Myocardial Infarction" contains more than 24 relevant ECG tracings; an echocardiogram depicting Takotsubo syndrome is shown to remind readers that this syndrome mimics acute MI.
- Chapter 14: "Management of Cardiac Arrhythmias" provides more than 24 ECG samples.
- Chapter 22: "Hallmark Clinical Trials" has been expanded to accommodate the wealth of practical information derived from recent randomized clinical trials.

As in all previous editions, therapeutic strategies and advice are based on a thorough review of the scientific literature, applied logically:

- Scientific documentation regarding which drugs are superior.
- Information on which cardiovascular drugs to choose and which agents to avoid in various clinical situations.
- Information that assists with the rapid writing of prescriptions. To write a prescription accurately, a practitioner needs to know how a drug is supplied and its dosage. Thus, supply and dosage are given first, followed by action and pharmacokinetics, and then advice as to efficacy and comparison with other drugs, indications, adverse effects, and interactions.

The text contains practical advice, such as the following: *The life-saving potential of 160–240 mg chewable aspirin is denied to many individuals who succumb to an acute coronary syndrome because of poor dissemination of clinically proven, documented facts.* The text advises: three ~80 mg chewable aspirins should be placed in the cap of a nitrolingual spray container to be used before proceeding to an emergency room. *Clinicians should inform patients that rapidly acting chewable aspirin may prevent a heart attack or death but that nitroglycerin does not.* The world faces an epidemic of heart failure [HF].

Although medical therapy for acute HF has improved dramatically from 1990, unfortunately more than 50 % of patients require readmission within 6 months of discharge. Several of these patients are not administered appropriate medications to prevent a recurrence. The chapter on heart failure gives practical advice as do other chapters on what drugs are best for a given situation.

Notable physicians have stated that the beta-blockers should not be prescribed for primary hypertension because of their ineffectiveness. Many investigators have reported in peer-reviewed journals that diuretics and beta-blockers cause diabetes and their use should be restricted for the management of hypertension. Chapter 2 discusses these controversies and gives clear answers to clinicians worldwide.

The information provided in the eighth edition should serve as a refresher for cardiologists and internists. The information should improve the therapeutic skills of interns, medical residents, generalists, and all who care for patients with cardiac problems.

Ottawa, ON   *M. Gabriel Khan*

Acknowledgment

I have quoted the published works of several investigators. These persevering women and men of medicine deserve my respect and my thanks.

A special, thank you, to my wife Brigid, who has allowed me to be a student of the science of Medicine to this day.

Ottawa, ON   **M. Gabriel Khan**

Contents

About the Author

Dr. M. Gabriel Khan is a cardiologist at the Ottawa Hospital and an Associate Professor of Medicine, at the University of Ottawa. Dr. Khan graduated MB, BCh, with First-Class Honors at The Queen's University of Belfast. He obtained, by thesis, the Degree of Doctor of Medicine with Honors [QUB].

Gabriel is a clinical Professor who loves teaching and was appointed Staff Physician in charge of a Clinical Teaching Unit at the Ottawa General hospital and is a Fellow of the American College of Cardiology, the American College of Physicians, and the Royal College of Physicians of London and Canada.

He is the author of *Encyclopedia of Heart Diseases* (2006), Academic Press/Elsevier; *Encyclopedia of Heart Diseases*, 2nd ed., Springer, New York. Online 2011; *Rapid ECG Interpretation*, 3rd ed., Humana Press New York 2008; *Cardiac Drug Therapy*, 7th ed., Humana Press 2007; *On Call Cardiology*, 3rd ed., Elsevier, Philadelphia (2006); *Heart Disease Diagnosis and Therapy*, 2nd ed., Humana Press (2006); *Cardiac and Pulmonary Management* (1993); *Medical Diagnosis and Therapy* (1994); *Heart Attacks, Hypertension and Heart Drugs* (1986); and *Heart Trouble Encyclopedia* (1996).

Dr. Khan's books have been translated into Chinese, Czech, Farsi, French, German, Greek, Italian, Japanese, Polish, Portuguese, Russian, Spanish, and Turkish. He has built a reputation as a clinician-teacher and has become an internationally acclaimed cardiologist through his writings.

Here is an excerpt from the foreword, written by a renowned cardiologist and author, Dr. Henry J. L. Marriott for the book, *Heart Disease Diagnosis and Therapy*:

> Whenever I read Khan, I am affected as the rustics were by Oliver Goldsmith's parson:
> And still they gaz'd, and still the wonder grew
> That one small head could carry all he knew.
> Khan's knowledge is truly encyclopedic and, for his fortunate readers, he translates it into easily read prose.

His peers have acknowledged the merits of his books by their reviews of *Cardiac Drug Therapy, the Encyclopedia of Heart Diseases, and Rapid ECG Interpretation.*

1

Beta-Blockers
The Cornerstone of Cardiac Drug Therapy

THIS CHAPTER TELLS YOU

- Which beta-blocker is best for your patients.

  The pharmacodynamic reasons why atenolol is a relatively ineffective beta-blocker and why the vast worldwide use of atenolol should be curtailed.

- More about the important indication for heart failure (HF), for New York Heart Association (NYHA) class II and III and compensated class IV, and for all with left ventricular (LV) dysfunction regardless of functional class; thus, in class I patients with an ejection fraction (EF) <40 % and in those with myocardial infarction (MI) with HF or LV dysfunction without HF, beta-blockers are recommended at the same level as angiotensin-converting enzyme (ACE) inhibitors. Beta-blockers are the mainstay of therapy for heart failure. They decrease total mortality, an effect only modestly provided by ACE inhibitors, and marginally by angiotensin receptor blockers [ARBS]. See discussion under ARBs.

- *Why beta-blockers should be recommended for diabetic patients with hypertension with or without proteinuria* and for diabetic patients with coronary heart disease (CHD). From about 1990 to 2007, most internists proclaimed in editorials and to trainees that these agents were a poor choice in this setting.

© Springer Science+Business Media New York 2015
M. Gabriel Khan, *Cardiac Drug Therapy*, Contemporary Cardiology,
DOI 10.1007/978-1-61779-962-4_1

- More recently, their use as initial agents for the treatment of primary hypertension has been criticized, particularly for diabetics with hypertension; do beta-blocking drugs cause diabetes or is the condition observed, simply, benign glucose intolerance in some? *(see* Chap. 2)
- Why is it incorrect to say that *beta-blockers are not advisable for hypertensive patients over age 70,* as many teachers, textbooks, and editorials state.
- The results of randomized clinical trials (RCTs) that prove the lifesaving properties of these agents.
- All their indications.
- Salient points that relate to each beta-blocker and show the subtle and important differences confirming that beta-blockers are not all alike. Beta-blockade holds the key, but lipophilic vs. hydrophilic features may be important, and brain concentration may enhance cardioprotection.

BETA-BLOCKERS AND CARDIOPROTECTION

Sufficient attention has not been paid by the medical profession and researchers regarding the subtle differences that exist amongst the available beta-blocking drugs (Khan 2005). The subtle differences in beta-blockers may provide the solution for the apparent lack of protection of some beta-blockers (Khan and Topol 1996).

- The common threads for enhanced cardioprotection are beta1, beta2, and lipophilicity that augment brain concentration and may protect from sudden death. In the timolol study, there was a 67 % reduction in sudden death (The Norwegian Multicenter Study Group 1981).
- Timolol is non-cardioselective and lipophilic. No other cardiovascular agent has produced such an outstanding reduction in cardiac sudden deaths, yet the drug is rarely prescribed worldwide.
- Propranolol, a beta1, beta2 lipophilic drug, caused a 56 % decrease in early morning sudden death from acute myocardial infarction [MI]; see later discussion of BHAT (1982), and Peters et al. (1989)

- Atenolol, a non-lipophilic agent, has been the most pre-scribed beta-blocker in the USA and worldwide from 1980 to 2007 with more than 44 million prescriptions in the USA annually. The drug is a poorly effective beta-blocker and its use should become obsolete. Unfortunately, investigators and trialists not noticing the subtle differences that exist among the beta-blocking drugs have used atenolol in the majority of large RCTs of hypertension conducted from 1980 to the present time (see Beta-Blocker Hypertension Controversy). Lindholm et al. (2005) from a meta-analysis of hypertension RCTs without regard for beta-blockers' subtle differences described above reached a conclusion, which was printed on the front cover of the Lancet: "beta-blockers should not remain first choice in the treatment of primary hypertension" (Lindholm et al. 2005). Atenolol was the beta-blocker used in the majority of RCTs analyzed by Lindholm et al.

- A rebuttal stated, "by lumping together all randomized hypertension trials involving beta-blockers, Lars Lindholm and colleagues have arrived at misleading conclusions" (Cruickshank 2000). But rebuttals are observed by few cli-nicians. Many notable physicians have endorsed the find-ings of Lindholm and colleagues and the misleading information has been disseminated worldwide.

- Lipophilicity allows a high concentration of drug in the brain. This appears to block sympathetic discharge in the hypothalamus and elevate central vagal tone to a greater extent than water-soluble, hydrophilic agents (Pitt 1992). This may relate to the prevention of sudden cardiac death. Highly lipid-soluble, lipophilic beta-blockers—carvedilol, propranolol, nebivolol, timolol, and metoprolol—reach high concentrations in the brain and are metabolized in the liver.

- Atenolol, nadolol, and sotalol are lipid insoluble, show poor brain concentration, and are not hepatic metabolized; they are water soluble, are excreted by the kidneys, and have a long half-life. Pindolol and timolol are about 50 % metabo-lized and about 50 % excreted by the kidney. Importantly, brain:plasma ratios are ~15:1 for propranolol and timolol, 3:1 for metoprolol, and 1:8 for atenolol.

- Lipid-soluble beta-blocking agents with high brain concentration block sympathetic discharge in the hypothalamus better than water-soluble agents (Pitt 1992) and they are more effective in the prevention of cardiac deaths. Bisoprolol is 50 % lipophilic and liver metabolized but does not involve the cytochrome P-450 3A4 pathway. Nebivolol is highly lipophilic. Propranolol and metoprolol have high first-pass liver metabolism. Acebutolol is metabolized to an active metabolite diacetolol, which is water soluble and is excreted by the kidneys. Atenolol, nadolol, and sotalol are not metabolized in the liver. First-pass metabolism varies greatly among patients and can alter the dose of drug required, especially with propranolol.
- Cigarette smoking interferes with drug metabolism in the liver and reduces the efficacy of propranolol, other hepatically metabolized beta-blockers, and calcium antagonists (Deanfield et al. 1984).

Beta-blockers are now recommended and used by virtually all cardiologists because they are necessary for the management of acute and chronic ischemic syndromes, manifestations of CHD.

Many internists and family physicians, however, remain reluctant to prescribe beta-blockers in many cardiovascular situations including HF, in hypertension in patients aged >65 years, and in diabetic patients.

Fears that beta-blockers influence lipid levels unfavorably are unfounded. Beta-blocking drugs do not alter low-density lipoprotein (LDL) levels; they may cause a mild increase in levels of triglycerides and may produce a 1 % to ~ 6 % lowering of high-density lipoprotein cholesterol (HDL-C) in fewer than 10 % of patients treated *(3)*. The alteration in HDL-C levels is of minimal clinical concern because the effect is so small, if it occurs at all (Frishman 1997). The clinical importance of this mild disturbance in lipid levels is of questionable significance and should not submerge the prolongation of life and

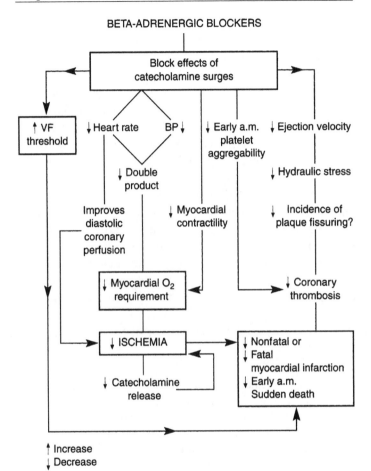

Fig. 1-1. Salutary effects of beta-adrenergic blockade.

other salutary effects obtained with the administration of beta-blocking drugs (Fig. 1-1).

Since their original discovery by Sir James Black at Imperial Chemical Industries in the UK (Black et al. 1964) and the introduction of the prototype, propranolol, for the treatment of hypertension in 1964 by Prichard and Gillam (1964), more than 12 beta-blocking drugs have become available.

The first edition of *Cardiac Drug Therapy* in 1984 included a table entitled "Beta-blockers: first-line oral drug treatment in angina pectoris" (Table 1-1); this table indicated the superiority of beta-blockers over calcium antagonists and nitrates. Calcium antagonists were down rated because they decreased blood flow to subendocardial areas; in addition, in the condition for which they were developed, coronary artery spasm (CAS), they were not shown to decrease mortality. This table has never been altered. The 1990s have shown the possible adverse effects and potential dangers of dihydropyridine calcium antagonists. Dihydropyridines increase the risk of death in patients with unstable angina; these agents are not approved for use in unstable angina in the absence of beta-blockade.

The cardiovascular indications for beta-blockers are given in Table 1-2 and allow the author to proclaim that beta-blockers are the cornerstone of cardiac drug therapy.

BETA-RECEPTORS

The beta-receptors are subdivided into

- The $beta_1$-receptors, present mainly in the heart, intestine, renin-secreting tissues of the kidney, those parts of the eye responsible for the production of aqueous humor, adipose tissue, and, to a limited degree, bronchial tissue.
- The $beta_2$-receptors, predominating in bronchial and vascular smooth muscle, gastrointestinal tract, the uterus, insulin-secreting tissue of the pancreas, and, to a limited degree, the heart and large coronary arteries. Metabolic receptors are usually $beta_2$. In addition, it should be noted that

  (a) None of these tissues contains exclusively one subgroup of receptors.
  (b) The beta-receptor population is not static, and beta-blockers appear to increase the number of receptors during long-term therapy. The number of cardiac $beta_2$-receptors increases after $beta_1$-blockade (Kaumann 1991).
  (c) The population density of receptors decreases with age

Table 1-1
**Beta-blockers: first-line oral drug treatment
in angina pectoris**

Effect on	Beta-blocker	Calcium antagonist	Oral nitrate
Heart rate	↓	↑↓	↓
Diastolic filling of coronary arteries	↑	−	−
Blood pressure	↓↓	↓↓	−
Rate pressure product (RPP)	↓	−[a]	−
Relief of angina	Yes	Yes	Variable
Blood flow (subendocardial ischemic area)[b]	↑	↓	Variable
First-line treatment for angina pectoris	Yes	No	No
Prevention of recurrent ventricular fibrillation	Proven	No	No
Prevention of cardiac death	Proven	No	No
Prevention of pain owing to CAS	No	Yes	Variable
Prevention of death in patient with CAS	No	No	No

[a]RPP variable decrease on exercise, but not significant at rest or on maximal exercise

[b]Distal to organic obstruction (Weintraub et al. 1982)

CAS, coronary artery spasm; ↓, decrease; ↑, increase; −, no significant change

The beta-receptors are situated on the cell membrane and are believed to be a part of the adenyl cyclase system. An agonist acting on its receptor site activates adenyl cyclase to produce cyclic adenosine-5′-monophosphate, which is believed to be the intracellular messenger of beta-stimulation.

The heart contains $beta_1$- and $beta_2$-adrenergic receptors in the proportion 70:30. Normally, cardiac $beta_1$-adrenergic

Table 1-2

Cardiovascular indications for beta-blockers

1.	Ischemic heart disease
	Stable angina
	Unstable angina
	Acute Ml
	Ml, long-term prevention
	Silent ischemia
2.	Arrhythmias
	VPBs
	AVNRT
	Atrial fibrillation
	Nonsustained VT
	VT
	Recurrent VF
3.	Hypertension
	Isolated
	With IHD, diabetes*, LVH, dyslipidemia[a]
	With arrhythmias
	Perioperative and on intubation
	Severe, urgent
	Pheochromocytoma (on alpha-blocker)
4.	Heart failure:
5.	Prolonged QT syndrome
6.	Aortic dissection
7.	Valvular heart disease
	Mitral stenosis? tachycardia in pregnancy*
	Mitral valve prolapse
	Mitral regurgitation
8.	To decrease perioperative mortality
9.	Cardiomyopathy
	Hypertrophic
	Dilated
10.	Marfan's syndrome
11.	Neurocardiogenic syncope
12.	Tetralogy of Fallot
13.	Aneurysm
14.	For coronary CT angiogram

[a]*See* text; 10-year CHD event risk score >20 %; *see* Chap. 17

AVNRT atrioventricular nodal reentrant tachycardia, *CHD* coronary heart disease, *IHD* ischemic heart disease, *LVH* left ventricular hypertrophy, *VPB* ventricular premature beat, *VF* ventricular fibrillation, *VT* ventricular tachycardia receptors appear to regulate heart rate and/or myocardial contractility, but in situations of stress, with the provocation of epinephrine release, stimulation of cardiac $beta_2$-receptors may contribute to additional increases in heart rate and/or contractility (Motomura et al. 1990). In HF, cardiac $beta_1$- but not $beta_2$-adrenergic receptors are reduced in number and population, and the myocardium may be less responsive to $beta_1$-inotropic agents.

MECHANISM OF ACTION

By definition, beta-blockers block beta-receptors. Structurally, they resemble the catecholamines. Beta-blockers are competitive inhibitors, their action depending on the ratio of beta-blocker concentration to catecholamine concentration at beta-adrenoceptor sites.

- Blockade of cardiac $beta_1$-receptors causes a decrease in heart rate, myocardial contractility, and velocity of cardiac contraction. The heart rate multiplied by the systolic blood pressure (i.e., the rate pressure product [RPP]) is reduced at rest and during exercise, and this action is reflected in a reduced myocardial oxygen demand (which is an important effect in the control of angina).
- The main in vitro antiarrhythmic effect of beta-blockers is the depression of phase 4 diastolic depolarization. Beta-blockers are effective in abolishing arrhythmias produced by increased catecholamines. Maximum impulse traffic through the atrioventricular (AV) node is reduced, and the rate of conduction is slowed. Paroxysmal supraventricular tachycardia (PSVT) caused by AV nodal reentry is often abolished by beta-blockers, which also slow the ventricular rate in atrial flutter and atrial fibrillation. There is a variable effect on ventricular arrhythmias, which may be abolished if induced by increased sympathetic activity, as is often seen in myocardial ischemia.
- Beta-blockers reduce the activity of the renin–angiotensin system by reducing renin release from the juxtaglomerular

cells. Also, beta-blockade augments atrial and brain natriuretic peptide (see next section and Suggested Reading).

- Beta-blockers interfere with sympathetic vasoconstrictor
nerve activity; this action is partly responsible for their
antihypertensive effect. Cardiac output usually falls and
remains slightly lower than normal with administration of
non-intrinsic sympathomimetic activity (ISA) agents.
Systemic vascular resistance increases acutely but falls to
near normal with long-term administration (Man in't Veld
et al. 1988).

Other Important Clinically Beneficial Mechanisms

Beta-Blockers

- Lower plasma endothelin-1 levels, as shown for carvedilol
(Krum et al. 1996), and inhibit catecholamine-induced cardiac necrosis (apoptosis) (Cruickshank et al. 1987).
- Stimulate the endothelial-*arginine/nitric oxide pathway*, as
shown for the interesting vasodilatory beta-blocker
nebivolol (Cockcroft et al. 1995).
- Augment atrial and brain natriuretic peptide, upregulate
cardiac beta$_1$-receptors, and inhibit stimulatory anti-beta$_1$-
receptor autoantibodies.

Beta-Blocker Effect on Calcium Availability

The slow channels represent two of the mechanisms by
which calcium gains entry into the myocardial cell. At least
two channels exist (Braunwald 1982), namely,

- A voltage-dependent channel blocked by calcium antagonists *(see* Chap. 8).
- A receptor-operated channel blocked by beta-receptor
blockers that therefore decrease calcium availability inside
the myocardial cell. The negative inotropic effect of beta-
blockers is probably based on this effect.

DOSAGE CONSIDERATIONS

- The **beta-blocking effect** is manifest as a blockade of tachycardia when induced by exercise or isoproterenol. The therapeutic response to beta-blockers does not correlate in a linear fashion with the oral dose or plasma level. Differences in the degree of absorption and variation in hepatic metabolism give rise to unpredictable plasma levels, but in addition the same blood level may elicit a different cardiovascular response in patients, depending on the individual's sympathetic and vagal tone and the population of beta-receptors.

- The **dose** of beta-blocker is titrated to achieve control of angina, hypertension, or arrhythmia. The dose is usually adjusted to achieve a heart rate of 50–60 per min and an exercise heart rate <110 per min. The dosage of propranolol varies considerably (120–480 mg daily) because of the marked but variable first-pass hepatic metabolism. There is a 20-fold variation in plasma level from a given dose of this drug. The proven **cardioprotective** (CP) dose may be different from the dose necessary to achieve control of angina or hypertension. The effective CP dose (i.e., the dose shown to prevent cardiac deaths in the post-MI patient) for timolol is 10–20 mg daily (Norwegian study 1981), and for propranolol it is within the range 160–240 mg daily. When possible, the dosage of beta-blocker should be kept within the CP range. Other experts are in agreement with this concern for use of the CP dose when possible (Pratt and Roberts 1983).

- An **increase in the dose** beyond the CP dosage (e.g., timolol >30 mg or propranolol >240 mg daily), for better control of angina, hypertension, or arrhythmia, may have a poor reward, that is, there could be an increase in side effects, especially dyspnea, HF, and distressing fatigue.

- A review of the clinical literature reveals that too large a dose of beta-blockers may be not only nonprotective but also positively harmful, and this is supported by studies on animals *(18)*. In some patients, one should be satisfied with 75 % control of symptoms and, if necessary, the addition of a further therapeutic agent. The patient is not fearful of anginal pain or high blood pressure—what the patient fears

Table 1-3
Beta-blockers: randomized controlled trials showing
significant reduction in mortality rate

| Trial | Drug | Mortality | | Relative risk reduction | |
		Placebo	Drug	%	P
APSI[a]	Acebutolol	34/309	17/298	48	0.019
		11.0 %	5.7 %		
BHAT[b]	Propranolol	188/1,921	138/1,916	26.5	<0.01
		9.8 %	7.2 %		
Norwegian Post-infarction Study[c]	Timolol	152/939	98/945	35.8	<0.001
		16.2 %	10.4 %		
Salathia	Metoprolol	43/364	27/391	41.5	<0.05
		11.8 %	6.9 %		
Hjalmarson et al. (1981)	Metoprolol Post-Ml	62/679	40/698	36.0	<0.03
		8.9 %	5.7 %		
COPERNICUS					
CAPRICORN					
CIBIS-II					
MERIT-HF					

[a]Boissel et al. (1990)
[b]Beta blocker Heart Attack Study Group
[c]The Norwegian multicenter study group (1981); sudden cardiac death was reduced 67 % by timolol administration

is death. *Beta-blockers do prevent cardiac deaths, but they have been shown to do so only at certain doses.* In addition, beta-blockers are not all alike; subtle differences can be of importance. Only bisoprolol, carvedilol, metoprolol, propranolol, and timolol have been shown to prolong life in RCTs (see Table 1-3).

- Patients may require different drug concentrations to achieve adequate beta-blockade because of different levels of sympathetic tone (circulating catecholamines and active beta-adrenoceptor binding sites). However, **plasma levels**

Table 1-4
Dosage of commonly used beta-blockers

Beta-blocker	Daily starting dose (mg)	Maintenance dose (mg)	Maximum suggested dose (mg)
Bisoprolol	5	5–10	15
Carvedilol	12.5	25–50	50
Metoprolol	50–100	100–200	300
Nadolol	20–80	20–160	160
Propranolol	40–120	40–240	320
Sotalol	80–160	60–320	320
Timolol	5–10	20–30	30

Atenolol is not recommended (see text)

do not indicate active metabolites, and the effect of the drug may last longer than is suggested by the half-life.

- Propranolol may take 4–6 weeks to achieve stable plasma levels because of the extensive hepatic metabolism, but timolol and pindolol undergo less than 60 % metabolism, and constant plasma concentrations are more readily achieved. Therefore, **propranolol** should be given three times daily for about 6 weeks and then twice daily, or propranolol long-acting (LA) 160–240 mg once daily.
- **Atenolol, nadolol,** and **sotalol** are excreted virtually unchanged by the kidneys and require alteration of the dosage in severe renal dysfunction, as follows:

  (a) Creatinine clearance of 30–50 mL/min, half the average dose per 24 h.
  (b) Creatinine clearance less than 30 mL/min, half the usual dose every 48 h.

The **oral doses** of commonly used beta-blockers are given in Table 1-4. The **intravenous (IV) doses** are as follows:

Esmolol: 3–6 mg over 1 min, then 1–5 mg/min.
Propranolol: up to 1 mg, at a rate of 0.5 mg/min, repeated if necessary at 2–5-min intervals to a maximum of 5 mg (rarely 10 mg): 0.1 mg/kg.

Metoprolol: up to 5 mg, at a rate of 1 mg/min, repeated if necessary at 5-min intervals to a maximum of 10 mg (rarely 15 mg).

Atenolol: up to 2.5 mg, at a rate of 1 mg/min, repeated if necessary at 5-min intervals to a maximum of 10 mg.

By IV infusion (atenolol): 150 mg/kg over 20 min repeated every 12 h if required.

PHARMACOLOGIC PROPERTIES AND CLINICAL IMPLICATIONS

A clinically useful classification of beta-blockers is given in Fig. 1-2, and their pharmacologic properties are summarized in Table 1-5.

Cardioselectivity

Cardioselectivity implies that the drug blocks chiefly the $beta_1$-receptors and therefore partially spares $beta_2$-receptors in the lungs and blood vessels. A small quantity of $beta_1$-receptors is present in the lungs. Large doses of all beta-blocking drugs block $beta_2$-receptors. Selectivity holds only for small doses and may be lost at the doses necessary for the relief of angina or for the control of hypertension. Atenolol, betaxolol, bisoprolol, metoprolol, bevantolol, esmolol, and, to a lesser degree, acebutolol have less of a blocking effect on $beta_2$-receptors in the lungs, so they are not cardiospecific. They can precipitate bronchospasm in susceptible individuals. Nebivolol is the most $beta_1$-selective, followed by bisoprolol, which is highly selective; the others are moderately to weakly selective.

1. **Bronchospasm**. Cardioselective agents may precipitate bronchospasm in a susceptible patient, and this is no different from that of nonselective drugs, **except** when bronchospasm occurs the patient will **respond to a beta$_2$-stimulant** such as albuterol (salbutamol) if a cardioselective

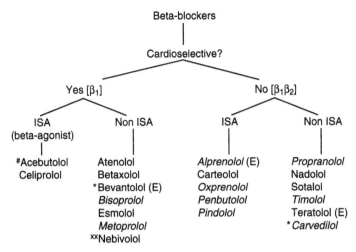

All available in the United States except if labeled (E)

ISA = Intrinsic sympathomimetic activity
E = Europe
* added weak alpha-blocker
Italic = lipid soluble
\# weak β_1 selectivity, weak ISA
xx = vasodilatory beta blocker
a unique highly lipophilic beta blocker:
stimulates β_3-adrenergic receptor-mediated
production of nitric oxide

Fig. 1-2. Classification of beta-blockers.

drug was administered. When bronchospasm occurs with the use of nonselective drugs, including pindolol, the spasm may be more resistant to beta-stimulants. Beta-blockers should not be given to patients with **bronchial asthma** or severe chronic bronchitis or emphysema. It is wise in such patients to choose alternative therapeutic agents. *Mild chronic bronchitis* is indicated by the following:

- Forced expiratory volume greater than 1.5 L.
- No hospital emergency room or office treatments for bronchospastic disease.

Table 1-5
Pharmacologic properties of beta-adrenoceptor blockers

Beta-blocker	Propranolol	Timolol	Metoprolol	Nadolol	Atenolol	Carvedilol	Bisoprolol	Acebutolol	Sotalol
Equivalent dose (mg)	80	10	100	60	50	12.5	10	400	80
Potency ratio Relative	1	6–8	1	1–1.5	1–2	?		0.3	0.5–1
Cardioselectivity	No	No	Yes, Moderate	No	Yes, Strong	No	Strong	Yes, Mild	No
Partial agonist activity (ISA)	0	0	0	0	0	0	Nil	Mild	0
Half-life(h)	2–6	2–6	2–6	14–24	7–20		14	2–6	7–20
Variation in plasma level	20-fold	Sevenfold	Sevenfold	Sevenfold	Fourfold			?	Fourfold
Lipid solubility	Strong	Moderate	Strong	Nil	Nil	Moderate	Moderate	Weak	Nil
Absorption (%)	90	90	95	30	50			75	90
Bioavailability (%)	30	75	50	30	50			40	90
Hepatic metabolism (HM)	HM	60 % HM	HM	No	No	HM	50 %	HM	No
Renal excretion (RE)		40 % RE		RE	RE		50 % RE	60 % RE	RE

ISA intrinsic sympathomimetic activity

If a patient with mild chronic bronchitis requires treatment with a beta-blocker for angina, treatment should begin with bisoprolol or metoprolol. If bronchospasm occurs, albuterol (salbutamol) should be added, or the beta-blocker should be discontinued. Bisoprolol is the most cardioselective beta-blocker available and is safer than metoprolol for patients with chronic obstructive pulmonary disease (COPD). In humans, the drug has a twofold higher beta1-selectivity than atenolol.

2. **Peripheral vascular disease** (PVD). If a beta-blocker is necessary in a patient with PVD, some clinical trials indicate that it is safer to use a cardioselective drug, atenolol or metoprolol; agents such as carvedilol or bucindolol that cause vasodilation may have a role. Analysis of 11 randomized trials of beta-blockers in patients with PVD showed no worsening of intermittent claudication. Patients with PVD are at high risk for CHD events, and beta-blockers are recommended for all indications. In the United Kingdom Prospective Diabetes Study Group (UKPDS) *(19),* atenolol did not worsen PVD, and there was a nonsignificant 48 % excess of amputations in the captopril group.

3. **Hypoglycemia** stimulates an increase in catecholamine release, which increases blood glucose. The recovery from hypoglycemia may be delayed by nonselective beta-blockers. The incidence of hypoglycemia is higher in insulin-dependent diabetic patients treated with nonselective beta-blockers, whereas both selective and nonselective varieties modify the symptoms of hypoglycemia (with the exception of sweating). Glycolysis and lipolysis in skeletal muscles are mediated mainly by $beta_2$-receptors. Hypoglycemia induced by exercise is more likely to occur with a nonselective beta-blocker. However, evidence to support a greater benefit of selective beta-blockers in joggers is lacking (Breckenridge 1982). **Insulin** secretion is probably $beta_2$-mediated. Glucose-sulfonylurea-stimulated insulin secretion is inhibited by beta-blockers. Beta-blockers may increase blood glucose by 1.0–1.5 mmol/L, but this glucose intolerance is not type 2 diabetes.

The following points deserve consideration:

- Catecholamine stimulation of beta$_2$-receptors produces transient hypokalemia. Thus, cardioselective drugs that spare beta$_2$-receptors may fail to maintain constancy of serum potassium in response to increase in epinephrine and norepinephrine during acute MI (Johansson 1986).
- *Non-cardioselective agents are superior to selective agents in preventing fluctuations of serum potassium concentration during stress and possibly during acute MI.*
- *Nonselective drugs should confer a greater degree of cardioprotection; carvedilol, propranolol, and timolol have been shown to prevent total mortality and cardiac death in well-controlled RCTs.*

Intrinsic Sympathomimetic Activity

Intrinsic Sympathomimetic Activity (ISA) indicates partial agonist activity, the primary agonists being epinephrine and isoproterenol. Beta-blockers that cause a small agonist response (i.e., stimulate as well as block the beta-receptors) include pindolol, alprenolol, acebutolol, celiprolol, carteolol, oxprenolol, and practolol. The last drug has been removed from medical practice because it produced the oculomucocutaneous syndrome. Beta-blockers with ISA cause a slightly lower incidence of bradycardia compared with non-ISA drugs. In practice, this is a minor advantage in the choice of a beta-blocker. The heart rate at rest may be only slightly lowered or unchanged; in patients with angina, a slower heart rate is conducive to less pain on activity.

The RPP at rest is not significantly reduced. Myocardial oxygen consumption is therefore not usually reduced at rest by ISA beta-blockers. Beta-blockers with ISA, therefore, carry **no advantage** in angina at rest or in angina occurring at low exercise levels; in particular, they do not have a beneficial effect on cardioprotection. The ISA of beta-blockers produces adverse effects on ventricular fibrillation (VF) threshold (Raeder et al. 1983). Acebutolol with weak

ISA, however, has been shown to prevent cardiac death. Because they limit exercise tachycardia, these drugs do have a **minor role** to play in the treatment of patients who have a relatively low resting heart rate (50–60 per min) and in whom further bradycardia may not be acceptable. Even in this subgroup, it is still important to exclude patients with sick sinus syndrome because all beta-blockers are contraindicated here. **Renin** secretion may remain unaltered or may even be increased by agents with ISA. There may be added sodium and water retention, causing edema. There is no clear-cut evidence that peripheral vascular complications are less frequent when beta-blockers with partial agonist activity are used. *Agents with ISA, except acebutolol (very weak ISA), are not recommended by the author because of the aforementioned points; these are not CP drugs.*

Membrane-Stabilizing Activity

The quinidine-like or local anesthetic action, membrane-stabilizing activity (MSA), is of no clinical importance, except perhaps for its effect on platelets and in the treatment of glaucoma. It is not related to the antiarrhythmic, antianginal, or CP properties of beta-blockers. Unlike most available beta-blockers, timolol and betaxolol have no MSA. Because of high potency and lack of anesthetic effect, these drugs are the only beta-blockers that have been proved safe and effective in the treatment of glaucoma when used topically.

MSA appears to be important in the management of thyrotoxic crisis, and propranolol has been shown to be more effective than nadolol in this condition.

Effects on Renin

Renin release from the juxtaglomerular cells is suppressed by $beta_1$-receptor blockade; this results in reduced activity of the renin–angiotensin system. Beta-blockers enhance the lifesaving effects of ACE inhibitors in patients with HF or MI (Pitt 1998).

Lipid Solubility

- Highly lipid-soluble, lipophilic beta-blockers—carvedilol, propranolol, timolol, and metoprolol—reach high concentrations in the brain and are metabolized in the liver.
- Atenolol, nadolol, and sotalol are lipid insoluble, show poor brain concentration, and are not metabolized by the liver; they are water soluble, are excreted by the kidneys, and have a long half-life. Pindolol and timolol are about 50 % metabolized and about 50 % excreted by the kidney.
- Brain:plasma ratios are 15:1 for propranolol, 3:1 for metoprolol, and 1:8 for atenolol.
- Lipid-insoluble, hydrophilic beta-blockers appear to have a lower incidence of central nervous system (CNS) side effects such as vivid dreams, significant effects on sleep (Kostis and Rosen 1987), impairment of very fast mental reactions (Engler et al. 1986), depression, fatigue, and impotence. Depending on dosage, even the lipid-insoluble drugs can achieve sufficient brain concentration to impair very fast mental reactions. There is little doubt, however, that atenolol causes fewer central side effects than propranolol (Engler et al. 1986). Timolol has been shown to cause less bizarre dreams than pindolol or propranolol in small groups of patients.
- **Lipid-soluble beta-blocking agents with high brain concentrations block sympathetic discharge in the hypothalamus better than water-soluble agents (Pitt 1992), and they are more effective in the prevention of cardiac deaths.**
- Bisoprolol is 50 % lipophilic and liver metabolized but does not involve the cytochrome P-450 3A4 pathway; renal elimination is ~50 %.

Plasma Volume

A reduction in cardiac output is usually followed by an increase in plasma volume. Beta-blockers cause a reduction in plasma volume; the exact reason for this is unknown. Pindolol (ISA) may increase plasma volume.

Hepatic Metabolism

Propranolol, oxprenolol, and metoprolol have high first-pass liver metabolism. Timolol and acebutolol have modest lipid solubility and undergo major hepatic metabolism. Acebutolol is metabolized to an active metabolite, diacetolol, which is water soluble and is excreted by the kidneys. Atenolol, nadolol, and sotalol are not metabolized in the liver. First-pass metabolism varies greatly among patients and can alter the dose of drug required, especially with propranolol. Cigarette smoking interferes with drug metabolism in the liver and reduces the efficacy of propranolol, other hepatically metabolized beta-blockers, and calcium antagonists (Deanfield et al. 1984).

Effects on Blood and Arteries

1. **Platelets**. Platelet hyperaggregation seen in patients with angina or induced by catecholamines can be normalized by propranolol. The second stage of platelet aggregation, induced by adenosine diphosphate, catecholamines, collagen, or thrombin, can be abolished or inhibited by propranolol. Propranolol is able to block [^{14}C]serotonin released from platelets and inhibits platelet adherence to collagen; these favorable effects can be detected with the usual clinical doses of propranolol and other beta-blocking drugs.

2. **HDL-C**. It has been suggested that beta-blockers may increase atherosclerosis by decreasing HDL levels. Propranolol causes a mild decrease in HDL levels of ~7 %. There is at present no proof that decreasing HDL values from, for example, 55 to 50 mg/dL (i.e., from 1.4 to 1.3 mmol/L) will have any adverse effect on the progression of atherosclerosis. Some studies suggest that HDL_2 remains unaltered (Valimaki and Harno 1986; Pasotti et al. 1986). There is little doubt that in some patients HDL_2 is slightly lowered. In one study, there was an 8 % lowering of HDL_2 and a rise in triglycerides produced by both propranolol and pindolol at 6 weeks. Beta-blockers do not decrease total serum cholesterol. The effect of beta-blockers on

triglycerides is variable, and the evidence associating raised triglycerides with ischemic heart disease (IHD) is weak. Acebutolol with weak ISA causes no significant disturbance of lipid levels. **Bisoprolol**, being highly $beta_1$-selective, does not significantly decrease HDL-C.

3. **Arteries**. Beta-blockers decrease the force and velocity of cardiac contraction, decrease RPP and heart rate × peak velocity, and therefore decrease hemodynamic stress on the arterial wall, especially at the branching of arteries. This action may decrease the atherosclerotic process and *plaque rupture*. This beneficial hemodynamic effect, and that described on blood coagulation, may favorably influence atherosclerotic CHD and subsequent occlusion by platelets or thrombosis.

4. **Coronary blood flow**. Beta-blockers increase diastolic coronary perfusion time and coronary blood flow because bradycardia lengthens the diastolic filling time. Thus, these agents produce beneficial effects in angina and IHD by increasing coronary blood supply while reducing myocardial oxygen demands; the reduction of hydraulic stress in the coronary arteries appears to *provide protection from plaque fissuring and rupture (see* Fig. 1-1).

Effect on Serum Potassium

- Beta-blockade causes a mild increase in serum potassium because of blockade of the $beta_2$-mediated epinephrine activation of the Na^+, K^+—ATPase pump, which transports potassium from extracellular fluid into cells.

- During stress, serum potassium has been observed to decrease up to 1.0 mEq (mmol)/L; this fall in serum potassium concentration can be prevented by blockade of $beta_2$-receptors.

- *Non-cardioselective agents are superior to selective agents in preventing fluctuations of serum potassium concentration during stress and possibly during acute MI.*

- Among inpatients with AMI, the lowest mortality was observed in those with post-admission serum potassium levels between 3.5 and <4.5 mEq/L compared with those who had higher or lower potassium levels (Goyal et al. 2012).

SALUTARY EFFECTS OF BETA-ADRENERGIC BLOCKADE

These beneficial effects include the following:

- A decrease in heart rate increases the diastolic interval and allows for improved diastolic filling of the coronary arteries. This effect is especially important during exercise in patients with angina.
- The RPP is decreased, so there is less myocardial demand for oxygen, resulting in an improvement of ischemia.
- A decrease in sudden cardiac death has been documented in several studies. *An impressive 67 % reduction in sudden death was observed in smokers and nonsmokers in the Timolol Norwegian Reinfarction Study (16):* timolol decreased the overall mortality rate by 36 %, $p < 0.001$.
- This beneficial effect of beta-blockers in post-infarction patients was reconfirmed in the Beta-Blocker Heart Attack Trial (BHAT). This well-run trial randomized 16,400 post-MI patients to propranolol or placebo and after 2-years follow-up showed a 26 % reduction in the mortality rate with propranolol.
- A decrease in fatal arrhythmias and an increase in VF threshold, as well as amelioration of bothersome benign ventricular and supraventricular arrhythmias, have been established by several clinical studies.
- A decrease in the velocity and force of myocardial contraction results in a decrease in myocardial oxygen requirement and also reduces the rate of rise of aortic pressure, which is important in the prevention and treatment of aortic dissection. Beta-blockade is effective in slowing the rate of aortic dilation and reducing the development of aortic complications in patients with Marfan's syndrome (Shore et al. 1994)
- A decrease in ejection velocity reduces hydraulic stress on the arterial wall that could be crucial at the site of atheroma. This mechanism of action may reduce the incidence of plaque rupture and may thus protect patients from coronary thrombosis and fatal or nonfatal infarction.

- Beta-blockers may prevent early morning platelet aggregation induced by catecholamines and may decrease the early morning peak incidence of acute MI (Peters et al. 1990).

The favorable effect of beta-blockade on sudden death relative to reduction in heart rate is observed only with the use of beta-blockers that reduce heart rate (Singh 1990). Beta-blockers such as pindolol with marked ISA and no bradycardic response at rest cause no reduction in sudden death or mortality rates Acebutolol with mild ISA, however, caused a 48 % reduction in overall mortality rate and a 58 % reduction in cardiovascular mortality rate in post-infarction patients (Boissel et al. 1990).

BETA-BLOCKERS VERSUS CALCIUM ANTAGONISTS AND ORAL NITRATES

The clinical effects of beta-blockers compared with calcium antagonists and oral nitrates are shown in Table 1-1.

1. **A decrease in heart rate** by beta-blockers allows for a **longer diastolic filling** time and therefore **greater coronary perfusion.**
2. It is often stated that beta-blockers may decrease coronary blood flow, but this is secondary to the reduction in myocardial work; in practice, this effect is not harmful. A decrease in blood flow does not occur if there is ischemia, and therefore it is not of importance in occlusive coronary disease. If you need less oxygen, you will need less blood flow; this fact is often misinterpreted. The RPP at rest and on maximal exercise is reduced by beta-blockers, but it is not decreased by calcium antagonists or oral nitrates.
3. Both beta-blockers and calcium antagonists have been proved to be more effective than nitrates when they are used alone in the relief of angina pectoris.
4. In animals, **blood flow** to the subendocardial ischemic myocardium distal to an organic obstruction is improved by beta-blockers, and it may be decreased by calcium antago-

nists (Weintraub et al. 1982). Beta-blockers divert blood from the epicardium to the ischemic subendocardium by activation of autoregulatory mechanisms. Calcium antagonists may have the opposite effect and can cause deterioration in patients with critical coronary artery stenosis (Warltier et al. 1983). Unfortunately, calcium antagonists, when used without a beta-blocker in patients with unstable angina, can increase chest pain and infarction, and they appeared to increase mortality in the largest subgroup of patients with unstable angina. Oral nitrates have an effect similar to that of calcium antagonists.

5. Beta-blockers can prevent **recurrent VF** in animals and in patients (Sloman et al. 1965), whereas calcium antagonists do not significantly alter VF threshold.

6. Beta-blockers have been shown to prevent cardiac death in patients after MI, followed for 2 years (The Norwegian Multicenter Study Group 1981; BHAT 1982). There is no reason to suppose that the same favorable effect is absent in the patient with angina pectoris or hypertension, provided an appropriate beta-blocker is used at CP doses (timolol, or metoprolol, and propranolol in nonsmokers). In contrast, calcium antagonists provide only symptomatic relief. There are good reasons, therefore, for employing beta-blockers as first-line drugs in the treatment of **angina pectoris,** and this should remain the case until other therapeutic maneuvers are proved conclusively to prevent sudden and other cardiac deaths. Current evidence clearly indicates that calcium antagonists do not prevent cardiac deaths. *There has been a misguided tendency to replace beta-blockers in the management of angina pectoris with calcium antagonists. Calcium antagonists cannot be regarded as alternative therapy; they constitute suitable therapy when beta-blockers are contraindicated.*

Occasionally, **CAS** can be made worse in allowing unopposed alpha-vasoconstriction. *It is emphasized that variant angina resulting from CAS is rare*, and only the occasional patient may have an increase in chest pain secondary to beta-blockers (Julian 1983). Usually, this is not dangerous, and it gives an indication that CAS may be present. In patients in whom the mechanism of unstable angina is unclear, beta-blockers should be used combined with calcium antagonists or nitrates (Julian 1983).

INDICATIONS FOR BETA-BLOCKERS

Angina

The use of beta-blockers in the management of angina pectoris and silent ischemia is discussed in Chap. 10 (see Table 1-2).

Arrhythmias

- Ventricular premature beats that are symptomatic in patients with normal hearts and in those with a history of cardiac disease benefit from treatment with a beta-blocker. In the acute phase of MI, ventricular premature beats and ischemia caused by catecholamine surge respond favorably.
- AV nodal reentrant tachycardia may be aborted by beta-blocker therapy.
- Atrial fibrillation: rate control is best achieved with a small dose of a beta-blocking drug: bisoprolol 2.5–5 mg is often sufficient to maintain a controlled ventricular response 70–100 per min. Digoxin does not decrease heart rate adequately in patients during exercise, but is sometimes necessary to combine digoxin and a beta-blocker at small doses. Sotalol may decrease the recurrence of paroxysmal atrial fibrillation. Other beta-blockers do not possess class III activity and are not recommended for the maintenance of sinus rhythm in patients with paroxysmal atrial fibrillation. In patients converted to sinus rhythm by DC shock, maintenance of sinus rhythm with the use of sotalol is as good as quinidine.
- Esmolol IV may be used instead of diltiazem or verapamil, particularly in the perioperative period for most supraventricular tachycardias (SVTs) including atrial fibrillation.

- Nonsustained ventricular tachycardia (VT) is more appropriately treated with a beta-blocker than with antiarrhythmic agents. The use of most antiarrhythmics has dwindled because of the increased mortality attributed to these agents.
- Recurrent episodes of VT may be prevented in some patients. In the management of life-threatening arrhythmias in patients after cardiac arrest, metoprolol has been shown to be as good as amiodarone. When amiodarone and a beta-blocker combination is used, it appears that the prolongation of life observed is caused mainly by the addition of the beta-blocker. A European trial has shown that empiric use of metoprolol was as effective as electrophysiologically guided antiarrhythmic therapy (Steinbeck et al. 1992).
- Recurrent VF is unique among cardiac arrhythmias because the management is immediate countershock. Antifibrillatory drugs can be useful in the prevention of recurrent VF. Beta-blockers have long been known to have a role in the management of patients with persistently recurring VF (Sloman et al. 1965; Rothfield et al. 1968). Beta-blockers decrease the incidence of VF in patients with acute MI (Ryden et al. 1983). Beta-blockers increase VF threshold and should be given by the IV route in patients with recurrent VF.

HYPERTENSION

- **Young patients.** A beta-blocker is the drug of choice in younger and older white patients with or without comorbid con*ditions, par*ticularly IHD, MI, diabetes, and hyperlipidemia. Beta-blockers are generally known to be effective in white people aged less than 65 years. In a study by Matterson et al. (1993) in African-American patients younger than 60 years, atenolol was, surprisingly, the second most effective drug, after diltiazem, and it was more effective than hydrochlorothiazide (HCTZ). *See* treatment algorithms in Chap. 9.
- **Elderly patients.** *Contrary to common opinion, beta-blockers have been proved effective in older white patients*

(Matterson et al. 1993). **The statement that beta-blockers are not advisable in elderly hypertensive patients, as given in textbooks and excellent editorials, review articles, and JNC and WHO guidelines, is false because it is based on the results of the Medical Research Council (MRC) trial in the elderly** (Medical Research Council Working Party 1992) (*see* Chaps. 8 and 9). Unfortunately, of the 4,396 elderly hypertensive patients **in this trial, 25 % were lost to follow-up, and the 63 % randomized to a beta-blocker either withdrew or were lost to follow-up**. More than half the patients were not taking their assigned therapy by the end of the study. Cruickshank's review (2000) quotes these relevant statistics.

- *The misleading MRC trial rings out this statement: elderly hypertensive patients respond best to diuretic-based rather than beta-blocker-based therapy in terms of fewer heart attacks.*

- The JNC8 and 2014 hypertension panelists believe this unsound study and advise against the use of beta-blocking drugs as first or second line to treat hypertension.

- If this poorly conducted MRC trial carries so much credibility, then diuretics should be used instead of beta-blockers to prevent heart attacks in all cardiac patients (hypertensive and normotensive) with high risk for CHD events. However, every practitioner knows that diuretics are not prescribed for prevention of CHD events in patients at risk for CHD events. Why prescribe them in place of beta-blockers in elderly hypertensive patients based on one unsound RCT? In the HANE (HCTZ, atenolol, nitrendipine, enalapril) study *(50),* at 8 weeks the blood pressure response rate was significantly higher for atenolol (64 %) than for enalapril (50 %), HCTZ (46 %), or nitrendipine (45 %). Effectivity was maintained at the end of 1 year. **A beta-blocker was as effective in elderly patients as in younger ones.**

- In patients with hypertension or angina with LV dysfunction, a beta-blocker used in combination with an ACE inhibitor improves outcome.

- For prevention and regression of LVH, a beta-blocker or ACE inhibitor is more effective than a diuretic or calcium antagonist (Pitt 1998; Devreux 1997).

Acute Myocardial Infarction

For the **first 7 days**, beta-blockers given within 4 h of an acute MI slightly reduce the 7-day mortality rate. There is evidence that beta-blockers can lower the incidence of acute MI, decrease the size of infarction, reduce the incidence of VF, and reduce the incidence of early cardiac rupture. Reduction of infarct size has been documented with the early use of timolol in acute MI (International Collaborative Study Group 1984). Beta-blockers are recommended from day 1 and for 2 years or more. During this period, these agents prevent sudden death and nonfatal and fatal MI and reduce overall mortality.

In the **CAPRICORN** (2001) study, carvedilol produced an outstanding reduction in cardiac deaths and events in early post-MI patients *(see* the discussion of study results in Chap. 22).

- Caution is needed because beta-blockers may increase cardiac mortality when used indiscriminately in patients in whom the drugs are contraindicated, particularly IV use in patients who are hemodynamically unstable, with impending cardiogenic shock, pulmonary edema, or acute MI with HF *(see* COMMIT, Chap. 22).

Elective Percutaneous Coronary Intervention (PCI)

Beta-blocker therapy is associated with a marked long-term survival benefit among patients undergoing successful PCI (Chan et al. 2002)*;* beta-blocker therapy was associated with a reduction from 6.0 to 3.9 % at 1 year ($p = 0.0014$).

- The benefit of beta-blocker therapy in patients in Korea receiving primary percutaneous coronary intervention after ST-elevation myocardial infarction was examined by Lee et al. (2012). Between November 2005 and January 2008, 2,688 hospital survivors who had an STEMI with a symptom-to-door time of 12 h and underwent primary PCI were analyzed from the Korean Acute MI registry. Patients who received BB therapy before hospitalization were excluded from this study. Results: The 12-month mortality was significantly lower in beta-blocker patients compared with no beta-blocker (2.0 % vs. 3.9 %; crude HR 0.498, 95 % CI 0.302–0.820; $p = 0.006$). There was no significant difference in the 12-month MACE [defined as a composite of death, non-fatal MI, and revascularizations] between BB patients and no-BB patients (9.9 % vs. 11.1 %; crude hazard ratio [HR] 0.864 (Lee et al. 2012). In patients with anterior Killip class < or equal to 11 ST elevation MI undergoing PCI, early IV metoprolol before reperfusion resulted in higher long-term left ventricular ejection fraction. This administration reduced the incidence of severe left ventricular dysfunction and implantable cardioverter defibrillator indications and fewer admissions for heart failure (Pizarro et al. 2014).

The METOCARD-CNIC Effect of Metoprolol in Cardioprotection During an Acute Myocardial Infarction trial:

- The study randomized 270 patients Killip class II anterior STEMI presenting early after symptom onset (<6 h) to pre-reperfusion IV metoprolol or control group.
- The proportion of patients fulfilling Class I indications for an implantable cardioverter-defibrillator (ICD) was significantly lower in the IV metoprolol group (7 % vs. 20 %, p ¼ 0.012). At a median follow-up of 2 years, occurrence of the prespecified composite of death, heart failure admission, reinfarction, and malignant arrhythmias was 10.8 % in the IV metoprolol group vs. 18.3 % in the control group. Heart

failure admission was significantly lower in the IV metoprolol group" (Pizarro et al. 2014).
- See Chap. 22.

Heart Failure

The potentially deleterious effects of overactivation of
the sympathetic nervous system in HF are now well established; beta-blockers curb this sympathetic overactivation,
hence the rationale for the judicious use of titrated doses of
beta-blockers in patients with impaired LV function (see
Chap. 12 for a discussion of the Second Cardiac Insufficiency
Bisoprolol Study (CIBIS II, 1998) and COPERNICUS
(2001), which showed a significant reduction in overall
mortality with bisoprolol and carvedilol therapy). Beta-
blockers are the mainstay of therapy for heart failure. They
decrease total mortality, an effect only modestly provided by
ACE inhibitors, and not at all by ARBS. See discussion
under ARBS.

- Carvedilol has been shown in an RCT in patients with class
  II and III HF to decrease mortality and the risk of hospitalization for recurrent HF. Thus, approved beta-blockers have
  a new indication for the management of patients with LV
  dysfunction or class I–III HF.
- In **COPERNICUS** (2001), carvedilol produced a
  significant reduction in serious events in patients with
  compensated class IV HF, and the indication has been
  extended from class I to *compensated class IV* patients (*see*
  Chaps. 12 and 22).
- *Most important, in MERIT-HF (2002), only a small dose of
  a beta-blocking drug administered to patients in the low-
  dose subgroup achieved risk reduction similar to that
  observed in the high-dose subgroup.*
- Nebivolol: The SENIORS Study 2009. These investigators
  studied 2,111 patients; 1,359 (64 %) had impaired (35 %)
  EF (mean 28.7 %) and 752 (36 %) had preserved (>35 %)

EF (mean 49.2 %). During a follow-up of 21 months, the primary end point occurred in 465 patients (34.2 %) with impaired EF and in 235 patients (31.2 %) with preserved EF. The effect of nebivolol on the primary end point (hazard ratio [HR] of nebivolol vs. placebo) was 0.86 (95 % confidence interval: 0.72–1.04) in patients with impaired EF and 0.81 (95 % confidence interval: 0.63–1.04) in preserved EF ($p = 0.720$ for subgroup interaction). Effects on all secondary end points were similar between groups (HR for all-cause mortality 0.84 and 0.91, respectively), and no p value for interaction was <0.48. Conclusions: The effect of beta-blockade with nebivolol in elderly patients with HF in this study was similar in those with preserved and impaired EF (Flather et al. 2005; van Veldhuisen et al. 2009). Nebivolol is a unique, highly selective beta-blocker with vasodilatory properties mediated through the nitric oxide pathway. This cardioactive agent is a highly selective beta1-adrenergic receptor blocker and is the only beta-blocker known to induce vascular production of nitric oxide, the main endothelial vasodilator. Nebivolol induces nitric oxide production via activation of beta3-adrenergic receptors and stimulates the beta3-adrenergic receptor-mediated production of nitric oxide in the heart; this stimulation results in a greater protection against heart failure (Maffei and Lembo 2009).

- Although Nebivolol combined with valsartan was shown in a small trial to significantly lower systolic blood pressure, it is not advisable to combine a beta-blocker with valsartan because an increase in mortality and cardiac events occurred in an HF RCT. Among those who were receiving both drugs at base line, valsartan had an adverse effect on mortality ($P = 0.009$) and was associated with a trend toward an increase in the combined end point of mortality and morbidity (Cohn and Tognoni 2001). The combination of nebivolol and ramipril is advisable.

Prolonged QT Interval Syndromes

Congenital syndromes are rare, but they do respond to beta-blockers. These agents appear to restore an imbalance between the left and right stellate ganglia. If recurrent episodes of torsades de pointes develop in a patient with a prolonged QT interval, the condition usually responds to propranolol and acutely to pacing. Propranolol has been proved to be useful in the congenital long-QT syndromes. Chockalingam et al. (2012) **based on a multicenter study recommend treatment of symptomatic long QT [LQT1] and LQT2 patients with propranolol, as clearly not all beta-blockers are equal in their antiarrhythmic efficacy in LQTS. Propranolol was superior to both nadolol and metoprolol in terms of shortening the cardiac repolarization time, particularly in high-risk patients with markedly prolonged QTc; Propranolol and nadolol were clinically effective in preventing events, metoprolol was not.**

Dissecting Aneurysm

A beta-blocker is the drug of choice to reduce the rate of rise of aortic pressure, which increases dissection. Even if the systolic blood pressure is 100–120 mmHg, propranolol or another IV preparation should be commenced. If the blood pressure exceeds 130 mmHg, a careful infusion of nitroprusside, or trimethaphan along with furosemide, is given to maintain systolic blood pressure at 100–120 mmHg. Labetalol has both beta- and alpha-blocking properties and has a role in therapy.

Note: The important effect of a beta-blocker in the treatment of dissecting aneurysm is not to lower blood pressure, but to decrease the force and velocity of myocardial contraction *(dp/dt)* and thus to arrest the progress of the dissection (Wheat 1973). The drug decreases the reflex tachycardia provoked by nitroprusside. The aforementioned beneficial effects of beta-blocking drugs can be translated to protection of arteries in patients with moderate to severe hypertension and in those with aneurysms. These agents are useful during the surgical clipping of intracranial aneurysms.

Mitral Valve Prolapse

Patients who have palpitations respond favorably to beta-blockers. These drugs should not be prescribed routinely, however, if the patient has only the occasional brief episode of palpitations. Asymptomatic atrial or ventricular ectopic beats require no medication. Chest pain in mitral valve prolapse syndrome is usually noncardiac. Care should be taken not to overtreat with medications and to avoid cardiac neurosis because this syndrome is usually benign. A beta-blocker can be tried if symptoms are distressing.

Mitral Regurgitation and Mitral Stenosis

Clinical trials with the use of carvedilol in patients with mitral regurgitation have shown salutary effects that include improved geometry of the left ventricle. Beta-blockers are the cornerstone of treatment for pregnant patients with mitral stenosis. These agents may prevent fulminant pulmonary edema.

Tetralogy of Fallot

Propranolol, by inhibiting right ventricular contractility, is of value in the acute treatment and prevention of prolonged hypoxic spells (Ponce et al. 1973).

- IV propranolol is used only for severe hypoxic spells.
- Oral propranolol for the prevention of hypoxic episodes is useful in centers where surgical correction is not available or the surgical mortality rate is greater than 10 % (Ponce et al. 1973).

Hypertrophic Cardiomyopathy

Medical management remains poor and does not significantly alter the mortality rate. Propranolol is effective for the relief of symptoms such as dizziness, presyncope, *angina, and dyspnea, but* the dose may need to be as high as 160–480 mg daily. Beta-blockers possessing ISA do not have a role here. **Verapamil** is a useful alternative if beta-blockers are contraindicated or have failed to relieve symptoms. **Disopyramide** appears to be of value in patients with hypertrophic cardiomyopathy, but it needs further randomized studies for confirmation. **Amiodarone** is useful for the control of arrhythmias associated with this condition, but it must not be combined with verapamil. See Chap. 23.

Marfan's Syndrome

Progressive dilation of the aorta, culminating in aortic dissection, is the most dreaded complication in patients with Marfan's syndrome. Prophylactic beta-blockade slows the rate of aortic dilation and retards the development of aortic complications (Kleiger et al. 1987). Propranolol has been shown to increase cross-linking of collagen in animals known to have a higher rate of aortic dissection (Brophy et al. 1989; Boucek et al. 1983).

- **Pyeritz (2007) indicated that beta-blocker therapy currently remains the "standard of care," and all patients should receive treatment, regardless of the presence or absence of aortic dilatation. "Atenolol administered twice daily is currently the drug of choice of many practitioners because it has long half-life and is relatively cardioselective, with fewer central nervous system and other side effects" (Pyeritz 2007).**
- **Lacro and colleagues state that an NIH clinical trial should provide some answers (Lacro et al. 2007). But unfortunately, these learned investigators choose to study atenolol, a poorly effective beta-blocker (▶Beta-Blockers).**
- *The choice of atenolol by Lacro et al. (2007) for an important RCT, Pyeritz (2007), and most Trialists is unfortunate. It must be emphasized that atenolol is a poorly effective beta-blocker because it is non-lipophilic and thus gains low brain concentration. The drug is not advisable and its use*

for all cardiac indications should be curtailed (Khan 2003).
The subtle differences in beta-blockers may provide the
solution for the apparent lack of cardioprotection of some
beta-blockers (Khan 1996a, b).

- **Atenolol is a hydrophilic beta-blocker that attains low**
brain concentration. Increased brain concentration and
elevation of central vagal tone confer cardiovascular
protection (Pitt 1992). Lipid-soluble beta-blockers (biso-
prolol, carvedilol, metoprolol, propranolol, and timolol)
with high brain concentration block sympathetic dis-
charge in the hypothalamus better than water-soluble
agents (atenolol, nadolol, and sotalol).

Subarachnoid Hemorrhage

Arrhythmias and other electrocardiographic abnormalities, LV dysfunction with reduced EF (Handlin et al. 1993),
and myocardial damage including subendocardial necrosis
have been documented in patients with subarachnoid
hemorrhage. These changes are believed to be caused by the
release of sympathetic outflow that occurs with CNS damage and by local norepinephrine release from sympathetic
nerves in the heart. Beta-blockers are indicated in individual
patients with subarachnoid hemorrhage in conjunction with
nimodipine therapy.

Perioperative Mortality

Optimization of cardiac medications in cardiac patients
undergoing noncardiac surgery requires the addition of a
beta-blocker. Beta-blockade allows safer induction of
anesthesia and prevents the hypertensive response to endotracheal intubation; also, these agents prevent recurrent
arrhythmias and have been shown to improve morbidity and
mortality.

Perioperative Protection Bisoprolol, in an RCT of 1,351
high-risk patients undergoing vascular surgery, significantly
reduced events ($p < 0.001$). Bisoprolol was started 1 week

preoperatively and continued for 30 days postoperatively; there were two deaths and no MIs vs. nine deaths and nine MIs in the untreated group (Poldermans et al. 1999).

- Beta-blocker administration should be used judiciously if needed, perioperatively in noncardiac patients undergoing noncardiac surgery. Some of these patients are at risk for cardiac events. POISE Trial: In the POISE trial (2008) patients were randomized in a double-blind manner to treatment with extended-release metoprolol ($n=4,174$) or placebo ($n=4,177$).
- A dose of the study drug (metoprolol 100 mg controlled release or placebo) was given 2–4 h prior to surgery and again 0–6 h after surgery. Daily doses of study drug (metoprolol 200 mg or placebo) were then taken for the next 30 days. At study entry, 43 % of patients had coronary artery disease, 41 % had peripheral vascular disease, and 15 % had a prior stroke. Type of surgery performed was vascular in 42 % of patients, intraperitoneal in 22 %, orthopedic in 21 %, and other types in 15 %. The primary end point of CV death, MI, or cardiac arrest was reduced in the metoprolol group compared with placebo (5.8 % vs. 6.9 %, hazard ratio [HR] 0.84, $p=0.04$), driven by a reduction in nonfatal MI (3.6 % vs. 5.1 %, HR 0.70, $p=0.0008$). There were also reductions with metoprolol in revascularization (0.3 % vs. 0.6 %, $p=0.012$) and new-onset atrial fibrillation (2.2 % vs. 2.9 %, $p=0.044$). However, total mortality was increased in the metoprolol group (3.1 % vs. 2.3 %, HR 1.33, $p=0.032$), as was stroke (1.0 % vs. 0.5 %, HR 2.17, $p=0.0053$).

Results

- The metoprolol group treated with **an inappropriately large dose of metoprolol** had increased rates of significant iatrogenic hypotension (15.0 % vs. 9.7 %, $p<0.0001$) and significant bradycardia (6.6 % vs. 2.4 %, $p<0.0001$), which contributed to the increase in mortality.
- Among patients undergoing noncardiac surgery, treatment with the beta-blocker metoprolol was associated with a

reduction in the primary end point of CV death, MI, or cardiac arrest at 30 days compared with placebo, but total mortality was higher in the metoprolol group (POISE trial 2008).

- This trial unfortunately selected a dose of metoprolol that was excessive.
- A significant excess of hypotension and bradycardia was caused by the large dose.
- See earlier discussion regarding the appropriate dose of beta-blockers.
- Too large a dose increases mortality.
- When beta-blockers are administered perioperatively, it is advisable to commence the drug >1 week before to obtain a heart rate of 55–60 per min and not <54min. Patients with blood pressure in the low normal range (systolic 105–115 mmHg) need a lower dose. Guidance is provided in the 2009 ACCF/AHA Focused Update on Perioperative Beta Blockade: a report of the American College of Cardiology Foundation/American Heart Association Task Force on Practice Guidelines (Fleischmann et al. 2009). This update of the ACCF/AHA 2007 guidelines on perioperative cardiovascular evaluation and care for noncardiac surgery addresses predominantly the use of perioperative beta-blockers to reduce cardiac risk.
- All recommendations for perioperative beta-blockade now also include the wording "titrated to heart rate and blood pressure," suggesting that, rather than a standard dose, perioperative beta-blocker therapy should be tailored to tolerated blood pressure and documented heart rate control.

Neurocardiogenic Syncope (Vasovagal/Vasodepressor Syncope)

If syncopal episodes are bothersome, a beta-blocking drug is advisable. Cardiac sympathetic overstimulation, vigorous LV contraction, and stimulation of intramyocardial mechanoreceptors (C fibers) are underlying mechanisms in the causation of unexplained syncope in patients with a normal heart (Theodorakis et al. 1993); a beta-blocker or disopyramide is the logical therapy and appears to be beneficial in patients with disabling syncope. Esmolol IV can be used to predict the outcome of oral beta-blocker therapy. Although a small trial has shown no beneficial effect for some beta-blockers, a non-cardioselective agent with greater vasoconstrictive properties such as timolol should be tested in RCTs.

Diabetic Patients

Diabetic patients at risk are a new indication for beta-blockers.

The UKPDS results (1998) confirm that in type 2 diabetes, beta-blockers significantly reduced all-cause mortality, risk for MI, stroke, PVD, and microvascular disease (Fig. 1-3). In addition, over the 9 years follow-up, the change in albuminuria and serum creatinine was the same in the captopril and beta-blocker groups: although the number of subjects in the study was small the follow-up was longer than most RCTs [9 years], atenolol produced salutary effects that were equal to that of captopril (Fig. 1-3). Importantly atenolol is a poorly effective beta-blocker, yet equaled ACE inhibitor therapy in type 2 diabetes. **Bisoprolol, carvedilol, and nebivlolol are first-choice beta-blockers recommended for the treatment of diabetic patients**. *See* Chap. 2.

Chronic Obstructive Pulmonary Disease

There is no longer a hesitation to prescribe a cardioselective beta-blocker (preferably bisoprolol, or nebivolol) to patients with stable chronic obstructive pulmonary disease (COPD). Short et al. (2011) examined the effect of β-blockers in the management of COPD assessing their effect on mortality, hospital admissions, and exacerbations of COPD when added to established treatment for COPD, in a population of 5,977 patients aged >50 years with a diagnosis of COPD.

Clinical end point	Patients with aggregate end points		Absolute risk (events per 1000 patient yr)			Relative risk for
	Captopril (n=400)	Atenolol (n=358)	Captopril	Atenolol	p value	captopril (95% CI)
Any diabetes-related end points	141	118	53.3	48.4	0.43	1.10 (0.86 – 1.41)
Deaths related to diabetes	48	34	15.2	12.0	0.28	1.27 (0.82 – 1.97)
All-cause mortality	75	59	23.8	20.8	0.44	1.14 (0.81 – 1.61)
Myocardial infarction	61	46	20.2	16.9	0.35	1.20 (0.82 – 1.76)
Stroke	21	17	6.8	6.1	0.74	1.12 (0.59 – 2.12)
Peripheral vascular disease	5	3	1.6	1.1	0.59	1.48 (0.35 – 6.19)
Microvascular disease	40	28	13.5	10.4	0.30	1.29 (0.80 – 2.10)

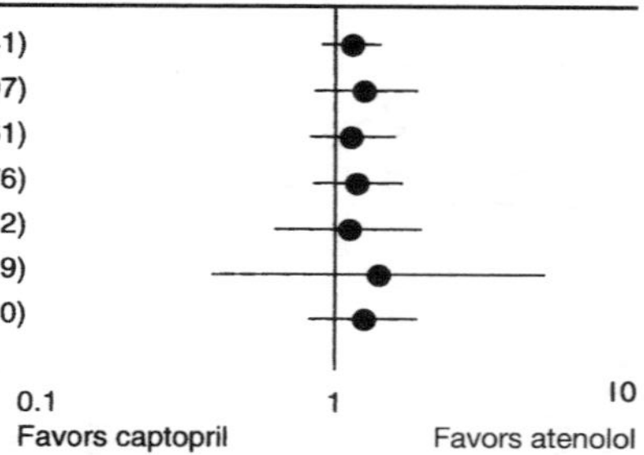

Fig. 1-3. Numbers of patients who attained one or more clinical end points in aggregates representing specific types of clinical complications, with relative risks comparing captopril with atenolol. Reproduced from United Kingdom Prospective Diabetes Study Group (1998) with permission from BMJ Publishing Group Ltd.

Results: Mean follow-up was 4.35 years, and 88 % of β-blockers used were cardioselective. There was a 22 % overall reduction in all-cause mortality with β-blocker use. In addition, there were significant reductions in oral corticosteroid use and hospital admissions for respiratory disease. Beta-blocker use did not show any deleterious effects on pulmonary function testing. The study findings suggest that β-blockers have effects on reducing mortality in COPD in addition to the benefits gained by reducing cardiovascular risk (Short et al. 2011). Similar findings have been observed by others.

Bisoprolol and nebivolol are the beta-blockers of choice for patients with COPD.

Noncardiac Indications

Noncardiac indications for beta-blockers are given in Table 1-6.

ADVICE AND ADVERSE EFFECTS

Warnings

Beta-blockers are relatively safe if the *warnings and contraindications* are carefully respected.

1. Beta-blockers are not advisable in patients with decompensated class IV HF (see discussions on the special use of these drugs in Chap. 12) (HF in the presence of acute MI with complete clearing of failure in a few days is not a contraindication). RCTs have established that these agents save lives in patients with class I–III HF and are strongly indicated.
2. **Severe cardiomegaly** is a relative contraindication.
3. They are not advisable in patients with EF <20 %.
4. They are not advisable in symptomatic bradycardia or chronotropic incompetence.
5. They are not advisable in conduction defects, or second- or third-degree AV block.

Table 1-6
Noncardiac indications for beta-blockers?

Situational anxiety (e.g., preoperative)
Essential tremor
Alcohol withdrawal: delirium tremens
Bartter's syndrome (juxtaglomerular hyperplasia)
Insulinoma
Glaucoma
Migraine prophylaxis
Narcolepsy
Thyrotoxicosis (arrhythmias)
Portal hypertension
Tetanus

6. Bronchial asthma is a contraindication. Chronic obstructive
   pulmonary disease [COPD] is not a contraindication. In
   fact these agents may decrease mortality in patients with
   COPD; see earlier discussion. Chronic bronchitis and
   emphysema are relative contraindications depending on
   their severity and the necessity for beta-blockade.
7. Severe allergic rhinitis is a relative contraindication.
8. **Avoid abrupt cessation** of therapy. A worsening of angina
   or precipitation of acute MI has occurred on abrupt withdrawal of therapy. Although this happens only rarely, the
   patient must be warned. The incidence of this syndrome is
   said to be infrequent with pindolol because of ISA. Do not
   discontinue suddenly before surgery. When it is necessary
   to discontinue beta-blockers, the dosage should be reduced
   gradually over 2–3 weeks, and the patient should be
   advised to minimize exertion during this period. Added
   therapy or nitrates and/or calcium antagonists are required
   during the withdrawal phase.
9. Insulin-dependent diabetes prone to hypoglycemia represents a relative contraindication.
10. Severe PVD, including Raynaud's disease, is a
    contraindication.

Side Effects

Cardiovascular

Precipitation of HF, AV block, hypotension, severe bradycardia, intermittent claudication, cold extremities,
Raynaud's phenomenon, and dyspnea may occur.

Central Nervous System

Depression may occur, especially with propranolol, and
psychosis can occur (Cunnane and Blackwood 1987).
Dizziness, weakness, fatigue, vivid dreams, insomnia,
and rare loss of hearing may occur.

Gastrointestinal

Nausea, vomiting, and epigastric distress are possible.

Respiratory

Bronchospasm, laryngospasm, respiratory distress, and
respiratory arrest (rare—with overdose) may occur.
Cardioselective agents are useful, however, in patients
with stable COPD; see earlier discussion under COPD.

Skin, Genitourinary

Rashes, exacerbation of psoriasis (Savola et al. 1987),
reduction of libido, and impotence. A clinical trial comparing propranolol with diuretics showed that impotence
was significantly more common in the diuretic-treated
group (MRC 1981) are possible.

Very rare cases of retroperitoneal fibrosis have been
reported with oxprenolol, atenolol, metoprolol, timolol,
propranolol, sotalol, pindolol, and acebutolol. The muco-
cutaneous syndrome observed with practolol has not
been reported with other beta-blockers. Positive antinuclear factor has been reported, however, with acebutolol,
pindolol, and labetalol. A lupus-like syndrome has been
seen rarely with the use of practolol, and a case has been
reported with the use of acebutolol. Labetalol can cause
a lupus syndrome and hepatic necrosis (Wallin and
O'Neill 1983).

INDIVIDUAL BETA-BLOCKERS

Drug name:	Acebutolol [**not a recommended beta-blocker**]
Trade names:	
Supplied:	100, 200, 400 mg
Dosage:	100–400 mg twice daily, max. 1,000 mg daily

Acebutolol is a relatively cardioselective and hydrophilic agent that possesses mild ISA and mild membrane-stabilizing activities (*see* Table 1-5). The very mild ISA activity prevents undue symptomatic bradycardia. Also, no significant decrease in HDL cholesterol occurs with long-term administration. In the Treatment of Mild Hypertension Study, acebutolol caused no significant change in HDL after 1 year of therapy.

Weak cardioselectivity and moderate lipid solubility are CP features. Mild ISA does not appear to negate the CP potential of acebutolol. It is possible that strongly cardioselective, water-soluble agents render less cardioprotection, and moderate or strong ISA is counterproductive.

The drug appears to have CP properties and caused about a 48 % decrease in cardiac deaths in a randomized post-MI study (Boissel et al. 1990). Clearly, a moderate degree of ISA is a disadvantage and destroys several salutary effects of beta-blockade (Khan 1996a, b), but mild ISA is an advantage in patients who require beta-blockade and demonstrate bothersome sinus bradycardia when they are given small doses of a non-ISA beta-blocker.

Drug name:	Atenolol [not a recommended beta-blocker]
Supplied:	25, 50, 100 mg
Dosage:	Initial: 25–50 mg once daily

This drug was a favorite of trialists from 1980 to 2007 but has often proved ineffective in decreasing CVD outcomes compared with newer agents. One notable exception is the UKPDS study; see Fig. 1-3 (1998). In these diabetic patients, renal dysfunction may have increased the serum levels of the drug, thus increasing effectiveness. In this small but long-term follow-up study in high-risk patients, atenolol was as effective as captopril in reducing CVD outcomes.

The drug is almost totally excreted by the kidney.

The author has discontinued use of atenolol since 2001 because the drug has lower CVD protective effects compared with other proven beta-blockers. THIS WIDELY USED BETABLOCKER SHOULD BECOME obsolete (Khan 2011). The use of atenolol in clinical trials should be curtailed (Khan 2003); see discussion under Marfan's syndrome. **Experts at the NIH recently conducted an RCT in patients with Marfan's syndrome, but unfortunately selected atenolol as the beta-blocker of choice.**

Drug name:	**Bisoprolol**
Trade names:	Zebeta, Monocor, Emcor
Supplied:	5–10 mg
Dosage:	5–10 mg daily, max. 20 mg
	Ziac, Monozide: bisoprolol and hydrochlorothiazide 6.25 mg

This agent is highly $beta_1$-selective, and it is more cardioselective than metoprolol; in humans, the drug has a twofold higher $beta_1$-selectivity than atenolol. A 10-mg dose is equivalent to atenolol 100 mg. The drug has a half-life of 12–14 h and thus has a long duration of action beyond 24 h.

Bisoprolol is 50 % lipophilic, metabolized by the liver, and 50 % hydrophilic, excreted by the kidney. The concentration of unchanged bisoprolol in rat brain is lower than that of metoprolol or propranolol but higher than that of atenolol after dosing. A study *(54)* in patients with LV dysfunction, CIBIS II, showed a markedly significant reduction in overall mortality with bisoprolol therapy; the study was stopped because of significant favorable effects. Bisoprolol treatment reduced all-cause mortality by 32 % ($p = 0.00005$) and sudden death by 45 % ($p = 0.001$). There was a 30 % reduction in hospitalization caused by worsening HF (*see* Chap. 12).

The combination of bisoprolol and 6.25 mg HCTZ (Ziac) has been approved by the U.S. Food and Drug Administration (FDA) as first-line initial therapy for hypertension (Monozide 10 in the UK).

The blood pressure-lowering effect is superior to that of atenolol (Neutel et al. 1993). The 5-mg dose seems equipotent to atenolol 50 mg. Most important, this is a genuine 24-h acting, once-daily drug.

Bisoprolol has been shown to *reduce ambulatory systolic and diastolic pressures by 43 % and 49 %, respectively, more than atenolol during the early morning hours, 4–10* am. *During this time frame, catecholamine surge causes an increased risk of ischemia and sudden death*. In response to pressure stimuli and increased catecholamines, there is less rise in blood pressure, *and excessive increase in exercise blood pressure is controlled*. Renal blood flow is enhanced.

Perioperative Protection: Bisoprolol, in an RCT of 1,351 high-risk patients undergoing vascular surgery, significantly reduced events ($p < 0.001$). Bisoprolol was started 1 week preoperatively and continued for 30 days postoperatively; there were two deaths and no MIs vs. nine deaths and nine MIs in the untreated group (Poldermans et al. 1999).

Drug name:	**Carvedilol**
Trade names:	Coreg, Eucardic
Supplied:	6.25, 12.5, 25 mg
Dosage:	Heart failure: 3.125 mg, then 6.25 mg twice daily; titrate over weeks to 25 mg twice daily; see text for further advice
	Hypertension: 12.5 mg daily; titrate over weeks to 25–50 mg daily, max. 50 mg
	Angina: 12.5 mg twice daily; titrate over days to weeks to 25 mg twice daily

For the beneficial results observed in the CAPRICORN and COPERNICUS trials, *see* Chap. 22. **Carvedilol is one of the most effective beta-blockers available and is a good choice for use in acute MI and post-MI prophylaxis particularly if LV dysfunction is present**. It is also recommended for hypertension, particularly in diabetics or prediabetics, because it has been shown to improve insulin sensitivity compared with metoprolol (GEMINI: Bakris et al. 2004) *(see* Chap. 2 and also the last section of this chapter, Which Beta-Blocker Is Best for Your Patients?).

Dosage (Further Advice)

The dosage must be individualized during up-titration. Titration also depends on the occurrence of hypotension and bradycardia. The dose of digoxin, diuretic, and ACE inhibitor or angiotensin II receptor blocker must be stabilized before commencing carvedilol. The initial dose is 3.125 mg twice daily for 2 weeks and then, if tolerated, 6.25 mg twice daily. The dose can be doubled every 4 weeks to the highest level tolerated by the patient. Observe the patient for dizziness, light-headedness, and hypotension for 1 h after the initiation of each new dose. The maximum dose is 25 mg twice daily in patients weighing less than 85 kg and 50 mg twice daily in those weighing over 85 kg. Carvedilol should be administered with food to slow the rate of absorption and to reduce the incidence of orthostatic effects. If symptoms of vasodilation occur (e.g., dizziness and light-headedness), reduce the dose of diuretic and then, if necessary, the ACE inhibitor. If symptoms do not resolve, reduce the carvedilol dosage. Symptoms of worsening HF (e.g., edema, weight gain, and shortness of breath) should be treated with increased doses of diuretic. The carvedilol dose should be reduced if symptoms persist.

Action

The ratio of alpha$_1$- to beta-blockade for carvedilol is 1:10, compared with 1:4 for labetalol, a more powerful alpha$_1$-blocker that causes a greater degree of vasodilation and orthostatic hypotension; antioxidant and antiproliferative properties have been reported. The drug improves ventricular function without upregulating downregulated myocardial beta-receptors in the failing heart.

Indications

The drug is approved by the FDA for the management of class I–III HF. The U.S. Carvedilol Heart Failure Study (Packer et al. 1996) in patients with NYHA class II and III HF showed a 27 % reduction in hospitalization and a 65 % reduction in mortality risk.

- The drug is contraindicated in patients with decompensated class IV HF.
- As with other beta-blockers, the drug is contraindicated in patients with asthma, severe COPD, second- or third-degree AV block, and sick sinus syndrome. Carvedilol is not advisable in patients with clinically manifest *hepatic impairment. Mild hepatic injury has been noted.* Stop the drug and do not restart if the patient has evidence of liver injury.

- *Class IV patients,* when stabilized and *free of fluid overload,* can be started on 3.125 mg, a dose titrated slowly up over several weeks.
- Ejection fraction and myocardial energetics take about 8 weeks to improve as a biologic effect with beta-blocker therapy. The ventricle goes from a more spherical shape to a more normal elliptical shape, and LV mass decreases; these changes indicate that the pathologic remodeling process is being attenuated and in many cases reverts back to normal. It is important to initiate therapy as early as possible while there is myocardial viability left and it is possible to recover a biologic effect on myocytes.
- End-diastolic volume decreases; myocardial contractility increases, after about 3 months of therapy; mechanical work improves, as reflected by stroke work; and myocardial O_2 consumption decreases.
- Myocardial efficiency increases in patients who receive a beta-blocker as well as an ACE inhibitor. Plasma norepinephrine increases over time in patients treated with an ACE inhibitor. *The combination of a beta-blocker and ACE inhibitor is complementary and cardioprotective in patients with MI, HF, diabetes, hypertension, and LVH.*

Drug name:	**Esmolol**
Trade name:	Brevibloc
Dosage:	IV infusion within range 50–200 µg/kg/min; *see* text for further advice

Dosage (Further Advice)

The dose is 5–40 mg, usually 3–6 mg IV infusion over 1 min (30–300 µg to maximum of 500 µg/kg over 1 min) and then maintenance infusion 1–5 mg/min (maximum 50 µg/ kg/min). If control of the clinical situation is not achieved and more rapid titration is necessary, a further bolus may be given followed by an increase in the maintenance infusion rate. If mild hypotension is present, the maintenance dose should be reduced to 1–3 mg/min. Hypotensive effects of the drug usually disappear within minutes of cessation of the infusion.

Esmolol IV 50–200 μg/kg/min has an effect equivalent to that of propranolol 3–6 mg IV.

Action

Esmolol is a cardioselective ultrashort-acting beta-blocker that is quickly converted by esterases of red blood cells to inactive metabolites (Gorczynski 1985). The drug has a short half-life of about 9 min *(74)* that is stable in patients with mild HF, hepatic dysfunction, or renal failure. The drug action dissipates within 20–30 min of administration.

Indications

1. The drug is used for SVT in the perioperative period (Cray et al. 1985) and for SVT not terminated by adenosine or in patients with contraindications to the use of adenosine or verapamil, especially during acute MI or other ischemic syndromes.
2. **Contraindications** include

   - Severe hypotension or cardiogenic shock.
   - Asthma or severe COPD.
   - Other contraindications to the use of beta-blocking agents.

Drug name:	**Labetalol**
Trade names:	Normodyne, Trandate
Supplied:	50, 100, 200, 400 mg
Dosage:	50–100 mg twice daily; titrate over weeks to 200–400 mg twice daily;
	see text for IV dosage

A combined alpha- and beta-blocker: this drug is useful in the management of hypertension of all grades including hypertensive emergencies.

Disadvantages: Labetalol causes significant postural hypotension and must be given two or three times daily in large doses. Side effects include a lupus-like illness, a lichenoid rash, impotence (Wallin and O'Neill 1983), and, very rarely, hepatotoxicity manifesting as raised levels of transaminases, abnormal liver function test results, hepatitis, and fatal or nonfatal hepatic necrosis (Clark et al. 1990) .

Drug name:	**Metoprolol**
Trade names:	Betaloc, Betaloc SR, Lopressor, Toprol-XL
Supplied:	50, 100 mg
	Betaloc SR: 200 mg
	Toprol-XL: 50, 100, 200 mg
Dosage:	50–200 mg twice daily
	Long-acting: 50–200 g once daily, max. 300 mg

Toprol XL, with its 24-h duration of action, is important for coverage of early morning catecholamine surge and early morning fatal MI. **This drug is superior to other sustained-release metoprolol tartrate formulations, whose action may not continue throughout the 24-h period.**

Metoprolol is beta$_1$-cardioselective. In patients with bronchospastic disease, metoprolol, in doses lower than 150 mg daily, causes less bronchospasm than a nonselective beta-blocker at equivalent beta-blocking dose. If bronchospasm is precipitated, it will respond to beta$_2$-stimulants, whereas there would be a poor response if a nonselective beta-blocker were used. Cardioselectivity confers advantages when beta-blockers are given to patients with labile diabetes.

Metoprolol has been shown to reduce the incidence of VT during acute MI (Ryden et al. 1983). The Göteborg metoprolol trial has documented the beneficial effect of metoprolol on survival during the early phase of MI (from day 1 for 90 days). Metoprolol caused a 36 % reduction in mortality rate during the 90 days of therapy, and benefit was maintained for 1 year.

Metoprolol causes less sedation and drowsiness than atenolol. In addition, *metoprolol is lipid soluble and appears to be more cardioprotective than water-soluble beta-blockers, which achieve lower concentration in the brain.*

The MERIT-HF study (MERIT-HF Study Group 1999, 2002) has established metoprolol as indicated in patients with class I–III HF. It is most important to start with small doses: metoprolol succinate (CR/XL) controlled-release 12.5 mg once daily, and titrate up slowly over 4–8 weeks to a target dose of 150–200 mg.

Drug name:	**Nadolol**
Trade name:	Corgard
Supplied:	40, 80, 120, 160 mg
Dosage:	40–80 mg once daily, max. 160 mg; *see* text for further advice

Dosage (Further Advice)

The manufacturers suggest a maximum of 240 mg for angina and 320 mg for hypertension. These high doses are not recommended by the author. Because the drug has a very long half-life and is excreted entirely by the kidneys, accumulation commonly occurs in patients with mild renal dysfunction and in patients over 65 years of age. In practice, a dose of 80 mg is equivalent to ~160 mg of propranolol. The dose must be reduced in renal failure and in the elderly. Also, the time interval between doses should be increased, that is, one tablet every 36 or 48 h may suffice in renal failure. Use a nonrenally excreted beta-blocker in the presence of severe renal failure.

Like propranolol, nadolol is a nonselective beta-blocker. It has a weak lipid solubility and therefore is almost completely excreted by the kidney. No large RCT has been done to prove its effectiveness in reducing CVD mortality or morbidity. Because of its long half-life it is given as a one-a-day tablet; this may be important when compliance is a problem.

Insomnia and **vivid dreams** occur much less frequently with nadolol and atenolol compared with propranolol and other lipid-soluble beta-blockers, but they can occur with sotalol.

The dose of atenolol, nadolol, and sotalol should be reduced in renal failure, and with severe renal failure, the time interval between doses should be increased.

Drug name:	**Nebivolol**
Trade name:	Bystolic, Nebilet/I in UK, Australia; Nebilong, Nebicard, Nubeta in India; Nodon in Italy and Greece; Byscard in Pakistan; Lobivon in Middle East
Dosage:	For hypertension: 5 mg daily; elderly initially 2.5 mg daily, increased if necessary to 5 mg daily. For mild to moderate heart failure, mainly in patients 70 years and older: initially 1.25 mg once daily, then if tolerated increased at intervals of 1–2 weeks to 2.5 mg once daily, then to 5 mg once daily, and then to max. 10 mg once daily. Manufacturer advises avoid if serum creatinine greater than 250 micromol/L. Cautions: reduce dose in renal impairment, in the elderly, and in hepatic dysfunction.

- Nebivolol is a novel beta-blocker with several important pharmacologic properties that distinguish it from traditional beta-blockers (Gray and Ndefo 2008).
- This highly selective beta1-adrenergic receptor blocker is the only beta-blocker known to induce vascular production of nitric oxide, the main endothelial vasodilator. Nebivolol stimulates the beta3-adrenergic receptor-mediated production of nitric oxide in the heart; this stimulation results in a greater protection against heart failure (Maffei and Lembo 2009).
- In addition, nebivolol increases NO by decreasing its oxidative inactivation (Cominacini et al. 2003). The drug stimulates the endothelial L-arginine/nitric oxide pathway and thus causes vasodilation (Cockcroft et al. 1995). Nebivolol should find a role in the management of heart failure, particularly in patients with normal or slightly reduced EF.
- In the small ENECA study in 260 elderly patients (>65 years) with chronic heart failure (CHF), nebivolol significantly improved cardiac function and proved to be safe and well tolerated in elderly patients with signs of heart failure and an impaired EF (EF: nebivolol 25.41 7.09 % and control 26.41 5.55 %. The EF improved significantly ($p=0.027$) more in the nebivolol group (6.51 9.15 %) than in the control group (3.97 9.20 %)) (Edes et al. 2005).
- In the SENIORS study (Flather et al. 2005; van Veldhuisen et al. 2009) of 2,111 patients, 1,359 (64 %) had impaired (35 %) EF (mean 28.7 %) and 752 (36 %) had preserved (>35 %) EF (mean 49.2 %).
- During follow-up of 21 months the primary end point occurred in 465 patients (34.2 %) with impaired EF and in 235 patients (31.2 %) with preserved EF. The effect of nebivolol on the primary end point (hazard ratio [HR] of nebivolol vs. placebo) was 0.86 (95 % confidence interval: 0.72–1.04) in patients with impaired EF and 0.81 (95 % confidence interval: 0.63–1.04) in preserved EF ($p=0.720$ for subgroup interaction). Effects on all secondary end points were similar between groups (HR for all-cause mortality 0.84 and 0.91, respectively). Conclusions: The effect

of beta-blockade with nebivolol in elderly patients with HF in ·this study was similar in those with preserved and impaired EF (van Veldhuisen et al. 2009).

- Nebivolol reduces P-wave dispersion on the electrocardiogram, which would attenuate the risk of atrial fibrillation (Tuncer et al. 2008).
- Time to maximum concentration is 0.5–2 h, and half-life is 11 h in extensive metabolizers; these values are about three times longer in poor metabolizers.
- Nebivolol appears to have a minor, if any, effect on libido and sexual performance, which likely ensues from a compensatory effect of the increased NO release (Boydak et al. 2005). In contrast with metoprolol, nebivolol improves secondary sexual activity and erectile dysfunction scores (Brixius et al. 2007).
- An extensive review article was forwarded by Münzel and Gori (2009). Although a decade of clinical experience with this drug in Europe provides support to its blood pressure-lowering and anti-ischemic effects, further clinical trial data are necessary. Particularly, comparative trials on the efficacy of nebivolol vs. other beta-blockers and/or other antihypertensive drugs are awaited (Münzel and Gori 2009).
- Maffei and Lembo provided informative information on nitric oxide mechanisms of nebivolol in an article: Therapeutic Advances in Cardiovascular Disease (Maffei and Lembo 2009).

Nebivolol, but not metoprolol, inhibited cardiac NADPH oxidase activation after MI. The drug, but not metoprolol, improved LV dysfunction 4 weeks after MI (LV ejection fraction: nebivolol vs. metoprolol vs. placebo: 32 ± 4 % vs. 17 ± 6 % vs. 19 ± 4 %; nebivolol vs. metoprolol: $p < 0.05$) and was associated with improved survival 4 weeks post-MI compared with placebo. Nebivolol had a significantly more pronounced inhibitory effect on cardiomyocyte hypertrophy after MI compared with metoprolol (Sorrentino et al. 2011).

Drug name:	**Propranolol**
Trade name:	Inderal
Supplied:	Inderal: 10, 20, 40, 80, 120 mg
	Inderal LA: 80, 120, 160 mg capsules
Dosage:	40–80 mg twice daily; titrate over weeks to 80–120 mg twice daily
	LA: 80–160 mg once daily, max. 240 mg; *see* text for further advice. *Do not use in smokers; the drug loses effectiveness.

Indications

This beta-blocker has been in use since 1964 and is still a frequently prescribed beta-blocker worldwide. Unlike other beta-blockers, the drug is approved by the FDA for many indications: angina, acute MI, post-infarction prevention, arrhythmias, hypertension, IV use, anesthetic arrhythmias, hypertrophic cardiomyopathy, syncope, anxiety and essential tremor, migraine prophylaxis, and thyrotoxicosis.

The long-acting preparation provides full 24-h coverage. The BHAT study (1982) proved the beneficial effects of propranolol in post-MI patients for the prevention of reinfarction, sudden death, and fatal and nonfatal MIs. *Cigarette smoking alters blood levels of propranolol and may mask CP effects.* In nonsmokers, however, the drug has been proved effective, whereas only timolol has been proved effective in RCTs and in the post-MI patient.

The drug is strongly lipid soluble and therefore has a high uptake in the brain; this may be the reason for fatigue, the rare occurrence of depression, and vivid dreams. Lipid solubility, brain concentration, and $beta_1$- and $beta_2$-blockade provide cardioprotection. In smokers, the salutary effects of propranolol are masked (Deanfield et al. 1984) .

If depression, fatigue, or mild memory impairment occurs, switch to bisoprolol, metoprolol, or timolol.

Drug name:	**Sotalol**
Trade names:	Sotacor, Betapace, Beta-Cardone
Supplied:	80, 160, 240 mg
Dosage:	40–80 mg once daily; increase over days to weeks to 80–160 mg once or twice daily

Indications

In the USA, this drug is approved for oral use in patients with life-threatening ventricular arrhythmias (nonsustained VT). This agent is not recommended for the treatment of hypertension or asymptomatic ventricular premature beats.

Sotalol is unique among the approved beta-blockers. The drug has all the effects of a nonselective beta-blocker plus an added class III antiarrhythmic effect: the drug lengthens the duration of the cardiac action potential and prolongs the QTc interval of the surface electrocardiogram.

The drug appears to be more effective than other beta-blockers in the control of numerous bothersome ventricular premature beats and sustained VT. However, some studies indicate no difference in efficacy. The drug has been shown to cause an 88 % reduction in ventricular ectopic beat frequency at the optimal titrated dosage.

Torsades de pointes have been precipitated as a rare complication, mainly in patients with hypokalemia. Torsades occurred, however, despite therapeutic plasma sotalol concentration and normal serum potassium level in the absence of diuretics. **Caution** is necessary: do not administer sotalol with nonpotassium-sparing diuretics and drugs that cause QT prolongation.

The drug represents a significant advance in the management of some ventricular tachyarrhythmias, including recurrent VT tachycardia or VF.

Contraindications

Congenital or acquired long QT syndromes are contraindications, low serum potassium, as well as other contraindications to beta-blockade.

Drug name:	**Timolol**
Trade names:	Blocadren, Betim
Supplied:	5, 10 mg
Dosage:	5–10 mg twice daily, max. 20 mg twice daily

This non-cardioselective drug has some advantages over propranolol. First-pass hepatic metabolism is 60, and 40 % of the drug is excreted unchanged in the urine. Variation in plasma level is only sevenfold. The drug is six times more potent than propranolol, so for a given dose, a better plasma level is achieved with less variation. It has moderate lipid solubility.

Timolol can be given twice a day with a fair certainty that plasma levels will be adequate. It has proved to be efficacious and safe in the reduction of raised intraocular pressure when used topically.

• Timolol is the first beta-blocker to have been shown beyond reasonable doubt to reduce cardiac mortality in the post-MI patient. A remarkable 67 % reduction in sudden cardiac deaths was achieved by timolol in the post-MI study (The Norwegian Multicenter Study Group 1981); unfortunately it is rarely used in the USA or Canada.

WHICH BETA-BLOCKER IS BEST FOR YOUR PATIENTS?

Sufficient attention has not been paid by the medical profession and researchers regarding the subtle differences that exist amongst the available beta-blocking drugs (Khan 2005, p. 55).

Agents with ISA are not cardioprotective drugs and should be avoided. For cardioselective agents, only bisoprolol and metoprolol (both lipophilic) have been shown to reduce CHD mortality and events significantly in the following well-conducted RCTs: CIBIS II (1998), MERIT-HF (2002), and SOLVD (beta-blocker) (1992).

- The non-cardioselective, lipophilic agents, carvedilol, propranolol, and timolol, are without doubt proven cardioprotective.
- Propranolol was shown in BHAT 1982.
- Carvedilol was studied in the successful CAPRICORN and COPERNICUS trials (see earlier discussion of the beta2-effect on potassium homeostasis). The common threads for reduction in mortality in post-MI patients are beta1, beta2, and lipophilicity that augment brain concentration and may protect from sudden death.
- *In the timolol study, there was a 67 % reduction in sudden death (timolol is beta1- and beta2-selective and lipophilic). No other cardiovascular agent has produced such an outstanding reduction in cardiac sudden deaths, yet the drug is rarely prescribed worldwide.* **A long-acting once-daily formulation is required.**
- Of the agents—timolol, nebivolol, bisoprolol, carvedilol, metoprolol, and propranolol [in nonsmokers] should be recommended based on the aforementioned logical approach.
- Bisoprolol has shown some advantages for the hypertensive and heart failure patient: genuine one-a-day administration, quelling of early morning catecholamine surge, and better control of early morning and exercise-induced excessive rise in blood pressure than atenolol (Kokkinos et al. 2006). Bisoprolol is highly cardioselective of the three and therefore safe to use in diabetes, COPD, and perioperatively, as Toprol XL a proven 24 h metoprolol formulation has been well tested for hypertension and heart failure.
- Nebivolol has several advantages over all beta-blocking drugs discussed for the management of heart failure and hypertension and results of large outcome trials are awaited (see discussion under nebivolol).

- For hypertension: bisoprolol, or metoprolol sustained-release (Toprol XL) given once daily; or carvedilol, which usually should be administered twice daily, is most useful if LV dysfunction is present.
- A once-daily formulation of carvedilol would be an advance because the drug is beta1 beta2, has antioxidant properties, and does not unfavorably alter insulin resistance as does metoprolol. See Chap. 2
- For diabetics: carvedilol, bisoprolol, or nebivolol are the preferred beta-blockers in patients with no risk of hypoglycemia for hypertension management or other indication for the use of a beta-blocker.
- For heart failure: carvedilol showed marked benefit and safety in the CAPRICORN post-MI study and the COPERNICUS HF study, and is the beta-blocker of choice for patients with HF or and post-MI patients with LV dysfunction. **Nebivolol has proved effective for heart failure preserved EF**.

Nebivolol, but not metoprolol, improved LV dysfunction 4 weeks after MI (LV ejection fraction: nebivolol vs. metoprolol vs. placebo: 32 ± 4 % vs. 17 ± 6 % vs. 19 ± 4 %; nebivolol vs. metoprolol: $p < 0.05$) and was associated with improved survival 4 weeks post-MI compared with placebo (Sorrentino et al. 2011). See discussion under nebivolol.

- Metoprolol tartrate slow release formulations may not have a full 24 h action).
- For ventricular arrhythmias: the choice of propranolol is appropriate in nonsmokers because it may prevent sudden cardiac death; bisoprolol or metoprolol is commonly prescribed.
- For thyrotoxicosis: propranolol is advisable.
- For Marfan's syndrome: propranolol or other lipophilic agent is recommended; the commonly used atenolol is not advisable; see earlier discussion under Marfan's syndrome.

Chockalingam et al. (2012) based on a multicenter study "recommend treatment of symptomatic long QT [LQT1] and LQT2 patients with propranolol or nadolol, as clearly not all beta-blockers are equal in their antiarrhythmic efficacy in LQTS. Propranolol was superior to both nadolol and metoprolol in terms of shortening the cardiac repolarization time, particularly in high-risk patients with markedly prolonged QTc."

- This finding is not surprising because propranolol is more liphophilic than nadolol and metoprolol and thus attains higher brain concentration than nadolol, metoprolol, and the commonly used atenolol, a hydrophilic drug that attains poor brain concentration. Atenolol is therefore not recommended by the author for all cardiac problems including for the management of hypertension.
- For HCM propranolol [in nonsmokers] or other lipophilic agent is advised [not atenolol]

REFERENCES

BHAT;β-Blocker Heart Attack Trial Research Group. A randomised trial of propranolol in patients with acute myocardial infarction. I: mortality results. JAMA. 1982;247:1707–14.

Black JW, Crowther AF, Shanks RG, et al. A new adrenergic beta-receptor-antagonist. Lancet. 1964;2:1080.

Boissel JP, Leizorovicz A, Picolet H, et al. Efficacy of acebutolol after acute myocardial infarction (the APSI Trial). Am J Cardiol. 1990; 66:24C.

Boucek RJ, Gunja-Smith Z, Noble NL, et al. Modulation by propranolol of the lysyl cross-links in aortic elastin and collagen of the aneurysm-prone turkey. Biochem Pharmacol. 1983;32:275.

Boydak B, Nalbantgil S, Fici F, et al. A randomised comparison of the effects of nebivolol and atenolol with and without chlorthalidone on the sexual function of hypertensive men. Clin Drug Investig. 2005; 25:409–16.

Braunwald E. Mechanism of action of calcium-channel-blocking agents. N Engl J Med. 1982;307:1618.

Breckenridge A. Jogger's blockade. Br Med J. 1982;284:532.

Brixius K, Middeke M, Lichtenthal A, et al. Nitric oxide, erectile dysfunction and beta-blocker treatment (MR NOED study): benefit of nebivolol versus metoprolol in hypertensive men. Clin Exp Pharmacol Physiol. 2007;34:327–31.

Brophy CM, Tilson JE, Tilson MD. Propranolol stimulates the crosslink-
    ing of matrix components in skin from the aneurysm-prone blotchy
    mouse. J Surg Res. 1989;46:330.

CAPRICORN: The Capricorn Investigators. Effect of carvedilol on out-
    come after myocardial infarction in patients with left-ventricular dys-
    function. Lancet. 2001;357:1385.

Chan AW, Quinn MJ, Bhatt DL, et al. Mortality benefit of beta-blockade
    after successful elective percutaneous coronary intervention. J Am
    Coll Cardiol. 2002;40:669–75.

Chockalingam P, Crotti L, Girardengo G, et al. Not all beta-blockers are
    equal in the management of long qt syndrome types 1 and 2: higher
    recurrence of events under metoprolol. J Am Coll Cardiol. 2012;
    60(20):2092–9.

Clark JA, Zimmerman HF, Tanner LA. Labetalol hepatotoxicity. Ann
    Intern Med. 1990;113:210.

Cockcroft JR, Chowienczyk PJ, Brett SE, et al. Nebivolol vasodilates
    human forearm vasculature: evidence for a L-arginine/No-dependent
    mechanism. J Pharmacol Exp Ther. 1995;274:1067–71.

Cominacini L, Pasini AF, Garbin U, et al. Nebivolol and its 4-keto deriva-
    tive increase nitric oxide in endothelial cells by reducing its oxidative
    inactivation. J Am Coll Cardiol. 2003;42:1838–44.

COPERNICUS, Packer M, Coast JS, Fowler MB, et al. Effect of carvedilol
    on survival in severe chronic heart failure. N Engl J Med. 2001;
    344:1651.

Cray RJ, Bateman TM, Czer LS, et al. Esmolol: a new ultrashort-acting
    beta-adrenergic blocking agent for rapid control of heart rate in post-
    operative supraventricular tachyarrhythmias. J Am Coll Cardiol.
    1985;5:1451.

Cruickshank JM, Degaute JP, Kuurne T, et al. Reduction of stress/cate-
    cholamine induced cardiac necrosis by B1 selective blockade. Lancet.
    1987;2:585.

Cruickshank JM. Beta-blockers continue to surprise us. Eur Heart
    J. 2000;21:355.

Cunnane JG, Blackwood GW. Psychosis with propranolol: still not recog-
    nized? Postgrad Med J. 1987;63:57.

Deanfield J, Wright C, Krikler S. Cigarette smoking and the treatment of
    angina with propranolol, atenolol and nifedipine. N Engl J Med.
    1984;310:951.

Devreux RB. Do antihypertensive drugs differ in their abilities to regress
    left ventricular hypertrophy? Circulation. 1997;95:1983.

Edes I, Gasior Z, Wita K. Effects of nebivolol on left ventricular function
    in elderly patients with chronic heart failure: results of the ENECA
    study. Eur J Heart Fail. 2005;7(4):631–9.

Engler RL, Conant J, Maisel A, et al. Lipid solubility determines the relative CNS effects of beta-blocking agents. J Am Coll Cardiol. 1986;7:25A.

Flather MD, Shibata MC, Coats AJ, et al. Randomized trial to determine the effect of nebivolol on mortality and cardiovascular hospital admission in the elderly patients with heart failure (SENIORS). Eur Heart J. 2005;26:215–25.

Fleischmann KE, Beckman JA, Buller CE, et al. 2009 ACCF/AHA focused update on perioperative beta blockade: a report of the American College of Cardiology Foundation/American Heart Association Task Force on Practice Guidelines. J Am Coll Cardiol. 2009;54:2102–28.

Frishman WH. Beta-adrenergic blocking drugs. Am Coll Cardiol Curr J Rev. 1997;23.

GEMINI, Bakris GL, Fonseca V, Katholi RE, et al. Metabolic effects of carvedilol vs. metoprolol in patients with type 2 diabetes mellitus and hypertension: a randomized controlled trial. JAMA. 2004;292:2227–36.

Gorczynski RJ. Basic pharmacology of esmolol. Am J Cardiol. 1985; 56:3F.

Goyal A, Spertus JA, Gosch K, et al. Serum potassium levels and mortality in acute myocardial infarction. JAMA. 2012;307(2):157–64.

Gray CL, Ndefo UA. Nebivolol: a new antihypertensive agent. Am J Health Syst Pharm. 2008a;65(12):1125–33.

Handlin LR, Kindred LH, Beauchamp GD, et al. Reversible left ventricular dysfunction after subarachnoid hemorrhage. Am Heart J. 1993; 126:235.

Hjalmarson A, Herlitz J, Malek I. Effect on mortality of metoprolol in acute myocardial infarction. Lancet. 1981;2:823.

International Collaborative Study Group. Reduction of infarct size with early use of timolol in acute myocardial infarction. N Engl J Med. 1984;310:9.

Johansson BW. Effect of beta-blockade on ventricular fibrillation and tachycardia induced circulatory arrest in acute myocardial infarction. Am J Cardiol. 1986;57:34F.

Julian DG. Is the use of beta-blockade contraindicated in the patient with coronary spasm? Circulation. 1983;67(Suppl):1.

Kaumann AJ. Some aspects of heart beta adrenoceptor function. Cardiovasc Drugs Ther. 1991;5:549.

Khan MG. Clinical trials. In: Khan MG, Cardiac Drug Therapy. Philadelphia: WB Saunders; 2003. p. 502.

Khan MG. Hypertension. In: Khan MG, Encyclopedia of heart diseases. New York: Springer; 2011. p. 556.

Khan MG. Which beta blocker to choose. In: Khan MG, Heart disease diagnosis and therapy. 2nd ed. Totowa, NJ: Humana Press; 2005.

Khan MG. Angina. In: Khan MG. Heart disease, diagnosis and therapy. Baltimore, MD: Williams & Wilkins; 1996a.

Khan MG. Hyperlipidemia. In: Khan MG. Heart disease, diagnosis and therapy. Baltimore, MD: Williams & Wilkins; 1996b. p. 384.

Khan MG, Topol EJ. Angina. In: Khan MG. Heart disease, diagnosis and therapy, a practical approach. Baltimore, MD: Williams and Wilkins; 1996. p. 157.

Khan MI, Hamilton JT, Manning GW. Protective effect of beta adrenoceptor blockade in experimental coronary occlusion in conscious dogs. Am J Cardiol. 1972;30:832.

Kjekshus JK. Importance of heart rate in determining beta-blocker efficacy in acute and long-termmyocardial infarction intervention trials. Am J Cardiol. 1986;57:43F.

Kleiger RE, Miller JP, Bigger JT, et al. Decreased heart rate variability and its association with increased mortality after acute myocardial infarction. Am J Cardiol. 1987;59:256.

Kokkinos P, Chrysohoou C, Panagiotakos D, et al. Beta-blockade mitigates exercise blood pressure in hypertensive male patients. J Am Coll Cardiol. 2006;47:794–8.

Kostis JB, Rosen RC. Central nervous system effects of beta-adrenergic blocking drugs: the role of ancillary properties. Circulation. 1987; 75:204.

Krum H, Gu A, Wiltshire-Clement M, et al. Changes in plasma endothelin-1 levels reflects clinical response to β-blockade in chronic heart failure. Am Heart J. 1996;131:337.

Lacro RV, Dietz HC, Wruck LM, et al. Rationale and design of a randomized clinical trial of beta-blocker therapy (atenolol) versus angiotensin II receptor blocker therapy (losartan) in individuals with Marfan syndrome. Am Heart J. 2007;154:624–31.

Lee JH, Bae MH, Chae SC, et al. The benefit of beta-blocker therapy in hospital survivors receiving primary percutaneous coronary intervention after ST-elevation myocardial infarction from the Korea acute myocardial infarction registry. J Am Coll Cardiol. 2012;60(17_S). doi:10.1016/j.jacc.2012.08.753.

Lindholm LH, Carlberg B, Samuelsson O. Should β blockers remain first choice in the treatment of primary hypertension? A meta-analysis. Lancet. 2005;366:1545–53.

Maffei A, Lembo G. Nitric oxide mechanisms of nebivolol. Ther Adv Cardiovasc Dis. 2009;3(4):317–27.

Man in't Veld AJ, Van den Meiracker AH, Schalekamp MA. Do beta-blockers really increase peripheralvascular resistance? Review of the literature and new observations under basal conditions. Am J Hypertens. 1988;1:91.

Matterson BJ, Reda DJ, Cushman WC, et al. Single drug therapy for hypertensive men: a comparison of 6 hypertensive agents with placebo. N Engl J Med. 1993;328:914.

Medical Research Council Working Party on Mild to Moderate Hypertension. Bendrofluazide and propranolol for the treatment of mild hypertension. Lancet. 1981;2:359.

Medical Research Council Working Party. MRC trial of treatment of hypertension in older adults: principal results. BMJ. 1992;304:405.

MERIT-HF Study Group. Dose of metoprolol CR/XL and clinical outcomes in patients with heart failure. Analysis of the experience in metoprolol CR/XL randomized intervention trial in chronic heart failure (MERIT-HF). J Am Coll Cardiol. 2002;40:491–8.

MERIT-HF Study Group. Effect of metoprolol CR/XL in chronic heart failure: metoprolol CR/XL Randomized Trial in Congestive Heart Failure (MERIT-HF). Lancet. 1999;353:2001.

Motomura S, Zerkowski HR, Daul A, et al. On the physiologic role of beta-2 adrenoceptors in the human heart: in vitro and in vivo studies. Am Heart J. 1990;119:608.

Münzel T, Gori T. Nebivolol. The somewhat-different b-adrenergic receptor blocker. J Am Coll Cardiol. 2009;54:1491–9.

Multi Center Diltiazem Postinfarction Trial Research Group. The effect of diltiazem on mortality and reinfarction after myocardial infarction. N Engl J Med. 1988;319:385.

Neutel JM, Smith DHG, Ram CVS. Application of ambulatory blood pressure monitoring in differentiating between antihypertensive agents. Am J Med. 1993;94:181.

Packer M, Bristol MR, Cohn JN, et al. The effect of carvedilol on morbidity and mortality in patients with chronic heart failure. N Engl J Med. 1996;334:1349.

Pasotti C, Zoppi A, Capra A. Effect of beta-blockers on plasma lipids. Int J Clin Pharmacol Ther Toxicol. 1986;24:448.

Peters RW, Muller JE, Goldstein S, et al. Propranolol and the morning increase in the frequency of sudden cardiac deaths (BHAT Study). Am J Cardiol. 1989;63:1518.

Phillips T, Anlauf M, Distler A, et al. Randomised, double blind, multicentre comparison of hydrochlorothiazide, atenolol, nitrendipine, and enalapril in antihypertensive treatment: results of the HANE study. BMJ. 1997;315:154.

Pitt B. Regression of left ventricular hypertrophy in patients with hypertension: blockade of the reninangiotensin- aldosterone system. Circulation. 1998;98:1987.

Pitt B. The role of beta-adrenergic blocking agents in preventing sudden cardiac death. Circulation. 1992;85(Suppl I):I107.

POISE trial, Devereaux PJ, Yang H, Yusuf S, et al. Effects of extended-release metoprolol succinate in patients undergoing non-cardiac surgery; a randomised controlled trial. Lancet. 2008;371:1839–47.

Pizarro G, Fuster F-FL, et al. Long-term benefit of early pre-reperfusion metoprolol administration in patients with acute MI: results from the METOCARD-CNTC trial (effect of metoprolol in cardioprotection during an acute myocardial infarction. J Am Coll Cardiol. 2014; 63(22):2356–62.

Poldermans D, Boersma E, Bax JJ, et al. The effect of bisoprolol on perioperative mortality and myocardial infarction in high-risk patients undergoing vascular surgery. N Engl J Med. 1999;341:1789.

Ponce FE, Williams LC, Webb HM, et al. Propranolol palliation of tetralogy of Fallot: experience with long-term drug treatment in pediatric patients. Pediatrics. 1973;52:100.

Pratt CM, Roberts R. Chronic beta-blockade therapy in patients after myocardial infarction. Am J Cardiol. 1983;52:661.

Pritchard BNC, Gillam PMS. The use of propranolol in the treatment of hypertension. BMJ. 1964;2:725.

Pyeritz RE. Marfan syndrome and related disorders. In: Rimoin DL, Connor JM, Pyeritz RE, Korf BR, editors. Emery and Rimoin's principles and practice of medical genetics, vol. 3. 5th ed. London: Churchill Livingstone; 2007. p. 3579–624.

Raeder EA, Verrier RL, Lown B. Intrinsic sympathomimetic activity and the effects of beta-adrenergic blocking drugs on vulnerability to ventricular fibrillation. J Am Coll Cardiol. 1983;1:1442.

Rothfield EL, Lipowitz M, Zucker IR, et al. Management of persistently recurring ventricular fibrillation with propranolol hydrochloride. JAMA. 1968;204:546.

Ryden L, Ariniego R, Arnman K, et al. A double-blind trial of metoprolol in acute myocardial infarction: effects on ventricular tachyarrhythmias. N Engl J Med. 1983;308:614.

Savola J, Vehvilainen O, Vaatainen NJ. Psoriasis as a side effect of beta-blockers. BMJ. 1987;295:637.

Second Cardiac Insufficiency Bisoprolol Study (CIBIS II). Presented by E. Merck at the 20th Congress of the European Society of Cardiology, Aug 1998, Vienna, Austria.

Shore SJ, Berger KR, Murphy EA, et al. Progression of aortic dilation and the benefit of long-term betaadrenergic blockade in Marfan's syndrome. N Engl J Med. 1994;330:1335.

Short et al. Effect of β blockers in treatment of chronic obstructive pulmonary disease: a retrospective cohort study. BMJ. 2011;342:d2549.

Singh BN. Advantages of beta-blockers versus antiarrhythmic agents and calcium antagonists in secondary prevention after myocardial infarction. Am J Cardiol. 1990;66:9C.

Sixth Report of Joint National Committee on Prevention, detection, evaluation and treatment of high blood pressure. Arch Intern Med. 1997; 157:2413.

Sloman G, Robinson JS, McLean K. Propranolol (Inderal) in persistent ventricular fibrillation. BMJ. 1965;5439:895.

SOLVD Investigators. Effect of enalapril on mortality and the development of heart failure in asymptomatic patients with reduced left ventricular ejection fractions. N Engl J Med. 1992;327:685–91.

Sorrentino SA, Doerries C, Manes C, et al. Nebivolol Exerts Beneficial Effects on Endothelial Function, Early Endothelial Progenitor Cells, Myocardial Neovascularization, and Left Ventricular Dysfunction Early After Myocardial Infarction Beyond Conventional $\beta1$-Blockade. J Am Coll Cardiol. 2011;57:601–11.

Steinbeck G, Andresen D, Bach P, et al. A comparison of electrophysiologically guided anti-arrhythmic drug therapy with beta-blocker therapy in patients with symptomatic sustained ventricular tachyarrhythmias. N Engl J Med. 1992;327:987.

The Norwegian Multicenter Study Group. Timolol-induced reduction in mortality and reinfarction in patients surviving acute myocardial infarction. N Engl J Med. 1981;304:801.

Theodorakis JM, Kremastinos T, Stephanokis GS, et al. The effectiveness of beta-blockade and its influence on heart rate variability in vasovagal patients. Eur Heart J. 1993;14:1499.

Tuncer M, Fettser DV, Gunes Y, et al. Comparison of effects of nebivolol and atenolol on P-wave dispersion in patients with hypertension [in Russian]. Kardiologiia. 2008;48:42–5.

United Kingdom Prospective Diabetes Study Group. Tight blood pressure control and risk of microvascular and microvascular complications in type 2 diabetes: UKPDS 38. BMJ. 1998;317:703.

Valsartan Heart Failure Trial Investigators, Cohn JN, Tognoni G. A randomized trial of the angiotensin-receptor blocker valsartan in chronic heart failure. N Engl J Med. 2001;345:1667–75.

Valimaki ML, Harno K. Lipoprotein lipids and apoproteins during beta-blocker administration: comparison of penbutolol and atenolol. Eur J Clin Pharmacol. 1986;30:17.

van Veldhuisen DJ, Cohen-Solal A, Bohm MA, Seniors Investigators, et al. Beta-blockade with nebivolol in elderly heart failure patients with impaired and preserved left ventricular ejection fraction: data from SENIORS (Study of Effects of Nebivolol Intervention on Outcomes and Rehospitalization in Seniors with Heart Failure). J Am Coll Cardiol. 2009;53:2150–8.

Wallin JD, O'Neill WM. Labetalol: current research and therapeutic status. Arch Intern Med. 1983;143:485.

Warltier DC, Hardman HJ, Brooks HL, et al. Transmural gradient of coronary blood flow following dihydropyridine calcium antagonists and other vasodilator drugs. Basic Res Cardiol. 1983;78:644.

Weintraub WS, Akizuki S, Agarwal JB, et al. Comparative effects of nitroglycerin and nifedipine on myocardial blood flow and contraction during flow-limiting coronary stenosis in the dog. Am J Cardiol. 1982;50:281.

Wheat Jr MW. Treatment of dissecting aneurysms of the aorta: current status. Prog Cardiovasc Dis. 1973;16:87.

2   Beta-Blocker Controversies

BETA-BLOCKERS ARE NOT A GOOD INITIAL CHOICE FOR HYPERTENSION: TRUE OR FALSE?

A meta-analysis (Lindholm et al. 2005) concluded that beta-blockers should not remain the first choice in the treatment of primary hypertension. This analysis included randomized controlled trials (RCTs) with poor methodology.

- In most of the RCTs analyzed by these investigators, atenolol was the beta-blocker used for comparison. Worldwide, atenolol is one of the most prescribed beta-blockers.
- Their analysis indeed suggests that atenolol does not give hypertensive patients adequate protection against cardiovascular disease (CVD). These investigators failed to recognize that beta-blockers possess important and subtle clinical properties. Their analysis does not indicate that other beta-blockers provide the same poor CVD protection as atenolol.

In the second edition of Cardiac Drug Therapy (*1988*), *this author emphasized that beta-blockers are not all alike:*

- Those with ISA activity (oxprenolol, pindolol) are not cardioprotective; *see* discussion of ISA activity in Chap. 1.
- Propranolol proved cardioprotective in BHAT (1982), and in the Medical Research Council (*MRC 1985*) trial of treatment of mild hypertension, but only in nonsmokers (*see* the last section of Chap. 1, Which Beta-Blocker Is Best for Your Patients?)

© Springer Science+Business Media New York 2015
M. Gabriel Khan, *Cardiac Drug Therapy*, Contemporary Cardiology,
DOI 10.1007/978-1-61779-962-4_2

- Bucindolol, a vasodilatory beta-blocker, surprisingly proved to be of no value for the treatment of heart failure (HF) (Beta-Blocker Evaluation of Survival Trial Investigators 2001) whereas carvedilol (in COPERNICUS (Packer et al. 2002) and CAPRICORN (The CAPRICORN Investigators 2001) significantly *decreased coronary heart disease (CHD) outcomes.*

- Bisoprolol (in CIBIS [*CIBIS-II Investigators and Committees* 1999]) and metoprolol succinate (in MERIT/HF [MERIT-HF *Study Group 1999*]) significantly reduced fatal and nonfatal myocardial infarction (MI) and recurrence of HF.

- In CAPRICORN, carvedilol achieved a 50 % reduction in nonfatal MI patients aged mainly >55 years. There was a 30 % reduction in total mortality and nonfatal MI. Carvedilol decreased CHD events in elderly normotensive and hypertensive patients.

- The causation of a fatal or nonfatal MI in patients with CHD is the same in a hypertensive and nonhypertensive individual. Thus calcium antagonist or diuretic therapy used for management of hypertension cannot give more cardioprotection (decrease in fatal and nonfatal MI) than treatment with beta-blockers that are proven in RCTs to prevent outcomes.

- Newer beta-blockers have other possible benefits. Carvedilol and nebivolol are beta-blockers with direct vasodilating and antioxidant properties. Nebivolol stimulates the endothelial L-arginine/nitric oxide pathway and produces vasodilation; the drug increases nitric oxide (NO) by decreasing its oxidative inactivation (Cominacini et al. 2003).

- These two beta-blockers should be subjected to long-term outcome trials in the treatment of primary hypertension.

Atenolol is a hydrophilic beta-blocker that attains low brain concentration. Most important, increased brain concentration and elevation of central vagal tone confers cardiovascular protection (Pitt 1992). **Lipid-soluble** beta-blockers (bisoprolol, carvedilol, metoprolol, propranolol, and timolol) have all been proven in large RCTs to significantly decrease cardiac deaths; they all attain high brain concentration block sympathetic discharge in the hypothalamus better than water-soluble agents (atenolol and sotalol) (Pitt 1992) Timolol in the Norwegian trial (1981) caused an astounding 67 % reduction in sudden cardiac deaths.

- Äblad et al. (1991), in a rabbit model, showed that although metoprolol (lipophilic) and atenolol (hydrophilic) caused equal beta-blockade, only metoprolol caused a reduction in sudden cardiac death. Metoprolol, but not atenolol, caused a significant increase, which indicates an increase in sympathetic tone.
- Importantly, only the lipophilic beta-blockers (carvedilol, bisoprolol, propranolol, and timolol) have been shown in large RCTs to prevent fatal and nonfatal MI and sudden cardiac death. In the timolol infarction RT, the drug caused a 67 % reduction in sudden deaths. These agents have been shown to quell early morning catecholamine surge and control early morning and exercise-induced excessive rise in blood pressure better compared with atenolol (Neutel et al. 1993; Kokkinos et al. 2006).

It is surprising that the experts who constructed the recent hypertensive guidelines (JNC8 et al. 2014) fail to understand the subtle but important differences that exist between the available beta-blocking agents. These experts do not recommend a beta-blocking drug for the management of hypertension based on an unsound study in which the poorly effective atenolol was administered.

- "The panel did not recommend beta-blockers for the initial treatment of hypertension because in one study use of beta-blockers "atenolol" resulted in a higher rate of the primary composite outcome of cardiovascular death, MI, or stroke compared to use of an ARB", (JNC8 2014). These experts state "a finding that was driven largely by an increase in stroke (Dahlöf et al. 2002).

The study by Dahlöf et al. did not reveal a significant change in cardiovascular deaths or occurrence of fatal and nonfatal MI as claimed by this expert panel. 204 losartan and 234 atenolol patients died from cardiovascular disease $(0 \cdot 89, 0 \cdot 73$—$1 \cdot 07, p = 0 \cdot 206)$; 232 and 309, respectively, had fatal or nonfatal stroke $(0 \cdot 75, 0 \cdot 63$—$0 \cdot 89, p = 0 \cdot 001)$; and myocardial infarction (nonfatal and fatal) occurred in 198 and 188, respectively $(1 \cdot 07, 0 \cdot 88$—$1 \cdot 31, p = 0 \cdot 491)$.(Dahlöf et al. 2002) the poorly effective atenolol (see chapter 1) was not a failure.

- To deny the use of a more effective beta-blocking drug [bisoprolol, carvedilol, nebivolol, Toprol Xl] as first line or second line in some patients is illogical thinking.
- **Importantly, the duration of action of atenolol varies from 18 to 24 h and fails in some individuals to provide 24 h of CVD protection. The drug leaves an early morning gap, a period crucial for the prevention of fatal MI and sudden cardiac death, information that escapes panel members**.
- The observation that atenolol is less effective than other antihypertensives including vasodilatory beta-blockers at lowering aortic pressure despite an equivalent effect on brachial pressure may partly explain the poor cardioprotection. In the Conduit Artery Function Evaluation (CAFÉ 2006) study, brachial and aortic pressures were measured in a subset of 2,199 patients from ASCOT (PBLA 2005). Despite virtually identical reductions in brachial pressure, the aortic systolic pressure was 4.3 mmHg lower in the amlodipine/perindopril arm versus those on atenolol/bendroflumethiazide.
- **It is clear that beta-blockers are not all alike with regard to their salutary effects, and older beta-blocking drugs including atenolol should become obsolete** (Khan 2003). Beta-blockers are CVD protective provided that bisoprolol, carvedilol, metoprolol, propranolol, or timolol are chosen and not atenolol (Khan 2005). Chockalingam et al. (2012), based on a multicenter study "recommend treatment of symptomatic long QT (LQT1) and LQT2 patients with either propranolol or nadolol, as clearly not all beta-blockers

are equal in their antiarrhythmic efficacy in LQTS. **Propranolol was superior to both nadolol and metoprolol in terms of shortening the cardiac repolarization time, particularly in high-risk patients with markedly prolonger QTc**. A New York–based LQTS Registry indicated that nadolol was the only beta-blocker associated with a significant risk reduction in patients with LQT2 (Abu-Zeitone 2014).

It is poor logic to accept the conclusions drawn from the Lindholm et al. (2005) meta-analysis and the JNC 8 recommendations. In the majority of clinical trials analyzed, atenolol was the beta-blocker administered.

- Nebivolol, bisoprolol carvedilol, or metoprolol succinate extended release [ToprolXL] are recommended for the initial management of mild primary hypertension *depending on the age and ethnicity* of the individual (*see* treatment tables and algorithms in Chap. 9, Hypertension Controversies).

BETA-BLOCKERS ARE NOT RECOMMENDED FOR TREATMENT OF ELDERLY HYPERTENSIVES: TRUE OR FALSE?

Messerli et al. (1998) concluded that this statement is truely based on their meta-analysis, which included the poorly run MRC trial in the elderly (1992).

- **The MRC Working Party** (1992) **confirmed that 25 % of patients were lost to follow-up and more than half the patients were not taking the therapy assigned by the end of the study**.
- **How can a learned expert use this unsound study result? But nonetheless it has convinced the world not to use beta-blockers in the elderly hypertensive. This statement is in major textbooks and editorials are taught to students and interns.**
- There was no difference in total mortality between atenolol and diuretic therapy, but, surprisingly, diuretics reduced

coronary heart disease (CHD) events, and atenolol did not. This is a spurious finding; to this date we do not use diuretics to effectively treat patients with CHD, but we do use beta-blockers. Atenolol, the beta-blocker used, is a poorly effective beta-blocker as outlined earlier in this chapter, and its use should be curtailed (Khan 2003).

- **The spurious and misleading finding nevertheless led Messerli et al.** (1998) **to publish an article in the Journal of the American Medical Association entitled "Are β-Blockers Efficacious as First-Line Therapy for Hypertension in the Elderly?"**
- These analysts concluded that beta-blockers should not be first-line therapy for elderly hypertensives. Unfortunately, this faulty expert opinion of Messerli and colleagues (1998) has gained access to notable textbooks and journals. It appears that virtually all internists and guideline providers (UK and USA) share this faulty opinion, which has been spread worldwide.

The beta-blocker hypertension controversy, including appropriate use in elderly hypertensive patients, is discussed fully in Chaps. 8 and 9, and algorithms are provided indicating which initial drug is best depending on the age and ethnicity of the hypertensive patient.

BETA-BLOCKERS CAUSE GENUINE DIABETES MELLITUS: TRUE OR FALSE?

A small presumed increased risk for the development of type 2 diabetes caused by beta-blocker therapy in hypertensive individuals has become a concern. Many national guidelines have been changed based on this notion. Thus, worldwide, many hypertensive patients and diabetics are denied treatment with a beta-blocking drug.

- Insulin secretion is probably partly $beta_2$ mediated. Glucose-sulfonylurea–stimulated insulin secretion is partially inhibited by beta-blockers (Loubatiere et al. 1971).

- Clinically, however, no significant worsening of glycemic control is seen when beta-blockers are combined with these agents.
- Long-term beta-blocker therapy may increase blood glucose concentration by approximately 0.2–0.5 mmol/L (~3–9 mg/dL), as observed in RCTs with follow-up beyond 5 years, but this mild increase in fasting glucose levels does not prove a diagnosis of type 2 diabetes.
- The increase in blood glucose observed in some subjects may be due to *benign reversible glucose intolerance or genuine diabetes in prediabetics.*

In **ASCOT-BPLA** (2005), baseline glucose concentration for amlodipine and the atenolol-based regimen was 6.24 versus 6.4 mmol/L.

- At follow-up 5 years later, levels for the atenolol regimen were only 0.2 mol/L higher than in the amlodipine group.
- Without clearly confirming a diabetic state, the investigators proclaimed that beta-blockers caused a 30 % increase in diabetes.
- The diagnosis of diabetes mellitus was not confirmed by a 2 h glucose assessment.
- It is surprising that *The Lancet*, a peer-reviewed journal, would print such erroneous conclusions.
- Physicians who incorrectly label individuals as diabetics are in line for medicolegal action.

UKPDS (1998) studied 1,148 hypertensive patients with type 2 diabetes to determine whether tight control of blood pressure with either a beta-blocker or an ACE inhibitor has a specific advantage or disadvantage in preventing the macrovascular and microvascular complications of type 2 diabetes.

- At 9-year follow-up, blood pressure lowering with captopril or atenolol was similarly effective in reducing the incidence of major diabetic complications.
- Glycated hemoglobin concentration was similar in the two groups over the second 4 years of study (atenolol 8.4 % versus captopril 8.3 %; *see* Figs. 1–3 and Chaps. 9 and 22).

- Clearly, beta-blocker therapy did not cause worsening of diabetes control during the lengthy 9-year follow-up. Importantly, for most clinical trials, follow-up is usually 1–4, rarely 5 years.

Gress et al. (2000) conducted a prospective study of 12,550 adults 45–64 years old who did not have diabetes. A health evaluation conducted at baseline included assessment of medication use. The incidence of type 2 diabetes was assessed after 3 and 6 years by assessment of fasting serum glucose. Individuals with hypertension treated with beta-blockers had a 28 % higher risk of subsequent diabetes.

- The diagnosis of diabetes mellitus versus *benign reversible glucose intolerance* was not clarified. Thus this analysis is flawed.

Padwal and colleagues (2004) conducted a systematic review of antihypertensive therapy and the incidence of type 2 diabetes.

- Data from the highest quality studies indicated that diabetes incidence is unchanged or increased by beta-blocker and thiazide diuretics and unchanged or decreased by ACE inhibitors and calcium antagonists.
- **The authors concluded that current data are far from conclusive. These investigators warned that poor methodologic quality limits the conclusions that can be drawn from the several nonrandomized studies quoted by many.**
- Most important, in the studies analyzed by Padwal et al., the increase in diabetic incidence reported is presumptive because type 2 diabetes was not proved by appropriate diagnostic testing.

In most studies, including LIFE (Lindholm et al. 2002), post hoc analysis suggests that increased risk of new-onset diabetes is confined to individuals with an elevated blood glucose at baseline and family predisposition to diabetes.

This finding strongly suggests that in prediabetics, beta-blockers bring to light type 2 diabetes at an earlier point in time but do not cause diabetes in nondiabetic individuals.

STOP-2 (Hansson et al. 1999), a large RCT, showed no difference between ACE inhibitors and beta-blockers in preventing cardiovascular events and no difference in incidence of diabetes.

- **Clinicians and Trialists should ask whether the reported increased incidence of diabetes is real, or are there other explanations for the observed minimal increase in fasting glucose concentrations observed. Murphy et al. (1982) holds the key.** Murphy et al. (1982) completed a lengthy 14-year follow-up in hypertensive patients treated with diuretics that caused a major increase in the incidence of glucose intolerance.
- *This effect, however, was promptly reversed in most (60%) of the patients on discontinuation of the diuretic.* **Thus, these individuals developed *benign reversible glucose intolerance*.**
- **It is important for clinicians to note that these patients were not classified as diabetics by these learned investigators. Similar findings have been reported when beta-blocker therapy is discontinued.**
- The study of Murphy et al. shows without doubt that diuretics do not cause genuine diabetes mellitus and this information should be made known to Trialists and experts in the field who continue to issue misleading medical reports.
- Trialists and those who claim to be experts in the field must be warned not to label individuals as diabetic solely on a fasting glucose level range of 6.4–7.0 mmol/L (115–125 mg/ dL) without further diagnostic confirmation in patients treated with a beta-blocker, a diuretic, or a combination of both.
- ACE inhibitors do not reduce diabetic risk as proclaimed by some (*see* Chap. 3).
- It is unclear whether long-term treatment with beta-blockers and diuretics increases glucose levels 0.2–0.9 mmol/L (3–10 mg/dL) in normal subjects or mainly in prediabetics.

- **In some subjects with prediabetes or a positive family history of type 2 diabetes, beta-blockers and diuretics might bring the diabetic state to light at an earlier point in time, and thus energetic treatment can commence. This presents a reassuring, rather than alarming, scenario.**
- It must be reemphasized that the finding of glucose intolerance does not necessarily mean a diabetic state exists. Beta-blockers do not cause type 2 diabetes, as proclaimed by several trialists and notable clinicians.
- In non-prediabetics, beta-blockers may cause mild glucose intolerance that is benign and reversible on discontinuation of these agents.

DO ALL BETA-BLOCKERS CAUSE BENIGN GLUCOSE INTOLERANCE?

The GEMINI trial (2004) compared the effects of two different beta-blockers on glycemic control as well as other cardiovascular risk factors in a cohort with glycemic control similar to the UKPDS.

- Carvedilol stabilized HbA_{1c}, improved insulin resistance, and slowed development of micro-albuminuria in the presence of renin-angiotensin system (RAS) blockade compared with metoprolol.
- Carvedilol treatment had no effect on HbA_{1c} (mean [SD] change from baseline to end point, 0.02 % [0.04 %]; 95 % CI, −0.06–0.10 %; $p = 0.65$), whereas metoprolol increased HbA_{1c} (0.15 % [0.04 %]; 95 % CI, 0.08–0.22 %; $p < 0.001$).
- HOMA-IR was reduced by carvedilol and increased with metoprolol, which resulted in a significant improvement from baseline for carvedilol (−9.1 %, $p = 0.004$) but not metoprolol which lowers insulin resistance (GEMINI 2004), an effect that correlated with HbA_{1c}. This finding supports the effect of carvedilol on reducing insulin resistance, which has been previously shown by Giugliano et al. (1997) in more time-intensive insulin clamp studies.

- Treatment with carvedilol was associated with improvement in total cholesterol and a smaller increase in triglyceride levels relative to metoprolol (GEMINI 2004).

BETA-BLOCKERS SHOULD NOT BE GIVEN TO PATIENTS DURING THE EARLY HOURS OF ACUTE MI: TRUE OR FALSE?

The results of COMMIT/CCS-2: Clopidogrel and metoprolol in Myocardial Infarction Trial/Second Chinese Cardiac Study (2005) may cause changes in the American College of Cardiology/American Heart Association (ACC/AHA) guidelines. In this huge RC, patients received aspirin and were randomized to receive clopidogrel 75 mg/day or placebo; within these two groups, patients were then randomized to inappropriately large doses of metoprolol (*15 mg IV in three equal doses followed by 200 mg/day orally*) or placebo. Patients were randomized within 24 h of suspected acute MI and demonstrating ST elevation or other ischemic abnormality.

- Metoprolol produced a significant 18 % reduction in reinfarction (2.0 % versus 2.5 %; $p=0.001$) as well as a 17 % reduction in ventricular fibrillation (2.5 % versus 3.0 %; $p=0.001$); there was no effect on mortality. Metoprolol, however, significantly increased the relative risk of death from cardiogenic shock, by 29 %, with the greatest risk of shock occurring primarily on d 0–1.
- Cardiogenic shock was understandably more evident in patients in Killip class II and III; this adverse effect was largely iatrogenic because the dose of metoprolol was excessive and given to patients in whom these agents are contraindicated.
- Oral beta-blocker therapy is preferred, and IV use is cautioned against, particularly in patients with pulmonary edema or systolic blood pressure (BP)<100 mmHg. In this study, a large dose of metoprolol was given IV to patients with systolic BP<95 mmHg and in those with Killip class II and III.

- Study cochair Rory Collins emphasized that it may generally be prudent to wait until a heart attack patient's condition has stabilized before starting beta-blocker therapy. This RCT persuaded some nonthinking cardiologists to not use metoprolol in patients with acute MI.
- The advice should be restated: do not give beta-blockers to patients who are hemodynamically unstable or in whom heart failure is manifest. Most patients with acute MI can be given metoprolol at an appropriate dose within the early hours of onset of acute MI (Khan Khan 2007)
- The METOCARD-CNIC: Effect of metoprolol in cardioprotection during an acute myocardial infarction trial
- The study randomized 270 patients with Killip class II anterior STEMI presenting early after symptom onset (<6 h) to pre-reperfusion IV metoprolol or control group
- In patients with anterior Killip class < or equal to 11 ST elevation MI undergoing PCI, early IV metoprolol before reperfusion resulted in higher long-tem left ventricular ejection fraction.
- This administration reduced the incidence of severe left ventricular dysfunction and implantable cardioverter defibrillator indications and fewer admissions for heart failure (Pizarro et al. 2014). See Chap. 22.

REFERENCES

Abu-Zeitone A, Peterson DR, Polonsky B, et al. Efficacy of different beta-blockers in the treatment of long QT syndrome. J Am Coll Cardiol. 2014;64:1352–8.

Äblad B, Bjurö T, Björkman JA, Edström T, Olsson G. Role of central nervous beta-adrenoceptors in the prevention of ventricular fibrillation through augmentation of cardiac vagal tone. J Am Coll Cardiol. 1991;17(Suppl):165.

Beta-Blocker Evaluation of Survival Trial Investigators. A trial of the beta-blocker bucindolol in patients with advanced chronic heart failure. N Engl J Med. 2001;62:1659–67.

BHAT:β-Blocker Heart Attack Trial Research Group. A randomised trial of propranolol in patients with acute myocardial infarction I: Mortality results. JAMA. 1982;247:1707–14.

CAFE investigators for the Anglo-Scandinavian Cardiac Outcomes Trial (ASCOT) investigators. Differential impact of blood pressure-lowering drugs on central aortic pressure and clinical outcomes: principal results of the conduit artery function evaluation (CAFE) study. Circulation. 2006;113:1213–25.

Chockalingam P, Crotti L, Girardengo G, et al. Not all beta-blockers are equal in the management of long QT syndrome types 1 and 2: higher recurrence of events under metoprolol. J Am Coll Cardiol. 2012;60:2092–9.

CIBIS-II Investigators and Committees. The cardiac insufficiency bisoprolol study II (CIBIS-II): a randomised trial. Lancet. 1999;353: 9–13.

Cominacini L, Fratta Pasini A, Garbin U, et al. Nebivolol and its 4-keto derivative increase nitric oxide in endothelial cells by reducing its oxidative inactivation. J Am Coll Cardiol. 2003;42:1838–44.

COMMIT (Clopidogrel and Metoprolol in Myocardial Infarction Trial) Collaborative Group. Early intravenous then oral metoprolol in 45,852 patients with acute myocardial infarction: randomised placebo-controlled trial. Lancet. 2005;366:1622–32.

COPERNICUS, Packer M, Fowler MB, Roecker EB, et al. Effect of carvedilol on the morbidity of patients with severe chronic heart failure: results of the Carvedilol Prospective Randomized Cumulative Survival (COPERNICUS) study. Circulation. 2002;106:2194–9.

Dahlöf B, Devereux RB, Kjeldsen SE, LIFE Study Group, et al. Cardiovascular morbidity and mortality in the Losartan Intervention For Endpoint reduction in hypertension study (LIFE): a randomised trial against atenolol. Lancet. 2002;359(9311):995–1003.

Dahlöf B, Sever PS, Poulter NR, et al. for the ASCOT investigators. Prevention of cardiovascular events with an antihypertensive regimen of amlodipine adding perindopril as required versus atenolol adding bendroflumethiazide as required, in the Anglo-Scandinavian cardiac outcomes trial-blood pressure lowering arm (ASCOT-BPLA): a multicentre randomised controlled trial. Lancet. 2005;366:895–906.

GEMINI, Bakris GL, Fonseca V, Katholi RE, et al. Metabolic effects of carvedilol vs metoprolol in patients with type 2 diabetes mellitus and hypertension: a randomized controlled trial. JAMA. 2004;292: 2227–36.

Giugliano D, Acampora R, Marfella R, et al. Metabolic and cardiovascular effects of carvedilol and atenolol in non-insulin-dependent diabetes mellitus and hypertension: a randomized, controlled trial. Ann Intern Med. 1997;126:955–9.

Gress TW, Nieto FJ, Shahar E, et al. The atherosclerosis risk in communities study: hypertension and antihypertensive therapy as risk factors for type 2 diabetes mellitus. N Engl J Med. 2000;342:905–12.

Hansson L, Lindholm LH, Ekbom T, et al. Randomised trial of old and new antihypertensive drugs in elderly patients: cardiovascular mortality and morbidity. The Swedish trial in old patients with hyper-tension-2 study. Lancet. 1999;354:1751–6.

JNC8, James PA, Oparil S, Carter BL. Evidence-based guideline for the management of high blood pressure in adults report from the panel members appointed to the eighth joint national committee (JNC 8). JAMA. 2014;311(5):507–20.

Khan MG. Hypertension. In: Khan MG. Cardiac drug therapy. 6th ed. Philadelphia: WB Saunders; 2003. p. 46–8.

Khan MG. Hallmark clinical trials. In: Khan MG. Cardiac drug therapy. 7th ed. New York: Springer; 2007. p. 391.

Khan MG. Which beta blocker to choose. In: Khan MG. Heart disease diagnosis and therapy, a practical approach. 2nd ed. Totowa: Humana Press; 2005. p. 311–4.

Kokkinos P, Chrysohoou C, Panagiotakos D, et al. Beta-blockade mitigates exercise blood pressure in hypertensive male patients. J Am Coll Cardiol. 2006;47:794–8.

Lindholm LH, Carlberg B, Samuelsson O. Should β blockers remain first choice in the treatment of primary hypertension? A meta-analysis. Lancet. 2005;366:1545–53.

Lindholm LH, Ibsen H, Borch-Johnsen K, et al. Risk of new-onset diabetes in the Losartan Intervention For Endpoint reduction in hypertension study. J Hypertens. 2002;20:1879–86.

Loubatiere A, Mariani MM, Sorel G, et al. The action of beta adrenergic blocking drugs and stimulating agents on insulin secretion. Characteristic of the type of beta receptor. Diabetologica. 1971;7: 127–32.

MERIT-HF Study Group. Effect of metoprolol CR/XL in chronic heart failure: metoprolol CR/XL randomised intervention trial in congestive heart failure (MERIT-HF). Lancet. 1999;353:2001–7.

Messerli FH, Grossman E, Goldbourt U. Are β-blockers efficacious as first-line therapy for hypertension in the elderly? JAMA. 1998;279: 1903–7.

MRC Working Party. Medical research council trial of treatment of hypertension in older adults: principal results. BMJ. 1992;304:405–12.

Murphy MB, Lewis PJ, Kohner E, Schumer B, Dollery CT. Glucose intolerance in hypertensive patients treated with diuretics: a fourteen-year follow-up. Lancet. 1982;2:1293–5.

Neutel JM, Smith DHG, Ram CVS. Application of ambulatory blood pressure monitoring in differentiating between antihypertensive agents. Am J Med. 1993;94:181.

Norwegian Multicentre Group. Timolol induced reduction in mortality and reinfarction in patients surviving acute myocardial infarction. N Engl J Med. 1981;304:801–7.

Padwal R, Laupacis A. Antihypertensive therapy and incidence of type 2 diabetes. A systematic review. Diabetes Care. 2004;27:247–55.

Pitt B. The role of beta-adrenergic blocking agents in preventing sudden cardiac death. Circulation. 1992;85(I Suppl):107.

Pizarro G, Fernandez-Friera L, Fuster V, et al. Long-term benefit of early pre-reperfusion metoprolol administration in patients with acute MI: results from the METOCARD-CNTC trial (effect of metoprolol in cardioprotection during an acute myocardial infarction. J Am Coll Cardiol. 2014;63(22):2356–62.

The CAPRICORN Investigators. Effect of carvedilol on outcome after myocardial infarction in patients with left-ventricular dysfunction: the CAPRICORN randomised trial. Lancet. 2001;357:1385–90.

Treatment of hypertension: the 1985 results. Lancet 1985;2:645–647

UK Prospective Diabetes Study Group. Efficacy of atenolol and captopril in reducing risk of macro-vascular and microvascular complications in type 2 diabetes: UKPDS. Br Med J. 1998;317:713–20.

3 Angiotensin-Converting Enzyme Inhibitors and Angiotensin II Receptor Blockers

Angiotensin-converting enzyme (ACE) inhibitors and angiotensin II receptor blockers (ARBs) play a pivotal role in the management of heart failure (HF) and hypertension. These agents are mildly *cardioprotective* and increase survival in patients with:

- HF.
- Left ventricular (LV) dysfunction.
- Acute myocardial infarction (MI). The Survival of Myocardial Infarction Long-Term Evaluation (SMILE) study (Ambrosioni et al. 1995) showed that zofenopril administered to patients with acute anterior infarction improved survival.
- Hypertension with LV hypertrophy (LVH).
- Hypertension with diabetes and proteinuria.
- Patients at high risk for cardiovascular events, as indicated by the Heart Outcomes Prevention Evaluation (HOPE) study (HOPE Investigators 2000). But in this hallmark RCT, unfortunately, optimal therapy (beta-blockers, aspirin, and statins) was administered to too few patients. One may question whether the benefits associated with ramipril in this study would have been maintained if patients had been

© Springer Science+Business Media New York 2015
M. Gabriel Khan, *Cardiac Drug Therapy*, Contemporary Cardiology,
DOI 10.1007/978-1-61779-962-4_3

treated with appropriate regimens of aspirin, beta-blockers, and lipid-lowering agents (Weinsaft et al. 2000). (See HOPE study under ramipril.)

Cardioprotection appears to be exaggerated and many people at low risk are prescribed these agents, in particular ARBs, which are not adequately proven to save lives or reduce stroke rates significantly; see discussion under TRANSCEND and **PRoFESS** (2008) trials.

Tissue angiotensin II production appears to be an important modulator of tissue function and structure. Angiotensin II produced in cardiac myocytes has been shown to play a role in stretch-induced hypertrophy and in the process of myocardial remodeling post infarction (Pfeffer and Braunwald 1990).

Three classes of ACE inhibitors have been developed. Most ACE inhibitors except captopril and lisinopril possess a carboxylic radical, are transformed in the liver to the active agent, and are thus prodrugs.

Class I: Captopril is not a prodrug; it is the active drug, but with metabolism, the metabolites are also active. Only captopril and zofenopril contain a sulfhydryl (SH) group.

Class II: All other available agents except lisinopril are prodrugs and become active only after hepatic metabolism to the diacid (Table 3-1).

Class III: Lisinopril is not a prodrug and is the only water-soluble agent; it is excreted unchanged by the kidneys. Lipid solubility does not confer clinical benefits beyond those observed with lisinopril.

The pharmacologic features and dosages of ACE inhibitors are given in Tables 3-1 and 3-2 and in Chap. 8.

MECHANISM OF ACTION

Vascular stretch of the renal afferent arteriole and the sodium concentration in the distal tubule, sensed by the macula densa and an interplay of beta-adrenergic receptors,

Table 3-1
Pharmacologic profile and dosages of ACE inhibitors

	Benazepril	Captopril	Cilazapril	Enalapril	Fosinopril	Lisinopril	Perindopril	Quinapril	Ramipril	Trandolapril
USA + Canada	Lotensin	Capoten	Inhibace	Vasotec	Monopril	Prinivil	Aceon Zestril	Accupril	Altace	Mavik
UK	–	Capoten	Vascace	Innovace	Staril	Carace, Zestril	Aceon	Accuprin	Tritace	Gopten/ Odrik
Europe	Cibace	Lopril, Lopirin	Inibace	Xanef, Renitec		Carace, Zestril	Acertil	Accupro	Tritace	Gopten
Prodrug Action	Yes	No	Yes	Yes	Yes	No	Yes	Yes	Partial	Yes
Apparent (h)	1	0.5	>24	2–4		2–4			3–6	
Peak effect (h)	2	1–2	>40	4		4–8			3–6	
Duration (h)	12–24	8–12		12–24		24–30			24–48	
Half-life (h)	10–11	2–3		11	>24	13	>24	>24	14–30	24
Metabolism	–	Partly hepatic		Hepatic	Renal + heptatic	None			Partial	
Elimination	Renal	Renal	Renal	Renal		Renal	Renal	Renal	Renal	Renal
SH group	No	Yes	No	No	No	No	No	No	No	No

(continued)

Table 3-1 (Continued)

	Benazepril	Captopril	Cilazapril	Enalapril	Fosinopril	Lisinopril	Perindopril	Quinapril	Ramipril	Trandolapril
Tissue specificity	No	No	Yes	No	Yes	No	Yes	Yes	Yes	Yes
Equivalent dose	10 mg	100 mg	2.5	20 mg	10	20 mg	3	15	10 mg	2
Initial dose Total daily dose	5–10 mg	6.25 mg	1.5	2.5 mg	5	2.5 mg	2	2.5–5	2.5–5	0.5
Hypertension	10–20 mg	25–150 mg	1.5–5 mg	5–40 mg	5–40 mg	5–40 mg	2–8 mg	5–40 mg	2.5–15 mg	1–4 mg
Heart failure	–	75–150 mg	–	10–35 mg	–	10–35 mg				
Dose frequency[a]	1 daily	2–3 daily	1 daily	1–2 daily	1 daily	1 daily	1 daily	1 daily	1 daily	1 daily
Supplied, tabs	5, 10, 20, 40 mg	12.5, 25, 50, 100 mg	1, 2.5, 5 mg	2.5, 5, 10, 20 mg	10, 20 mg	2.5, 5, 10, 20, 40 mg	2, 4 mg	5, 10, 20, 40 mg	1.25, 2.5, 5, 10 mg	0.5, 1, 2 mg

[a]Increase dosing interval with renal failure or in the elderly

Table 3-2
Profile of angiotensin II receptor blockers

Drug	Active metabolite	Bioavail- ability (%)	Half- life (h)	Food effect	Dose once daily (mg)
Candesartan	No	15	9	None	4–16
Irbesartan	No	60–80	11–15	None	150–300
Losartan	Yes	33	6–9	Minimal	50–100
Valsartan	No	25	6	50 %	80–160

control the release of renin from the juxtaglomerular cells located in the media of the afferent renal arteriole (Davis and Freeman 1976; Torretti 1982; Reid 1985).

Stimuli to the release of renin include:

- A decrease in renal blood flow (ischemia), hypotension, and reduction of intravascular volume
- Sodium depletion or sodium diuresis
- Beta-adrenoceptor activation

The enzyme renin is a protease that cleaves the leucine 10–valine 11 bond from angiotensinogen to form the decapeptide angiotensin I (Ganong 1984). ACE now cleaves histidine–leucine from angiotensin I, resulting in the formation of angiotensin II, which causes:

- Vasoconstriction about 40 times more intense than that caused by norepinephrine. Vasoconstriction occurs predominantly in arterioles and, to a lesser degree, in veins; this action is more pronounced in the skin and kidney, with some sparing of vessels in the brain and muscle.
- Renal effects: marked sodium reabsorption occurs in the proximal tubule.
- Adrenal effects: aldosterone release enhances sodium and water reabsorption and potassium excretion in the renal tubule distal to the macula densa. Angiotensin II also promotes release of catecholamines from the adrenal medulla.

- Increased sympathetic outflow and facilitated ganglionic stimulation of the sympathetic nervous system (Ganong 1984; Munzel and Keaney 2001).
- Modest vagal inhibition, which may explain the lack of tachycardia in response to the marked vasodilator effect of ACE inhibitors.
- Enhanced antidiuretic hormone secretion, resulting in free water gain.

ACE inhibitors are competitive inhibitors of angiotensin-converting enzyme, and therefore they prevent the conversion of angiotensin I to angiotensin II (see Fig. 3-1). The consequences of this action are as follows.

Arteriolar dilation causes a fall in total systemic vascular resistance, blood pressure, and afterload; these three terms are interrelated but are not synonymous (Burnier 2001).

- **Sympathetic activity decreases** because of attenuation of angiotensin-related potentiation of sympathetic activity and release of norepinephrine. The diminished sympathetic activity causes further vasodilation with additional reduction in afterload and some decrease in preload. It is because of this further indirect antisympathetic and vagal effect that heart rate is not increased by ACE inhibitors, as opposed to several other groups of vasodilators.
- Reduction in aldosterone secretion promotes sodium excretion and potassium retention.
- **Vascular oxidative stress is favorably influenced** (Munzel and Keaney 2001) because vascular superoxide is reduced. Thus, ACE inhibitors are believed to have important antioxidant properties superior to those of vitamin E and other antioxidants. A review by Burnier (2001) gives details and relevant references. Vascular wall endothelium, smooth muscle, and fibroblasts contain enzyme systems that use nicotinamide adenine dinucleotide and its reduced form (NADH and NADPH) for the production of superoxide anion that is increased in response to angiotensin II. ACE activity has been noted to increase in atheromatous plaques, and inhibition appears to influence inflammatory reaction

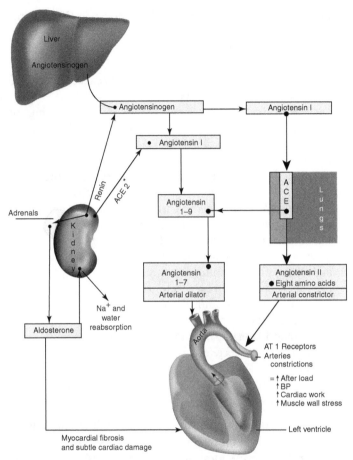

Fig. 3-1. Renin–angiotensin–aldosterone system: action on the heart and arterial system. *Asterisk*: ACE 2 may counteract some of the effects of ACE activity. Angiotensin II action, however, must prevail to maintain adequate blood pressure to the brain and vital organs during catastrophic events: nature's way of survival; ACE, angiotensin-converting enzyme. Angiotensin II activates two subtypes of angiotensin II receptors: AT1 and AT2, but only AT1 mediates clinical effects of angiotensin. Reproduced with permission from Khan MG, *Encyclopedia of Heart Diseases*, 2nd edition. New York: Springer Science + Business Media; 2011, p. 2. With kind permission from Springer Science + Business Media.

favorably within the arterial wall. Angiotensin II is a mitogen for vascular smooth muscle cells that can be inhibited. Superoxide is a major source of hydrogen peroxide; thus, smooth muscle cell proliferation may be limited. Also, nitric oxide (NO) activity appears to improve because superoxide reacts with NO (Burnier 2001).

- **Increased free water loss is caused** by blocking of angiotensin-mediated vasopressin release, resulting in some protection from dilutional hyponatremia. This action is important in patients with severe HF.

- **Increased bradykinin-converting enzyme** is the same as kinase II, which causes degradation of bradykinin. *The accumulation of bradykinin stimulates release of vasodilatory NO and prostacyclin that may protect the endothelium and contribute to arterial dilation and to a decrease in peripheral vascular resistance.* Thus, indomethacin and other prostaglandin inhibitors reduce the effectiveness of ACE inhibitors. Captopril has been shown to be uricosuric (Leary and Reyes 1987), and it reduces hyperuricemia.

- **Arteriolar hyperplasia is decreased.** ACE inhibitors have been shown to decrease arteriolar hyperplasia caused by hypertension. Therapy with cilazapril for 1 year appears to correct the structural and functional abnormalities in the resistance arteries of patients with mild essential hypertension.

ACE gene polymorphism contributes to the modulation and adequacy of the neurohormonal response to ACE inhibitor long-term administration in HF (Cicoira et al. 2001). Patients with HF with aldosterone escape have been shown to have a higher prevalence of DD genotype compared with patients with normal aldosterone levels (Cicoira et al. 2001). The antihypertensive response to ACE inhibition has also been shown in a small series to be more pronounced in subjects with ACE DD genotype than in those with the ACE-11 genotype (Cicoira et al. 2001). Genetic screening of large populations of patients, however, remains controversial.

ACE INHIBITORS VERSUS OTHER VASODILATORS

The reversal of iatrogenic hypokalemia caused by ACE inhibition is an important asset in the management of patients with hypertension and HF, who often require diuretic therapy.

The suppression of ADH activity by ACE inhibitors decreases free water gain, which is useful in the management of the hyponatremic patient with HF. This salutary effect is not observed with other vasodilators.

- Both **ACE inhibitors** and calcium antagonists are effective in preventing LVH and also cause it to regress when present, but other vasodilators do not consistently prevent hypertrophy or cause regression. LVH is an independent risk factor for sudden death, and its prevention is therefore an important aspect of pharmacologic therapy. ACE inhibitors are generally well tolerated, with few adverse effects, whereas fewer than 33 % of patients tolerate hydralazine or alpha$_1$-blockers after 6 months of therapy at doses sufficient to achieve goal blood pressure. ACE inhibitors cause marked arteriolar vasodilation and a significant decrease in venous tone, resulting in a decrease in afterload and preload. In contrast with other vasodilators, with the exception of calcium antagonists, they cause afterload reduction, but their administration sets in motion compensatory mechanisms that have several effects tending to counteract their beneficial action.
- **Prazosin** and other alpha$_1$-blockers cause a decrease in afterload and a mild decrease in preload, but they increase heart rate and cardiac ejection velocity, resulting in a deleterious rate of rise of aortic pressure. These agents cause sodium and water retention that necessitates an increase in prazosin dosage and often requires added diuretic therapy. Tachyphylaxis occurs, and clinical trials have proved prazosin to be ineffective for prolonging life in the setting of HF.
- **Hydralazine** has had extensive clinical testing. The Veterans Administration Vasodilator Heart Failure Trial (V-HeFT II) (Cicoira 2001) showed the drug to be effective in HF when

combined with the venodilator effect of nitrates. Hydralazine causes a marked enhancement in heart rate and cardiac ejection velocity. This action is undesirable in patients with ischemic heart disease and limits the usefulness of this agent. Other vasodilators of this class, including alpha$_1$-adrenergic receptor blockers (trimazosin, indoramin, terazosin), cause undesirable effects similar to those of prazosin and hydralazine. Other vasodilators, except for those that have a primary renal and adrenal action, of necessity cause a stimulation of the renin–angiotensin system as well as an adrenal release of catecholamine and sympathetic stimulation to compensate for the arteriolar dilation. These untoward effects, however, allow for the occasional combination of one of the aforementioned vasodilators with an ACE inhibitor.

- **Nitroglycerin** is predominantly a venous dilator and decreases preload. A minimal decrease in afterload occurs with the use of intravenous (IV) nitroglycerin but not oral nitrates. These agents are useful in the management of chronic HF only when they are added to arteriolar vasodilators.

CLINICAL INDICATIONS

Hypertension

ACE inhibitors and selected ARBs are indicated for hypertension of all grades (telmisartan and olmesartan are not recommended). Some would argue that there are many ACE inhibitors and ARBs that have not been associated with a signal of increased cardiovascular death, so why not prescribe one of those agents (Ingelfinger 2011)? Their low side effect profile, especially with the quality-of-life advantages over some other antihypertensive agents, has resulted in their inappropriately widespread use.

- But compared with calcium antagonists, they are surprisingly weak antihypertensive agents; they achieve reasonable reduction in blood pressure in <45 % of individuals and reach ~66 % only when a diuretic is added.

As outlined earlier, their built-in protection from reflex sympathetic stimulation, resulting in an increase in heart rate and the rate of rise of aortic pressure, is a major advantage over alpha$_1$-adrenergic receptor antagonists (alpha-blockers) and similar vasodilators. ACE inhibitors and ARBs retain potassium and avoid the need for gastric-irritating potassium supplements.

Rebound hypertension observed after withdrawal of clonidine, guanabenz, guanfacine, methyldopa, and, rarely, calcium antagonists and beta-blockers is not a feature of ACE inhibition.

ACE inhibitors are most effective in young patients, aged less than 55 years, with essential hypertension, who usually have increased renin activity. In this subset of patients, ACE inhibitors or ARBs prescribed as monotherapy are effective in about 45 % of cases. In patients with more severe hypertension, ACE inhibitors in combination with diuretics are effective in up to 70 %. ACE inhibitors are slightly less effective in reducing blood pressure in nonwhite patients and in the elderly, although studies indicate a sufficiently good response to justify a trial of ACE inhibitors or ARBs as monotherapy in the elderly when other agents are contraindicated or poorly tolerated. The antihypertensive action of ACE inhibitors is multifactorial and partially depends on the renin and sodium status. Thus, it is not surprising that ACE inhibitors have been shown to be effective in elderly patients with low renin status.

ACE inhibitors and ARBs are particularly effective in lowering blood pressure in patients with high renin–angiotensin states, such as:

- In combination with moderate to high doses of diuretics and calcium antagonists for the management of resistant hypertension.
- In malignant hypertension.
- In hypertension resulting from oral contraceptive use.
- In coarctation of the aorta.

- Immediately after dialysis in patients with chronic renal failure, when sodium and volume depletion is associated with enhancement of the renin–angiotensin system and responds to ACE inhibition (Weber 1999).
- For the management of hypertensive patients with concomitant HF, for which ACE inhibitors are ideal. In this subset of patients, the systolic blood pressure should be maintained at less than 140 mmHg. The use of ACE inhibitors complements therapy with diuretics because diuretic use in this context stimulates the renin–angiotensin system.

ACE inhibitors are highly recommended in the following clinical situations:

- In the hypertensive diabetic patient, ACE inhibitors are first-choice agents because they do not adversely affect glucose metabolism, they have a proven effect in reducing diabetic proteinuria, and there is some evidence suggesting prolongation of nephron life. ACE inhibition enhances insulin-mediated uptake of glucose, and this effect may be important in the management of hypertensives with diabetes.
- These drugs are useful in hypertensive patients with hyperlipidemia because these agents produce no change in lipid parameters. When needed, a combination with a beta-blocking drug may provide cardioprotection.
- Tissue ACE inhibition allows for the use of ACE inhibitors to decrease blood pressure in patients who have undergone nephrectomy.

Although these agents are very effective in patients with renovascular hypertension, they must be used, if at all, with extreme caution because severe renal insufficiency may occur in patients with bilateral renal artery stenosis or stenosis in a solitary kidney. Because ACE inhibitors cause dilation of the efferent arteriole, they may precipitate renal failure or the loss of a kidney.

CLINICAL TRIALS

PROGRESS: The Perindopril Protection Against Recurrent Stroke Study was a large, well-run RCT of 6,105 individuals with hypertension and previous stroke or transient ischemic attack.

- **The ACE inhibitor perindopril attained blood pressure goal in only about 42 % of trial patients**. The addition of a diuretic was required in the majority of patients. No discernible reduction in the primary outcome, reduction in the risk of stroke, was observed for perindopril monotherapy (PROGRESS Collaborative Group 2001).

ACCOMPLISH: In a large RCT, a benazepril–amlodipine combination was superior to the benazepril–hydrochlorothiazide combination in reducing cardiovascular events (Jamerson et al. for the ACCOMPLISH Trial Investigators 2008). This is not surprising because diuretics are weak antihypertensive agents and calcium antagonists are the most powerful agents currently available. (See Chap. 22 for details.)

- **The post hoc observation of an adverse effect on mortality and morbidity in the subgroup receiving valsartan, an ACE inhibitor, and a beta-blocker raises concern about the potential safety of this specific combination** (Cohn and Tognoni 2001).

Heart Failure

ACE inhibitors have provided a major improvement in the management of HF, resulting in both amelioration of symptoms and an increase in survival when they are used in combination with diuretics and digoxin (Cohn et al. 1991). The fall in cardiac output with HF triggers a compensatory response that involves enhancement of the sympathetic nervous system and the renin–angiotensin–aldosterone system. As a result of these adjustments, systemic vascular resistance and afterload are increased inappropriately, with further deterioration in cardiac performance, and a vicious circle ensues (*see* Chap. 12). ACE inhibitors play a vital role in halting the counterproductive pathophysiologic events that tend to perpetuate, rather than correct, cardiac decompensation.

The beneficial effects of diuretics in the management of HF are limited by excessive stimulation of the renin–angiotensin system; the addition of ACE inhibitors results in further amelioration. This improvement is partly the result of reduced arterial and venous tone, but changes in fluid and electrolyte balance are also important.

Stimulation of the sympathetic and the renin–angiotensin-aldosterone system causes intense sodium and water retention in the proximal and distal nephron. Also, an increase in venous tone occurs. Both adjustments result in an increase in filling pressure, which enhances preload. ACE inhibitors partially inhibit sodium and water retention and decrease venous tone, which produces a decrease in preload, an improvement or decrease in symptoms and signs of pulmonary congestion, and an increase in exercise tolerance. The improvement in functional capacity is superior to that observed with hydralazine and is similar to the combination of hydralazine and isosorbide dinitrate.

CLINICAL TRIALS

CONSENSUS: The Cooperative North Scandinavian Enalapril Survival Study (CONSENSUS 1987) indicated an increased survival in New York Heart Association (NYHA) class IV patients treated for over 6 months with enalapril added to diuretics and digoxin. The 6-month mortality rate was 26 % in patients treated with enalapril, versus 44 % in those given diuretic and digoxin alone ($P<0.001$). Forty-two percent of the group treated with enalapril showed functional class improvement compared with 22 % in the control group ($P=0.001$).

SOLVD Investigators (1991): Patients with chronic heart failure and EF < or equal to 0.35 (New York Heart Association functional classes II and III), receiving conventional treatment for heart failure, were randomly assigned to receive either placebo ($n = 1,284$) or enalapril ($n = 1,285$) at doses of 2.5–20 mg/day in a double-blind trial. Results were as follows:

- At 41.4 months, there were 510 deaths in the placebo group (39.7%), as compared with 452 in the enalapril group (35.2%), a modest 11.4 % reduction (reduction in risk, 16%; $P = 0.0036$).
- Fewer patients died or were hospitalized for worsening heart failure (736 in the placebo group and 613 in the enalapril group; risk reduction, 26 % [95 % confidence interval, 18–34%; $P < 0.0001$]) (SOLVD Investigators 1991). But the exact reduction in hospital admissions for heart failure should be separated.
- Although these agents have provided much relief for suffering patients and have significantly decreased the mortality, the effect is still modest and newer agents must be sought.

In **Val-HeFT** valsartan when combined with a beta-blocker caused significantly more cardiac events. A total of 5,010 patients with HF class II, III, or IV were randomly assigned to receive 160 mg of valsartan or placebo twice daily. There was no reduction in all-cause mortality. The incidence of the combined end point, however, was a modest 13.2 % lower with valsartan than with placebo $P = 0.009$), predominantly because of a lower number of patients hospitalized for heart failure: 455 (18.2%) in the placebo group and 346 (13.8%) in the valsartan group ($P < 0.001$). "**Overall mortality was not reduced by valsartan administration**" (Cohn and Tognoni 2001).

Unfortunately, less than 36 % of subjects received a beta-blocker and ~68 % received digoxin.

The post hoc observation of an adverse effect on mortality and morbidity in the subgroup receiving valsartan, an ACE inhibitor, and a beta-blocker raises concern about the potential safety of this specific combination

(Cohn and Tognoni 2001).

V-HeFT 11: The V-HeFT II trial, at an average 2.5-year follow-up, showed a modest improvement in survival, the mortality rate being 33 % for enalapril added to diuretics and digoxin versus 38 % in patients given a diuretic and digoxin along with hydralazine and isosorbide dinitrate (Cicoira 2001).

It is clear that ACE inhibitors improve survival in certain categories of patients, and benefit is beyond question for patients with NYHA class IV HF (15). There is as yet no convincing evidence that these drugs decrease mortality in patients with NYHA class II HF, and although V-HeFT II results suggest some benefit in class II patients, this is not statistically significant (*see* Chap. 12).

In the management of patients with HF, it is of paramount importance to commence with the smallest dose of ACE inhibitor, enalapril 2.5 mg or captopril 6.25 mg once or twice daily, and to titrate the dose slowly over several days, to avoid relative hypovolemia and hypotension, which can worsen cerebral and coronary perfusion. In a randomized study, patients with HF and concomitant angina showed an increase in angina and a reduced exercise tolerance when treated with captopril (Cleland et al. 1991). The deleterious effects were related to the hypotensive effect of captopril. Poor diastolic coronary perfusion to contractile myocardial segments supplied by arteries with significant stenosis may precipitate angina in patients with HF. Caution is therefore especially necessary when ACE inhibitors are combined with calcium antagonists, nitrates, or other agents that may result in the lowering of blood pressure.

Acute Myocardial Infarction

After acute MI, there is stimulation of the renin–angiotensin system resulting in increased myocardial wall stress, as well as cardiac dilation that may ultimately increase morbidity and mortality. The process by which the left ventricle dilates and progressively enlarges after infarction is called ventricular remodeling. After MI, some patients develop an increase in LV size and an increase in end-systolic and end-diastolic volumes. ACE inhibitors cause favorable myocardial remodeling. These agents have been shown to decrease the incidence of HF and the rate of hospitalization in postinfarction patients with ejection fraction <40 in the Survival and Ventricular Enlargement (SAVE) and Acute Infarction Ramipril Efficacy (AIRE) studies (*see* Chap. 12).

In the SMILE trial (Ambrosioni et al. 1995), patients with anterior MI were treated early with zofenopril regardless of HF. Treatment lasted only 6 weeks and resulted in a significant reduction in deaths and HF. After 1 yr, mortality was lower in the treated group than in the placebo group. In the AIRE trial, ramipril administered to patients within 3–10 days of acute MI with transient signs and symptoms of HF caused a significant 27 % reduction in the risk of death at 15 months, a benefit that was maintained for 5 years.

Renoprotection

Based mainly on retrospective studies, ACE inhibitors were noted to slow the progression of renal disease in nondiabetic patients. In the African American Study of Kidney Disease and Hypertension, an ACE inhibitor was shown to be more effective than a calcium antagonist in retarding the progression of renal disease. The ACE inhibitor captopril has been shown in an RCT to slow progression in patients with type 1 diabetes with microalbuminuria. Captopril therapy was associated with a 50 % reduction in the risk of the combined end points of death, dialysis, and transplantation that was independent of the small disparity in blood pressure between the groups (Lewis et al. 1993). Two hundred seven patients received captopril, and 202, placebo. Serum creatinine concentrations doubled in 25 patients in the captopril group, as compared with 43 patients in the placebo group ($P=0.007$). But the investigators do not give the mean systolic pressure in each group. The beneficial effect observed with captopril could be due to mild lowering of blood pressure and not proven to be caused by a specific action of the ACE inhibitor. In the UKPDS study with a long follow-up of 9 years, atenolol therapy was as beneficial as captopril therapy in significantly reducing the incidence of major diabetic complications (see Chap. 4). A small study of 92 patients comparing enalapril and losartan in hypertensive type 2 diabetes indicated equal protection.

CLINICAL TRIALS

Results of two large randomized controlled trials (RCTs) with ARBs are now available: both losartan and irbesartan retarded the progression of nephropathy caused by type 2 diabetes independent of reduction in blood pressure. The average blood pressure during the course of the irbesartan trials was 144/83 mmHg with placebo and 143/83 mmHg in the treated group (see Chap. 22).

Brenner et al. (2001): A total of 327 patients in the losartan group reached the primary end point, as compared with 359 in the placebo group (risk reduction, 16%; $P=0.02$). Losartan reduced the incidence of a doubling of the serum creatinine concentration (risk reduction, 25%; $P=0.006$) and end-stage renal disease (risk reduction, 28%; $P=0.002$) but had no effect on the rate of death. The benefit exceeded that attributable to changes in blood pressure. The composite of morbidity and mortality from cardiovascular causes was similar in the two groups, although the rate of first hospitalization for heart failure was significantly lower with losartan (risk reduction, 32%; $P=0.005$). The level of proteinuria declined by 35 % with losartan ($P<0.001$ for the comparison with placebo) (Brenner et al. 2001).

Parving et al. (2001): A total of 590 hypertensive patients with type 2 diabetes and microalbuminuria were enrolled in a double-blind, placebo-controlled study of irbesartan, at a dose of either 150 mg daily or 300 mg daily, and were followed for 2 years. The primary outcome was the time to the onset of diabetic nephropathy, defined by persistent albuminuria in overnight specimens, with a urinary albumin excretion rate that was greater than 200 μg/min and at least 30 % higher than the baseline level. The difference between the placebo group and the irbesartan 150 mg group was not significant ($P = 0.08$ by the log-rank test), but the difference between the placebo group and the irbesartan 300 mg group was significant ($P < 0.001$ by the log-rank test). Irbesartan is renoprotective independently of its blood-pressure-lowering effect in hypertensive patients with type 2 diabetes and microalbuminuria (Parving et al. 2001).

Lewis et al. randomly assigned 1,715 hypertensive patients with nephropathy due to type 2 diabetes to treatment with irbesartan (300 mg daily), amlodipine (10 mg daily), or placebo. Follow-up was 2.6 years. Irbesartan therapy was associated with a risk of the primary composite end point [the composite of a doubling of the baseline serum creatinine concentration, the onset of end-stage renal disease (as indicated by the initiation of dialysis, renal transplantation, or a serum creatinine concentration of at least 6.0 mg per deciliter [530 μmol/L]), or death from any cause]. That was 20 % lower than that in the placebo group ($P = 0.02$) and 23 % lower than that in the amlodipine group ($P = 0.006$) (Lewis et al. 2001).

The risk of a doubling of the serum creatinine concentration was 33 % lower in the irbesartan group than in the placebo group ($P = 0.003$) and 37 % lower in the irbesartan group than in the amlodipine group ($P < 0.001$). Treatment with irbesartan was associated with a relative risk of end-stage renal disease that was 23 % lower than that in both other groups ($P = 0.07$ for both comparisons). These differences were not explained by differences in the blood pressures that were achieved. The serum creatinine concentration increased 24 % more slowly in the irbesartan group than in the placebo group ($P = 0.008$) and 21 % more slowly than in the amlodipine group ($P = 0.02$). There were no significant differences in the rates of death from any cause or in the cardiovascular composite end point (Lewis et al. 2001).

In 2011 the FDA cautioned against using olmesartan to delay or prevent microalbuminuria in patients with diabetes. In the Randomized Olmesartan and Diabetes Microalbuminuria Prevention trial (ROADMAP), olmesartan was, as anticipated, associated with increased time to the onset of microalbuminuria. Nonfatal cardiovascular events occurred in 81 patients in the olmesartan group (3.6%) and 91 in the control group (4.1%); however, fatal cardiovascular events occurred in more patients in the olmesartan group than in the placebo group—15 (0.7%) as compared with 3 (0.1%) ($P = 0.01$). The Olmesartan Reducing Incidence of End Stage Renal Disease in Diabetic Nephropathy Trial (ORIENT). In ORIENT, 566 patients with type 2 diabetes, who differed from the patients in the ROADMAP trial in that they had overt nephropathy, were randomly assigned to olmesartan (at a dose of 10–40 mg daily) or to placebo. Additional antihypertensive medications were permitted, including ACE inhibitors but not including ARBs. The end point was a composite of the time to the first event of doubling of the serum creatinine level, end-stage renal disease, or death from any cause. In ORIENT, there were ten deaths in the olmesartan group and three in the control group.

Coarctation of the Aorta

In this condition, the renin–angiotensin system is especially active, and these agents have a role.

Pulmonary Hypertension

ACE inhibitors may lower pulmonary artery pressure and may increase cardiac output and functional capacity. As with other agents, the improvement is generally not spectacular.

Scleroderma Renal Crisis

This condition is associated with activation of the renin–angiotensin system with rapid progression of renal failure. ACE inhibitor therapy may prevent disease progression and improve survival (Ferner et al. 1987). An interesting case report (Caskey et al. 1997) indicates the failure of losartan to control blood pressure caused by scleroderma renal crisis but with excellent control achieved with an ACE inhibitor. Thus, there may be subtle differences between ACE inhibitors and ARBs that may be important in clinical management.

Bartter's Syndrome

Correction of hyperkalemia is achieved.

ACE Inhibitors/ARBs and Diabetes

DREAM Trial Investigators (2006): In a double-blind RCT with a 2-by-2 factorial design, the trialists randomly assigned 5,269 participants without cardiovascular disease but with impaired fasting glucose levels (after an 8 h fast) or impaired glucose tolerance to receive ramipril (up to 15 mg/day) or placebo (and rosiglitazone or placebo) and followed them for a median of 3 years. They assessed the effects of ramipril on the development of diabetes or death, whichever came first (the primary outcome), and on secondary outcomes, including regression to normoglycemia. Results are as follows:

- The incidence of the primary outcome did not differ significantly between the ramipril group (18.1%) and the placebo group (19.5%; hazard ratio for the ramipril group, 0.91; 95 % confidence interval [CI], 0.81–1.03; *P*=0.15). See Chap. 4 for further details.

CONTRAINDICATIONS

- **Renal artery stenosis** in a solitary kidney or significant bilateral renal artery stenosis (Hricik et al. 1983). In patients with tight renal artery stenosis, renal circulation is critically dependent on high levels of angiotensin II. A sharp decrease in angiotensin II concentration causes dilation of the glomerular efferent arteriole, resulting in a marked fall in renal blood flow that may cause the loss of a kidney. This catastrophic event is heralded by a sharp rise in serum creatinine concentration.
- **Significant aortic stenosis** is a contraindication.
- **Hypertrophic and restrictive cardiomyopathy, constrictive pericarditis,** and hypertensive hypertrophic "cardiomyopathy" of the elderly with impaired ventricular relaxation (Topol et al. 1985) are contraindications.
- **Severe carotid artery stenosis** is a contraindication.
- **Renal failure,** serum creatinine level greater than 2.3 mg/dL, 203 µmol/L (glomerular filtration rate [GFR] 40 mL/min). Caution is necessary when ACE inhibitors are used in patients with renal failure because worsening of renal failure or hyperkalemia may occur.
- **Angina** complicating HF or hypertension is a contraindication because, in these situations, ACE inhibitors may cause an increase in angina (Cleland et al. 1991).
- **Severe anemia** is a relative contraindication to the use of all vasodilators.
- **Preexisting neutropenia** is a contraindication because of the effect on white blood cell function.
- **Pregnancy and lactation** are contraindications.
- **Immune-related renal disease** or coadministration of agents that alter immune function, immunosuppressives, procainamide, tocainide, probenecid, hydralazine, allopurinol, and perhaps acebutolol and pindolol, which have

been reported to cause a lupus-like syndrome, are contraindications.
- **Porphyria** is a contraindication.
- **Uric acid renal calculi** are contraindications because these agents are uricosuric (Leary and Reyes 1987).

ADVICE, ADVERSE EFFECTS, AND INTERACTIONS

Hypotension

Symptomatic hypotension is not uncommon in patients with HF who are already being treated with diuretics or in patients with unilateral tight renal artery stenosis with high circulating renin levels.

Renal Failure

Development or worsening of renal failure may result from relative hypotension or in patients with tight renal artery stenosis.

Hyperkalemia

This may be precipitated by an increase in renal failure, by the use of potassium-sparing diuretics or potassium supplements or the use of salt substitutes, and in patients with hyporeninemic hypoaldosteronism.

Cough

A dry, ticklish, irritating, nonproductive cough occurs in up to 20 % of patients and is clearly dose related, occurring with equal frequency with captopril, enalapril, and lisinopril. ACE is the same as kinase II, which degrades bradykinin completely. The accumulation of bradykinin appears to be responsible for the cough. ARBs cause cough in less than 2 % of treated patients, and angioedema rarely occurs.

Loss of Taste Sensation

This side effect is uncommon and can occur with all ACE inhibitors because the effect appears to be related to the binding of zinc by the ACE inhibitor. A metallic or sour taste in the mouth occurs in some patients with most agents. Mouth ulcers are not uncommon.

Angioedema

This rare complication is important because it can be life-threatening, and deaths have occurred (Jett 1984; Giannoccaro et al. 1989). The occurrence appears to be slightly more common with longer-acting ACE inhibitors than with captopril. Bradykinin and kallidin mediate hereditary angioedema. Thus, ACE inhibition results in an accumulation of bradykinin, which can cause angioedema.

Angioedema is usually observed after the very first few doses or within the first month (Jett 1984), but it can occur after the first dose or after several months of therapy. Cases have been reported within the first year of therapy. Warning signs include localized facial swelling or unilateral facial edema and periorbital edema, which is usually mild and subsides with cessation of drug therapy. Swelling may progress over a few hours to the lips, tongue, and larynx, with obstruction to the airway, which may be resistant to antihistamines and IV epinephrine. The severity of laryngeal edema may render endotracheal intubation impossible, and it may necessitate emergency tracheostomy. Thus, all patients taking an ACE inhibitor who develop mild facial edema and initially respond to antihistamine should be hospitalized, given epinephrine and antihistamine, and observed in an intensive care setting, because, rarely, a rebound, worsening, life-threatening situation can ensue (Giannoccaro et al. 1989; Cameron 1990) and should be prevented. Antihistamines alone may not suffice, and whereas an injection of antihistamine may appear to cause relief over a few hours, severe angioedema may still develop (Cameron 1990).

Rash

A pruritic rash may occur in up to 10 % of patients, typically maculopapular on the arms and trunk, occasionally involving the face. Pruritus may be severe. An urticarial or erythematous eruption, sometimes associated with eosinophilia, may ensue, and, very rarely, pemphigus and onycholysis have been reported. Captopril and enalapril appear to exhibit the same incidence of rash.

Proteinuria

This occurs in fewer than 1 % of captopril-treated patients and mainly in those with underlying renal collagen vascular disease or other immunologic abnormality with a dose of captopril in excess of 150 mg/day. Proteinuria results from stimulation of immune mechanisms and relative hypotension.

Neutropenia and Agranulocytosis

This complication is very rare and occurs mainly in patients with collagen vascular disease and other immunologic disturbances. This complication usually manifests within the first 4 months of therapy and reverses about 3 weeks after cessation of ACE inhibitor therapy.

Mild Dyspnea and/or Wheeze

This may develop, particularly in some asthmatic patients, within the first few weeks of ACE inhibitor therapy (Lunde et al. 1994).

Anaphylactoid Reactions

In patients given ACE inhibitors, anaphylactoid reactions may occur during desensitization treatment with bee or wasp venom. Discontinuation of the ACE inhibitor for at least 24 h before treatment is advisable.

Uncommon Adverse Effects

These include headache, dizziness, fatigue, nausea, diarrhea, impotence, loss of libido, myalgia, muscle cramps, hair loss, hepatitis, cholestatic jaundice, acute pancreatitis, and the occurrence of antinuclear antibodies.

Interactions

- Interactions may occur with allopurinol, acebutolol, hydralazine, procainamide, pindolol, tocainide, and immunosuppressives because these drugs alter the immune response.
- With diuretics, hypotensive effects have been emphasized, and potassium-sparing diuretics or potassium supplements may cause life-threatening hyperkalemia.
- Lithium levels may increase, and toxicity has been reported.

INDIVIDUAL ACE INHIBITORS

Pharmacologic Profile and Individual Differences

The pharmacologic profiles of the commonly used ACE inhibitors are given in Table 3-1.

Subtle Differences

Short-acting ACE inhibitors such as captopril have obvious advantages in the treatment of hypertensive emergencies because the several hours' delay of peak action of other ACE inhibitors does not allow their use when blood pressure lowering is required urgently. Angioedema appears to be slightly more common with enalapril than is observed with captopril, and the longer-acting ACE inhibitors are not exempt from this life-threatening adverse effect. Quinapril, ramipril, and some other ACE inhibitors inhibit tissue renin production. The renin–angiotensin system not only is confined to blood vessels and the kidney but also exists in the heart, liver, adrenals, brain, pituitary glands, salivary glands, gut, uterus, ovaries, and other tissues. The possible theoretical benefit of inhibiting tissue renin–angiotensin systems, however, has not yet been translated into clearly defined clinical differences among the various ACE inhibitors. Quinapril and ramipril penetrate to myocardial ACE binding sites. Myocardial angiotensin has a minimal positive inotropic effect and thus could conceivably be implicated in the development of myocardial hypertrophy. Long-acting preparations with half-lives ranging from 24 to 48 h include cilazapril, perindopril, quinapril, ramipril, spirapril, and zofenopril. Zofenopril is five times more potent than captopril, but it is the only other compound of those mentioned that has an SH group.

Hypotension

Short-acting compounds have an advantage in the initial management of patients with HF. The observation period after the first dose is 1–2 h for captopril, 2–4 h for enalapril, and 2–10 h for longer-acting compounds. When hypotension occurs, cessation of the drug leads to quicker recovery with the shorter-acting compounds. Also, renal failure may be more protracted with longer-acting agents. The agents that are not prodrugs (Table 3-1) have a rapid onset of action. Lisinopril is not a prodrug, and its action is not affected by concurrent administration of food or liver transformation.

Drug name:	**Captopril**
Trade name:	Capoten
Supplied:	12.5, 25, 50 mg
Dosage:	Hypertension: 12.5–50 mg twice daily, max. 150 mg daily; *see* text for further advice Heart failure: 6.25 mg test dose, 6.25–12.5 mg twice daily; titrate over days to weeks to 25–50 mg twice daily; *see* text for further advice

Dosage (Further Advice)

Heart failure: When feasible, discontinue diuretics for 24 h before the initial dose of captopril 6.25 mg. Lower doses (e.g., 3 mg) have been used in special situations, including HF after MI. Observe the blood pressure every 15 min after dosing for 2 h. If hypotension does not occur, give 6.25 mg twice daily for 1–2 days and then, depending on the urgency of the situation, 12.5 mg twice daily, increasing, if needed, to 25 mg twice daily. Most patients require a dose of 37.5–50 mg daily. Maximum suggested dose is 100 mg daily in two or three divided doses if renal function is normal. If interrupted, diuretics should be recommenced approx 24–36 h after the initial dose of captopril. At times, it is not possible to discontinue diuretics completely, and the dose is halved. Also, nitrates should be withheld, to allow the introduction of captopril without producing hypotension or presyncope.

Hypertension: The initial dose is 12.5 mg on day 1 and then twice daily, increasing over the next days or weeks as needed, to a maintenance dose of 25–50 mg twice daily. The maximum dose is 150 mg daily in two divided doses in patients with normal renal function. In patients with renal dysfunction, the total dose should be decreased and the dosing interval increased. In elderly hypertensive patients and in patients with renal impairment or with concomitant diuretic use, the initial dose should be 6.25 mg.

The action, indications, contraindications, and adverse effects of captopril are given under the general discussion of ACE inhibitors.

Pharmacokinetics

Food has been shown to cause about a 33 % reduction in absorption of captopril, so the drug should be given 1 h before meals on an empty stomach. The effect on blood pressure, however, does not appear to be affected by giving the drug with food. About 50 % of the absorbed captopril is metabolized by the liver and is eliminated with the active drug by the kidney, with a plasma half-life of approximately 2–3 h. Captopril is 25–30 % albumin bound; some binding occurs to endogenous thiol compounds, and the drug does not cross the blood–brain barrier. An apparent action on blood pressure is observed within half an hour of oral inges-tion, with a peak effect in 1–2 h and duration of 8–12 h, so in the management of hypertension or HF, twice-daily dosage produces a 24 h therapeutic effect.

Drug name:	**Enalapril**
Trade names:	Vasotec, Innovace (UK)
Supplied:	2.5, 5, 10, 20 mg
Dosage:	Hypertension: 5–20 mg daily, max. 40 mg; *see* text for further advice
	Heart failure: 2.5 mg test dose, then 10–15 mg once or twice daily, max. 30 mg daily; see text for further advice

Dosage (Further Advice)

Heart failure: The dose of diuretics should be halved or held for 24 h to allow for the introduction of enalapril. This is sometimes not possible, and the initial dose of enalapril must be given under close hospital supervision. The initial dose is 2.5 mg orally; observe under close supervision with blood pressure monitoring for 2–6 h. In the absence of hypotension, give 2.5 mg twice daily for a few days, and reintroduce diuretics as soon as possible to prevent the recurrence or worsening of HF. The dose of enalapril is increased to 5 mg twice daily for several days and, if needed, to 7.5–10 mg twice daily, which is approximately equivalent to 75–100 mg captopril daily; the suggested maximum dose is 30 mg, preferably in two divided doses. Patients with HF often have concomitant renal dysfunction, and the once-daily dosing of enalapril is usually sufficient to produce a salutary response. A twice-daily enalapril dose, however, allows for finer titration and may avoid relative hypotension. The effective median dose in CONSENSUS was 18 mg, and in V-HeFT it was 15 mg.

Hypertension: Discontinue diuretics for 2–3 days, and then give 2.5 mg daily, increasing slowly over several weeks to 5–10 mg daily. With more severe hypertension, the starting dose could be 2.5 mg on the first day and then 5 mg daily. If blood pressure control is not achieved with a dose of 10 mg, increase the dose to 10 mg in the morning and 5 mg at night. Failure to control the condition with this dose should prompt the reintroduction of the diuretic. The maximum dose of enalapril should be kept to 30 mg daily, equivalent to 150 mg captopril. A dose of 40 mg is rarely necessary, except with severe or resistant hypertension requiring therapy.

Pharmacokinetics

After oral dosing, about 60 % of the drug is absorbed and is not influenced by ingestion of food. Enalapril is inactive and undergoes hepatic hydrolysis to the active enalaprilat. Peak effect of enalaprilat is at about 5 h; after multiple dosing, the plasma half-life is approx 11 h. The peak hypotensive effect is observed from 4 to 6 h after oral dosing, and excretion is virtually all renal. The dose of enalapril may need to be increased in patients with severe liver dysfunction.

The adverse effects and contraindications of enalapril have been given earlier under ACE inhibitors.

Drug name:	**Lisinopril**
Trade names:	Prinivil, Zestril, Carace
Supplied:	2.5, 5, 10, 20 mg
Dosage:	Hypertension: 5–20 mg once daily, max. 40 mg; *see* text for further advice Heart failure: 2.5–5 mg once daily, increasing over weeks to 10–20 mg daily, max. 40 mg daily

Dosage (Further Advice)

As with other ACE inhibitors, it is recommended, if feasible, to discontinue diuretics for at least 2 days before commencing lisinopril and to recommence diuretics a few days to weeks later, if needed. Initially, give 2.5 mg daily, increasing slowly over weeks with evaluation of blood pressure and renal function, to a maintenance dose of 5–20 mg once daily. The maximum suggested dose of lisinopril is 30 mg daily; doses in excess of 20 mg usually do not cause further lowering of blood pressure (Kochar et al. 1987). In the Assessment of Treatment with Lisinopril and Survival (ATLAS) trial (ATLAS; Packer et al. 1999), a daily dose of 30–35 mg versus 2.5–5 mg reportedly caused a significant decrease in hospitalizations, but the decrease was only 14%, with no reduction in total mortality.

Pharmacokinetics

The drug is well absorbed when given orally, and absorption is not influenced by food. Lisinopril is not a prodrug and does not undergo hepatic metabolism. The drug is hydrophilic and is completely eliminated by the kidney with a plasma half-life of 13 h, but the elimination half-life is long, up to 30 h. An apparent action is observed in 2–4 h with peak effect at 4–8 h and duration of action of 24–30 h. Lisinopril is the only water-soluble ACE inhibitor.

Drug name:	**Benazepril**
Trade name:	Lotensin
Supplied:	5, 10, 20, 40 mg
Dosage:	5 mg daily, increasing over weeks to 10–20 mg daily, max. 40 mg

The plasma half-life is about 11 h; the terminal half-life is 21–22 h.

Drug name:	**Cilazapril**
Trade names:	Inhibace, Vascace (UK)
Supplied:	1, 2.5, 5 mg
Dosage:	1–2, 5 mg daily, max. 5 mg

Cilazapril is a prodrug and undergoes hepatic metabolism to the active form cilazaprilat with a terminal half-life that exceeds 40 h.

Drug name:	**Fosinopril**
Trade names:	Monopril, Staril (UK)
Supplied:	10, 20 mg
Dosage:	5–10 mg once daily, increasing gradually to 20 mg daily, max. 40 mg; *see* text for further advice

Dosage (Further Advice)

Avoid taking within 2 h of antacids. Fosinopril undergoes hepatic and renal elimination. More of the drug is removed through the liver with increasing renal failure (30). Fosinopril appears to cause less cough than is observed with other ACE inhibitors. The terminal half-life is approximately 13 h, but inhibition of serum ACE lasts 24 h after a 40 mg dose of the drug.

Drug name:	**Perindopril**
Trade name:	Aceon
Supplied:	2, 4, 8 mg
Dosage:	2 mg daily; maintenance 4 mg, max. 8 mg

The drug is long acting, given once daily. The terminal half-life is 27–33 h.

Drug name:	**Quinapril**
Trade names:	Accupril, Accupro (UK)

Supplied:	5, 10, 20, 40 mg
Dosage:	2.5–5 mg initially, increasing to 10–40 mg daily, max. 60 mg

Drug name:	**Ramipril**
Trade names:	Altace, Tritace (UK)
Supplied:	1.25, 2.5, 5, 10 mg
Dosage:	1.25–2.5 mg daily, increasing over weeks to 5–10 mg; max. 15 mg once daily or two divided doses

The drug is partially metabolized to the active form, ramiprilat, and is partially a prodrug. Ramiprilat is about 70 % and ramipril approximately 50 % protein bound. The effective half-life is 14–18 h, but accumulation of the drug occurs resulting in a terminal half-life of up to 110 h. The maximal effect is observed in about 6 h, with duration of action exceeding 24 h. The drug has tissue-specific ACE inhibitor activity.

The HOPE study showed that in a high-risk group of patients (81 % ischemic heart disease, 11 % stroke, 38 % diabetes), 10 mg of ramipril given for a mean of 4.5 years caused a modest reduction of 22 % in the primary outcome of MI, stroke, or death from cardiovascular diseases (HOPE Investigators 2000).

• Unfortunately optimal therapy was not given to patients. Although, 65.4 % of the treated group had documented hyperlipidemia, only 28.4 % were taking statins. In addition 51.9 % had had a documented MI and 54.8 % had a history of stable angina, only 39.2 % were taking beta-blockers. Thus, one may question whether the benefits associated with ramipril in this study would have been maintained if patients had been treated with appropriate regimens of aspirin, beta-blockers, and lipid-lowering agents (Weinsaft et al. 2000).

In diabetic patients after adjustment for the changes in systolic (2.4 mmHg) blood pressure, ramipril lowered the risk of the combined primary outcome by 25%.

Drug name:	**Spirapril**
Trade names:	Renpress, Sandopril
Supplied:	12.5 mg
Dosage:	6.5–12.5 mg daily, max. 30 mg

The drug is well absorbed when given orally. The onset of action occurs in 1 h after ingestion, with a prolonged duration of action reflecting a half-life of about 72 h. The drug is eliminated by the liver and kidney.

Drug name:	**Trandolapril**
Trade names:	Mavik, Gopten (UK)
Supplied:	0.5, 1, 2 mg
Dosage:	0.5–1 mg daily, max. 4 mg

This agent without SH moiety has a long plasma half-life of 24 h. It is rapidly hydrolyzed to trandolaprilat, the active compound, which has high lipophilicity.

Drug name:	**Zofenopril**
Dosage:	Initially 7.5 mg every 12 h; titrate slowly to 15–30 mg daily

The dose outlined under dosage was administered for 6 weeks in the SMILE study (1). Patients with acute anterior infarcts were randomized at a mean of 15 h from the onset of symptoms. Therapy resulted in a significant reduction in the incidence of severe HF and improved survival at 1-year follow-up. Efficacy was observed mainly in patients with previous infarction. Further clinical trials with ACE inhibitors administered within 6 h of onset of symptoms are required to document the safety and efficacy of very early ACE inhibitor therapy.

ANGIOTENSIN II RECEPTOR BLOCKERS

There are two main types of angiotensin II receptor: AT_1 and AT_2. Most actions of angiotensin II are mediated through the AT_1 receptor. ARBs specifically block the angiotensin II receptor AT_1, and this causes blockade of the renin–angiotensin aldosterone system, although we know that the blockade is not complete. Because angiotensin can be synthesized outside the renin–angiotensin system, angiotensin receptor antagonists could produce more effective control of angiotensin II than ACE inhibitors. The major pathway for angiotensin II production in the heart is not ACE but a serine protease, chymase. Angiotensin I can be converted to angiotensin II by enzymes such as cathepsin, trypsin, and heart chymase, but the exact contribution of these alternative pathways to the generation of angiotensin II is unclear.

Angiotensin II blockade causes an increased flux of superoxide that improves NO bioactivity. Most important, AT_2 receptors are not blocked by ARBs. It appears that AT_2 receptors mediate a physiologic cardioprotective role: production of bradykinin, NO, prostaglandins in the kidney, inhibition of cell growth, promotion of cell differentiation, and apoptosis.

Their proven beneficial effect in type 2 diabetes (Brenner et al. 2001; Parving et al. 2001; Lewis et al. 2001), in which no proven effect of ACE inhibitors has emerged, will render ARBs (not olmesartan or telmisartan) a popular choice in diabetics, particularly because of the rare occurrence of cough and angioedema. There is proven clinical efficacy for ACE inhibitors in type 1 diabetes (Lewis et al. 1993). There has not been RCT comparisons of ARBs and ACE inhibitors in type 1 or type 2 diabetes.

Clinical Trials

ELITE 11: **Effect of losartan compared with captopril on mortality in patients with symptomatic heart failure: randomised trial—the Losartan Heart Failure Survival Study ELITE II.** Pitt et al. conducted a double-blind, RCT of 3,152 patients aged 60 years or older with New York Heart Association class II–IV heart failure and ejection fraction of 40 % or less. Patients, stratified for β-blocker use, were randomly assigned losartan ($n=1,578$) titrated to 50 mg once daily or captopril ($n=1,574$) titrated to 50 mg three times daily. The primary and secondary end points were all-cause mortality and sudden death or resuscitated arrest. Analysis was by intention to treat (Pitt et al. 2000). At 555 days, there were no significant differences in all-cause mortality (11.7 vs. 10.4 % average annual mortality rate) or sudden death or resuscitated arrests (9.0 vs. 7.3%) between the two treatment groups (hazard ratios 1.13 [95.7 % CI 0.95–1.35], $P=0.16$ and 1.25 [95 % CI 0.98–1.60], $P=0.08$). Significantly fewer patients in the losartan group (excluding those who died) discontinued study treatment because of adverse effects (9.7 vs. 14.7%, $P<0.001$), including cough (0.3 vs. 2.7%). Losartan was not superior to captopril in improving survival in elderly heart failure patients. ACE inhibitors should be the initial treatment for heart failure (Pitt et al. 2000). The results of CHARM indicated that the ARB candesartan is equal to ACE inhibitor therapy for the management of heart failure (see the results of CHARM in Chap. 22).

ONTARGET: The ONTARGET investigators conducted an RCT in patients with vascular disease or high-risk diabetes but absence of HF and assigned 8,576 patients to receive 10 mg of ramipril per day, 8,542 to receive 80 mg of the ARB telmisartan per day, and 8,502 to receive both drugs (combination therapy). The primary composite outcome was death from cardiovascular causes, myocardial infarction

(MI), stroke, or hospitalization for HF. The results are as follows:

- At a median follow-up of 56 months, the primary outcome was reported in 1,412 patients in the ramipril group (16.5%) and in 1,423 patients in the telmisartan group (16.7%); telmisartan was equivalent to ramipril in this study. The combination of the two drugs was associated with more adverse events with no improvement in outcomes (ONTARGET Investigators 2008).
- **Telmisartan was shown equivalent to ramipril in ONTARGET but without effect in TRANSCEND.** Yusuf et al. (2008b) and in PRoFESS: Yusuf et al. (2008a), it is important to reassess the benefits of ramipril in the HOPE study. **Weinsaft and colleagues indicated that the population studied in HOPE was one in which a considerable number of patients were being treated with suboptimal medication regimens, according to current treatment guidelines**.
- Although 65.4 % of the treated group had documented hyperlipidemia, only 28.4 % were taking statins. In addition 51.9 % had had a documented MI and 54.8 % had a history of stable angina; only 39.2 % were taking beta-blockers.
- **Thus, one may question whether the benefits associated with ramipril in this study would have been maintained if patients had been treated with appropriate regimens of aspirin, beta-blockers, and lipid-lowering agents** (Weinsaft et al. 2000).

Drug name:	**Candesartan**
Trade names:	Atacand, Amias (UK)
Supplied:	8, 16, 32 mg; 8, 16 mg; UK, 4, 8, 16 mg
Dosage:	Initially 8 mg once daily (4 mg in the elderly or in hepatic/renal impairment), then 8–16 mg; max. 32 mg daily

Half-life:	9 h, 9–12 h in elderly
Excretion:	60 % renal; 40 % bile

Drug name:	**Irbesartan**
Trade names:	Avapro, Aprovel (UK)
Supplied:	75, 150, 300 mg
Dosage:	150–300 mg once daily (initial dose 75 mg in the elderly)
Half-life:	11–15 h
Excretion:	80 % renal; 20 % bile

Drug name:	**Losartan**
Trade name:	Cozaar
Supplied:	25, 50 mg
Dosage:	25–50 mg once or twice daily (initially in the elderly and in those with hepatic or renal impairment 25 mg daily); max. 100 mg daily

HEAAL Study (2009): Losartan for heart failure. Three thousand four hundred and forty-six patients of New York Heart Association class II–IV with HF, left ventricular ejection fraction 40 % or less, and intolerance to (ACE) inhibitors were randomly assigned to losartan 150 mg ($n = 1,927$) or 50 mg daily ($n = 1,919$) and unfortunately none to placebo. With 4.7-year median follow-up in each group, 828 (43%) patients in the 150 mg group versus 889 (46%) in the 50 mg group died or were admitted for HF (hazard ratio [HR] 0.90, $P = 0.027$). For the two primary end point components, 635 patients in the 150 mg group versus 665 in the 50 mg group died (HR 0.94, 95 % CI 0.84–1.04; $P = 0.24$), and 450 versus 503 patients were admitted for HF (0.87, 0.76–0.98; $P = 0.025$). Renal impairment ($n = 454$ vs. 317), hypotension (203 vs. 145), and hyperkalemia

(195 vs. 131) were more common in the 150 mg group than in the 50 mg group.

- High-dose losartan 150 mg resulted in more adverse events: hyperkalemia, hypotension, renal insufficiency, and angioedema but with only a modest benefit compared with a low dose of 50 mg. The maximum losartan dose used in clinical practice is 100 mg.
- It is surprising and unfortunate that these investigators chose a dose higher than the manufacturer's suggested maximum dose.

See Table 3-2 for a comparison of ARBs.

Drug name:	**Valsartan**
Supplied:	40, 80 mg
Dosage:	80–160 mg once daily (initial dose in the elderly 40 mg); max. 320 mg

Caution: Neutropenia has been reported in 1.9 % of valsartan-treated patients. Increased hepatic enzymes and the rare occurrence of severe hepatic dysfunction with two fatalities have been reported in association with marketed ARBs. *Caution: valsartan interacts with beta-blockers.* (Val-HeFT (2001): But the efficacy of nebivolol and valsartan as fixed-dose combination was shown in hypertension: a randomised, multicentre study (Giles et al. 2014).

Drug name:	**Telmisartan**
Supplied:	40, 80 mg
Dosage:	20–80 mg once daily
Half-life:	24 h
Excretion:	98 % in the feces

- Telmisartan appears equivalent to ramipril as indicated by ONTARGET, yet telministan therapy failed. The TRANSCEND investigators studied the effects of the ARB telmisartan on cardiovascular events in 5,926 high-risk patients intolerant to ACE inhibitors (Yusuf et al. 2008b). Many patients receiving concomitant proven therapies were randomized to receive telmisartan 80 mg/day ($n=2,954$) or placebo ($n=2,972$). The primary outcome was the composite of cardiovascular death, MI, or hospitalization for HF. After a median duration of follow-up of 56 months, 465 (15.7%) patients experienced the primary outcome in the telmisartan group compared with 504 (17%) in the placebo group ($P=0.216$); a fallure even when combined endpoints used.

- **Telmisartan administration for 56 months in high-risk patients intolerant to ACE inhibitors surprisingly had no significant effect on the primary outcome, which included hospitalizations for HF** (Yusuf et al. 2008b). GFR decreased significantly more in the telmisartan group than placebo.

In the well-run RCT PRoFESS, telmisartan failed to decrease recurrent stroke (Yusuf et al. for the PRoFESS Study Group 2008).

- **The efficacy of the ARB telmisartan raises some concern because of poor efficacy in two large RCTs.**

Drug name:	**Eprosartan**
Trade name:	Teveten
Supplied:	400, 600 mg
Dosage:	300–400 mg twice daily or 300–800 mg once daily
Half-life:	7 h

REFERENCES

ACCOMPLISH: Jamerson K, Weber MA, Bakris GL et al For the ACCOMPLISH trial investigators (2008) Benazepril plus amlodipine or hydrochlorothiazide for hypertension in high-risk patients. N Engl JMed 359:2417–2428.

Ambrosioni E, Borghi C, Magnani B, for the Survival of Myocardial Infarction Long-term Evaluation (SMILE) Study Investigators, et al. The effect of the angiotensin-converting enzyme inhibitor zofenopril on mortality and morbidity after anterior myocardial infarction. N Engl J Med. 1995;332:80.

ATLAS Study Group, Packer M, Poole-Wilson PA, Armstrong PW, et al. Comparative effects of low and high doses of the angiotensin-converting enzyme inhibitor, lisinopril on morbidity and mortality in chronic heart failure. Circulation. 1999;100:2312.

Burnier M. Angiotensin II, type 1 receptor blockers. Circulation. 2001; 103:904.

Cameron DI. Near fatal angioedema associated with captopril. Can J Cardiol. 1990;6:265.

Caskey FJ, Thacker EJ, Johnston PA, et al. Failure of losartan to control blood pressure in scleroderma renal crisis. Lancet. 1997; 349:620.

Cicoira M, Zanolla L, Rossi A. Failure of aldosterone suppression despite angiotensin converting enzyme (ACE) inhibitor administration in chronic heart failure is associated with ACE DD genotype. J Am Coll Cardiol. 2001;37:1808.

Cleland JGF, Henderson E, McLenachan J, et al. Effect of captopril, an angiotensin converting enzyme inhibitor, in patients with angina pectoris and heart failure. J Am Coll Cardiol. 1991;17:733.

Cohn JN, Johnson G, Ziesche S, et al. A comparison of enalapril with hydralazine-isosorbide dinitrate in the treatment of chronic congestive heart failure. N Engl J Med. 1991;325:303.

CONSENSUS Trial Study Group. Effects of enalapril on mortality in severe congestive heart failure: results of the Cooperative North Scandinavian Enalapril Survival Study (CONSENSUS). N Engl J Med. 1987;316:1429.

Davis JO, Freeman RH. Mechanisms regulating renin release. Physiol Rev. 1976;56:1.

DREAM Trial Investigators. Effect of ramipril on the incidence of diabetes. N Engl J Med. 2006;355:1551–62.

ELITE II, Pitt B, Poole-Wilson PA, Segal R, et al. Effect of losartan compared with captopril on mortality on patients with symptomatic heart failure: randomized trial. The Losartan Heart Failure Study. Lancet. 2000;255:1582.

Ferner RE, Simpson JM, Rawlings MD. Effects of intradermal bradykinin after inhibition of angiotensin converting enzyme. BMJ. 1987;294: 1119.

Ganong WF. The brain renin-angiotensin system. Annu Rev Physiol. 1984;46:17.

Giannoccaro PJ, Wallace GJ, Higginson L, et al. Fatal angioedema associated with enalapril. Can J Cardiol. 1989;5:335.

Giles TD, Weber MA, Basile J, for the NAC-MD-01 Study Investigators, et al. Efficacy and safety of nebivolol and valsartan as fixed-dose combination in hypertension: a randomised, multicentre study. Lancet. 2014;383:1889–98.

HOPE Investigators, Yusuf S, Sleight P, Pogue J, et al. Effects of an angiotensin-converting enzyme inhibitor, ramipril, on death from cardiovascular causes, myocardial infarction, and stroke in high-risk patients. N Engl J Med. 2000;342:145.

Hricik DE, Browning PJ, Kopelman R, et al. Captopril-induced functional renal insufficiency in patients with bilateral renal-artery stenoses or renal-artery stenosis in a solitary kidney. N Engl J Med. 1983;308:373.

Ingelfinger JR. Editorial. Preemptive olmesartan for the delay or prevention of microalbuminuria in diabetes. N Engl J Med. 2011;364:970–1.

Jett GK. Captopril-induced angioedema. Ann Emerg Med. 1984;13:489.

Kochar MS, Bolek G, Kalbfleish JF, et al. A 52 week comparison of lisinopril, hydrochlorothiazide and their combination in hypertension. J Clin Pharmacol. 1987;27:373.

Leary WP, Reyes AJ. Angiotensin I converting enzyme inhibitors and the renal excretion of urate. Cardiovasc Drugs Ther. 1987;1:29.

Lewis EJ, Hunsicker LG, Bain RP, for the Collaborative Study Group, et al. The effect of angiotensin-converting-enzyme inhibition on diabetic nephropathy. N Engl J Med. 1993;329:1456–62.

Lewis EJ, Hunsicker LG, Clarke WR, for the Collaborative Study Group, et al. Renoprotective effect of the angiotensin receptor antagonist irbesartan in patients with nephropathy due to type 2 diabetes. N Engl J Med. 2001;345:851.

Lunde H, Hedner T, Samuelsson O, et al. Dyspnoea, asthma, and bronchospasm in relation to treatment with angiotensin converting enzyme inhibitors. BMJ. 1994;308:18.

McMurray JV, Swedberg K (2010) HEAAL: the final chapter in the story of angiotensin receptor blockers in heart failure–lessons learnt from a decade of trials. Eur J Heart Fail 12(2):99–103.

Munzel T, Keaney JF. Are ACE inhibitors a "magic bullet" against oxidative stress? Circulation. 2001;104:1571.

ONTARGET: The ONTARGET Investigators (2008) Telmisartan, ramipril, or both in patients at high risk for vascular events. N Engl J Med 358:1547–1559.

Parving H-H, Lehnert H, Brochner-Mortensen J, for the Irbesartan in Patients with Type 2 Diabetes and Microalbuminuria Study Group, et al. The effect of irbesartan on the development of diabetic nephropathy in patients with type 2 diabetes. N Engl J Med. 2001;345:870.

Pfeffer MA, Braunwald E. Ventricular remodelling after myocardial infarction: experimental observations and clinical implications. Circulation. 1990;81:1161.

PROGRESS Collaborative Group. Randomized trial of a perindopril-based blood pressure lowering regimen among, individuals with previous stroke or transient ischaemic attack. Lancet. 2001;358:1033.

PRoFESS, Yusuf S, Diener H-C, Sacco RL, et al. Telmisartan to prevent recurrent stroke and cardiovascular events. N Eng J Med. 2008a; 359(12):1225–37.

Reid IA. The renin-angiotensin system and body function. Arch Intern Med. 1985;145:1475.

RENAAL Study Investigators, Brenner BM, Cooper ME, de Zeeuw D, et al. Effects of losartan on renal and cardiovascular outcomes in patients with type 2 diabetes and nephropathy. N Engl J Med. 2001;345:861.

ROADMAP Trial Investigators, Haller H, Ito S, Izzo Jr JL, et al. Olmesartan for the delay or prevention of microalbuminuria in type 2 diabetes. N Engl J Med. 2011;364:907–17.

The ONTARGET Investigators (2008). Telmisartan, Ramipril, or Both in Patients at High Risk for Vascular Events Randomized,– April 10, 2008. N Engl J Med 2008; 358:1547-1559. http://www.nejm.org/doi/full/10.1056/NEJMoa0801317

SOLVD Investigators. Effect of enalapril on survival in patients with reduced left ventricular ejection fractions and congestive heart failure. N Engl J Med. 1991;325:293.

Topol EJ, Thomas A, Fortuin NJ. Hypertensive hypertrophic cardiomyopathy of the elderly. N Engl J Med. 1985;312:277.

Torretti J. Sympathetic control of renin release. Annu Rev Pharmacol Toxicol. 1982;22:167.

Val-HeFT, Cohn JN, Tognoni G. A randomized trial of the angiotensin-receptor blocker valsartan in chronic heart failure. N Engl J Med. 2001;345:1667–75.

Weber KT. Aldosterone and spironolactone in heart failure. N Engl J Med. 1999;341:753.

Weinsaft JW (2000) Effect of ramipril on cardiovascular events in highrisk patients. N Engl J Med 343:64–66.

Yusuf S, Teo K, Anderson C et al for the TRANSCEND Investigators (2008b) Effects of the angiotensin-receptor blocker telmisartan on cardiovascular events in high-risk patients intolerant to angiotensin-converting enzyme inhibitors: a randomised controlled trial. Lancet 372:1174–1183. TRANSCEND.

4   ACE Inhibitor ARB Controversies

ACE INHIBITORS VERSUS ARBS: DOES THE CHOICE MATTER?

Angiotensin-converting enzyme (ACE) inhibitors have been shown in large randomized controlled trials (RCTs) to prevent cardiovascular disease (CVD) outcomes significantly in patients with hypertension and heart failure (HF) and particularly in patients with LV dysfunction caused by acute myocardial infarction (MI).

- The results are not as good for angiotensin receptor blockers [ARBs] that are unfortunately now more widely used than ACE inhibitors.

In Val-HeFT (2001): mainly classes II and III were randomly assigned to receive 160 mg of valsartan or placebo twice daily. **There was no reduction in all-cause mortality**. The incidence of the combined end point was a modest 13.2 % lower with valsartan than with placebo, predominantly because of a lower number of patients hospitalized for heart failure: 455 (18.2 %) in the placebo group and 346 (13.8 %) in the valsartan group ($P<0.001$). This result is similar for that observed for digoxin. Yet digoxin is rarely used for HF.

In **Val-HeFT, valsartan when combined with a beta-blocker caused significantly more cardiac events**. A total of 5,010 patients with HF class II, III, or IV were randomly

© Springer Science+Business Media New York 2015
M. Gabriel Khan, *Cardiac Drug Therapy*, Contemporary Cardiology, DOI 10.1007/978-1-61779-962-4_4

assigned to receive 160 mg of valsartan or placebo twice daily. There was no reduction in all causes of mortality. The incidence of the combined end point, however, was a modest 13.2 % lower with valsartan than with placebo ($P = 0.009$), predominantly because of a lower number of patients hospitalized for heart failure: 455 (18.2 %) in the placebo group and 346 (13.8 %) in the valsartan group ($P < 0.001$). **Overall mortality was not reduced by valsartan administration** (Cohn and Tognoni 2001).

Unfortunately less than 36 % of subjects received a beta-blocker and ~68 % received digoxin.

Often in patients with HF, a beta-blocker is needed as proven therapy. Thus, an ACE inhibitor must be used, not an ARB; telmisartan also failed in HF trials [TRANSCEND].

Caution: valsartan must not be combined with a beta-blocker.

In **VALIANT** (2003): a clinical trial of valsartan, captopril, or both in MI complicated by HF, left ventricular dysfunction, or both, during a median follow-up of 24.7 months, **total mortality was not reduced by valsartan**: 979 patients in the valsartan group died, as did 941 patients in the valsartan-and-captopril group and 958 patients in the captopril group. **There was no placebo group.**

Caution: Valsartan is not advisable in HF patients because in this large number of patients, a beta-blocker is the needed therapy.

- **Significant mortality reduction remains unknown for ARBs.**

CHARM-Overall program (2003) compared candesartan with placebo in three distinct populations: patients with left ventricular ejection fraction (LVEF) 40 % or less who were not receiving ACE inhibitors because of previous intolerance or who were currently receiving ACE inhibitors and patients with LVEF higher than 40 %. Overall, 7,601 patients (7,599 with data) were randomly assigned candesartan ($n = 3,803$, titrated to 32 mg once daily) or matching placebo ($n = 3,796$); median follow-up was 37.7 months. The primary outcome of the overall program was all-cause mortality.

- **Total mortality was not reduced**; 886 (23 %) patients in the candesartan and 945 (25 %) in the placebo group died $p = 0.055$.

CHARM-Alternative trial (2003) enrolled 2,028 patients with symptomatic heart failure and left ventricular ejection fraction 40 % or less who were not receiving ACE inhibitors because of previous intolerance. Patients were randomly assigned candesartan (target dose 32 mg once daily) or matching placebo.

- **There was no reduction in total mortality**; 265 deaths occurred in the candesartan group and 296 in the placebo group $p = 0.11$. But 334 (33 %) of 1,013 patients in the candesartan group and 406 (40 %) of 1,015 in the placebo group had cardiovascular death or hospital admission for CHF $p = 0.0004$. Hospital admission for HF was modestly reduced. Only by combining events do these trials show positive results.

TRANSCEND (2008) investigators studied the effects of telmisartan on cardiovascular events in high-risk patients intolerant to ACE inhibitors. Telmisartan therapy for 56 months, although shown in ONTARGET to be equivalent to ramipril surprisingly:

- **Failed to decrease total mortality and had no significant effect on the primary outcome and hospitalizations for HF. Thus, telmisartan use should be avoided.**
- **In the large well-run PRoFESS RCT, telmisartan failed to decrease recurrent stroke** (Yusuf et al. 2008).

ARBs appear to be associated with a modestly increased risk for cancer, according to a meta-analysis published in the

Lancet Oncology (Sipahi et al. 2010). Researchers, examining data from five randomized trials comprising nearly 62,000 patients, found that those taking ARBs (85 % were using telmisartan) had a significantly greater risk for new cancer than did controls (7.2 % vs. 6 %). **Should we be concerned about all ARBs or a single drug, telmisartan?**

- **Angioedema**: ACE inhibitors cause cough in more than 20 % of treated individuals and produce a significantly higher incidence of angioedema vs. ARBs. This incidence is much higher in patients of African origin. Deaths owing to angioedema have been reported in several hypertension RCTs. In the well-run large Antihypertensive and Lipid-Lowering Treatment to Prevent Heart Attack Trial (ALLHAT 2002), significant differences for angioedema were seen for the lisinopril vs. chlorthalidone comparison overall ($p < 0.001$). In blacks angioedema was seen in 2 of 5,369 (<0.1 %) for chlorthalidone and 23 of 3,210 (0.7 %) for lisinopril ($p < 0.001$). In non-blacks angioedema was seen in 6 of 9,886 (0.1 %) for chlorthalidone and 15 of 5,844 for lisinopril (0.3 %); $p = 0.002$). The only death from angioedema was in the lisinopril group. Death should not occur in the treatment of healthy individuals; the patient with mild primary hypertension is invariably healthy and asymptomatic. Importantly, most patients with angioedema caused by an ACE inhibitor require emergency room treatment.

Conclusion: ACE inhibitors should be the first choice in all patients with a CVD problem. ARBs are indicated only if there is intolerance to ACE inhibitor use.

ACE INHIBITORS/ARBS CAUSE RENOPROTECTION: TRUE OR FALSE?

Experts and clinical teachers believe that ACE inhibitors and ARBs have specific renoprotective effects. Guidelines indicate that these are the drugs of choice for the treatment of hypertension in patients with renal disease with or without proteinuria. Casas et al. (2005) assessed electronic databases for RCTs of antihypertensive drugs and progression of renal disease. Effects on primary discrete end points (doubling of creatinine and end-stage renal disease) and secondary continuous markers of renal outcomes (creatinine, albuminuria, and glomerular filtration rate) were calculated with random-effect models. Comparisons of ACE inhibitors or ARBs with other antihypertensive drugs yielded a relative risk of 0.71 (95 % CI 0.49–1.04) for doubling of creatinine and a small benefit in end-stage renal disease (relative risk 0.87, 0.75–0.99). In patients with diabetic nephropathy, no benefit was seen in comparative trials of ACE inhibitors or ARBs on the doubling of creatinine (1.09, 0.55–2.15) or end-stage renal disease (0.89, 0.74–1.07), glomerular filtration rate, or creatinine amounts. These investigators concluded that:

The benefits of ACE inhibitors or ARBs on renal outcomes in placebo-controlled trials probably result from a blood-pressure-lowering effect (Casas et al. 2005). In 2011 the FDA cautioned against using olmesartan to delay or prevent microalbuminuria in patients with diabetes. In the Randomized Olmesartan and Diabetes Microalbuminuria Prevention (ROADMAP) trial, olmesartan was, as anticipated, associated with increased time to the onset of microalbuminuria. Nonfatal cardiovascular events occurred in 81 patients in the olmesartan group (3.6 %) and 91 in the control group (4.1 %); however, fatal cardiovascular events occurred in more patients in the olmesartan group than in the placebo group—15 (0.7 %) as compared with 3 (0.1 %) ($P = 0.01$). This possible cardiovascular safety signal, together with a similar signal from the Olmesartan Reducing Incidence of End-Stage Renal Disease in Diabetic Nephropathy Trial (ORIENT), has led to an ongoing investigation by the Food and Drug Administration (FDA). In ORIENT, 566 patients with type 2 diabetes, who differed from the patients in the ROADMAP trial in that they had overt nephropathy, were randomly assigned to olmesartan (at a dose of 10–40 mg daily) or to placebo. Additional anti-hypertensive medications were permitted, including ACE inhibitors but not including ARBs. The end point was a composite of the time to the first event of doubling of the serum creatinine level, end-stage renal disease, or death from any cause. In ORIENT, there were 10 deaths in the olmesartan group and 3 in the control group.

- The FDA is reviewing the safety of the ARB after two ongoing trials among patients with type 2 diabetes suggested increased risk for cardiovascular death with the drug.

ACE INHIBITORS DECREASE THE INCIDENCE OF DIABETES: TRUE OR FALSE?

In the Losartan Intervention for Endpoint (LIFE 2002) reduction in hypertension study, atenolol was compared with losartan. In a post hoc analysis it is claimed that there was a significant 15 % excess of new-onset diabetes over 5 years, but the absolute rise in glucose was not stated. A large number of patients in the beta-blocker group received diuretics, and the frequency of diuretic use in each study arm was not given. In most studies, including LIFE, post hoc analysis suggested that increased risk of new-onset diabetes was confined to individuals with an elevated blood glucose at baseline and family predisposition to diabetes (Lindholm et al. 2002).

In the Valsartan Antihypertensive Long-Term Use Evaluation (VALUE 2004) trial, new-onset type 2 diabetes was 25 % more frequent in the patients on amlodipine than in those on valsartan (13.1 % vs. 16.4 %; $p < 0.0001$). This is a spurious finding because amlodipine does not cause diabetes, and ACE inhibitors do not prevent the occurrence of diabetes. A genuine diabetic state was not confirmed.

Nathan (2010), in an editorial, emphasized that the only clinical trial that directly examined whether ACE

inhibition would prevent diabetes failed to show that diabetes was prevented.

Among persons with impaired fasting glucose levels or impaired glucose tolerance, the use of ramipril for 3 years did not significantly reduce the incidence of diabetes or death (DREAM Trial Investigators 2006)

The Nateglinide and Valsartan in Impaired Glucose Tolerance Outcomes Research (NAVIGATOR 2010) trial examined the effects of the approved diabetes medication nateglinide, a relatively weak, rapid-acting, sulfonylurea-like drug, and the ARB valsartan on the development of diabetes and cardiovascular disease in a high-risk population.

The NAVIGATOR (Study 2010) **results do not indicate a reduction in the incidence of diabetes mellitus. The extended cardiovascular outcome occurred in 672 patients (14.5 %) in the valsartan group and 693 patients (14.8 %) in the placebo group.**

COMBINATION OF ACE INHIBITOR AND ARB PROVEN EFFECTIVE: TRUE OR FALSE?

The search for virtually complete renin-angiotensin-aldosterone system (RAAS) blockade appears to make good sense. The combination of ACE inhibitor and ARB, however, did not result in satisfactory therapeutic goals in the valsartan RCT. **Combination therapy did not result in significant reduction in primary outcomes in patients with HF. Most important, the combination of valsartan with a beta-blocker needed for HF treatment increased mortality (Val-HeFT** 2001).

In CHARM-Added (Pfeffer et al. 2003), after 41 months of follow-up, addition of candesartan to an ACE inhibitor led to modest reduction in cardiovascular death and hospitalization for HF, **but total mortality was not reduced.**

Caution is needed when a combination of ACE inhibitor and ARB is administered because hyperkalemia may ensue, especially if renal dysfunction is present, a scenario that is common in the elderly. In the CHARM trial, hyperkalemia occurred in 2.7 %, and creatinine increased 3.7 % above placebo. It is preferable to add an aldosterone antagonist to an ACE inhibitor rather than adding an ARB. Caution is needed in HF patients treated with aldosterone antagonists because these agents may cause hyperkalemia, and the addition of an ARB would cause severe hyperkalemia. The strategy of complete RAAS blockade with the combination of ACE inhibitor and ARB remains controversial, particularly when the combination of an ACE inhibitor and an aldosterone antagonist has proved successful in RCTs [spironolactone in RALES (Pitt et al. 1999) and eplerenone in EPHESUS (Pitt et al. 2003)].

REFERENCES

ALLHAT Officers and Coordinators for the ALLHAT Collaborative Research Group. Major outcomes in high-risk hypertensive patients randomized to angiotensin-converting enzyme inhibitor or calcium channel blocker vs. diuretic: the antihypertensive and lipid-lowering treatment to prevent heart attack trial (ALLHAT). JAMA. 2002;288: 2981–97.

Casas JP, Chau W, Loukogeorgakis S, et al. Effect of inhibitors of the renin-angiotensin system and other antihypertensive drugs on renal outcomes: systematic review and meta-analysis. Lancet. 2005;366: 2026–33.

CHARM-Added trial, Swedberg K, Granger CB, McMurray JJV, et al. Effects of candesartan in patients with chronic heart failure and reduced left-ventricular systolic function taking angiotensin-converting-enzyme inhibitors. Lancet. 2003;362:767–71.

CHARM-Alternative, Granger CB, McMurray JJV, Yusuf S, et al. Effects of candesartan in patients with chronic heart failure and reduced left ventricular systolic function and intolerant to ACE inhibitors: the CHARM-alternative trial. Lancet. 2003;362(9386):772–6.

DREAM Trial Investigators. Effect of ramipril on the incidence of diabetes. N Engl J Med. 2006;355:1551–62.

LIFE, Dahlöf B, Devereux RB, Kjeldsen SE, for the LIFE Study Group, et al. Cardiovascular morbidity and mortality in the Losartan Intervention for Endpoint Reduction in Hypertension study: a randomised trial against atenolol. Lancet. 2002;359:995–1003.

Lindholm LH, Ibsen H, Borch-Johnsen K, et al. Risk of new-onset diabetes in the Losartan Intervention for Endpoint Reduction in Hypertension study. J Hypertens. 2002;20:1879–86.

Nathan DM. Navigating the choices for diabetes prevention. NEJM. 2010;362:1533–5.

NAVIGATOR Study Group. Effect of nateglinide on the incidence of diabetes and cardiovascular events. N Engl J Med. 2010a;362:1463–76.

NAVIGATOR Study Group. Effect of valsartan on the incidence of diabetes and cardiovascular events. N Engl J Med. 2010b;362:1477–90.

Pfeffer MA, McMurray JJV, Velazquez EJ, et al. Valsartan, captopril, or both in myocardial infarction complicated by heart failure, left ventricular dysfunction, or both. N Engl J Med. 2003;349:1893–906.

Pitt B, Remme W, Zannad F, for the Eplerenone Post-Acute Myocardial Infarction Heart Failure Efficacy and Survival Study Investigators, et al. Eplerenone, a selective aldosterone blocker, in patients with left ventricular dysfunction after myocardial infarction. N Engl J Med. 2003;348:1309–21.

Pitt B, Zannad F, Remme WJ, for the Randomized Evaluation Study Investigators, et al. The effect of spironolactone on morbidity and mortality in patients with severe heart failure. N Engl J Med. 1999; 341:709.

PRoFESS, Yusuf S, Diener H-C, Sacco RL, et al. Telmisartan to prevent recurrent stroke and cardiovascular events. N Eng J Med. 2008; 359(12):1225–37.

Sipahi I, Debanne SM, Rowland DY, Simon DI, Fang JC. Angiotensin-receptor blockade and risk of cancer: meta-analysis of randomised controlled trials. Lancet Oncol 2010;11:627–636.

TRANSCEND, Yusuf S, Teo K, Anderson C, et al. Effects of the angiotensin-receptor blocker telmisartan on cardiovascular events in high-risk patients intolerant to angiotensin converting enzyme inhibitors: a randomised controlled trial. Lancet. 2008;372:1174–83.

Val-HeFT, Cohn JN, Tognoni G, for the Valsartan Heart Failure Trial Investigators. A randomized trial of the angiotensin-receptor blocker valsartan in chronic heart failure. N Engl J Med. 2001;345:1667–675.

VALIANT, Pfeffer MA, McMurray JJ, Velazquez EJ, et al. Valsartan, captopril, or both in myocardial infarction complicated by heart failure, left ventricular dysfunction, or both. N Engl J Med. 2003;349: 1893–906.

VALUE Trial Group, Julius S, Kjeldsen SE, Weber M, et al. Outcomes in hypertensive patients at high cardiovascular risk treated with regimes based on valsartan or amlodipine. Lancet. 2004;363:2002–31.

5 Calcium Antagonists (Calcium Channel Blockers)

There are important, subtle differences among the available calcium antagonists that may affect the choice in treating individual patients. First generation dihydropyridines are short-acting agents that include felodipine, isradipine, nifedipine, and nitrendipine. These rapid-acting vasodilators are powerful antihypertensive agents, but their fast onset of action results in marked vasodilation that causes reflex stimulation of the sympathetic nervous system and hemodynamic adverse effects that include increased heart rate, increased cardiac workload, and an increased incidence of heart failure in patients with left ventricular dysfunction. The short-acting formulations of dihydropyridines, verapamil, and diltiazem are no longer recommended.

- Calcium antagonists are the most effective blood pressure-lowering agents currently available and have been proved in randomized clinical trials (RCTs) to decrease cardiovascular disease (CVD) outcomes in patients with hypertension but carry a significant risk for heart failure (HF) in the elderly. Available calcium channel blockers include: **amlodipine, diltiazem, felodipine, isradipine lacidipine, lercanidipine hydrochloride, nicardipine hydrochloride nifedipine, nimodipine, and verapamil hydrochloride.**

© Springer Science+Business Media New York 2015
M. Gabriel Khan, *Cardiac Drug Therapy*, Contemporary Cardiology,
DOI 10.1007/978-1-61779-962-4_5

- **It is important to know when to choose a calcium antagonist for the individual patient** and which one to choose.

Recommendations are given after discussion of the mechanism of action.

MECHANISM OF ACTION

Calcium antagonists influence the myocardial cells, the cells within the specialized conducting system of the heart, and the cells of vascular smooth muscle. Calcium antagonists act at the plasma membrane to inhibit calcium entry into cells by blocking voltage-dependent calcium channels. They interfere with the inward displacement of calcium ions through the slow channels of active cell membranes. Calcium ions play a vital role in the contraction of all types of muscle: cardiac, skeletal, and smooth. **Myoplasmic calcium** depends on calcium entry into the cell. Calcium binds to the regulatory protein troponin, removing the inhibitory action of tropomyosin, and in the presence of adenosine triphosphate allows the interaction between myosin and actin with consequent contraction of the muscle cell. During phase 0 of the cardiac action potential, there is a rapid inward current of sodium through so-called fast channels. During phase 2 (the plateau phase), there is a slow inward current of calcium through channels that are 100 times more selective for calcium than for sodium; these channels have been termed slow calcium channels.

Fleckenstein (1977) showed that **calcium channels** can be selectively blocked by a class of agents he termed calcium antagonists (also called calcium channel blockers, calcium channel antagonists, and calcium entry blockers).

There are at least two types of calcium channels: L and T. L channels are increased in activity by catecholamines. The calcium antagonists available for clinical use are mainly

L channel blockers. A second type of channel, termed the T channel, appears at more negative potentials and seems to play a role in the initial depolarization of the sinoatrial (SA) and atrioventricular (AV) nodal tissue. T channels are also present in vascular smooth muscle cells, Purkinje cells, and neurohormonal secretory cells. Mibefradil was touted as a T channel blocker; it caused bradycardia and has a host of adverse effects and interactions. The drug has been withdrawn from the market.

Calcium movement into the cell is mediated by at least seven mechanisms (Braunwald 1982). The slow channels represent two of these mechanisms. Two or more types of slow channels exist:

1. **Voltage-dependent** calcium channels are blocked by calcium antagonists.
   - **Nifedipine** is one of the most potent calcium antagonists and appears to act by plugging the calcium channels. It causes dilation of coronary arteries and arterioles and considerable peripheral arteriolar dilation. Nifedipine has a small and usually unimportant negative inotropic effect on the heart.
   - **Verapamil and diltiazem** cause distortion of calcium channels and also cause coronary artery dilation: there are additional effects on the SA and AV nodes; in addition, these drugs have a negative inotropic effect. Peripheral vasodilation is relatively milder than that noted after nifedipine administration.
2. **Receptor-operated** calcium channels are blocked by beta-adrenoceptor blockers. Beta-agonists increase calcium influx through such channels, and this effect is blocked by beta-adrenoceptor blocking agents, which cause the failure of a certain proportion of the calcium channels to open. Beta-adrenergic blockers reduce intracellular levels of cyclic adenosine monophosphate; this, in turn, decreases the number of receptor-operated calcium channels available for calcium influx and thus lowers intracellular calcium

Table 5-1
Clinical classification of calcium antagonists

Group	Characteristics
I	L channel blockers: no action on SA or AV nodes: no effect
	Dihydropyridines: amlodipine, felodipine, isradipine, nifedipine, nicardipine, niludipine, nimodipine, nisoldipine, nitrendipine, ryosidine
II	L channel blockers and probably some T channel blockade: additional action on SA and TV nodes: EP effects
	Phenylalkylamines: verapamil
	Benzothiazepines: diltiazem
III	Mainly T-type channel blocker: mibefradil (Posicor, withdrawn)

and actuates a decrease in heart rate and myocardial contractility. In other words, beta-adrenoceptor blockers have a calcium channel blocking property. In fact, verapamil was first investigated because its action resembled that of the beta-adrenoceptor blocking agents.

A clinical classification of calcium antagonists is given in Table 5-1.

The dihydropyridines (DHPs), phenylalkylamines, and benzothiazepines have vastly different actions (Table 5-2). Their indications are necessarily different, as well as several of their important adverse effects and cautions. They are interchangeable only in the management of coronary artery spasm. For use in other clinical situations (in angina, in hypertension, or in the elderly), care is necessary in their selection. Only amlodipine and felodipine have proved safe in patients with mild left ventricular (LV) dysfunction. (*See* Table 5-2 for a comparison of cardiac effects and peripheral dilation.)

Table 5-2
Hemodynamic and electrophysiologic effects
of calcium antagonists

	Nifedipine[a]	Diltiazem	Verapamil
Coronary dilation	++	++	+
Peripheral dilation	++++	++	+++
Negative inotropic	+	++	+++
AV conduction ↓	↔	+++	++++
Heart rate	↑↔	↓↔	↓↔
Blood pressure ↓	++++	++	+++
Sinus node depression	↔	++	++
Cardiac output ↑	++	↔	↔

+ minimal effect, ++++ maximal effect, ↔ no significant change, ↓ decrease, ↑ increase

[a]Or other dihydropyridines

The DHPs are discussed first because they were used in clinical practice much before the benzothiazepine diltiazem.

Drug name:	**Nifedipine**
Trade names:	Procarida XL, Adalat CC; Adalat XL (C), Adalat LA (UK)
Supplied:	Procardia XL 30, 60, 90 mg; Adalat XL 30, 60, 90 mg; Adalat LA 30, 60 mg
Dosage:	Extended release, 30 mg once daily; average maintenance dose 60 mg; max. 90 mg (rarely advisable); short-acting formulations not recommended; *see* text; avoid grapefruit juice

Action

Nifedipine is a DHP calcium antagonist. Nifedipine and most DHPs are primarily **powerful vasodilators** and are effective in all grades of hypertension at all ages. They possess negligible negative inotropic and electrophysiologic effects. In clinical practice, there is virtually no adverse effect on the sinus or AV nodes. The absence of significant electrophysiologic effect renders DHPs ineffective as antiarrhythmic agents.

- *Caution: Their minimal negative inotropic effect may precipitate pulmonary edema in patients with poor LV function.*

Adverse Effects and Interactions for DHPs

Contraindications include the following:

- Patients with **heart failure** or those with poor LV function, ejection fraction (EF) < 30 %, should not be given nifedipine or other calcium antagonists.
- **Significant aortic stenosis:** In severe aortic stenosis, impedance to LV ejection is fixed, and nifedipine, like other arteriolar vasodilators, will not reduce LV afterload. In such patients, the mild negative inotropic effect of nifedipine or DHPs may precipitate pulmonary edema, if the LV end-diastolic pressure is already increased. Nifedipine and DHPs should be avoided in the presence of a fixed obstruction to LV ejection. Other vasodilators are of limited value in this situation, and indeed any of these agents may be harmful when there is dynamic obstruction, as in aortic stenosis or in some patients with hypertrophic cardiomyopathy with severe obstructive features.
- **Bradycardia:** Patients with sick sinus syndrome and second- or third-degree AV block represent relative contraindications. It is preferable to pace such patients before using a DHP, although studies indicate that nifedipine has no electrophysiologic effects, causing no depression of SA or AV node function at conventional doses, 30–60 mg/day (Krikler et al. 1982). It is relatively safe to combine a DHP with beta-blockers, whereas it is necessary to select patients and to be careful when verapamil or diltiazem is added to a beta-blocker because of the tendency for the verapamil and diltiazem to exacerbate bradycardia or HF.

The **side effects** of nifedipine and verapamil are given in Table 5-3. Further clinical trials from 1984 to 1999 indicate that about 20 % of patients complain of side effects from nifedipine or DHP therapy, and in about 10 %, the agent has to be discontinued. Adverse effects are much less common with extended-release formulations such as Procardia XL, Adalat XL, or Adalat LA. **Rapid-release nifedipine capsules are no longer recommended.** *Flatulence and heartburn may be increased by all calcium antagonists because they cause relaxation of the lower esophageal sphincter.* A rebound increase in angina sometimes, but rarely, occurs on sudden discontinuation of nifedipine or other calcium antagonists, especially in patients with coronary artery spasm (Lette et al. 1984). Slow withdrawal with the addition of nitrates is advisable. A similar withdrawal phenomenon has been noted with nisoldipine in patients with stable angina.

Nifedipine, by increasing ventilation–perfusion imbalance, slightly reduces altered oxygen tension at rest and

Table 5-3
Side effects of dihydropyridines (DHPs) and verapamil

Side effect	DHPs (%)	Verapamil (%)
Dizziness	3	3.6
Edema	15	2
Headaches	5	1.8
Flushing and burning	8	2
Hypotension	0.5	2.9
Constipation	2	1.5
Upper GI upset	1.6	—
Heart failure	0.5	10
Prolonged PR interval	—	3.2
Second-degree AV block	—	0.4
Third-degree AV block	—	0.8
Intraventricular conduction defect	—	1.2
Bradycardia	—	1.1
Need to discontinue the drug because of side effects	4	4

during submaximal exercise in patients with stable angina (Choong et al. 1986). These effects are also observed with diltiazem and verapamil. It may be prudent to administer calcium antagonists with care in patients with compromised respiratory function. Although oral nifedipine significantly reduces airway reactivity in patients with asthma, it also lowers arterial oxygen tension because of a worsening ventilation–perfusion relationship (Ballester et al. 1986). Other very rare side effects of nifedipine and other calcium antagonists include shakiness, jitteriness, depression, psychosis, transient blindness at the peak of plasma level, arthritis, and muscle cramps.

* *Gingival hyperplasia occurred in 38 % of patients receiving nifedipine compared with 4 % for controls* (Steele et al. 1994).

Verapamil has a lower incidence of minor side effects, but it has the potential to produce more serious side effects including a high incidence of constipation, which is particularly bothersome in the elderly. Peripheral edema may occur during nifedipine or DHP therapy in the absence of HF. Edema is believed to result from an increase in capillary permeability. In patients developing bilateral leg edema, symptoms and signs of HF should be sought. All calcium antagonists can produce severe **hypotension.**

Interactions include:

* An interaction has been noted with **prazosin,** and hypotension can be precipitated.
* **Cimetidine and ranitidine** interfere with hepatic metabolism.
* **Phenytoin** blood levels have been noted to increase (see Chap. 21).

Drug name:	**Verapamil**
Trade names:	Isoptin SR, Securon SR, Cordilox (UK), Univer, Covera-HS-, Chronovera (C)

Supplied:	120, 180, 240 mg; *180, 240 mg
Dosage:	120–240 mg once daily; avoid grapefruit juice

Verapamil structurally is a phenylalkylamine calcium antagonist and is a derivative of papaverine.

Action

Verapamil is a moderately potent vasodilator. Peripheral vasodilation is much less conspicuous than that seen with nifedipine. Verapamil has a marked negative inotropic effect. The electrophysiologic effects are mild depression of the sinus node function and of conduction through the AV node.

Adverse Effects and Interactions

The side effects are illustrated in Table 5-3 and are compared with those of DHPs.

Contraindications include the following:

- **Bradycardia and sinus and AV node disease:** The drug is contraindicated in patients with bradycardia or AV block. Patients with sick sinus syndrome are often very sensitive to verapamil: sinus arrest and asystole unresponsive to atropine have been reported.
- **Heart failure:** The drug is contraindicated in patients with cardiomegaly or LV function, EF<40 %.
- **Acute myocardial infarction:** The drug should not be used in this condition. Earlier studies had suggested that verapamil could have salutary effects on jeopardized myocardium after coronary occlusion. It is now fairly clear that verapamil and other calcium antagonists do not salvage myocardium when they are given after arterial occlusion has occurred. *Patients with unstable angina, threatened infarction, or acute infarct appear to have an increased risk of death* (Scheidt et al. 1982). No routine role for verapamil in the management of patients with infarction is advised.
- **Hypotension:** Precautions similar to those for DHPs should be taken.

- The drug is contraindicated in patients with **Wolff–Parkinson–White (WPW) syndrome** associated with atrial fibrillation or flutter because ventricular fibrillation can be precipitated (Gulamhusein et al. 1983). Patients with WPW syndrome and AV nodal reentrant tachycardia may develop atrial fibrillation, so verapamil is best regarded as contraindicated in patients with WPW syndrome (*see* Chap. 14). The dose should be reduced in patients with liver dysfunction and in those treated with cimetidine.

Adverse effects include:

- Constipation may be distressing, especially in the elderly.
- Galactorrhea and minor degrees of hepatotoxicity may rarely occur.
- Rare occurrences include hepatotoxicity resulting from a hypersensitivity reaction.
- Respiratory arrest has been reported in a patient with muscular dystrophy (Zalman et al. 1983).

Interactions include the following:

- **Beta-blockers:** Oral administration of verapamil combined with beta-blockers should be used with caution and only in selected patients because the negative inotropic effect of both drugs may precipitate HF. Verapamil should not be given as an intravenous (IV) bolus to patients receiving beta-blockers. It is preferable to give an oral preparation that takes about 2 h to act, especially if the reduction of ventricular rate is not urgent. Interaction of verapamil and timolol eyedrops producing severe bradycardia may occur.
- **Digoxin:** Verapamil should never be given to a digitalized patient when digitalis toxicity is suspected. Serum digoxin levels may be increased 50–70 % by verapamil. Verapamil also reduces both the renal and nonrenal elimination of digoxin.
- **Amiodarone:** There have been reports of serious interactions between verapamil and amiodaone, which may also depress the SA and AV nodes. Verapamil is usually avoided in patients taking amiodarone.

- **Tranquilizers:** When verapamil is combined with tranquilizers, the patient should be warned about the possible sedative effect.
- **Oral anticoagulants:** There is some evidence that verapamil increases the effect of oral anticoagulants.
- **Disopyramide** and verapamil have added negative inotropic effects that can result in HF.
- **Prazosin** and similar alpha blockers used for prostatic problems and calcium antagonists have added vasodilator effects, and hypotension may be produced.

Drug name:	**Diltiazem**
Trade names:	Cardizem CD, Tiazac, Adizem-XL, <u>Tildiem LA</u> (UK), Viazem XL
Supplied:	Cardizem CD 120, 180, 240, 300 mg Tiazac 120, 180, 240, 300, 360 mg Adizem-XL 180, 240, 300 mg
Dosage:	Extended release 120–300 mg once daily. **Hepatic impairment:** reduce dose. **Renal impairment:** start with smaller dose. **Pregnancy:** avoid. Short-acting formulations not recommended; *see* text

Diltiazem has a structural relationship to benzothiazepine.

Action

Diltiazem causes moderate dilation of arteries. Its dilatory effect is not as powerful as that of nifedipine or other DHPs (*see* Table 5-2). The effect on the SA node is more powerful than that of verapamil, but its action on the AV node is less so. Thus, the drug is not as effective as verapamil in the termination of AV nodal reentrant tachycardia. The modest actions give the drug a balanced profile of action. Diltiazem causes a decrease in the rate pressure product at any given level of exercise. The drug has a mild negative inotropic effect.

Advice, Adverse Effects, and Interactions

The large multicenter study of 1998, including 2,466 patients randomized to diltiazem or placebo, showed no decrease in overall mortality and no significant decrease in reinfarction rates in patients with Q-wave versus non-Q-wave infarction (Multicenter Diltiazem Postinfarction Trial 1989). *A significant increase in mortality was observed resulting from diltiazem in patients with pulmonary congestion and LV dysfunction, EF < 40 %.* The increase in mortality persisted through long-term therapy beyond 1 year (*20*). Congestive HF occurred in 39 (12 %) patients receiving placebo and in 61 (21 %) patients given diltiazem.

Contraindications include HF, sick sinus syndrome, second- or third-degree AV block, hypotension, and pregnancy and lactation.

Interactions have been reported, with amiodarone producing sinus arrest and hypotension (Lee et al. 1985). Also, digoxin levels are increased by about 46 % (Kuhlmann 1985). In general, beta-blockers and diltiazem are a relatively safe and effective combination for the management of stable and unstable angina. In rare instances, the addition of diltiazem to a beta-blocker can decrease the pulse rate to low levels, and HF is occasionally precipitated. Interactions occur with cimetidine, cyclosporine, and carbamazepine (*see* Chap. 21).

Drug name:	**Amiodipine**
Trade names:	Norvasc, Istin (UK)
Supplied:	5, 10 mg
Dosage:	2.5 mg daily increasing to 5–7.5 mg; max. 10 mg

Amlodipine has a half-life of 35–50 h, and peak blood levels are reached after 6–12 h. Possible increased risk of myopathy when amlodipine given with simvastatin.

Caution: Reduce dosage in the elderly; avoid in LV dysfunction, pregnancy, and lactation.

Contraindications: cardiogenic shock, acute MI , unstable angina, significant aortic stenosis, acute porphyria.

Drug name:	**Isradipine**
Trade names:	DynaCirc, Prescal (UK)
Supplied:	2.5 mg
Dosage:	2.5 mg twice daily; max. 10 mg; avoid grapefruit juice; elderly (or in hepatic or renal impairment): 1.25 mg twice daily, increased if necessary after 3–4 weeks according to response, maintenance dose of 2.5 mg or 5 mg once daily

Indications: hypertension
Cautions: sick sinus syndrome (if pacemaker not fitted); avoid grapefruit juice

Drug name:	**Felodipine**
Trade names:	Plendil, Renedil
Supplied:	2.5, 5, 10 mg
Dosage:	Hypertension: 2.5–5 mg once daily; max. 10 mg; reduce dosage in the elderly: 2.5 mg daily; and in hepatic impairment, avoid grapefruit juice

Drug name:	Lacidipine
Trade name:	Motens [UK]
Dosage:	Initially 2 mg as a single daily dose, preferably in the morning; increased after 3–4 weeks to 4 mg daily, then if necessary to 6 mg daily; avoid grapefruit juice

Indications: hypertension

Drug name:	**Lercanidipine Hydrochloride**
Trade name:	Zanidip
Dosage:	Initially 10 mg once daily; increased, if necessary, after at least 2 weeks to 20 mg daily. Avoid if eGFR less than 30 mL/min/1.73 m^2; avoid grapefruit juice; **combination of lercanidipine with ciclosporin may increase plasma concentration of either drug (or both)— avoid concomitant use**

Indications: mild to moderate hypertension

Drug name:	**Nicardipine**
Trade name:	Cardene
Dosage:	5–30 mg twice or 3 times daily usual range 60–120 mg daily); Avoid grapefruit juice

Nicardipine has actions, effects, and indications similar to those of nifedipine.

Drug name:	**Nimodipine**
Trade name:	Nimotop
Dosage:	0.35 mg/kg four times hourly; by intravenous infusion via central catheter, initially 1 mg/h (up to 500 µg/h if body weight less than 70 kg or if blood pressure unstable), increased after 2 h to 2 mg/h if no severe fall in blood pressure; continue for at least 5 days (max. 14 days); if surgical intervention during treatment, continue for at least 5 days after surgery; max. total duration of nimodipine use 21 days; monitor renal function closely with intravenous administration; *see* text for further advice

Nimodipine is useful in the management of cerebral arterial spasm after subarachnoid hemorrhage (Allen et al. 1983).

Indications: prevention and treatment of ischemic neurological deficits following aneurysmal subarachnoid hemorrhage

Dosage (Further Advice)

For patients over 70 kg, use an IV central line, 1 mg/h initially, increasing after 2 h to 2 mg/h, if hypotension does not occur. Halve the dose in patients weighing less than 70 kg. Use the IV route for 5 days and then give orally 60 mg every 4 h starting within 4 days of subarachnoid hemorrhage and for 21 days.

INDICATIONS FOR CALCIUM ANTAGONISTS

Hypertension

Calcium antagonists , particularly long-acting dihydropyridines are commonly and appropriately administered for the management of hypertension of all grades because they are more powerful antihypertensive agents than beta-blockers , diuretics, or ACE inhibitors. The combination with an ACE inhibitor proved very effective (*see* ACCOMPLISH trial (2008) and Chap. 8).

- In older African-American people, an RCT by Matterson and associates (1993) showed that diltiazem was slightly more effective than hydrochlorothiazide (HCTZ). Thus, in older black patients *with isolated hypertension,* diltiazem or a DHP calcium antagonist is indicated if HCTZ does not achieve goal blood pressure.
- In younger black people, in the study by Matterson and colleagues *(38),* diltiazem was effective in 64 % compared with 47 % for atenolol and 40 % for HCTZ. Thus, diltiazem or amlodipine should be tried if a small dose of a beta-blocking agent fails to control blood pressure. Failure to reach goal blood pressure should prompt the combination of a DHP and a beta-blocker.

- In older white people with isolated systolic hypertension, diltiazem showed a 64 % effectiveness versus 68 % for atenolol.
- **Patients with severe, stage II and III, hypertension require the combination of several agents, and calcium antagonists are appropriate, except in patients with LV dysfunction.**

In this RCT, the ACCOMPLISH trial investigators assigned 11,506 patients with hypertension who were at high risk for cardiovascular events to receive treatment with either benazepril plus amlodipine or benazepril plus hydrochlorothiazide. The primary end point was the composite of death from cardiovascular causes, nonfatal MI, nonfatal stroke, hospitalization for angina, and coronary revascularization (ACCOMPLISH Trial Investigators, Jamerson et al. 2008).

- **After a mean follow-up of 36 months, the trail was halted. There were 552 primary-outcome events in the benazepril–amlodipine group (9.6 %) and 679 in the benazepril–hydrochlorothiazide group (11.8 %), representing an absolute risk reduction with benazepril–amlodipine therapy of 2.2 % and a relative risk reduction of 19.6 % (hazard ratio, 0.80, 95 % confidence interval [CI], 0.72–0.90; $p < 0.001$).**
- **For the secondary end point of death from cardiovascular causes, nonfatal MI, and nonfatal stroke, the hazard ratio was 0.79; $p = 0.002$). The benazepril–amlodipine combination was superior to the benazepril–hydrochlorothiazide combination in reducing cardiovascular events (ACCOMPLISH Trial Investigators 2008).**
- In the presence of renal disease or renal failure with or without proteinuria (nondiabetic), if ACE inhibitors are contraindicated or poorly effective, DHPs have a role.

Stable Angina

These drugs are considered second-line agents in

- The management of angina added to a beta-blocker or a nitrate.

- Silent ischemia: combined with a beta-blocker, they decrease the occurrence of silent ischemia.
- Prinzmetal's variant angina (coronary artery spasm). These agents are useful and are first-line drugs in the management of this category of patients; they may be used in combination with nitrates. This condition is rare, however. Because of the widespread discussion of coronary artery spasm in the 1980s, calcium antagonists became commonly used agents in patients with stable angina. Coronary artery spasm is no longer considered to play an important role in stable or unstable angina; thus, the role of these agents has been downgraded but when coronary artery spasm is present (Prinzmetal angina), calcium antagonists are first-line treatment.
- **Caution: DHPs are contraindicated in unstable angina.** Diltiazem is also contraindicated, but diltiazem may be tried if a beta-blocker is contraindicated. These agents are not recommended for acute MI. Diltiazem was thought to be useful following non-Q-wave MI. In a clinical trial, diltiazem decreased early reinfarction rates, but the incorrect use of a one-tailed probability test brought about statistical doubt. Further studies have not confirmed the usefulness of diltiazem in non-Q-wave MI. In addition, the drug increases the incidence of pulmonary edema in patients with acute MI and LV dysfunction. Verapamil is contraindicated in unstable angina or acute MI.
- Supraventricular tachycardia: Verapamil is well known for its excellent effect on AV nodal reentrant tachycardia.
- Diltiazem IV has a role for emergency ventricular rate control of atrial fibrillation.
- Hypertrophic cardiomyopathy: Verapamil is advisable in selected patients when beta-blockers are contraindicated.
- Pulmonary hypertension: Calcium antagonists have shown a variable response in patients with primary pulmonary hypertension. The beneficial effect of nifepidine and verapamil, however, carries a risk of causing HF.
- Raynaud's phenomenon.

The clinical application of calcium antagonists versus beta-blockers is shown in Table 5-4.

Table 5-4
Clinical applications of calcium antagonists versus beta-blockers

	Heart failure I–III	Hypertensive with nephropathy and proteinuria	Diabetics with hypertension	Diabetics with IHD	Lone systolic hypertension/ elderly	Angina	Unstable angina	Acute MI	Post-MI prevention
Amlodipine	Not FDA approved	Indicated if ACE inhibitor CI	Not advisable	Not advisable	Second-line therapy	Second-line therapy	CI Not FDA approved	Not FDA approved	Not FDA approved
Diltiazem	CI	CI	Not advisable	Not advisable	Second-line therapy	Second-line therapy	CI		
Nifedipine	CI	CI	Not advisable	Not advisable	Second-line therapy		CI	Not FDA approved	
Verapamil	CI	CI	Not advisable	Not advisable	Not advisable	Second-line therapy	CI	Not FDA approved CI	Not FDA approved

Isradipine	CI	CI	Not advisable	Not advisable	First-line therapy approved	Second-line therapy	CI	First-line therapy approved	First-line therapy approved
Beta-blocker	FDA approved[a]	Second-line therapy	Advisable if not prone to hypoglycemia	Advisable if not prone to hypoglycemia	First-line therapy approved	First-line therapy approved	First-line therapy approved	First-line therapy approved	First-line therapy approved

CI contraindicated, *ACE* angiotensin-converting enzyme, *IHD* ischemic heart disease, *MI* myocardial infarction

[a]Carvedilol

REFERENCES

ACCOMPLISH, Jamerson K, Weber MA, Bakris GL, (for the ACCOMPLISH Trial Investigators), et al. Benazepril plus amlodipine or hydrochlorothiazide for hypertension in high-risk patients. N Engl J Med. 2008;359:2417–28.

Allen GS, Ahn HS, Preziosi TJ, et al. Cerebral arterial spasm: a controlled trial of nimodipine in patients with subarachnoid hemorrhage. N Engl J Med. 1983;308:619.

Ballester E, Roca J, Rodriquez-Roisin R, et al. Effect of nifedipine hypoxemia occurring after metacholine challenge in asthma. Thorax. 1986; 41:468.

Braunwald E. Mechanism of action of calcium-channel-blocking agents. N Engl J Med. 1982;307:1618.

Choong CYP, Roubin GS, Shen WF, et al. Effects of nifedipine on arterial oxygenation at rest and during exercise in patients with stable angina. J Am Coll Cardiol. 1986;8:1461.

Fleckenstein A. Specific pharmacology of calcium in myocardium, cardiac pacemakers and vascular smooth muscle. Annu Rev Pharmacol Toxicol. 1977;17:149.

Gulamhusein S, Ko P, Klein GJ. Ventricular fibrillation following verapamil in the Wolff-Parkinson-White syndrome. Am Heart J. 1983; 106:145.

Krikler DM, Harris L, Rowland E. Calcium-channel blockers and beta blockers: advantages and disadvantages of combination therapy in chronic, stable angina pectoris. Am Heart J. 1982;104:702.

Kuhlmann J. Effects of nifedipine and diltiazem on plasma levels and renal excretions of beta-acetyldigoxin. Clin Pharmacol Ther. 1985; 37:150.

Lee TH, Friedman PL, Goldman L, et al. Sinus arrest and hypotension with combined amiodarone-diltiazem therapy. Am Heart J. 1985; 109:163.

Lette J, Gagnon RM, Lemire TG, et al. Rebound of vasospastic angina after cessation of long-term treatment with nifedipine. Can Med Assoc J. 1984;130:1169.

Matterson BJ, Reda DJ, Cushman WC, et al. Single-drug therapy for hypertension in men: a comparison of six hypertensive agents with placebo. N Engl J Med. 1993;328:914.

Multicenter Diltiazem Postinfarction Trial Research Group. The effect of diltiazem on mortality and reinfarction after myocardial infarction. N Engl J Med. 1989;319:385.

PRAISE, Packer M, O'Connor CM, Ghali JK, et al. Effect of amlodipine on morbidity and mortality in severe chronic heart failure: for the prospective randomised amlodipine survival evaluation study group. N Engl J Med. 1996;335:1107.

Scheidt S, Frishman WF, Packer M, et al. Long term effectiveness of verapamil in stable and unstable angina pectoris: one year follow-up of patients treated in placebo-controlled, double-blind randomized clinical trial. Am J Cardiol. 1982;50:1185.

Steele RM, Schuna AA, Schreiber RT. Calcium antagonist-induced gingival hyperplasia. Ann Intern Med. 1994;120:663–4.

Zalman F, Perloff TK, Durant NN, et al. Acute respiratory failure following intravenous verapamil in Duchenne's muscular dystrophy. Am Heart J. 1983;105:510.

6 Calcium Antagonist Controversies

CALCIUM ANTAGONISTS CAUSE AN INCREASED INCIDENCE OF HF AND MI: TRUE OR FALSE?

Calcium antagonists without doubt cause an increased incidence of heart failure (HF) as observed in several well-run randomized controlled trials (RCTs):

- Amlodipine in Antihypertensive and Lipid-Lowering Treatment (ALLHAT 2002): HF 38 % vs. diuretic.
- Nifedipine in Intervention as a Goal in Hypertension Treatment (INSIGHT 2000): HF 46 % vs. diuretic.
- Verapamil in Controlled Onset Verapamil Investigation of Cardiovascular End Points (CONVINCE 2003): HF 30 %.
- Amlodipine in Prospective Randomized Amlodipine Survival Evaluation (PRAISE 1996) caused significant increased pulmonary edema in patients with left ventricular (LV) dysfunction. These patients, however, did have left ventricular dysfunction.
- Diltiazem caused a significant increase in HF in a non-Q-wave infarction study (Multicenter Diltiazem Postinfarction Trial 1989).

  – The short-acting preparations of nifedipine and other dihydropyridines used (1985–1995) have been shown in RCTs to cause an increased incidence of myocardial infarction (MI). These formulations are no longer used.

© Springer Science+Business Media New York 2015
M. Gabriel Khan, *Cardiac Drug Therapy*, Contemporary Cardiology,
DOI 10.1007/978-1-61779-962-4_6

- Although the sustained release formulations have been shown to be much safer than the rapid-acting older preparations, these agents are contraindicated in patients with unstable angina or acute MI. *Verapamil is contraindicated in patients with acute ST elevation MI (STEMI) and non-STEMI.*
- Diltiazem is contraindicated in patients with LV dysfunction, prior heart failure, or EF <40 % but may be used in patients with unstable angina if beta-blockers are contraindicated and systolic function is normal.

NEWER CALCIUM ANTAGONISTS ARE BETTER THAN OLDER AGENTS: TRUE OR FALSE?

Lercanidipine was introduced into the United Kingdom a few years ago. It appeared to have advantages over amlodipine and older dihydropyridines. Because the drug dilates both afferent and efferent arterioles, the high incidence of peripheral edema caused by older calcium antagonists was reportedly reduced more than 50 %. The balanced effect of lercanidipine and manidipine on efferent and afferent arterioles was believed to be important in renoprotection; older calcium antagonists dilate only afferent arterioles.

Lercanidipine is only indicated for hypertension and is contraindicated in patients with LV dysfunction, sick sinus syndrome (if pacemaker not fitted), hepatic impairment, aortic stenosis, unstable angina, uncontrolled HF, within 1 month of MI, and renal impairment. Adverse effects include flushing, peripheral edema, palpitations, tachycardia, headache, dizziness, and asthenia, also gastrointestinal disturbances, hypotension, drowsiness, myalgia, polyuria, and rash.

Conclusion: newer agents are not more effective and do not possess more safety than older agents. Most importantly, the combination of lercanidipine and digoxin is potentially hazardous.

ARE CALCIUM ANTAGONISTS SAFE FOR HYPERTENSIVES WITH CAD?

Calcium antagonists are widely used in patients to treat coronary artery disease (CAD) events, particularly stable angina. Their role in patients with unstable angina is limited, and caution is required for acute MI. Post-MI prophylaxis with verapamil has been advocated by few in the field and remains controversial and is not recommended by the Author.

Their use in hypertensive patients with unsuspected or stable CAD has been widespread for more than two decades because they cause more effective and consistent lowering of blood pressure than angiotensin-converting enzyme (ACE) inhibitors/ARBs, beta-blockers, and diuretics.

Their salutary effects on adverse cardiovascular disease (CVD) outcomes appear similar to the other three classes in patients without CAD, **but caution is needed** in patients with known or suspected CAD. Two large RCTs, again atenolol is the beta-blocker chosen, give few answers.

INVEST

- The large RCT International Verapamil-Trandolapril (INVEST 2003) trial studied 22,576 hypertensive patients with CAD. Subjects were aged 50 years or older randomly assigned to **either CAS (verapamil-sustained release) or NCAS (atenolol).**
- Here is another atenolol trial.
- At 24 months, in the CAS group, 6,391 patients (81.5 %) were taking **verapamil**-sustained release, 4,934 (62.9 %) were taking **trandolapril**, and 3,430 (43.7 %) were taking **hydrochlorothiazide**. In the NCAS group, 6,083 patients (77.5 %) were taking **atenolol**, 4,733 (60.3 %) were taking **hydrochlorothiazide**, and 4,113 (52.4 %) were taking trandolapril. Primary outcomes: first occurrence of death (all cause), nonfatal MI, or nonfatal stroke; others: cardiovascular death, angina, adverse experiences, hospitalizations, and blood pressure control at 24 months.

Results: 2,269 patients had a primary outcome event with **no statistically significant difference between treatment strategies** (9.93 %) in CAS and 10.17 % in NCAS; relative risk (RR), 0.98). **It is impossible to draw conclusions about the contribution of any single agent in this complex, open-label study that used blunderbuss drug combinations. The exception was patients with prior HF: those assigned to the NCAS (atenolol) strategy appeared to have fewer events ($p = 0.03$ for interaction).**

- **Verapamil, as expected, because of its strong negative inotropic action, increased the incidence of HF even when combined with an ACE inhibitor and diuretic. Yet, this drug continues to be prescribed and unfortunately was administered to patients in a large RCT.**
- **Verapamil use should be restricted; it has a small role as an antihypertensive agent and for the management of stable angina in selected patients with proven normal LV function.**

CONVINCE

The principal results of the Controlled Onset Verapamil Investigation of Cardiovascular End Points (CONVINCE 2003) trial were as follows:

Aim: To determine whether initial therapy with **controlled onset extended-release (COER) verapamil** is equivalent to a **physician's choice of atenolol (another atenolol trial) or hydrochlorothiazide** in preventing cardiovascular disease. An RCT of 16,602 hypertensive patients who had one or more additional risk factors for CVD was conducted. After a mean of 3 years of follow-up, the sponsor closed the study before unblinding the results.

Initially, 8,241 participants received 180 mg of COER verapamil, and 8,361 received either 50 mg of atenolol or 12.5 mg of hydrochlorothiazide. Other drugs (e.g., a diuretic, beta-blocker, or ACE inhibitor) could be added in specified sequence if needed. Primary outcomes: first occurrence of stroke, MI, or cardiovascular disease (CVD)-related death.

Results: 364 primary CVD-related events occurred in the COER **verapamil** group versus 365 in the **atenolol** or hydrochlorothiazide group (hazard ratio [HR], 1.02; 95 % CI, 0.88–1.18; $p = 0.77$). Non-stroke hemorrhage was more common with participants in the COER verapamil group ($n = 118$) compared with the atenolol or hydrochlorothiazide group ($n = 79$) (HR, 1.54; 95 % CI, 1.16–2.04; $p = 0.003$).

- **Most importantly, verapamil caused a 30 % increase in HF. More CVD-related events occurred between 6 AM and noon in both the COER verapamil (99/277) and atenolol or hydrochlorothiazide (88/274) groups.**

It must be emphasized that atenolol often has a less than 22-h duration of action, and studies have shown that it fails to quell early morning catecholamine surge, which is suppressed by other beta-blockers including metoprolol, timolol, bisoprolol, and carvedilol (see Chaps. 1 and 2). Because most MIs occur during the hours of 6 AM and 11 AM, caution should be used with administration of poorly cardioprotective verapamil and atenolol.

- **Clinicians and expert trialists should recognize that both verapamil and atenolol are not suitable antihypertensive agents, particularly in patients with CAD; verapamil is potentially harmful in the elderly who are at high risk for HF, and atenolol has only mild cardiovascular-protective effects.**

See **the discussion of atenolol's poor effectiveness in Chaps. 2 and 9, Hypertension Controversies.**

REFERENCES

CONVINCE, Black HR, Elliott WJ, Grandits G, et al. for the CONVINCE Research Group. JAMA. 2003;289:2073–82.

INVEST, Pepine CJ, Handberg EM, Rhonda M, et al. for the INVEST Investigators. A calcium antagonist vs. a non-calcium antagonist hypertension treatment strategy for patients with coronary artery disease. The International Verapamil-Trandolapril Study. A randomized controlled trial. JAMA. 2003;290:2805–16.

Multicenter Diltiazem Postinfarction Trial Research Group. The effect of diltiazem on mortality and reinfarction after myocardial infarction. N Engl J Med. 1989;319:385.

PRAISE STUDY: Packer M, O'Connor CM, Ghali JK, et al. Effect of amlodipine on morbidity and mortality in severe chronic heart failure: for the prospective randomised amlodipine survival evaluation study group. N Engl J Med. 1996;335:1107.

The ALLHAT Officers and Coordinators for the ALLHAT Collaborative Research Group. Major out-comes in high-risk hypertensive patients randomized to angiotensin-converting enzyme inhibitor or calcium channel blocker vs. diuretic: the antihypertensive and lipid-lowering treatment to prevent heart attack trial (ALLHAT). JAMA. 2002;288:2981–97.

7 Diuretics

Diuretics have appropriately maintained a stable place in the management of hypertension and heart failure (HF) because of their proven efficacy and low cost. The aldosterone antagonists spironolactone and its analog eplerenone are diuretics but have added actions that improve myocardial function and are an important part of our armamentarium for the management of patients with HF and hypertension. Loop diuretics are a mainstay for the management of HF; they are powerful agents, however, and serum potassium must not be allowed to fall <3.5 mEq/L (mmol/L). The same caution is needed for thiazide use for the management of hypertension.

Aldosterone antagonists produce salutary effects in selected patients with HF but carry a risk of hyperkalemia that can be avoided by a watchful clinician. Importantly, among inpatients with acute myocardial infarction (MI), the lowest mortality was observed in those with postadmission serum potassium levels between 3.5 and <4.5 mEq/L compared with those who had higher or lower potassium levels. Rates of ventricular fibrillation or cardiac arrest were higher only among patients with potassium levels of less than 3.0 mEq/L and at levels of 5.0 mEq/L or greater (Goyal et al. 2012).

The generic and trade names of available diuretics are listed in Table 7-1.

© Springer Science+Business Media New York 2015
M. Gabriel Khan, *Cardiac Drug Therapy*, Contemporary Cardiology,
DOI 10.1007/978-1-61779-962-4_7

Table 7-1
Generic and trade names of diuretics

Generic name	Trade name	Tablets	Usual maintenance (mg daily)
Group I: thiazides			
Chlorothiazide	Diuril, Saluric	250, 500	500–1,000
Hydrochlorothiazide	Hydrodiuril, Hydrosaluric, Esidrix, Oretic, Direma	25, 50, 100	12.5–25
Bendrofluazide	Aprinox, Berkozide, Centyl, Neo-Naclex	2.5, 5	2.5–5
Bendroflumethiazide	Naturetin	2.5, 5, 10	2.5–10
Benzthiazide	Aquatag, Exna, Hydrex	50	50–100
Cyclothiazide	Anhydron	2	2
Hydroflumethiazide	Diurcardin, Hydrenox, Saluron	50	50
Chlorthalidone	Hygroton	25, 50, 100	25–50
Methyclothiazide	Enduron, Aquatensen, Diutensen-R	2.5, 5	2.5–5
Polythiazide	Renese, Nephril	1, 2, 4	0.5–4
Trichlormethiazide	Naqua, Metahydrin	2, 4	2–4
Cyclopenthiazide	Navidrex, Navidrix	0.5	0.5–1
Metolazone	Zaroxolyn, Metenix	2.5, 5, 10	2.5–5
Quinethazone	Aquamox, Hydromox	50	50–100

Drug	Trade names	Strengths (mg)	Dose (mg)
Indapamide	Lozol, Natrilix, Lozide (C)	2.5	2.5
Group II: loop diuretics			
Furosemide	Lasix, Dryptal	20, 40, 80	40–120
Frusemide (UK)	Frusetic, Frusid	500	50–150
Ethacrynic acid	Edecrin	25, 50	50–150
Bumetanide	Burinex, Bumex	0.5, 1, 5	1–2
Piretanide	Arlix	6 (capsule)	6–12
Torsemide	Demadex	5, 10, 20, 100	5–20
Group III: K⁺-sparing diuretics			
Spironolactone	Aldactone	25, 50 (UK), 100	25–100
Triamterene	Dyrenium, Dytac	50, 100	50–100
Amiloride	Midamor	5	5–10
Eplerenone	Inspra	25	50
Group IV			
Thiazide + K⁺ sparing	Aldactazide, Dyazide, Moduretic, Moduret		
Frusemide + K⁺ sparing	Frumil, Frusene, Lasoride		
Group V			
Acetazolamide	Diamox	250	—

INDICATIONS

Hypertension

- In ALLHAT (2002), 33,357 hypertensive patients of mean age 67 were randomized to receive the diuretic, chlorthalidone, 12.5–25 mg/day ($n=15,255$); amlodipine, 2.5–10 mg/day ($n=9,048$); or lisinopril, 10–40 mg/day ($n=9,054$) with a follow-up of 4.9 years. There was good representation for women (47 %) and blacks (35 %); 36 % were diabetics. The primary outcome combined fatal coronary heart disease (CHD) or nonfatal myocardial infarction (MI) occurred in 2,956 participants, with no difference between treatments:
  - All-cause mortality did not differ between groups. Diuretics proved as effective in controlling blood pressure to goal levels, and outcomes were similar to calcium antagonist or angiotensin-converting enzyme (ACE) inhibitor therapy (ALLHAT 2002).
  - A diuretic is the drug of choice for the initial treatment in individuals of African origin over age 60, because these agents have been shown to be more effective than the three other agents (calcium antagonists, beta-blockers, and ACE inhibitors or angiotensin receptor blockers) available for the management of hypertension. Diuretics are not as effective in the younger individuals of African origin. A diuretic is necessary for the management of hypertension in patients with HF or edema and in patients who have not responded adequately to one of the three commonly used antihypertensive agents.

- **Elderly hypertensives.**
- Diuretics have shown beneficial effects in elderly hypertensive patients beyond age 80.
- In HYVET, a double-blind, randomized, placebo-controlled clinical trial involving 3,845 **patients 80 years of age or older with hypertension**, the effect of stepped-care therapy, beginning with the diuretic indapamide and adding perindopril

as needed, was assessed. Active treatment, as compared with placebo, caused a modest reduction in risk.

– Treatment was associated with a 21 % reduction in the relative risk of death from any cause, a 64 % reduction in the relative risk of heart failure, and a 30 % reduction in the relative risk of stroke (Beckett et al. 2002).

Heart Failure

- Management and relief of symptoms of HF: dyspnea, orthopnea, paroxysmal nocturnal dyspnea, and edema.
- **Spironolactone and eplerenone** have been shown to have an important role in the management of class III and IV HF.
- Edema due to renal dysfunction or ascites due to cirrhosis.

Note: edema of the legs presumed to be caused by HF, edema resulting from obstruction of venous return, and dependent edema caused by lack of muscle pump action are some of the most common reasons for diuretic abuse.

CAUTIONS

- **Cardiac tamponade**: when the jugular venous pressure (JVP) is grossly raised (>7 cm) and the patient is not responding to conventional therapy for HF, before giving diuretics to such patients, consideration should be given to a diagnosis of cardiac tamponade or constrictive pericarditis.
- **Cardiomyopathy**: obstructive and restrictive.
- **Tight mitral stenosis** or aortic stenosis.
- **Ascites** with impending hepatic coma.
- **Edema** with acute renal failure.
- **Pulmonary embolism** with shortness of breath: edema caused by cor pulmonale should not be treated aggressively with diuretics. Correct the hypoxemia, and then try to accomplish a very mild diuresis over several weeks.

Monitor intensive diuretic therapy as follows: if any of the following six-point checklist occurs, discontinue diuretics for 24 h and then recommence at approximately half the dose.

1. Systolic blood pressure is <95 mmHg or orthostatic hypotension is present.
2. More than 2-kg weight loss per day is associated with symptoms (1 kg of water loss = 140–150 mEq (mmol) of Na^+ loss in the presence of normal serum Na^+).
3. Electrolytes:
    (a) Blood urea: >7.0 mmol/L from baseline.
    (b) Serum chloride (Cl^-): <94 mEq (mmol)/L.
    (c) Serum sodium (Na^+): <128 mEq (mmol)/L.
    (d) Serum potassium (K^+): <3.2 mEq (mmol)/L.
    (e) CO_2: >32 mEq (mmol)/L.
    (f) Uric acid: >8 mg/dL (464 mmol/L).
    (g) JVP is <1 cm if previously raised. The Frank–Starling compensatory mechanism is lost if diuresis is too excessive and filling pressures fall below a critical point, thereby causing cardiac output and tissue perfusion to fall.
4. Arrhythmias develop or worsen.
5. The 24-h urinary Na^+ excretion is >150 mEq (mmol).
    For the management of moderate-to-severe HF with bilateral edema and pulmonary crepitations, the goal should be
6. Weight loss, a little more than 1 kg/day for 3 days and then 0.5 kg/day for 7 days, with a minimum of 4 kg to a maximum of 10 kg in 10 days.

Note: a 24-h urinary Na^+ excretion < 20 mEq (mmol) indicates inadequate diuretic therapy; 24-h urinary excretion > 100 mEq (mmol), with no weight loss, requires reduction of Na^+ intake. This estimation is, however, seldom required.

THIAZIDES

The thiazide diuretics are shown in Table 7-1. They inhibit sodium reabsorption at the beginning of the distal convoluted tubule (see Fig. 7-1). Thiazides and related diuretics are ineffective if eGFR is less than 30 mL/min/1.73 m^2 and should be avoided; metolazone, however, remains effective. Metolazone is effective for resistant

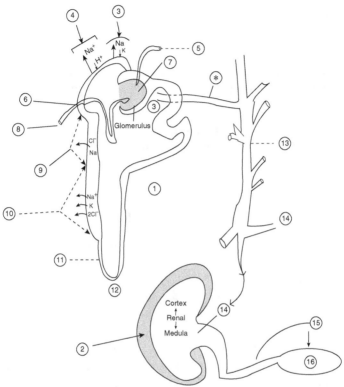

Fig. 7-1. The nephron and the site of action of diuretics. 1, single nephron; 2, the kidney: one million nephrons; 3, distal tubule site of action of aldosterone, spironolactone, and eplerenone; 4, amiloride and triamterene; 5, efferent arteriole; 6, macula densa; 7, glomerular capillaries; 8, afferent arteriole; 9, thiazides; 10, loop diuretics, distal tubule; 11, ascending limb; 12, loop of Henle; 13, collecting tubule; 14, to the renal pelvis; 15, to the ureter; 16, the bladder; *asterisk*, distal tubule: H$_2$O reabsorption under control of vasopressin. Reproduced with permission from Khan MG, *Encyclopedia of Heart Diseases*, 2nd edition. New York: Springer Science + Business Media; 2011, p. 417. With kind permission from Springer Science + Business Media.

edema or heart failure when combined with a loop diuretic, even in renal failure. Profound diuresis can occur, however; thus, the patient should be monitored closely.

- Chlorthalidone appears to have slightly more antihypertensive effects than hydrochlorothiazide (see chapter 8 discussion of resistant hypertension).

Indapamide and xipamide are chemically related to chlorthalidone. Indapamide is claimed to be effective with less metabolic disturbances.

Thiazides are further discussed in Chap. 8.

LOOP DIURETICS

The rapid onset of action of loop diuretics, together with their potency in the presence of normal and abnormal renal function and their venodilator effect, renders them more effective than thiazides for the management of acute and chronic HF and life-threatening pulmonary edema.

Mechanism of Action

Loop diuretics inhibit the $Na^+/K^+/Cl^-$ transport system of the luminal membrane in the thick ascending loop of Henle, and thus they block Cl^- reabsorption at the site where approximately 40 % of filtered Na^+ is normally reabsorbed (Fig. 7-1). Loop diuretics, through their action on $Na^+–Cl^-$ cotransport, inhibit Ca^{2+}, K^+, and Mg^{2+} reabsorption in the loop where some 25 % of filtered K^+, 25 % of Ca^{2+}, and 65 % of Mg^{2+} are normally reabsorbed.

Drug name:	**Furosemide; frusemide**
Trade name:	Lasix
Supplied:	20, 40, 80, 500 mg
Dosage:	20, 40, or 80 mg **after food each morning**; maintenance 20–40 mg daily or every second day; *see* text for further advice

Dosage (Further Advice)

Patients with severe HF may require between 80 and 160 mg furosemide daily, rarely 240 mg daily for a few days, and then a lower maintenance dose. In such patients, it is preferable to give the total dose of furosemide as **one dose each morning**. If a second dose is necessary, this should be given before 2 PM to avoid bothersome nocturia. Hypokalemia is more common with twice-daily dosage. Also, if the patient was formerly resistant to 80 mg, the renal tubule may be resistant to the 80 mg given later in the day. If a dose of furosemide >60 mg/day is predicted to be necessary for several weeks, then it is advisable to add a K^+-sparing diuretic or ACE inhibitor. This will increase diuresis by inhibiting aldosterone and at the same time will conserve K^+.

- **The addition of spironolactone or eplerenone to the HF regimen of beta-blocker, ACE inhibitor, and furosemide has been shown to improve survival**.

Intravenous (IV) Dosage Ampules are available in 10 mg/mL, 20 mg/2 mL, 40 mg/4 mL, and 250 mg/25 mL. The IV dose is given slowly (20 mg/min), and if renal failure is present, it should not exceed 4 mg/min (to prevent ototoxicity).

Action and Pharmacokinetics

Furosemide inhibits Na^+ and Cl^- reabsorption from the ascending limb of the loop of Henle with, in addition, weak effects in the proximal tubule and the cortical diluting segment. The drug is excreted by the proximal tubule. Because of the site and potency of action, loop diuretics are much more effective than thiazides when the glomerular filtration rate (GFR) is markedly reduced. Loop diuretics remain effective even at GFRs as low as 10 mL/min (Maclean and Tudhope 1983). If a diuretic is required in a patient with a serum creatinine level > 2.3 mg/dL (203 μmol/L), it is reasonable to choose furosemide. Furosemide is also used in preference to thiazide as maintenance therapy in patients with moderate-to-severe or recurrent HF, that is, in patients in whom further episodes may be predicted because of the extent of cardiac disease. IV furosemide has a **venodilator** effect, and, when it is given to patients with pulmonary edema, relief may appear in 5–10 min.

Intravenous Indications This route is indicated in emergency, life-threatening situations, such as the following:

- Pulmonary edema or interstitial edema resulting from left ventricular failure
- Severe HF. with poor oral absorption
- Hypertensive crisis
- Hypercalcemia and hyperkalemia

In addition to the mechanism of action of loop diuretics outlined earlier, furosemide causes venodilation. This action involves prostaglandins and can be inhibited by nonsteroidal antiinflammatory drugs (NSAIDs). Furosemide has a half-life of 1.5 h and a duration of action of 4–6 h. Diuresis commences some 15–20 min after IV administration, but relief of shortness of breath may be apparent within 10 min because of an increase in systemic venous capacitance, reduced cardiac preload, and a decrease in left atrial pressure. After oral administration, diuresis peaks in 60–90 min.
   Contraindications:

- Hepatic failure.
- Hypokalemia or electrolyte depletion, hyponatremia, or hypotension.
- Hypersensitivity to furosemide or sulfonamides.
- In women of child-bearing potential, except in life-threatening situations, in which IV furosemide may be

absolutely necessary. Furosemide has caused fetal abnormalities in animal studies.

Warnings:

- Commence with a minimum dose of 20–40 mg, especially in the elderly.
- Monitor electrolytes, blood urea, creatinine, complete blood counts, and uric acid, especially when the dose exceeds 60 mg daily.

Adverse Effects Hypokalemia, dehydration, anemia, leukopenia, thrombocytopenia, rare agranulocytosis, and thrombophlebitis have been noted, but aplastic anemia seems to be more common with thiazides than with furosemide. Hypotension, hyperuricemia and precipitation of gout, and hypocalcemia and precipitation of nonketotic hyperosmolar diabetic coma may occur. Table 7-2 summarizes the metabolic adverse effects.

Table 7-2
Diuretic-induced metabolic adverse effects

- Hypokalemia
- Hyponatremia
- Hypochloremic metabolic alkalosis:
  $Cl^- < 94$ mEq (mmol)/L
  $CO_2 > 32$ mEq (mmol)/L
- Azotemia
- Hyperuricemia
- Hypomagnesemia
- Dyslipidemia
- Glucose intolerance
- Nonketotic hyperosmolar coma
- Hypocalcemia (loop diuretics)
- Hypercalcemia (thiazides)
- Hyperkalemia (K^+-sparing diuretics)

DRUG INTERACTIONS

1. Use carefully in the presence of renal dysfunction when combined with **cephalosporin** or **aminoglycoside antibiotics**, because increased nephrotoxicity has been noted.

2. Care should be taken when loop diuretics or thiazides are given to **lithium-treated** patients. The decreased Na⁺ reabsorption in the proximal tubules causes an increased reabsorption of lithium and may cause **lithium toxicity** (Kerry et al. 1980). Patients receiving concomitant chloral hydrate may experience hot flushes, sweating, and tachycardia. Prostaglandin inhibitors indomethacin and other NSAIDs antagonize the actions of loop diuretics as well as thiazides (Yeung Laiwah and Mactier 1981).

3. The effects of tubocurarine may be increased.

Drug name:	**Bumetanide**
Trade names:	Burinex, Bumex
Supplied:	Tablets: 0.5, 1, and 5 mg Ampules: 2, 4, 10 mL; 500 mg/mL
Dosage:	Oral: 0.5–1 mg daily, increased if required to 2–4 mg; 5 mg in oliguria IV: 1–3 mg over 1–2 min, repeated after 20 min

Bumetanide is as effective as furosemide, and it has a similar site of action in the medullary diluting segment (Puschett 1981). The drug is excreted along with its metabolites in the urine and is believed to cause less Mg^{2+} loss than furosemide during long-term administration. Bumetanide and furosemide have similar pharmacokinetic characteristics. Bumetanide is more potent than furosemide: 1 mg bumetanide = 40 mg furosemide. The drug is absorbed more rapidly in patients with HF and has a bioavailability twice that of furosemide. Bumetanide is more nephrotoxic but appears to be less ototoxic than furosemide, so it is prudent not to use the drug with aminoglycosides or other potentially nephrotoxic drugs. Indications are as listed for furosemide. The drug is not approved in the United States for hypertension.

Drug name:	**Torsemide; torasemide (UK)**
Trade names:	Demadex, Torem (UK)
Supplied:	Tablets: 5, 10, 20, 100 mg Ampules: 50 mg
Dosage:	Oral: 2.5–40 mg once daily; HF dose 20–200 mg IV: 5–50 mg

Torasemide given orally achieves high bioavailability, and a 10-mg dose produces diuresis equivalent to 40 mg furosemide (Sherman et al. 1986).

Dosage: edema, 5 mg once daily, preferably in the morning, increased if required to 20 mg once daily; usual max. 40 mg daily.

Hypertension, 2.5 mg daily, increased if necessary to 5 mg once daily.

POTASSIUM-SPARING DIURETICS

Mechanism of Action Increased renin release from the juxtaglomerular cells is caused by several conditions:

- Reduction in renal blood flow from HF, blood loss, hypotension, or ischemia
- Na^+ diuresis
- Beta-adrenergic stimulation

Renin converts liver angiotensinogen to angiotensin I. Angiotensin II and adrenocorticotropic hormone stimulate adrenal aldosterone production.

The "aldosterone antagonists" are very weak diuretics. Aldosterone handles approximately 2 % of filtered Na^+ at the distal tubule, so only a small diuresis is achieved. Diuretics that block aldosterone or act at the same site distal to the macula densa cause a small amount of Na^+ excretion and prevent exchange of K^+. Only spironolactone and potassium canrenoate antagonize aldosterone. Spironolactone interferes with the effect of aldosterone to increase the rate of Na^+–K^+ exchange at the basolateral surface (Narins 1994). Amiloride and triamterene interact with lumen membrane transporters to prevent urinary Na^+ entry into the cytoplasm (Narins 1994). They are direct inhibitors of K^+ secretion.

K^+-sparing diuretics play a vital role in conserving K^+ and Mg^{2+} in patients treated with thiazides or loop diuretics. The addition of a K^+-sparing drug to low-dose thiazide therapy results in a reduced risk of cardiac arrest (Siscovick 1994).

The available K^+-sparing diuretics are **amiloride** (Midamor), **eplerenone** (Inspra), **spironolactone** (Aldactone), and **triamterene** (Dyrenium, Dytac).

These weak diuretics are very important in the following situations:

1. **Spironolactone** 25 mg added to an ACE inhibitor in patients with HF causes a more complete block of aldosterone production than is achieved with ACE inhibition and reduces mortality and morbidity in these patients. The salutary effects are related not only to Na^+ loss but also to a decrease in cardiac fibrosis, retardation of endothelial dysfunction, and increased nitric oxide production caused by inhibition of aldosterone. Aldosterone, a compensatory "good" hormone, appears to have fibrogenic and other deleterious properties. Tissue collagen turnover and fibrosis appear to be important facets of HF, and spironolactone may attenuate deleterious structural remodeling (Webert 2001).

2. When added to thiazides or loop diuretics, diuresis is greatly augmented. The serum K^+ often remains within the normal range.

3. Clinical situations in which secondary aldosteronism is involved. The "aldosterone antagonists" are first-line diuretics in conditions associated with secondary aldosteronism:
   - Cirrhosis with ascites
   - Nephrotic syndrome
   - **Recurrent HF** (they can be extremely effective and beneficial when added to loop or to thiazide diuretics and ACE inhibitors)
   - Cyclical edema
   - Renovascular hypertension

Spironolactone is also of value in the diagnosis of primary aldosteronism and in treatment of Bartter's syndrome.

The following are suggested **guidelines** for the diuretic management of the patient with marked ascites caused by cirrhosis. Ensure that

- Hepatic encephalopathy is not present.
- The patient can sign his or her name and constructional apraxia is not present.
- The patient can tolerate a 60–80-g protein diet for 1 week without the precipitation of encephalopathy.
- Jaundice is either not present or not increasing.

If these four assessments are passed for more than 7 days, then commence spironolactone 25–100 mg twice daily. Some 2–8 weeks later, if there is no encephalopathy, add 25 mg of hydrochlorothiazide (HCTZ) every second day and then if needed daily or furosemide 40 mg daily. It may be necessary to wait 2–3 months to achieve a 75 % reduction in the ascites.

Contraindications/Warnings The following are contraindications and warnings for the use of K^+-sparing diuretics or combinations with thiazides or furosemide:

1. Acute or chronic renal failure. These drugs should be avoided if there is any evidence of renal failure, in particular a serum creatinine level >1.3 mg/dL (115 µmol/L) in patients aged <70 years, and >1.0 mg/dL (88 µmol/L) for those >70 years, or urea >7 mmol/L. These ground rules should be

broken only if the patient is under strict observation in hospital and an order is written to discontinue the medications if the serum K^+ level is >5 mEq (mmol)/L.

2. Do not use in conjunction with K^+ supplements or ACE inhibitors or in patients who have metabolic acidosis because these diuretics may themselves increase acidosis by retaining H^+ along with K^+.

3. Do not use triamterene combined with indomethacin or other NSAIDs; acute renal failure may be precipitated (Favre et al. 1982; Weinberg et al. 1985). **Triamterene is relatively insoluble and may precipitate as renal calculi** (Ettinger et al. 1980). This agent is contraindicated in patients who have had a renal stone.

Spironolactone is a competitive inhibitor of aldosterone.

Drug name:	**Spironolactone**
Trade names:	Aldactone, Spiroctan (UK)
Dosage:	25–100 mg daily in single or two divided doses

Advantages

- The drug appears to decrease cardiac fibrosis (Weber 1999) and endothelial dysfunction (Farquharson and Struthers 2000) and to increase nitric oxide bioactivity (*see* Chap. 12, Management of Heart Failure). These actions appear to explain the beneficial effects of the drug in patients with HF, as shown in the Randomized Aldactone Evaluation Study (RALES 1999).

- Spironolactone is metabolized in the liver, whereas amiloride is excreted by the kidney, so if renal dysfunction supervenes, the risk of hyperkalemia is less with spironolactone.

- Spironolactone does not cause aplastic anemia or have any other serious hematologic effects. Amiloride and triamterene have been associated with aplastic anemia (although rarely).

- The drug does not cause megaloblastic anemia, seen rarely with triamterene.

Table 7-3
Interactions of spironolactone

- Aspirin antagonizes the diuretic effect of spironolactone
- ACE inhibitors and spironolactone both cause hyperkalemia
- Digoxin levels are increased (laboratory reaction)
- NSAIDs combined with spironolactone may precipitate acute renal failure

- Spironolactone has a positive inotropic effect independent of and additive to that of digitalis. Stroke volume is increased.

Disadvantages

- Gynecomastia. This depends on the dose and its duration. Keep the maintenance dose at less than 50 mg/day. Eplerenone is as effective as spironolactone. Most important, the drug does not cause gynecomastia and will replace spironolactone.
- **Caution**: potential human metabolic products are carcinogenic in rodents and tumorigenic in rats.

Interactions are summarized in Table 7-3.

Drug name:	**Eplerenone**
Trade name:	Inspra
Dosage:	12.5–25 mg once daily, max. 50 mg daily

Indications: left ventricular dysfunction with evidence of HF following MI (start therapy within 3–14 days of event).

Caution: increased risk of hyperkalemia—close monitoring required especially if ACE inhibitor or ARB used concomitantly; avoid if eGFR less than 50 mL/min and in patients over age 75 because renal dysfunction may exist in the face of a normal serum creatinine.

Eplerenone is an important addition to our therapeutic armamentarium for the management of HF, acute MI, and hypertension.

This selective aldosterone blocker has been shown to provide the same clinical benefits as spironolactone, but with a mild decrease in the incidence of two main adverse effects: gynecomastia and hyperkalemia. In the eplerenone post-myocardial infarction and heart failure efficacy and survival study (EPHESUS: Pitt et al. 2003), 6,632 patients 3–14 days post-acute MI with an ejection fraction of less than 40 % with heart failure and diabetes were randomized. Patients with a serum creatinine greater than 2.5 mg/dL (220 µmol/L) or serum potassium greater than 5 mmol/L were excluded. At 1-year follow-up, eplerenone-treated patients had an all-cause mortality of 14.45 % versus 16.7 % for spironolactone-treated patients (one life saved for every 100 patients treated). But eplerenone-treated patients had slightly and significantly higher rates of worsening renal function (creatinine increased 0.06 mg/dL vs. 0.02 mg/dL) and of serious hyperkalemia (5.5 % vs. 3.9 %). Because eplerenone was not shown to be significantly more effective than spironolactone, the drug may not replace the well-known spironolactone, except in men who show early signs of gynecomastia. Eplerenone has been shown to be as effective as losartan in reducing blood pressure in patients with high plasma renin activity and more effective than losartan in patients with low plasma renin activity.

This agent is proven effective in post-MI patients with heart failure or left ventricular (LV) dysfunction. It is estimated that more than 30 % of post-MI patients have LV dysfunction, but on hospital discharge and on follow-up, less than 5 % are prescribed with eplerenone or Aldactone (*see* Chaps. 12 and 22).

Combination of a Thiazide or Furosemide and Potassium-Sparing Diuretic

It is now well established that thiazide diuretics cause significant **K⁺ loss**, which increases the incidence of arrhythmias, cardiac arrest (Siscovick et al. 1994), and cardiac mortality. **Among inpatients with AMI, the lowest mortality was observed in those with postadmission serum potassium levels between 3.5 and <4.5 mEq/L compared with those who had higher or lower potassium levels** (Goyal et al. 2012).

Conservation or replacement of K⁺ is therefore essential and has been proved to decrease the risk of cardiac arrest. K⁺-sparing diuretics are useful and can prevent the use of gastric-irritating potassium chloride (KCl) preparations in most patients if these drugs are used with careful restrictions:

Dyazide: tablets (capsules, USA) of 50 mg triamterene and 25 mg HCTZ. **Triamterene use should be curtailed.**

Dytide: tablets of triamterene 50 and 25 mg benzthiazide. *Dosage*: one tablet each morning or every second day; for mild to moderate hypertension, a dose of one tablet daily for maintenance; **contraindicated** in patients who have had a **renal stone** (Ettinger et al. 1980) or renal failure.

Aldactazide: tablets of 25 mg spironolactone and 25 mg HCTZ.

Aldactide: tablets of 25 mg spironolactone and 25 mg hydroflumethiazide; tablets of 50 mg spironolactone and 50 mg hydroflumethiazide.

Moduretic (Moduret): tablets of 50 mg HCTZ and 5 mg amiloride hydrochloride (the thiazide dosage of 50 mg is excessive).

Moduret 25 or nonproprietary in the United Kingdom, co-amilozide = HCTZ 25 mg, amiloride 2.5 mg; *dosage*: 1 tablet each morning; **not advisable to use more than 1 tablet daily**.

Frumil (Lasoride): tablets of 40 mg frusemide and 5 mg amiloride, given 1–2 tablets daily.

Frusene: tablets of 40 mg frusemide and 50 mg triamterene.

WARNINGS

- K^+-sparing diuretics must not be given concomitantly with K^+ supplements or ACE inhibitors except under strict supervision; severe hyperkalemia may result.
- Elderly diabetic patients may develop hyporeninemic hypoaldosteronism and may therefore retain K^+ despite a normal serum creatinine level.
- If the patient develops gynecomastia during spironolactone therapy, then triamterene or amiloride can replace the spironolactone because these two agents do not cause gynecomastia. They are devoid of the hormonal effects of spironolactone. Triamterene, however, is slightly insoluble and can precipitate as renal calculi.
- K^+-sparing diuretics may rarely produce mild metabolic acidosis.

OTHER DIURETICS

Drug name:	**Metolazone**
Trade names:	Zaroxolyn, Metenix (UK)
Supplied:	2.5, 5, 10 mg
Dosage:	2.5–5 mg once daily; rarely 10 mg

Metolazone has a prolonged action of up to 24 h. The drug acts in both the proximal convoluted tubule and the distal nephron, similar to thiazide. Both thiazides and metolazone have secondary effects in the proximal tubule that are not usually manifested because the proximally rejected ions are ordinarily reabsorbed in the loop. **Thus, combinations of metolazone and loop diuretics are very effective in the management of intractable HF**. Sequential nephron blockade is a proven concept.

Thiazides become ineffective when the GFR falls to <30 mL/min, whereas loop diuretics and metolazone retain effectiveness. **The combination of metolazone and a loop diuretic is very potent** and useful, but K^+ loss is often pronounced.

Drug name	**Acetazolamide**
Trade name	Diamox
Supplied	250 mg
Dosage	250 mg three times daily, max. 4 days; treatment can be repeated once or twice in a month

This drug is a carbonic anhydrase inhibitor. It causes excretion of HCO_3^-, retention of Cl^-, and, consequently, metabolic acidosis and hyperchloremia. Acetazolamide is a very weak diuretic, and the action is lost after 4 days. It is of importance only in the management of hypochloremic metabolic alkalosis in the presence of a normal serum K^+ level (Khan 1980). The typical case is one of refractory HF in a patient taking furosemide and K^+-sparing diuretics. The electrolyte picture shows $Cl^- < 92$ mEq (mmol)/L, $CO_2 > 30$ mEq (mmol)/L, and K^+ 3.5–5 mEq (mmol)/L. In such cases, acetazolamide, added to the spironolactone with the furosemide dose discontinued or halved, results in continued diuresis and correction of the normokalemic hypochloremic metabolic alkalosis.

Acetazolamide is contraindicated in patients with renal failure, renal calculi, metabolic acidosis, and severe cirrhosis.

POTASSIUM CHLORIDE SUPPLEMENTS

To physicians caring for cardiac and hypertensive patients, diuretics are the commonest cause of hypokalemia. The incidence of hypokalemia is about 5–30 % with HCTZ and 5–20 % with loop diuretics, but as high as 50–% with chlorthalidone (Whelton 1986).

Mild hypokalemia of 3–3.5 mEq (mmol)/L is of concern
and must be corrected if the patient is taking digoxin or has
arrhythmias, cardiac disease, or weakness. If metabolic acidosis is present, a serum K^+ level <3.5 mEq (mmol)/L
constitutes a definite total body K^+ deficit. It is a relatively
useless exercise to tell the patient to take an extra glass of
orange juice, as is commonly done (6 oz=8.4 mEq K^+).
Note that salt substitutes, such as Cosalt, Nosalt, and other
brands, also aid in increasing serum K^+ levels. However, salt
substitutes contain KCl and may therefore cause gastric
irritation in some patients.

It is important **not** to give KCl mixtures along with K^+-
sparing diuretics or an ACE inhibitor and then continue with
enriched diets and salt substitutes without knowledge of
renal function, because this occasionally causes hyperkalemia. Patients taking thiazide diuretics should be allowed to
continue for at least 1–2 months and the electrolytes reassessed. Depending on the dose, hypokalemia occurs in
30–50 % of patients. If, however, patients are instructed to
follow a diet containing K^+-rich foods, such as those outlined in Table 7-4, the incidence of hypokalemia can be
reduced. Patients showing even mild hypokalemia should be
given KCl supplements or preferably taken off thiazides and
given a thiazide K^+-sparing diuretic.

As an alternative, patients may be started on Moduretic
(Moduret) if renal function is normal. If the serum K^+ concentration is <2.5 mEq (mmol)/L, IV K^+ is given. In the range of
2.5–3.5 mEq (mmol)/L, oral K^+ is usually sufficient, but it
must always be in the form of Cl^- except in renal tubular acidosis, in which citrates and bicarbonates can be used.

Diuretics cause significant hypokalemia, but only rarely
do they cause a significant fall in total body K^+. Compare
extracellular 65 mEq (mmol) with 4,000 mEq (mmol) intracellular total K^+. Thus, the importance of determining the
serum K^+ level is emphasized, because it is the abnormalities at this level that dictate alterations of the K^+ gradient

Table 7-4
K⁺-enriched foods

Food	Amount	K^+ (mEq)
Orange juice	Half cup	6
Milk (skim powdered)	Half cup	27
Milk (whole powdered)	Half cup	20
Melon (honeydew)	Quarter	13
Banana	One	10
Tomato	One	6
Celery	One	5
Spinach	Half cup	8
Potato (baked)	Half	13
Beans	Half cup	10
Strawberries	Half cup	3
Meats, shellfish, and avocado	All contain increased K^+	K^+

across the myocardial cell membrane and that can result in severe electrical changes and cardiac arrhythmias. Fluctuations of the serum K^+ concentration are often exaggerated by acidosis, causing hyperkalemia, and by alkalosis, causing hypokalemia. It is necessary to watch for the occurrence of the two conditions because they can be altered within minutes (e.g., metabolic acidosis during seizures, diabetic ketoacidosis, cardiac arrest, or respiratory hyperventilation causing respiratory alkalosis and perhaps triggering ventricular tachycardia or ventricular fibrillation). **A low serum K^+ level reduces ventricular fibrillation threshold** and therefore increases the potential for sudden death (Hohnloser et al. 1986):

1. Hypokalemia produced by catecholamines is mediated by beta2-adrenoceptors (Clausen 1983). The increase in catecholamines that occurs during acute MI can cause a significant decrease in serum K^+ concentration. Catecholamine-induced hypokalemia may be prevented by beta2-blockade.

2. The beta2-stimulants salbutamol (including long acting formulations), terbutaline, and pirbuterol may precipitate hypokalemia that is transient but perhaps important.

Potassium Chloride

1. Mixtures: patients dislike the taste of these costly mixtures.
   A dose of 20 mEq (mmol)/L is given twice daily, and it is
   usually adequate, along with a K^+-rich diet. Patients in
   whom the serum K^+ level consistently falls to <3 mEq
   (mmol)/L, despite this regimen, and who are taking necessary doses of diuretics may require as much as 40 mEq KCl
   three times daily. It is preferable in these patients to add a
   K^+-retaining diuretic rather than using KCl.
2. The **effervescent** potassium preparations contain very little
   KCl and are not recommended.
3. KCl **tablets**, **capsules**, or **slow-release wax matrix** are not
   completely satisfactory because there is a significant incidence of ulceration of the gastrointestinal tract, including
   perforations (Farquharson-Roberts et al. 1975). Controlled-
   release preparations, K-Dur 20 (USA) and K-Contin (UK),
   are safer than wax matrix KCl. Nonwax matrix preparations
   include Micro-K and K-Dur 20. The dispersion and slow-
   release characteristics of these preparations are believed to
   minimize contact between erosive K^+ and the mucosal lin-
   ing, but caution is required (Mahon et al. 1982). Diuretic-K^+
   combinations are not recommended.

Salt Substitutes

The patient who has edema, HF, or hypertension must be
on a restricted Na^+ diet. There is a definite case, therefore,
for salt substitutes in which K^+ takes the place of Na^+. There
are many such products on the market—Nosalt, Cosalt,
Morton's salt substitute, and Featherweight-K all have a
reasonable taste. It is important, however, to recognize that
the occasional patient may develop gastric discomfort.
Thiazide and loop diuretics cause K^+ and Mg^{2+} losses. Some
patients with severe K^+ deficiency may require supplemental

Mg^{2+} to achieve correction of the K^+ and Mg^{2+} deficiency. The Mg^{2+} deficiency often continues undetected. Importantly, K^+-sparing diuretics are also Mg^{2+} sparing.

Intravenous Potassium Chloride Care should be taken with IV KCl because death from **iatrogenic hyperkalemia** is not uncommon:

- Use IV KCl only when necessary, that is, when $K^+ < 2.5$ mEq (mmol)/L.
- Ensure an adequate urine output and that renal failure is absent.
- Do not give along with K^+-sparing diuretics, captopril, or enalapril.
- Correct metabolic acidosis or alkalosis.
  1. In the presence of **metabolic alkalosis** with a pH > 7.5 and $CO_2 > 30$ mEq (mmol)/L, smaller amounts of KCL are required.
  2. **Metabolic acidosis**, with a pH < 7.3 and serum K^+ level < 3 mEq (mmol)/L, means a major K^+ deficit and therefore the need for correction over several days.

Dilute KCl as much as possible: 40–60 mEq (mmol)/L. In noncardiac patients, dilute KCl in **normal saline**, especially if severe hypokalemia is present. In life-threatening situations, dilute in saline for all patients.

Dilute in dextrose:

- If aggressive therapy is not required and there is a need to limit Na^+ load, as in the presence of HF or poor cardiac contractility in patients with recurrent or past HF.
- If on the first day of therapy the KCl was diluted in saline.

WARNINGS
- The container must not usually contain >40 mEq (mmol) KCl.
- The rate should not exceed 10 mEq (mmol)/h, except in severe hypokalemia <2.5 mEq (mmol)/L or when symptoms or arrhythmias are present.

- If the rate must exceed 10 mEq (mmol)/h, an electrocardio-graphic monitor is necessary with observations every 15 min. The maximum rate of 30 mEq (mmol)/h is rarely necessary.

FURTHER ADVICE

Torsemide

- The loop diuretic **torsemide** (torasemide, UK) is completely absorbed and appears to have higher reliability and predict-ability compared with furosemide. The variability of absorp-tion is 9 for torsemide and 30 for furosemide.
- Torsemide has been shown in a small study to cause a dra-matic decrease in hospitalization and reduced mortality in patients with class III and IV HF compared with furosemide (Sherman et al. 1986). The simple expedient of the choice of a diuretic can result in a decrease in hospitalization for HF of >33 %.
- **Food further reduces absorption of furosemide, and not many physicians recognize that this well-known drug must be taken on an empty stomach.**

Aldosterone Antagonists

The therapeutic value of aldosterone antagonists used judiciously must not be underestimated in the management of HF of all grades. The drug should not be reserved for class IV HF.

- A therapeutic dose of loop diuretic must reach the kidney site of action. A small dose of a poorly absorbed drug has no effect; a large dose loses effect later and also stimulates the renin–angiotensin aldosterone system that causes Na^+ and water retention, hence the not surprising proven value of **spironolactone** (Aldactone) in the RALES study (1999) in patients with class III and IV HF, in whom this agent is strongly recommended.

- In more than 55 % of patients admitted with CHF, the pre-cipitating factor is Na^+ and water retention. Consequently, we must focus on a better choice of loop diuretic and insist on combination with an aldosterone antagonist in virtually all patients admitted for HF.
- Patients with Class II–III HF can benefit from a smaller main-tenance dose of loop diuretic: 20 mg furosemide (instead of 40–60 mg) plus spironolactone 25–50 mg or eplerenone 25 mg daily, with monitoring of serum potassium.
- Importantly, aldosterone antagonists are administered not only for the enhancement of diuresis but also because of their beneficial actions on cardiac myocytes. Spironolactone blockade of aldosterone actions appears to decrease cardiac fibrosis (Weber 1999) and endothelial dysfunction (Farquharson and Struthers 2000) and to increase nitric oxide bioactivity.
- Aldosterone blockade prevents ventricular remodeling and collagen formation in patients with left ventricular (LV) dysfunction after acute myocardial infarction (MI) (Rodríguez et al. 1997).
- Because ACE inhibitors only partially block aldosterone activity, and aldosterone causes myocardial and other dele-terious effects in patients with HF, the use of aldosterone antagonists or receptor blockers constitutes a major addition to our effective armamentarium. In the RALES study, there was a 30 % reduction in the rate of death **and a similar reduction in sudden deaths and** hospitalizations among class III and IV patients with HF who were treated with spironolactone 25 mg in combination with an ACE inhibitor loop diuretic, compared with patients who received placebo. Baseline serum creatinine was <2.5 mg/dL (221 μmol/L); severe hyperkalemia occurred in 2 % of patients. Importantly, 75 % of patients received digoxin.
- Only 11 % received a beta-blocker.
- *See* cautions given earlier for use in patients with GFR<50 mL/min.
- The derivative compound of spironolactone, eplerenone (Inspra), does not cause gynecomastia and impotence. In the

Eplerenone Post-Acute Myocardial Infarction Heart Failure Efficacy and Survival Study (EPHESUS 2003), the drug reduced adverse outcomes in patients with acute MI and LV dysfunction. This agent binds more specifically to the aldosterone receptor and does not bind as avidly to the androgen receptor. It blocks the mineralocorticoid receptor and not glucocorticoid, progesterone, or androgen receptors (de Gasparo et al. 1987).

- In EPHESUS (2003), patients 3–14 days post-acute MI were randomly assigned to eplerenone (25 mg daily titrated to a maximum of 50 mg (3,313 patients) or placebo (3,319 patients) in addition to optimal medical therapy.
- The primary end points were death from any cause and death from cardiovascular causes or hospitalization for HF acute MI. At 16-month follow-up, there were 478 deaths in the eplerenone group and 554 deaths in the placebo group (relative risk [RR], 0.85; 95 % confidence interval [CI], 0.75–0.96; $p = 0.008$).
- Cardiovascular deaths were 407 in the eplerenone group and 483 in the placebo group (RR, 0.83; 95 % CI, 0.72–0.94; $p = 0.005$).
- The cardiovascular mortality reduction observed was caused mainly by a 21 % reduction in the rate of sudden death from cardiac causes. A significant reduction in the rate of hospitalization for cardiovascular events was caused by a 15 % reduction in the risk of hospitalization for HF and a 23 % reduction in the number of episodes of hospitalization for HF.
- The risk of serious hyperkalemia was significantly increased in patients with significant renal dysfunction: creatinine clearance at baseline < 50 mL/min.
- Eplerenone reduces coronary vascular inflammation and the risk of subsequent development of interstitial fibrosis in animal models of myocardial disease (Rocha et al. 2002; Sun et al. 2002). Eplerenone also reduces oxidative stress, improves endothelial dysfunction (Struthers and MacDonald 2004; Rajagopalan et al. 2002), attenuates platelet aggregation, decreases activation of matrix metalloproteinases, and improves ventricular remodeling (Suzuki et al. 2002). In addition, aldo-

sterone blockade decreases sympathetic drive in rats through direct actions in the brain (Zhang et al. 2002) and improves norepinephrine uptake in patients with HF (Barr et al. 1995).

Francis and Tang (2005) emphasized the following:

- In animal studies, excessive aldosterone has been associated with collagen deposition, myocardial fibrosis, and myocardial remodeling (Struthers and MacDonald 2004).
- Blocking the synthesis or function of aldosterone has also been demonstrated to improve diastolic dysfunction in hypertensive patients with diastolic heart failure (Mottram et al. 2004).
- In EPHESUS, eplerenone was beneficial in patients who were receiving optimal therapy including an ACE inhibitor or an ARB, a beta-blocker, aspirin, a lipid-lowering agent, and coronary reperfusion therapy.
- Rassi et al. emphasized that The American College of Cardiology/American Heart Association ST-segment myocardial infarction (STEMI) guidelines published after the EPHESUS trial gave the use of aldosterone inhibitors in post-STEMI patients with a decreased EF and either symptomatic heart failure or diabetes without contraindications (renal dysfunction, hyperkalemia) a Class I recommendation. Non-STEMI guidelines are similar.
- From a data-based study, Rassi et al. indicated that among eligible post-MI patients, only 9.1 % were prescribed an aldosterone antagonist at discharge. These investigators concluded that although rates of aldosterone antagonist use are increasing slightly over time, the vast majority of acute MI patients eligible for treatment fail to receive it at hospital discharge. "The reason for this discrepancy between guideline-based therapy and actual prescribing patterns is unclear and should be further studied" (Rassi et al. 2013).

REFERENCES

ALLHAT Officers and Coordinators for the ALLHAT Collaborative Research Group. Major outcomes in high-risk hypertensive patients randomized to angiotensin-converting enzyme inhibitor or calcium channel blocker vs. diuretic: the antihypertensive and lipid-lowering treatment to prevent heart attack trial (ALLHAT). JAMA. 2002;288:2981–97.

Barr CS, Lang CC, Hanson J, Arnott M, Kennedy N, Struthers AD. Effects of adding spironolactone to an angiotensin-converting enzyme inhibitor in chronic congestive heart failure secondary to coronary artery disease. Am J Cardiol. 1995;76:1259–65.

Clausen T. Adrenergic control of Na+-K+-homoeostasis. Acta Med Scand Suppl. 1983;672:111.

de Gasparo M, Joss U, Ramjoue HP, et al. Three new epoxy-spirolactone derivatives: characterization in vivo and in vitro. J Pharmacol Exp Ther. 1987;240:650–6.

EPHESUS, Pitt B, Remme W, Zannad F, for the Eplerenone Post-Acute Myocardial Infarction Heart Failure Efficacy and Survival Study Investigators, et al. Eplerenone, a selective aldosterone blocker, in patients with left ventricular dysfunction after myocardial infarction. N Engl J Med. 2003;348:1309–21.

Ettinger B, Oldroyd NO, Sorgel F. Triamterene nephrolithiasis. JAMA. 1980;244:2443.

Farquharson CAJ, Struthers AD. Spironolactone increases nitric oxide bioactivity, improves endothelial vasodilator dysfunction, and suppresses vascular angiotensin I/angiotensin II conversion in patients with chronic heart failure. Circulation. 2000;101:594.

Farquharson-Roberts MA, Giddings AEB, Nunn AJ. Perforation of small bowel due to slow release potassium chloride (Slow-K). BMJ. 1975;3:206.

Favre L, Glasson P, Vallotton MB. Reversible acute renal failure from combined triamterene and indomethacin: a study in healthy subjects. Ann Intern Med. 1982;96:317.

Francis GS, Tang WHW. Should we consider aldosterone as the primary screening target for preventing cardiovascular events? J Am Coll Cardiol. 2005;45:1249–50.

Goyal A, Spertus JA, Gosch K, et al. Serum potassium levels and mortality in acute myocardial infarction. JAMA. 2012;307(2):157–64.

Hohnloser SH, Verrier RL, Lown B, et al. Effect of hypokalemia on susceptibility to ventricular fibrillation in the human and ischemic canine heart. Am Heart J. 1986;112:32.

HYVET: Beckett NS, Peters R, Fletcher AE, et al. for the HYVET Study Group. Treatment of hypertension in patients 80 years of age or older. N Engl J Med. 2008;358:1887–98.

Kerry RJ, Ludlow JM, Owen G. Diuretics are dangerous with lithium. BMJ. 1980;281:371.

Khan MG. Treatment of refractory congestive heart failure and normokalemic hypochloremic alkalosis with acetazolamide and spironolactone. Can Med Assoc J. 1980;123:883.

Maclean D, Tudhope GR. Modern diuretic treatment. BMJ. 1983;286:1419.

Mahon FG, Ryan JR, Akdamar K, et al. Upper gastrointestinal lesions after potassium chloride supplements: a controlled clinical trial. Lancet. 1982;2:1059.

Mottram PM, Haluska B, Leano R, Cowley D, Stowasser M, Marwick TH. Effect of aldosterone antagonism on myocardial dysfunction in hypertensive patients with diastolic heart failure. Circulation. 2004;110:558–65.

Narins RG, editor. Maxwell & Kleeman's clinical disorders of fluid and electrolyte metabolism. 5th ed. New York: McGraw-Hill; 1994.

Puschett JB. Renal effects of bumetanide. J Clin Pharmacol. 1981;21:575.

Rajagopalan S, Duquaine D, King S, Pitt B, Patel P. Mineralocorticoid receptor antagonism in experimental atherosclerosis. Circulation. 2002;105:2212–6.

RALES, Pitt B, Zannad F, Remme WJ, for the Randomized Aldactone Evaluation Study Investigators, et al. The effect of spironolactone on morbidity in patients with severe heart failure. N Engl J Med. 1999;341:709.

Rassi AN, Cavender MA, Fonarow GC, et al. Temporal trends and predictors in the use of aldosterone antagonists post-acute myocardial infarction. J Am Coll Cardiol. 2013;61(1):35–40.

Rocha R, Rudolph AE, Frierdich GE, et al. Aldosterone induces a vascular inflammatory phenotype in the rat heart. Am J Physiol Heart Circ Physiol. 2002;283:H1802–10.

Rodríguez JA, Godoy I, Castro P, et al. Ramipril vs. espironolactona en el remodelamiento ventricular izquierdo post-infarto: randomizado y dobleciego. Rev Med Chile. 1997;125:643–52.

Sherman LG, Liang C, Baumgardner S, et al. Piretanide, a potent diuretic with potassium-sparing properties, for the treatment of congestive heart failure. Clin Pharmacol Ther. 1986;40:587.

Siscovick DS, Raghunathan TE, Psaty BM, et al. Diuretic therapy for hypertension and the risk of primary cardiac arrest. N Engl J Med. 1994;330:1852.

Struthers AD, MacDonald TM. Review of aldosterone- and angiotensin II-induced target organ damage and prevention. Cardiovasc Res. 2004;61:663–70.

Sun Y, Zhang J, Lu L, Chen SS, et al. Aldosterone-induced inflammation in the rat heart: role of oxidative stress. Am J Pathol. 2002;161:1773–81.

Suzuki G, Morita H, Mishima T, et al. Effects of long-term monotherapy with eplerenone, a novel aldosterone blocker, on progression of left ventricular dysfunction and remodeling in dogs with heart failure. Circulation. 2002;106:2967–72.

Weber KT. Aldosterone and spironolactone in heart failure. N Engl J Med. 1999;341:753.

Webert KT. Aldosterone in congestive heart failure. N Engl J Med. 2001;345:1689.

Weinberg MS, Quigg RJ, Salant DJ, et al. Anuric renal failure precipitated by indomethacin and triamterene. Nephron. 1985;40:216.

Whelton A. An overview of national patterns and preferences in diuretic selection. Am J Cardiol. 1986;57:2A.

Yeung Laiwah AC, Mactier RA. Antagonistic effect of non-steroidal anti-inflammatory drugs on frusemide-induced diuresis in cardiac failure. BMJ. 1981;283:714.

Zhang ZH, Francis J, Weiss RM, Felder RB. The renin-angiotensin-aldosterone system excites hypothalamic paraventricular nucleus neurons in heart failure. Am J Physiol Heart Circ Physiol. 2002;283:H423–33.

8   Hypertension

RELEVANT KEY ISSUES

There are more than one billion individuals with hypertension worldwide; the number is predicted to grow to 1.56 billion by 2025 (Kearney et al. 2005).

Unfortunately there are only four classes of antihypertensive agents available (only four drugs with many reduplications) and the old well-tried agent beta-blockers have been retired by the JNC8 (2014) mainly because of the results of RCTs in which the most ineffective beta-blocker, atenolol, was used. There are > 6 beta-blockers available, but of the 10 or more hypertensive randomized clinical trials (RCTs), atenolol was the choice beta-blocker in >90 % of trials (see Table 9-1). The JNC8 panelist and guideline providers in many countries fail to understand that beta blockers have subtle and important differences (Khan 2005) The author stated in the sixth edition of this book (2003) "the use of atenolol in clinical trials should be curtailed". Diuretics are no longer first line according to the JNC8 because of the notion they cause diabetes and are mildly acting antihypertensive agents. In essence two agents to treat the many. This chapter gives practical guidance to clinicians that should prove helpful in clinical practice. Fortunately, calcium antagonists are very effective anti-hypertensive agents.

© Springer Science+Business Media New York 2015
M. Gabriel Khan, *Cardiac Drug Therapy*, Contemporary Cardiology,
DOI 10.1007/978-1-61779-962-4_8

- More than 60 million Americans, 20 % of the population, have hypertension that requires drug therapy. At age 65–75, more than 40 % of individuals worldwide have hypertension. The prevalence of hypertension in industrialized countries in general is similar to that in the white population of the United States.

- Most important, we only have four groups of drugs: diuretics, beta-blockers, angiotensin-converting enzyme (ACE) inhibitors, [or angiotensin 11 receptor blockers (ARBs)], and calcium antagonists to treat this most common condition that leads to devastating events, particularly cardiovascular death and disability. I have purposely left out centrally acting agents (methyldopa and clonidine) and alpha-blockers because their use is limited to a few selected individuals. Methyldopa is used mainly in pregnancy.

- **It must be emphasized that ACE I/ARBs are excellent, well-tested, but mild antihypertensive agents, and that calcium antagonists are the most powerful of the four antihypertensive agents available** for management of moderate and severe hypertension. We would be lost if these agents were not part of our antihypertensive armamentarium but it is illogical to demote beta-blockers to third or 4th line therapy they can be used as first or second line in many depending on age and ethinicity.

- ACE inhibitors and the identically acting ARBs are a major advance but represent a single class of agent. Importantly some ARBs (telmisartan, olmesartan) have come under scrutiny; see later discussion and Chap. 4.

- Calcium antagonists are the most effective antihypertensive agent available but are not superior to the two older classes of agents, beta-blockers and diuretics, when used as monotherapy to treat mild hypertension **depending on the age and ethnicity of the individual.** Mild hypertension is common and treatment choice can be individualized.

- *Alpha-blockers cause heart failure (HF) and are not recommended agents* because they cause heart failure (ALHAT 2000)

- In clinical practice, patients who cannot tolerate one or two of the four types of agents are frequently encountered, and many patients require three agents to attain adequate control.

- Thus, drug choice is limited. **This situation will change only if pharmaceutical companies and experts who formulate hypertension therapeutic guidelines will admit that after more than 60 years of intensive research and numerous RCTs, only four antihypertensive agents are available.** The recognition of the truth should promote more intensive research to discover new groups of agents or innovative strategies to add to our present armamentarium of four drug classes.

- The organizers of RCTs must provide sound methodology, which has been lacking in many such trials (see the later criticisms of RCTs).

- For example, the beta-blocker atenolol is the main beta-blocker that has been compared with other agents in RCTs done from 1984 to 2005.

- Most important, Trialists and the JNC8 expert panelists (2014) have failed to recognize that **the non-lipid-soluble atenolol is not as cardioprotective <u>as timolol, carvedilol, bisoprolol, propranolol or metoprolol; the only beta-blockers shown in RCTs to be cardioprotective</u>. Beta-blockers have subtle and important differences (Khan 2005, p 150). The use of atenolol in clinical trials should be curtailed (Khan 2003 p 502); this widely prescribed beta-blocker should become obsolete** (Khan 2011 p 556) (*see* Chaps. 1 and 2).

- The author often used atenolol from 1974 to 1984 and has nothing to gain from asking clinicians not to prescribe atenolol (except for selected cases of hypertension in pregnancy).

- It is surprising that the experts who constructed the recent hypertensive guidelines, (JNC8 2014), fail to understand the subtle but important differences that exist between the available beta-blocking agents.

- "The JNC8 panel did not recommend beta-blockers for the treatment of hypertension (first, second, or third line) because in one study use of the beta-blocker atenolol "resulted in a higher rate of the primary composite outcome of cardiovascular death, MI, or stroke compared to use of an ARB a finding that was driven largely by an increase in stroke" (Dahlöf 2002 Life study). In that study (LIFE), 204 losartan and 234 atenolol patients died from cardiovascular disease ($p = 0.206$); a nonsignificant change in cardiovascular death. Myocardial infarction (nonfatal and fatal) occurred in 198 and 188, respectively (1.07, 0.88–1.31, $p = 0.491$), a nonsignificant finding (Dahlöf et al. 2002).

- Yet another misguided recommendation by the JNC8
- In the large Captopril Prevention Project (CAPP 1999) study of captopril versus diuretic and beta-blocker, fatal and **nonfatal stroke was increased in the captopril group ($p = 0.044$)**, with no significant differences in other events. **A result perhaps as spurious as the LIFE study.**
- **In the large well-run PRoFESS RCT, telmisartan failed to decrease recurrent stroke** (Yusuf et al. 2008). **ARBs are not as useful as proclaimed.**
- **(See Chap. 4 controversies)**

Others have stated their surprise at both the JNC8 and UK guidelines. Results from LIFE cannot be extrapolated to the general population; the mean age in THE LIFE STUDY was 66.9 years (Morales-Salinas et al. 2014). Beta-blockers are effective in white patients with age less than and older than 60 years and in older black patients with hypertension.

Dickerson et al. (1999) showed in an excellent study that beta-blocker therapy was equal to that of ACE inhibitor monotherapy in younger white patients.

In the ACCOMPLISH RCT trial, investigators assigned 11,506 patients with hypertension who were at high risk for cardiovascular events to receive treatment with either benazepril plus amlodipine or benazepril plus hydrochlorothiazide. The primary end point was the composite of death from cardiovascular causes, nonfatal MI, nonfatal stroke, hospitalization for angina, and coronary revascularization (ACCOMPLISH Trial Investigators, Jamerson et al. 2008).

- **After a mean follow-up of 36 months, the trail was halted. There were 552 primary-outcome events in the benazepril–amlodipine group (9.6 %) and 679 in the benazepril–hydrochlorothiazide group (11.8 %), representing an absolute risk reduction with benazepril–amlodipine therapy of 2.2 % and a relative risk**

reduction of 19.6 % (hazard ratio, 0.80, 95 % confidence interval [CI], 0.72–0.90; p < 0.001).

For the secondary end point of death from cardiovascular causes, nonfatal MI, and nonfatal stroke, the hazard ratio was 0.79; (p = 0.002). The benazepril–amlodipine combination was superior to the benazepril–hydrochlorothiazide combination in reducing cardiovascular events (ACCOMPLISH Trial Investigators 2008).

There is little doubt that the combination of the calcium antagonist amlodipine and ACE inhibitor is most useful but treatment must still be individualized.

Consider the following:

- Hypertension is the leading cause of cardiovascular disease (CVD) morbidity and mortality.
- The prevalence of left ventricular hypertrophy (LVH) as a function of blood pressure (BP) has been proved. The incidence of myocardial infarction (MI) in Framingham subjects with hypertension shows a stepwise increase in risk as BP rises. In more than 40 % of patients with acute MI, an antecedent history of hypertension is obtained. MI is a critical factor in the development of heart failure (HF).
- Renal failure caused by renal diseases is often nonpreventable, but that caused by hypertension is. The risk of renal failure is increased in patients with diabetes and in patients of African origin. In virtually all patients with renal failure regardless of cause, antihypertensive agents are administered to maintain a goal BP less than 130 mmHg. Often three or four agents are required.

Most physicians are cognizant of the aforementioned statements, but few are aware of the following distressing facts:

- Studies indicate that about 66 % of elderly patients with HF had antecedent hypertension. The bulk of HF is related to hypertension and MI. The message is that effective hypertension control is the single greatest means to prevent diastolic and systolic HF (Fig. 8-1). Heart failure with preserved ejection fraction (HFPEF) has no effective therapy, and

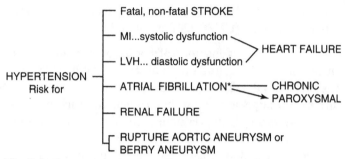

Fig. 8-1. Common detrimental effects of hypertension. *Asterisk*: Not well appreciated: epidemic of atrial fibrillation with its management problems.

prevention is the key (see Chaps. 12 and 13). Interestingly the unique beta-blocker nebivolol in the SENIORS (2009) study has shown salutary effects in patients with HFPEF.

- Hypertension is a common underlying cause of atrial fibrillation, which is the most common sustained arrhythmia encountered in the office and emergency room.

- In North America, <40 % of hypertensive patients have their BP controlled to goal.

This chapter discusses antihypertensive agents and emphasizes

- Which drugs are best for the management of mild hypertension in younger and older white and black patients. BP reductions caused by antihypertensive agents differ in different ethnic groups and in younger and older patients.

- Which drugs are best for patients with major risk factors, target organ damage, and coexisting disease: ischemic heart disease (IHD), diabetes, and hyperlipidemia. These three conditions markedly increase the risk of cardiovascular death. The risk of cardiovascular morbidity and mortality is determined not only by the BP but also by the presence or absence of these coexisting diseases, target organ damage, and risk factors (Table 8-1). Risk stratification is necessary for the formulation of appropriate antihypertensive therapy.

Table 8-1
Major risk factors, target organ damage, and coexisting disease

Major risk factor	Target organ damage	Coexisting disease
Smoking	Heart failure	Diabetes
Age	LV dysfunction	Hyperlipidemia
Men >45 years	LV hypertrophy	IHD
Women > 55 years	Retinopathy	Angina
Family history of IHD or stroke	Renal insufficiency	Silent ischemia
Men <55 years		MI
Women < 65 years		Previous CABG
		LV dysfunction
		Stroke or TIA
		Nephropathy
		Peripheral vascular disease

IHD ischemic heart disease, *LV* left ventricular, *MI* myocardial infarction, *TIA* transient ischemic attack

CONTROVERSIES

ARBs may not be as cardioprotective as shown for ACE inhibitors.

- The widely held notion that ACE inhibitors or ARBs reduce the incidence of diabetes and beta-blockers and diuretics increase the incidence is false. See Chaps. 2, 4, and 9. The results of the Dream trial and the study by Hanley et al. (2010) should provide core knowledge for Trialists who have incorrectly reported an increase incidence of diabetes caused by some drugs and a reduction caused by ACE inhibitors and ARBs.
- **Telmisartan therapy for 56 months, although shown in ONTARGET (2008) to be equivalent to ramipril surprisingly, had no significant effect on the primary outcome, hospitalizations for HF in TRANSCEND** (Yusuf et al.

2008). **In addition, there was no reduction in total mortality**. In the large well-run PRoFESS RCT, telmisartan failed to decrease recurrent stroke (Yusuf et al. 2008).

- **ARBs appear to be associated with a modestly increased risk for cancer, according to a meta-analysis published in the Lancet Oncology** (Sipahi et al. 2010). **Should we be concerned about all ARBs or a single drug, telmisartan?** (Nissen 2010).

The safety of the angiotensin receptor blocker olmesartan is questionable after two ongoing trials among patients with type 2 diabetes suggested increased risk for cardiovascular death with the drug.

DEFINITIONS

It is generally accepted that systolic hypertension is as important as diastolic hypertension.

Isolated Systolic Hypertension in Older Patients

Isolated systolic hypertension is defined as systolic BP > 140 mmHg and diastolic BP < 90 mmHg present in the absence of target organ damage and coexisting disease (*see* Table 8-1). Systolic hypertension in individuals aged over 65 years is a major cause of stroke, left ventricular failure (LVF), and mortality from IHD.

- The prevalence of high BP in African Americans is among the highest in the world, and organ damage occurs earlier in these patients than in whites.
- In approximately 95 % of individuals, hypertension exists without a known cause and is termed primary (essential) hypertension. In the remaining 5 %, hypertension is secondary to known causes (Table 8-2).
- Proper technique for BP measurement is essential for adequate diagnosis and patient care.
- The results of the Hypertension Optimal Treatment (HOT) trial (Hansson et al. 1999) indicate that, in patients with diastolic BP mean 105 mmHg, it is safe to decrease the

Table 8-2
Causes of secondary hypertension

Cause	%
Renal parenchymal disease	3
Renal vascular disease	1
Cushing's syndrome	0.1
Pheochromocytoma	0.1
Primary hyperaldosteronism	0.1
Coarctation of the aorta	0.1
Estrogens	0.4
Alcohol	0.2 or more

diastolic BP to <90 mmHg; further lowering to <85 mmHg did not result in a significant decrease in mortality or event rates but was not harmful. In diabetic patients, a decrease in diastolic BP to ≤80 mmHg resulted in a 51 % reduction in major cardiovascular events compared with target group ≤90 mmHg.

Pseudohypertension

Pseudohypertension is a false reading of high blood pressure. It is not unusual for this to occur in patients with arteriolosclerosis, calcification, and diffuse hardening of the arteries, particularly in the upper limbs. With hardening of the arteries, the rigid, pipe-like arteries resist compression by the sphygmomanometer cuff, and the pressure in the cuff wrapped around the arm fails to constrict and collapse the brachial artery. Because of this, blood continues to flow through the artery into the forearm, causing a false high reading. A reading in the range of 180–220 mmHg is not unusual (Zweifler and Shahab 1993).

Pseudohypertension should be excluded in elderly individuals whose brachial arteries characteristically feel rigid and pipe-like and in individuals who have no effects of hypertension after several years of abnormal readings, such as evidence of hypertension in the retina or cardiovascular or renal disease.

Pseudohypertension may also be suspected in these individuals with blood pressure apparently resistant to therapy and in those who develop dizziness and lightheadedness related to change in posture. Recordings over a period of weeks in the home, particularly with a simple finger or wrist blood pressure measurement, should resolve the diagnosis of pseudohypertension in virtually all patients.

Home Measurements

Home measurements of blood pressure are crucial for the adequate management of hypertension in more than 33 % of hypertensives. A record of home measurements verified by measurements outside the physicians' office is an important strategy to prevent overmedication. Measurements in the home have been shown to give virtually all of the information provided by ambulatory blood pressure monitoring. Home blood pressure measurements are strongly indicated for the following:

- To assist the physician with the diagnosis of borderline or stage 1 hypertension (see stages and classification given above)
- To exclude short-term hypertension that may occur for a few months because of stressful situations at work or at home and do not require lifelong medications
- To exclude white-coat hypertension
- To exclude pseudohypertension in the elderly
- To monitor response to therapy to avoid the addition of another antihypertensive agent to achieve control.

NONDRUG THERAPY

Nondrug therapy should be tried rigorously before drug therapy in all patients with mild hypertension. Nondrug therapy—low-sodium diet, weight reduction, cessation of smoking, reduction in alcohol intake, removal of stress and/ or learning to deal with stress, relaxation, exercises, and a potassium-enriched diet—may result in adequate control of hypertension in up to 40 % of patients with stage 1 or isolated systolic hypertension in the elderly. In addition, low saturated fat intake is often necessary because of coexisting hyperlipidemia, which increases risk.

WHICH DRUGS TO CHOOSE

- The physician should strive for monotherapy in the treatment of mild primary hypertension whenever possible. If the choice of initial agent is based on age and ethnicity, about 45 % of patients attain goal BP < 140 mmHg systolic with monotherapy. There is no justification to strive for a systolic blood pressure <130. A goal of 130–140 is acceptable.
- *The JNC8 advises a goal <150 mmHg. A state-of-the-art review emphasizes that this new goal has been criticized by many. Certain groups have opposed the decision to initiate pharmacologic treatment to treat to a goal systolic BP of <150 mmHg in the general population age >60 years* (Krakoff et al. 2014)

The association of Black cardiologists issued a statement "we strongly disagree with the new 2014 recommendations to raise the threshold for initiating drug treatment and systolic blood pressure goal for older persons, specifically because of the implications for women who comprise the majority of this elderly hypertensive population" (Gillespie et al. 2014).

- **It is advisable to give a trial of individual agents before using combinations of drugs or fixed-dose combinations**. *A combination, however, of two agents at low dose may achieve the therapeutic goal with less potential for adverse effects.*
- The patient should have a thorough understanding of the problems associated with drug therapy to facilitate acceptance and compliance during medication changes.

- It is important for the physician to consider the efficacy and the pharmacologic and adverse effects of the antihypertensive agent to be chosen, as well as the cost to the patient and the ability of the drug to prolong life.

Recommendations for Patients Without Coexisting Disease

MILD PRIMARY HYPERTENSION IN YOUNGER PATIENTS: BP 140–160 SYSTOLIC

There is abundant evidence from RCTs that whites and African Americans differ in their response to antihypertensive agents. Materson and Reda (1993, 1994) from their study concluded that the effective response to treatment with diltiazem, atenolol, diuretic, and captopril were as follows:

- Younger blacks 70, 51, 47, 43;
- Older blacks 84, 44, 63, 33;
- Younger whites 57, 64, 32, 61 ;
- Older whites 71, 72, 68, 61
- the weakly effective beta-blocker, atenolol, gave the best response in younger and older white patients.

Deary et al. (2002) completed a double-blind placebo-controlled crossover comparison of five antihypertensive drugs (amlodipine, doxazosin, lisinopril, bisoprolol, and bendrofluazide) and placebo in 34 young nonblack hypertensives and showed that **bendrofluazide performed significantly worse ($p = 0.0016$) and a beta-blocker, bisoprolol, significantly better ($p = 0.004$)**. Note the beta-blocker used was not atenolol, the favorite of Trialists; this drug that has given beta-blockers a foul name and conjured incorrect notions in the heads of experts who attempt to produce guidelines for clinicians worldwide.

Dickerson et al. (1999) undertook a crossover rotation of the four main classes of **antihypertensive drugs in 40 untreated young white hypertensive patients < age 55** to assess the response rate with monotherapy achieved by a systematic rotation 36 patients completed all four cycles. Success of monotherapy was achieved ($p=0.0001$); in half the patients, BP on the best treatment was 135/85 mmHg or less.

The responses to the ACE inhibitor or beta-blocker pair were, on average, at least 50 % higher than those to the calcium antagonist/diuretic pair.

• Thus beta-blockers are proven antihypertensive agents with effectiveness equal to that of ACE inhibitors or diuretics, depending on age and ethnicity. ACE inhibitors and ARBs are weak antihypertensive agents, and achieve control in <45 % of patients with mild hypertension; the addition of a diuretic improves effectiveness to ~66 %. These agents are overused instead of a beta-blocker or diuretic as first line; it is still useful in clinical practice to think of first or second line choices.

RECOMMENDATIONS FOR WHITE PATIENTS YOUNGER THAN AGE 65

It may appear old fashioned to recommend beta-blockers and diuretics as first-line agents, but the scientific evidence gleaned from the aforementioned three sound studies and carefully conducted meta-analysis of RCTs reemphasizes their efficacy, safety, and costs (Staessen et al. 2001).

• A meta-analysis by Staessen et al. (2001) and ALLHAT (2002) indicates that new drugs are not more effective; they do not have more beneficial effects.

Importantly, calcium antagonists significantly increase the risk of HF in patients older than age 70 (ALLHAT 2002); see Chap. 9 and Table 9-2.

Alpha-blockers increase the risk of HF (ALLHAT 2000) and have deleterious effects on the cardiovascular system. **A warning was issued by the American College of Cardiology following the ALLHAT findings in 2000.**

• ACE inhibitors are more effective than diuretics in younger whites. Recommendations are given in Table 8-3.

Table 8-3
Choice of drug for the treatment of mild primary hypertension based on age and ethnicity

White patients *younger than age 65*
1. Beta-blocker: bisoprolol, carvedilol, metoprolol (Toprol XL), or nebivolol preferred over other beta-blockers: monotherapy success in ~50 % in this age and ethnic category: *Warning*: avoid atenolol, see text.
   ACE inhibitor: monotherapy success in ~45 %; often requires combination with diuretic to achieve goal BP
   But addition of amlodipine is advisable; see ACCOMPLISH trial 2008 success with amlodipine benazepril combination
2. Diuretic: monotherapy success in ~33 %
3. Beta-blocker or ACE Inhibitor/ + diuretic
4. Calcium antagonist: success in ~50 %
5. Combinations at smaller doses advisable

Black patients *younger than age 65*
1. Calcium antagonist: monotherapy success in ~70 %
2. Beta-blocker (bisoprolol, carvedilol, metoprolol extended release [Toprol XL]): success in ~50 %; avoid atenolol
3. Calcium antagonist + beta-blocker success in >90 % (avoid verapamil[b])
4. Diuretic: success in ~33 %

White patients *older than age 65*
1. Diuretic: monotherapy success in ~50 % (first choice because of safety) older than 80, diuretic first choice
2. Beta-blocker: carvedilol, bisoprolol, metoprolol extended release, or nebivolol; avoid atenolol; success expected in ~ 60 %; second choice because safer than calcium antagonists in the elderly
3. ACE inhibitor: success in > 50 %[a]
4. Calcium antagonist (avoid verapamil): success in ~60 %
5. Calcium antagonist + ACE inhibitor useful as shown in ACCOMPLISH trial

Black patients *older than age 65*
1. Calcium antagonist (avoid verapamil): success in ~70 %[c]
2. Diuretic: success in ~50 %; safe agent tried first

(continued)

Table 8-3 (continued)

3. Betablocker + diuretic ~70 %
   Diuretic + calcium antagonist ~80 %
4. ACE inhibitor ~50 % but risk angioedema
AGE. 80–85: small dose diuretic Indapamide : see HYVET study
But beta-blocker has a definite role: e.g., bisoprolol 2.5–5 mg
daily, see text

ARB preferred over ACE INHIBITOR in view of angioedema risk
[a]PROGRESS only 42 % goal BP achieved in mixed population
[b]Severe bradycardia risk
[c]See Table 9.2; HF risk

Recommendations for Younger Black Patients. Calcium
antagonists are the most effective agents, followed by a non-
atenolol beta-blocker; *the latter may be tried first because
these agents are safe and inexpensive and are particularly
useful in patients with diabetes; they do not cause diabetes
as proclaimed by experts* [*see* the United Kingdom
Prospective Diabetes Study Group (UKPDS) and discussion
in Chaps. 2, 9, and 22].

MILD PRIMARY HYPERTENSION IN OLDER PATIENTS

***Recommendations for White Patients Age 65–80. Goal
systolic <140; but caution is needed to prevent falls and in
some patients a treatment goal to <150 is acceptable.***
There is no sound evidence to support national committees' choice of calcium antagonists for the management of
isolated hypertension in elderly whites. Beta-blockers are as
effective (Materson et al. 1993; HANE 1997) and are safer
and much less expensive. Beta-blockers are safe in patients
aged 65–85 years, and the safety and ability of these drugs
in very elderly post-MI patients, and to prevent HF
(CAPRICORN 2001; COPERNICUS 2001), have been
endorsed in RCTs. Also beta-blockers are widely used in
patients of age 65–85 with atrial fibrillation. Thus safety is
assured, whereas calcium antagonists may cause heart

failure and falls causing serious injuries. Calcium antagonists the most effective antihypertensive agents do cause
heart failure, a condition not uncommon in the elderly.

- **The JNC8 experts have ignored the sound findings of
  ALLHAT in which amlodipine and nifedipine carried
  a 32 and 46 % risk for heart failure compared with
  diuretic therapy** (Table 9-2)

Staessen et al. (2001) analyzed nine randomized trials
comparing treatments in 62,605 hypertensive patients.
Results:

- Compared with old drugs (diuretics and beta-blockers),
  calcium-channel blockers and ACE inhibitors offered similar overall cardiovascular protection.
- There was a higher risk of stroke in patients for whom captopril was randomly assigned .
- Increase in fatal myocardial infarction on treatment with
  nifedipine GITS.
- Overall cardiovascular risk did not differ between patients
  randomized to diuretics or beta-blockers compared with
  those allocated initial treatment with calcium-channel blockers or ACE inhibitors.
- In patients randomized to calcium-channel blockers, reduction in risk of stroke was greater, $p=0.03$ than in those in
  whom treatment was started with old drugs.

In this excellent meta-analysis by Staessen and associates, the authors concluded: "All antihypertensive drugs
have similar long-term efficacy and safety," *but in the same
article indicated that new drugs significantly increased the
risk of HF.*

- HF is a common cause of morbidity, hospitalization, and
  death; effective control of hypertension is necessary to
  stem the epidemic of HF. In the Intervention as a Goal in
  Hypertension Treatment (INSIGHT 2000) study, among
  primary end points HF and MI were statistically more
  frequent in the Adalat XL group. In the Prospective

Randomized Amlodipine Survival Evaluation (PRAISE study 1996), pulmonary edema was more frequent in the amlodipine-treated group. In the Multicenter Diltiazem Postinfarction Trial of non-Q-wave MI (1988), diltiazem increased the risk of HF.

These findings are not surprising because calcium antagonists possess significant negative inotropic effects. Elderly hypertensive patients are at a higher risk of HF and MI than younger patients; thus, although calcium antagonists are highly effective antihypertensives in the elderly, beta-blockers, diuretics, and ACE inhibitors are *preferred because these drugs have proved useful in the prevention and management of HF*. The combination of ACE inhibitor and beta-blocker is not considered complementary, because these drugs do not enhance antihypertensive effects. However, they are both cardioprotective and deserve a clinical trial. **Nebivolol and valsartan fixed-dose combination proved to be an effective and well-tolerated treatment option for patients with hypertension** (Giles et al. 2014). **But it is not advisable to combine valsartan with a beta-blocker because mortality and morbidity are increased as shown in an RCT.** In **Val-HeFT**, valsartan when combined with a beta-blocker caused significantly more cardiac events. A total of 5,010 patients with HF class II, III, or IV were randomly assigned to receive 160 mg of valsartan or placebo twice daily. There was no reduction in all cause mortality. The incidence of the combined end point, however, was a modest 13.2 % lower with valsartan than with placebo ($p = 0.009$), predominantly because of a lower number of patients hospitalized for heart failure: 455 (18.2 %) in the placebo group and 346 (13.8 %) in the valsartan group ($p < 0.001$). **Overall mortality was not reduced by valsartan administration** (Cohn and Tognoni 2001).

In **VALIANT** (2003): a clinical trial of valsartan, captopril, or both in MI complicated by HF, left ventricular dysfunction, or both, during a median follow-up of

24.7 months, **total mortality was not reduced by valsartan**: 979 patients in the valsartan group died, as did 941 patients in the valsartan-and-captopril group and 958 patients in the captopril group. **There was no placebo group.**

- The JNC8 (2014) guidelines are flawed and should be revised.
- In the SHEP study, atenolol was the second agent used, after a diuretic. After 5 years of follow-up, IHD was reduced by 25 %, with a major reduction in stroke. The Swedish Trial in Old Patients with Hypertension (STOP 2 1999) in the elderly showed a significant reduction in mortality and strokes as a result of beta-blocker therapy.

Recommendations for Elderly Patients of African Origin. Goal in the majority should be <140 systolic and in all ethnic groups, selected individuals over age 75 a goal of <150 is acceptable in the absence of heart or renal failure.

A diuretic and calcium antagonists have been shown to have better antihypertensive effects than beta-blockers and ACE inhibitors and are recommended. However, caution is required in patients with ejection fraction <45 % because the risk of HF may increase with long-term calcium antagonist therapy. Thus, <u>a diuretic is the first choice in elderly patients of African origin.</u>

Recommendations for All Elderly Over Age 80. Advice is based on HYVET, a double-blind RCT of 3,845 hypertensive patients 80 years of age or older (Beckett et al. 2008).

Stepped-care therapy began with indapamide with addition of perindopril as needed. At 2 years, the trial was halted because active treatment, as compared with placebo, was associated with a 21 % reduction in the relative risk of death from any cause, a 64 % reduction in the relative risk of heart failure, and a 30 % reduction in the relative risk of stroke (Beckett et al. 2008).

- Small dose diuretic: indapamide 1.25 mg or chlorthalidone 25 mg, alternate day should suffice in the majority but serum potassium must be maintained >3.9 mmol/l.
- *Prospective data suggest that in older men and women, the use of thiazide diuretic agents is associated with a reduction of approximately one-third in the risk of hip fracture.*

  Selected elderly over age 80 in whom systolic pressure is constantly greater than 170 mmHg (in the absence of pseudohypertension) may require the following:

- In the presence of coronary artery disease, heart failure in past, atrial fibrillation, palpitations (premature beats) or renal dysfunction, TIA or post stroke; a small dose of a beta-blocking drug [nebivolol 2.5 mg. bisoprolol 2.5 to maximum 5 mg once daily; is strongly advisable; **the widely used atenolol is not recommended.** In SHEP (65–85 year old) a beta-blocker was added to diuretic with salutary results.

Clinicians worldwide should not be reluctant to add a small dose of an appropriate beta-blocker to small dose diuretic in the elderly. **The notion that beta-blockers are not effective or harmful or cause genuine diabetes is false. Nonetheless this is a notion held by many experts who write guidelines (UK and USA).**

A small dose of a beta-blocking drug, e.g., bisoprolol 2.5–5 mg (not atenolol), is successfully administered for the commonly occurring atrial fibrillation of the elderly or for angina or post-MI and should be just as safe for the elderly hypertensive whose blood pressure must not be aggressively lowered by an ACE inhibitor or calcium antagonist resulting in falls. Amlodipine 2.5 mg or ramipril added to the beta-blocker often suffices. Diuretics are effective in the elderly and with beta-blockers should be preferred therapy because they do not result in falls compared with ACE inhibitor or calcium antagonist therapy. But some individuals older than age 75, particularly women, may be bothered by frequency of micturition.

Thus some may be controlled with 5 mg of bisoprolol only. ACE inhibitors are contraindicated in patients with anemia, a not uncommon finding in the elderly. Much thought must be given in writing the final prescription.

- Failure to maintain BP < 150 mmHg may require amlodipine 2.5 to maximum 5 mg daily. *Avoid diltiazem and verapamil in elderly because of bothersome constipation and increased HF rate.*
- *Goal BP 130–150 mm in patients age >75 if HF and renal failure are not present. Falls are not infrequent in the elderly who are overtreated with calcium antagonists and ACE inhibitors.*
- An RCT with nisoldipine in patients with hypertension and non-insulin-dependent diabetes was terminated early because nisoldipine-treated patients had a higher risk of fatal and nonfatal acute MI than observed in the enalapril group: 25/235 versus 5/235 ($p < 0.001$).
- Sustained-release calcium antagonists may increase the risk of cardiac mortality in patients who are at risk of IHD events, particularly in those with diabetes, dyslipidemia, and coexisting IHD and in the elderly with silent ischemia or undetected IHD. Long-term RCTs in the elderly age of 75–84 are necessary before calcium antagonists may be considered safe alternatives to diuretics and beta-blockers.
- *Beta-blockers*: The Swedish STOP 2 study (1999) in the elderly showed a significant reduction in mortality and strokes as a result of beta-blocker therapy. Newer agents were not superior to beta-blockers or diuretics. *The beta-blockers used were atenolol (a poorly effective beta-blocker) and the non-cardioprotective pindolol.*
- Some RCTs used propranolol, a beta-blocker influenced unfavorably by cigarette smoking. Smoking interferes with hepatic metabolism of propranolol and decreases blood levels of this agent (Materson et al. 1988). In the Beta-Blocker Heart Attack Trial (BHAT 1982), propranolol failed to prevent fatal and nonfatal MI in smokers but mortality and recurrent MI were significantly improved in nonsmokers.

- **Propranolol and oxprenolol lose their effects in smokers;**
- **Timolol** (Norwegian Multicentre Study Group 1981) **have been shown to prevent fatal MI, nonfatal MI, and sudden cardiac death in smokers and nonsmokers.** A remarkable 67 % reduction in sudden deaths was recorded in the well-run RCT.
- Yet this beta-blocker which caused an outstanding reduction in sudden death not matched by any other cardiac drug is rarely prescribed. *A long acting formulation should be developed.*
- *It is clear that beta-blockers are not all alike with regard to their salutary effects, and older agents including atenolol should become obsolete* (Khan 2011, 2007a); *use in clinical trials should be curtailed* (Khan 2003a) *and trials in which this drug has been administered should be suspected*
- **The reason why atenolol became the most widely prescribed beta-blocking drug is twofold**
  1. **It was one of the first agents available following the breakthrough good news provided by propranolol in 1970, and was used by the author.**
  2. **The drug was observed to have less adverse effects because it achieves a much lower brain concentration than propranolol and metoprolol. But, the beneficial effect depends on the brain concentration and this renders it much less effective, a fact that appears to have eluded teaching professors, clinical Trialist and guideline providers.**

In addition, the physician must be aware of the reasons for poor drug control of BP in the treated patient (Table 8-4).

RCTs of **ACE inhibitors** have not shown these drugs to be superior to beta-blockers or diuretics (Casas et al. 2005). Importantly, **RCTs have indicated that ACE inhibitors rarely achieve goal BP without the addition of a diuretic. In the large PROGRESS (2001) trial, only 42 % achieved goal BP; 58 % required addition of diuretics to achieve control in ~ 66 %.**

Table 8-4
Reasons for poor drug control of blood pressure

- Poor compliance
  Inconvenient drug dosing, e.g., b.i.d. or t.i.d.
  Inability to purchase drug (financial)
  Adverse effect of drug
- Related to drug
  Inappropriate drug selection or drug combination
  Interactions with NSAIDs, nasal decongestants, cocaine
- Salt intake; volume overload
  Diuretic required
  ↑Na+ intake
  Renal failure
- Weight gain
- Alcohol intake >4 oz/day
- Renovascular hypertension
- Other causes of secondary hypertension
- Cuff size
- White coat syndrome
- Pseudohypertension
- Primary hyperaldosteronism; see section "Resistant
  Hypertension"

Therapy for Patients with Coexisting Diseases

In the presence of coexisting disease and target organ damage with comorbid conditions (*see* Table 8-1), agents are recommended as follows:

- **Angina, after MI, or suspected IHD**: Beta-blockers are strongly recommended. Use diltiazem sustained-release preparation (e.g., or amlodipine if beta-blockers are contra-indicated. A DHP used without a beta-blocker may increase mortality if unstable angina or acute MI supervenes.
- Atrial fibrillation or other arrhythmias: Beta-blockers are strongly advisable. Hypertension is the leading cause of atrial fibrillation and HF (*see* Fig. 8-1).
- Aortic and other aneurysms: Beta-blockers are strongly indicated because they decrease ejection velocity and shearing

stress in arteries; thus, they may provide some protection from rupture or further expansion of the aneurysm.

- In the Antihypertensive and Lipid-Lowering Treatment to Prevent Heart Attack Trial (ALLHAT 2002), diuretics were as effective as ACE inhibitors and calcium antagonists in decreasing CVD outcome.
- Diabetic patients have a high incidence of MI and cardiac death; thus, both ACE inhibitors and beta-blockers are strongly recommended. The UKPDS study (1998) showed beta-blocker therapy to be as effective as captopril in reducing the risk of macrovascular and microvascular complications in type 2 diabetes . Importantly, glycemic control was not different between groups.
- Stroke or transient ischemic attack: BP must be cautiously reduced, if at all, in the acute stage. A beta-blocker or diuretic or combination is advisable.
- In the large PROGRESS (2001) RCT 6,105 patients with previous stroke or transient ischemic attack showed no reduction in the risk of cardiovascular events or stroke, but the combination with indapamide significantly reduced adverse events.
- In the large Captopril Prevention Project (CAPP 1999) study of captopril versus diuretic and beta-blocker, fatal and **nonfatal stroke was increased in the captopril group ($p = 0.044$)**, with no significant differences in other events. Primary endpoint events occurred in 363 patients in the captopril group and 335 in the conventional-treatment group $p=0.52$). Cardiovascular mortality was not significantly lower with captopril than with conventional treatment (76 vs 95 events; p=0.092), the rate of fatal and non-fatal MI was similar (162 vs 161), in addition, some captopril-treated patients required addition of diuretic to achieve goal BP.
- Alpha-blockers may increase cardiovascular mortality and have not been shown to prevent or reduce LVH. Patients with dyslipidemia are at high risk of IHD events. Beta-blockers are the logical choice. If beta-blockers are contraindicated, an ACE inhibitor and low-dose diuretic are advisable.
- Congestive heart failure (CHF) classes I–II and III: Diuretics plus ACE inhibitor plus a beta-blocker. In this subset, beta-

blockers have been shown in RCTs to prolong life and to reduce the risk of hospitalization.

- Thus, beta-blockers are strongly indicated for patients with LV dysfunction, ejection fraction 25–45 %. The combination of bisoprolol ,carvedilol or nebivolol and an ACE inhibitor is advisable.
- Renal insufficiency, except renovascular hypertension, creatinine clearance <265 µmol/L, 3 mg/dL: ACE inhibitor plus loop diuretic is indicated, but a beta-blocker and/or calcium antagonist may be necessary to achieve goal BP; see later discussion of metolazone.
- LVH: Beta-blockers and/or ACE inhibitors are preferred. Avoid alpha-blockers. Calcium antagonists and alpha-blockers have not shown to reduce LV mass consistently (Devereux 1985; Dunn et al. 1987).
- Liver disease: Avoid methyldopa and labetalol; the latter may cause hepatic necrosis (Clark et al. 1990).
- Severe depression: Diuretics or ACE inhibitors are recommended; a calcium antagonist may be used in the absence of diabetes. Beta-blockers may increase depression, but this effect is rare and does not contraindicate the use of beta-blocker therapy if needed. Reserpine, methyldopa, clonidine, and other central alpha-agonists are contraindicated.
- Stasis edema or varicose veins with edema: Avoid calcium antagonists, particularly the DHPs.
- Renal vascular hypertension or anemia: Avoid ACE inhibitors and ARBs.
- Gastroreflux syndrome: Avoid calcium antagonists because they may increase reflux.
- Gout: Avoid diuretics.
- Sensitivity to sulfonamides: Avoid all diuretics except ethacrynic acid and amiloride.
- Severe peripheral vascular disease: Avoid beta-blockers; these agents are not contraindicated in patients with mild or stable peripheral vascular disease because these patients often have coexisting IHD, and beta-blockers may ameliorate symptoms and prolong life in this subset.
- Renal calculi: Avoid triamterene because this agent may precipitate calculi (*see* Chap. 7).

- Migraine: A nonselective beta-blocker is the most logical agent because vasoconstriction may relieve symptoms.
- Osteoporosis: Thiazides have been shown to increase bone mass (Felson et al. 1991). *Prospective data suggest that in older men and women the use of thiazide diuretic agents is associated with a reduction of approximately one third in the risk of hip fracture* (LaCroix et al. 1990).
- Symptomatic mitral valve prolapse: Beta-blockers are the obvious choice.
- Hyperthyroidism: Beta-blockers are recommended for the management of arrhythmias.
- Cyclosporine-induced hypertension: Calcium antagonists are of value.
- Pregnancy: Avoid ACE inhibitors, ARBs and diuretics. A beta-blocking agent is used by some obstetricians depending on the timing (see Chap. 20).
- Methyldopa may be indicated at certain periods during pregnancy.
- For preeclampsia, a diuretic should be avoided. For eclampsia, hydralazine or labetalol is recommended (*see* Chap. 20).
- Subarachnoid hemorrhage: Nimodipine or a beta-blocking agent such as labetalol should suffice.
- Silent myocardial ischemia is commoner than nonsilent ischemia (angina): Beta-blockers are strongly indicated.

BETA-BLOCKERS

A beta-blocker is strongly recommended for the management of

- All hypertensive patients, white or black.

Dosage

The dosage of beta-blockers is given in Table 8-5. In the elderly, it is preferable to start with smaller doses, for example, bisoprolol 2.5–5 mg, nebivolol 2.5–5 mg daily, metoprolol succinate extended release (Toprol XL) 50 mg, carvedilol 12.5–25 mg, or timolol 5 mg daily. It is not advisable to use

Table 8-5
Doses[a] of beta-blockers

Drug	Before addition of diuretics (mg daily)	With diuretics (mg)
Bisoprolol[b]	5–10	5–10[b]
Carvedilol	12.5–50	12.5–50
Metoprolol	100–200	100–200
Nebivolol	2.5–10	2.5–10
Propranolol LA	120–180	120–160
Timolol	10–20	5–15

[a]Probable cardioprotective dose. See Chap. 9. Atenolol is not recommended

[b]Ziac: 5, 7.5, 10 mg bisorpolol with 6.25 mg HCTZ

a dose higher than that given in Table 8-5. If BP goal is not attained, a low-dose diuretic should be added or the beta-blocker should be discontinued and the patient commenced on a diuretic or other agent.

Action of Beta-Blockers

Beta-blockers lower BP by

- Decreasing cardiac output.
- Inhibiting the release of renin, thus decreasing angiotensin and aldosterone (*see* Chap. 1).
- Decreasing central vasomotor activity.
- Releasing norepinephrine from sympathetic neurons.

Drug name:	**Bisoprolol**
Trade names:	Zebeta, Monocor, Emcor
Supplied:	5, 10 mg
Dosage:	5–10 mg once daily

Ziac is a combination of bisoprolol 2.5-, 5-, and 10-mg tablets with HCTZ 6.25 mg. This combination showed response rates of up to 84 % in two well-controlled RCTs. Ziac has been approved by the U.S. Food and Drug Administration (FDA) as initial therapy; Monozide 10 = bisoprolol 10 mg, HCTZ 6.25 mg, in the UK.

Drug name:	**Carvedilol**
*Trade names*v	Coreg, Eucardic
Dosage:	Hypertension, initially 12.5 mg once daily, increased after 2 days to usual dose of 25 mg once daily; if necessary may be further increased at intervals of at least 2 weeks to max. 50 mg daily in single or divided doses; elderly initial dose of 12.5 mg daily may provide satisfactory control

Drug name:	**Metoprolol succinate**
Trade name:	Toprol XL
Supplied:	50, 100, 200 mg
Dosage:	50–200 mg once daily

Toprol XL has a 24-h duration of action. A combination of Toprol XL and low-dose HCTZ 6.25 mg should be appropriate for the control of more than 80 % of patients with stage 1 isolated hypertension. *Metoprolol tartrate* is not recommended by the author but dosage given: 50–100 mg twice daily.

Drug name:	**Nebivolol**
Trade names:	Bystolic; Nebilet, Nebilong, Lobivon
Supplied:	2.5, 5, 0, 20 mg
Dosage:	5 mg once daily, increasing at 2-week intervals up to 10 mg. max. 20 mg Elderly: start with 2.5 mg. Manufacturer advises to avoid if serum creatinine greater than 250 μmol/L; see Chap. 1

Nebivolol is a novel beta-blocker with several important pharmacologic properties that distinguish it from traditional beta-blockers (Gray and Ndefo 2008).This highly selective beta1-adrenergic receptor blocker is the only beta-blocker known to induce vascular production of nitric oxide, the main endothelial vasodilator. Nebivolol induces nitric oxide production via stimulates the beta3-adrenergic receptor-mediated production of nitric oxide in the heart; this stimulation results in a greater protection against heart failure (Maffei and Lembo 2009).

In addition, nebivolol increases NO by decreasing its oxidative inactivation (Cominacini et al. 2003). The drug stimulates the endothelial L-arginine/nitric oxide pathway and thus causes vasodilation (Cockcroft et al. 1995).

Nebivolol should find a role in the management of HF, particularly in patients with normal or slightly reduced EF. The effect of beta-blockade with nebivolol in elderly patients with HF in this study was similar in those with preserved and impaired EF (van Veldhuisen et al. 2009).

- Nebivolol reduces P-wave dispersion on the electrocardiogram, which would attenuate the risk of atrial fibrillation (Tuncer et al. 2008).
- Nebivolol appears to have a minor, if any, effect on libido and sexual performance, which likely ensues from a compensatory effect of the increased NO release (Boydak et al. 2005). In contrast with metoprolol, nebivolol improves secondary sexual activity and erectile dysfunction scores (Brixius et al. 2007). An extensive review article was forwarded by Münzel and Gori (2009). Although a decade of clinical experience with this drug in Europe provides support to its blood pressure-lowering and antiischemic effects, further clinical trial data are necessary.

Particularly, comparative trials on the efficacy of nebivolol versus other beta-blockers and/or other antihypertensive drugs are awaited (Münzel and Gori 2009). Maffei and Lembo provided informative information on nitric oxide mechanisms of nebivolol in an article: Therapeutic Advances in Cardiovascular Disease Maffei and Lembo (2009).

Nebivolol and valsartan fixed-dose combination proved to be an effective and well-tolerated treatment option for patients with hypertension (Giles et al. 2014). But the combination of beta-blocker and valsartan has caused increased cardiac events and is not recommended by the author (see Chaps. 1, 2, 4).

DIURETICS

Action

The exact mechanism of action and antihypertensive effect of thiazides are unknown, and the effect is believed to be related to decrease in vascular volume, negative sodium (Na+) balance, and arteriolar dilation, causing a decrease in total peripheral resistance.

Contraindications

Hypersensitivity to thiazides or sulfonamides; anuria or severe renal failure; pregnancy and breast-feeding (see Chap. 20); concomitant lithium therapy.

Adverse effects include the following:

1. Dehydration and electrolyte imbalance are the most common adverse effects. The dose is too large if signs of dehydration or orthostatic hypotension develop, or if the patient has increased urea >10.0 mmol/L or an increase of 7.0 mmol/L from baseline, chlorides <94 mEq (mmol)/L, total carbon dioxide >32 mEq (mmol)/L, and uric acid >7 mg/dL (420 µmol/L).
2. Hypokalemia occurs in a significant number of patients receiving thiazides and contributes to increased risk of

cardiac arrest (Siscovick et al. 1994). Chlorthalidone causes a greater loss of potassium (K+) than for equivalent doses of HCTZ. The incidence of hypokalemia can be decreased by the use of low-dose thiazide regimens with K+-sparing diuretics. It is advisable to use the following: A thiazide-K+-sparing diuretic, such as amiloride with HCTZ (Moduretic, Moduret), if renal function is normal. If mild renal dysfunction exists, hyperkalemia may occur with the use of K+-sparing diuretics; therefore, a plain thiazide is recommended without potassium supplements.

3. Gastrointestinal effects: anorexia, gastric irritation, intrahepatic cholestatic jaundice, and pancreatitis.

4. Central nervous system effects include dizziness, vertigo, paresthesia, and headache.

5. Hematology and blood disturbances include leukopenia, rare agranulocytosis, thrombocytopenia, aplastic anemia and hemolytic anemia, increased serum cholesterol, decreased HDL cholesterol, and increased blood viscosity.

6. Cardiovascular effects include orthostatic hypotension, low cardiac output, and arrhythmias from hypokalemia.

7. For use in pregnant or nursing mothers, thiazides cross the placental barrier, appear in breast milk, and can cause fetal or neonatal jaundice, thrombocytopenia, decreased vascular volume and placental perfusion, and acute pancreatitis.

8. Precipitation of gout and hyperuricemia is a well-known complication of all diuretics. If gout or hyperuricemia occurs, this is treated in the usual fashion, and the diuretic is discontinued. There is no reason to add allopurinol to the regimen to prevent further episodes of gout. This is commonly done and adds to polypharmacy and expense.

9. Acute allergic interstitial pneumonitis (Biron et al. 1991; Hoegholm et al. 1990) is an extremely rare, but life-threatening, complication.

10. Drug interactions with lithium, steroids, and oral anticoagulants have been reported.

Use Proven in Elderly

The Systolic Hypertension in the Elderly Program (SHEP 1991), in which a diuretic was used in patients aged 65–85 years, showed a 36 % reduction in the risk of stroke ($p=0.0003$), a 27 % decrease in IHD event rates, and a 54 % decrease in the risk of LVF. In the SHEP trial, a low-dose diuretic was used as initial therapy, and a beta-blocker was added if necessary. HYVET (2008): a double-blind, randomized, placebo-controlled clinical trial involving 3,845 patients 80 years of age or older with hypertension, the effect of stepped care therapy, beginning with the diuretic indapamide and adding perindopril as needed was assessed. Active treatment, as compared with placebo, caused a modest reduction in risk. Treatment was associated with a 21 % reduction in the relative risk of death from any cause, a 64 % reduction in the relative risk of heart failure, and a 30 % reduction in the relative risk of stroke (Beckett et al. 2008).

There is no question about the efficacy of diuretics in patients with mild to moderate hypertension, and, when they are combined with other antihypertensive agents, they can be used in all types and degrees of hypertension.

Recommendations for the use of diuretics are as follows:

- Low-dose diuretic therapy is strongly recommended as first-line therapy in older patients (age >70 years) of any ethnic group.
- If the diuretic was not the first-choice agent, it is logical to add a diuretic if goal BP has not been achieved.
- Diuretics are highly recommended in patients with coexisting disease (*see* Fig. 8-2) for special situations, in particular in combination with ACE inhibitors for HF. Renal failure with increased volume overload is a common cause of resistant hypertension that requires the addition of a diuretic to enhance the efficacy of other agents.

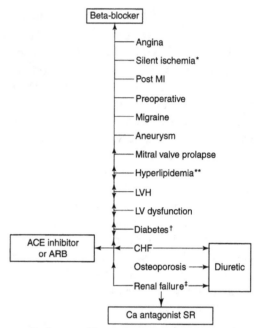

*More common than angina in men >50 yr.
**Statin and beta-blocker or ACE inhibitor, not alpha-blocker.
†Not prone to hypoglycemia.
‡Not renovascular.

Fig. 8-2. Choice of antihypertensive agent in patients with coexisting diseases. *Single asterisk*: More common than angina in men >50 years, *double asterisks*: statin and beta-blocker or ACE inhibitor, not alpha-blocker, *dagger symbol*: Not prone to hypoglycemia, *double dagger symbol*: Not renovascular.

- Thiazide diuretic agents lower the urinary excretion of calcium. Their use has been associated with increased bone density (Ray et al. 1989)
- LaCroix et al. (1990) prospectively studied the effect of thiazide diuretic agents on the incidence of hip fracture among 9,518 men and women 65 years of age or older residing in three communities. Prospective data suggest that in older men and women, the *use of thiazide diuretic agents is*

associated with a reduction of approximately one-third in the risk of hip fracture.

- **Metolazone** is a thiazide diuretic that has a unique property of retaining effectiveness when other thiazides become ineffective in patients with renal failure GFR < 30 mL/min. Dosage 2.5–7.5 mg daily.

Drug name:	**Hydrochlorothiazide**
Trade names:	HydroDIURIL, Esidrex, Hydro-Saluric
Supplied:	25, 50 mg
Dosage:	12.5–25 mg each morning; max. 50 mg daily

The 50-mg dose was necessary to achieve control of BP, and it was commonly used from 1965 to 1980, prior to newer agents.

Drug name:	**Bendrofluazide**
Trade names:	UK Aprinox, Berkozide, Centyl, Neo-Naclex, Urizide
Supplied:	2.5, 5 mg
Dosage:	2.5–5 mg daily
Advice and adverse effects	
Recommendations are the same as for HCTZ	

Chlorthalidone

Dosage 12.5–25 mg daily

This thiazide appears to cause better control of blood pressure compared with the commonly used hydrochlorothiazide (HCTZ) as indicated by a study completed by Ernst et al. (2006). The BP difference was particularly impressive in the evening hours. The reduction in systolic BP during nighttime hours was –13.5 to 1.9 mmHg for chlorthalidone versus –6.4 to 1.7 mmHg for HCTZ and was highly significant. If one believes that the degree to which BP is reduced is the most important variable in defining outcome then there is now better support for chlorthalidone as the preferred thiazide-type diuretic.

Chlorthalidone is distinguished from HCTZ in having an extremely long half-life and a very large volume of distribution, owing to its extensive partitioning into red blood cells. This latter feature creates a hefty depot for chlorthalidone, allowing for a slow streaming effect (red cell plasma) with subsequent gradual elimination from the plasma compartment by tubular secretion (Riess et al. 1977).

The extremely long half-life of 40–60 h for chlorthalidone differentiates it from HCTZ, which has a much shorter but wider variation in half-life, from 3.2 to 13.1 h (Chen and Chiou 1992). This plasma half-life difference can be expected to correlate with a more extended effect of chlorthalidone on diuresis and possibly BP.

In addition, chlorthalidone was used with beneficial effects that were equal to newer agents in the ALLHAT study: A study of 33,357 hypertensive patients of mean age 67 were randomized to receive chlorthalidone, 12.5–25 mg/day ($n=15,255$); amlodipine, 2.5–10 mg/day ($n=9,048$); or lisinopril, 10–40 mg/day ($n=9,054$) with a follow-up of 4.9 years. There was good representation for women (47 %) and blacks (35 %); 36 % were diabetics. The primary outcome combined fatal CHD or nonfatal MI occurred in 2,956 participants, with no difference between treatments. All-cause mortality did not differ between groups (ALLHAT 2002).

A study used 24-h ambulatory blood-pressure measurements to study the effects of 25 mg of chlorthalidone daily as compared with 50-mg hydrochlorothiazide daily. Although blood-pressure levels measured during the daytime in the clinician's office were similar, blood pressure levels measured during the nighttime and 24-h average blood pressures were considerably lower with chlorthalidone than with hydrochlorothiazide (Ernst et al. 2006).

Indapamide Natrilix 2.5 mg

Dose: 1.25–2.5 mg once daily

This agent is believed to cause slightly less metabolic derangements compared with other thiazides; this notion is mainly unproven. The results of HYVET provide evidence that antihypertensive treatment with indapamide 1.5 mg (sustained release), with or without perindopril, in persons 80 years of age or older is beneficial (Beckett et al. 2008).

Drug name:	**Hydrochlorothiazide and Amiloride**
Trade names:	Moduretic, Moduret (C)
Supplied:	Tablets containing 50 mg hydrochlorothiazide and 5 mg amiloride
Dosage:	Half a tablet daily; *see* text for further advice

The manufacturer indicates up to four tablets daily. The physician must insist on a lower dose of diuretics. *A more appropriate combination, co-amilozide, available in the United Kingdom and Europe, contains amiloride 2.5 mg, HCTZ 25 mg.*

Dyazide: Hydrochlorothiazide combined with triam-terene is not recommended. Triamterene may cause stone formation. It is avoided in patients with renal calculi.

Ziac (US) or Monocor (UK) is a combination of biso-prolol 2.5, 5, and 10 mg with 6.25 mg HCTZ. This is an appropriate combination of a diuretic and a beta-blocker. BP is lowered to goal levels in about 80 % of patients. This combination-type therapy with Ziac has shown consistently low discontinuation rates because of adverse effects, compared with enalapril.

Drug name:	**Furosemide; [Lasix]**
	Frusemide

Furosemide is less effective than thiazides in mild to moderate hypertension, and therefore it is not advisable to use this drug unless the patient has significant renal dysfunction, such as a creatinine level >2.3 mg/dL (203 µmol/L). Because furosemide inhibits the reabsorption of a very high percentage of filtered sodium, it is more effective than thiazides in patients with reduced glomerular filtration rate (GFR). As with thiazides, the combination with a K^+-sparing diuretic has proved to be useful in causing further diuresis and in reducing K^+ loss.

Drug name:	**Eplerenone** Inspra
Dosage:	25 mg once daily, max. 50 mg

This selective aldosterone blocker has proved effective in the management of hypertension, heart failure, and in the post-MI patient. See Chap. 7 and The EPHESUS trial (2003) in Chap. 22. Avoid if eGFR is less than 50 mL/min. Contraindications: hyperkalemia; concomitant use of potassium-sparing diuretics or potassium supplements. Assess serum potassium before treatment, during initiation, and when dose changed.

ACE INHIBITORS AND ANGIOTENSIN II RECEPTOR BLOCKERS

ACE inhibitors and ARBs play a major role in the management of hypertension, particularly in patients with target organ damage and coexisting diseases (*see* Table 8-1). The major advantage of ARBs over ACE inhibitors is the absence of cough and very rare occurrence of angioedema; these agents are as effective as ACE inhibitors for the control of hypertension and HF. The failure of losartan, however, to control BP in scleroderma renal crisis with responsiveness to lisinopril has been reported (Caskey et al. 1997).

Table 8-6
Rationale for not recommending alpha$_1$-blockers

- They cause an increase in cardiac ejection velocity, ↑ in heart rate. This action results in:

  ↑ in cardiac work and myocardial oxygen requirement

  Damage to arteries at branching points: may cause rupture of aneurysms. These agents are contraindicated in patients with CHD and aneurysms
- They cause an ↑ in circulating norepinephrine and activate the renin–angiotensin system, causing:

  Na$^+$ and water retention

  ↑ A serious risk for HF: in ALLHAT (2000) doxazosin showed a 82 % increased risk

  Their use often requires addition of a diuretic
- They may cause retrograde ejaculation
- They do not prevent or cause regression of left ventricular hypertrophy
- Rupture of aneurysms may occur; do not use in patients with aneurysms

---

- In patients with target organ damage and coexisting conditions and special situations (*see* Table 8-6), particularly HF, LVH, diabetes with proteinuria, and selected cases of nephropathy (excluding renovascular hypertension), these agents are indicated. They are, however, not superior to other agents in diabetic patients, as is often claimed (*see* Chap. 9).

ACE inhibitors prevent the conversion of angiotensin I to angiotensin II; ARBs block the effects of angiotensin II on blood vessel walls and do not interfere with the breakdown of bradykinin. These actions of ACE inhibitors and ARBs result in

- Arteriolar dilation, which causes a fall in total systemic vascular resistance.
- Attenuation of angiotensin potentiation of sympathetic activity and release of norepinephrine. The diminished sympathetic

activity causes vasodilation, reduction in afterload, and some decrease in preload. Also, heart rate is not increased by these agents, as opposed to other vasodilators.

- Reduction in aldosterone secretion. The latter action promotes Na^+ excretion and K^+ retention.
- Blocking of angiotensin-mediated vasopressin release, which appears to be important in HF.
- Converting enzyme (the same as kinase II), which causes degradation of bradykinin. The accumulation of bradykinin stimulates release of vasodilator prostaglandins that contribute to the decrease in peripheral vascular resistance. Thus, indomethacin and other prostaglandin inhibitors reduce the effectiveness of ACE inhibitors.

Adverse Effects and Interactions

ACE inhibitors may retain K^+, so these drugs should not be given with potassium supplements or K^+-sparing diuretics, Aldactazide (spironolactone and HCTZ), Dyazide (triamterene and HCTZ), Maxzide (triamterene and HCTZ), or Moduretic (Moduret) (amiloride and HCTZ). Hyperkalemia may also occur with renal failure. Cough occurs in up 20–40 % of patients; angioedema is discussed in Chap. 3.

Adverse reactions reportedly include severe pruritus and rash in 10 % and loss of taste in 7 % of patients (Jenkins et al. 1985), as well as mouth ulcers, neurologic dysfunction, and gastrointestinal disturbances. Occasionally, tachycardia, increased angina, and precipitation of MI may occur. Neutropenia and agranulocytosis are rare and occur mainly in patients with serious intercurrent illness, particularly immunologic disturbances, and in those with an altered immune response, in particular collagen vascular disease. Precipitation of renal failure in patients with tight renal artery stenosis has been reported. Uncommon side effects include fatigue, Raynaud's phenomenon, cough and/or wheeze, myalgia, muscle cramps, hair loss, angioedema of the face, mouth, or larynx, impotence or decreased libido, pemphigus, lichen planus, hepatitis, and the occurrence of antinuclear antibodies.

Contraindications

The use of ACE inhibitors and ARBs should be avoided in the following clinical situations:

- Hypotension: systolic pressures <100 mmHg.
- Renal artery stenosis
- Moderate or severe aortic stenosis.
- Severe renal failure; serum creatinine level >2.3 mg/dL, 203 μmol/L. If the use of an ACE inhibitor is necessary, alter the dose and dosing interval.
- Hyperkalemia or concomitant use of K+-sparing diuretics or potassium supplements.
- Renal artery stenosis or stenosis in a solitary kidney.
- Severe anemia.
- Immune problems, in particular collagen vascular disease and autoimmune disease; ACE inhibitors are necessary. Discontinue the following drugs, which alter immune response: steroids, procainamide, hydralazine, probenecid, tocainide, allopurinol, acebutolol, pindolol, and others.
- Patients known to have neutropenia or thrombocytopenia.
- Severe carotid artery stenosis.
- Restrictive, obstructive, or hypertrophic cardiomyopathies, constrictive pericarditis, cardiac tamponade, and hypertensive hypertrophic cardiomyopathy of the elderly with impaired ventricular relaxation.
- Pregnancy and breastfeeding.
- **Avoid in women aged <45 years who may wish to become pregnant**
- Chlorpromazine therapy because severe hypotension may occur.

Drug name:	**Captopril**
Trade name:	Capoten
Supplied:	12.5, 25, 50 mg
Dosage:	Hypertension: 12.5 mg twice daily for a few days and then three times daily for about 1 week, and then 25 mg three times daily; max. 75–100 mg daily; *see* text for further advice

Dosage (Further Advice)

The 75-mg dose appears to be as effective as higher doses. Do not exceed 150 mg daily. A twice-daily maintenance dose is effective for hypertension. If the BP is not excessively high (systolic >180 mmHg, diastolic >100 mmHg), it is advisable to discontinue diuretics 24–48 h before commencing the ACE inhibitor and to restart them a few days to weeks later, depending on BP response.

In renal failure, increase the dose interval depending on creatinine clearance (GFR):

GFR 75–35 mL/min dose every 12–24 h;
GFR 34–20 mL/min dose every 24–48 h

Drug name:	**Enalapril**
Trade names:	Vasotec, Innovace (UK)
Dosage:	Hypertension: 2.5 mg once daily for 1–2 days, and then 5 mg increasing over weeks or months to 10–20 mg; max. 30 mg (rarely 40 mg); *see* text for further advice

Occasionally, the daily dose must be given in two divided doses to achieve 24-h control of BP. The usual recommended initial dose in patients not taking a diuretic is 5 mg once daily, except in the elderly or in those with renal impairment, and in suspected high renin states as seen with renal artery stenosis, prior diuretic use, and low-sodium diets. Here 2.5 mg is advisable. Note that the serum creatinine level may be normal in patients aged >70 years with renal impairment, and caution with dosage is necessary.

The dosages of ACE inhibitors and ARBs are given in Tables 8-7 and 8-8, respectively. The maximum doses given in these tables are approximately 20 % lower than those stated by the manufacturer. The goal BP should be achieved with approximately 75 % of the maximum dose; if this is not achieved, the drug should be combined with a small dose of another agent.

Table 8-7
ACE inhibitors

Drug	Trade name	Dosage (mg)[a]	Max/day (mg)
Benazepril	Lotensin	5–30	30
Captopril	Capoten	25–100 (2)	100
Cilazapril	Inhibace, Vacase	1–5	5
Enalapril	Vasotec, Innovace	5–20 (1, 2)	30
Fosinpril	Monopril	10–30 (1, 2)	30
Lisinopril	Prinivil, Zestril	5–30 (1)	30
Moexipril	Perdix	7.5–15 (2)	15
Perindopril	Coversyl	2–8	8
Quinapril	Accupri, Accupro	5–40 (1, 2)	40
Ramipril	Altace, Tritace	1.25–15 (1)	15
Trandolapril	Mavik, Gotpen	1–4 (1)	4

(1) once daily; (2) two divided doses
[a]See text: suggested maximum is slightly lower than manufacturer's maximum

For other ACE inhibitors, the action, pharmacokinetics, and adverse effects of ACE inhibitors, and ARBs, *see* Chap. 2.

ACE Inhibitor-Diuretic Combination

Capozide: 15–30 mg contains 15 mg captopril with 30 mg HCTZ for twice-daily dosage. These preparations carry the disadvantages of fixed combinations.

Vaseretic: 10–25 mg contains enalapril 10 mg with HCTZ 25 mg and is effective when given once daily. The combinations are not recommended if there is moderate renal impairment: serum creatinine level >2.3 mg/dL, 203 µmol/L.

Hyzaar: This is a combination of losartan 50 mg and HCTZ 12.5 mg. **Combinations should not be prescribed as initial therapy but only after a trial of a diuretic or ACE inhibitor(ARB) independently.**

Table 8-8
Angiotensin II receptor blockers

Drug	Trade name	Dosage (mg)[a]	Max/day (mg)[a]
Candesartan	Atacand, Amias	4–10	32
Losartan	Cozaar	25–100 (1, 2)	100
Valsartan	Diovan	80–160 (1)	160
Irbesartan	Avapro, Aprovel	75–225 (1)	300
Eprosartan	Teveten	300–400 (2)	800

(1) once daily; (2) two divided doses. Halve the initial dose in elderly patients and in the presence of hepatic or renal impairment

[a]See text: suggested maximum is slightly lower than manufacturer's maximum telmisartan is not recomnded based on clinical trial results (PROFESS (2008) and TRANSCEND (2008); olmesartan is not recommended because of adverse events and probable cancer causation. ARBs appear to be associated with a modestly increased risk for cancer, according to a meta-analysis published in the Lancet Oncology. Sipahi et al. (2010). Should we be concerned about all ARBs or a single drug, telmisartan? Nissen 2010

CALCIUM ANTAGONISTS

Calcium antagonists are recommended for the following situations:

- In older African Americans or if diuretics are contraindicated or cause adverse effects (*see* Table 8-3).
- In younger African Americans if beta-blockers are contraindicated or not well tolerated.
- In older white patients with isolated systolic hypertension if beta-blockers or diuretics are contraindicated or cause adverse effects provided that left ventricular function is normal.
- As second-line therapy in combination with beta-blockers or other agents in patients with angina or renal dysfunction.

The calcium antagonists are used with caution in the following situations:

- Patients with IHD, with silent ischemia, and after MI: diltiazem is indicated if beta-blockers are contraindicated. DHPs may be used in this subset of patients if a beta-blocker is being used concomitantly.
- Patients with hypertension and diabetes: RCTs have shown an increase in mortality in patients treated with extended-release calcium antagonists.
- Patients with HF, LV dysfunction, or ejection fraction <45 %.

Drug name	**Amlodipine**
Trade names:	Norvasc, Istin (UK)
Supplied:	Tablets 5, 10 mg
Dosage:	5 mg, max. 10 mg once daily; initial 2.5 mg in the elderly

Drug name:	**Nifedipine**
Trade names:	Procardia XL, Adalat CC, Adalat LA (UK), Adalat XL (C)
Dosage:	30 mg daily increasing to 60 mg, max. 60 mg

DHPs cause a significant increase in sodium excretion, and a diuretic may not be necessary or may not lower BP further.

Nifedipine and other DHPs may cause rebound hypertension. A case of an increase from 170/100 to 300/200 mmHg has been reported on sudden cessation of nifedipine therapy (Bursztyn et al. 1986). The INSIGHT trial (2000) showed nifedipine equivalent to diuretic in preventing stroke, but it increased the risk of HF significantly.

Drug name:	**Diltiazem extended release**
Trade names:	Cardizem CD, Tiazac, Adizem-XL (UK)
Supplied:	Cardizem CD, Tiazac: 120, 180, 240, 300 mg
Dosage:	120 mg increasing to 240 mg daily, max. 300 mg

Diltiazem is a weak vasodilator, 50 % less potent than DHPs. Caution is needed when this drug is combined with a beta-blocker because bradycardia or LVF may ensue. Interactions occur with digoxin and amiodarone. *A diltiazem-lithium interaction causing psychosis has been reported* (Binder et al. 1991). The NORDIL trial (2000) indicated that diltiazem was as safe as a beta-blocker or diuretic, but there was a small increase in the combined end point of MI and HF.

Drug name:	**Verapamil extended release**
Trade names:	Covera-HS[a], Chronovera[a], Isoptin SR, Securon SR (UK)
Supplied:	120, 180, 240 mg
Dosage:	120 mg once daily, max. 240 mg. [a]180–240 mg daily; reduce the dose in liver disease, renal failure, or the elderly

Caution: Short-acting formulations are not recommended. Verapamil should not be used in patients with acute MI, cardiomegaly, or LV dysfunction. Also avoid in HF, conduction defects, and sick sinus syndrome. Constipation and bradycardia are limiting considerations, particularly in patients aged >70 years. **Combination with a beta-blocker is contraindicated.**

Drug name:	**Felodipine**
Trade names:	Plendil, Renedil
Supplied:	Extended-release tablets: 2.5, 5, 10 mg
Dosage:	2.5–10 mg once daily

Other calcium antagonists are discussed in Chap. 5.

ALPHA1-BLOCKERS

The ACC has issued a caution regarding the use of alpha-blockers for the management of hypertension (ALLHAT 2000). The author issued a caution in the 4 th edition of this book in 1995. Prazosin, terazosin, and doxazosin are not recommended.

Doxazosin, prazosin, terazosin, and vasodilators of this class are known to cause heart failure. In the large well-run ALLHAT hypertensive RCT, doxazosin caused a 82 % increased risk for heart failure versus diuretic therapy (ALLHAT 2000). In addition, they do not significantly prevent or reduce LVH, and have some nonbeneficial effects on the cardiovascular system (*see* Table 8-6).

Drug name:	**Phentolamine**
Trade name:	Rogitine
Supplied:	10 mg/dL; as 1- or 5-mL ampoules
Dosage:	IV: 10–20 µg/kg/min; average 5–10-mg dose IV repeated as necessary Infusion: 5–60 mg over 10–30 min at rate of 0.1–2 mg/min

Phentolamine and phenoxybenzamine block alpha$_1$-receptors and especially alpha$_2$-receptors. The drug is very expensive; action is rapid and lasts only minutes. Thus, nitroprusside is preferred for control of most hypertensive crises including pheochromocytoma.

Drug name:	**Phenoxybenzamine**
Supplied:	10-mg capsules
Dosage:	Pheochromocytoma: 10 mg every 12 h, increasing the dose every 2 days by 10 mg daily; usual dosage 1–2 mg/kg daily in divided doses; saline may be needed to prevent postural hypotension

The drug is given for 1–2 weeks before surgical removal of pheochromocytoma. Postoperative hypotension may be avoided by discontinuing the drug several days before operation and limited use in selected patients. Beta-blockers may be added after 1 week of alpha-blockade, but only if it is necessary to treat catecholamine-induced arrhythmias. HF is a contraindication.

CENTRALLY ACTING DRUGS

Drug name:	**Methyldopa**
Trade name:	Aldomet
Supplied:	125, 250, 500 mg
Dosage:	250 mg twice daily, increasing over days to weeks to 250 mg three times daily; max. 500 mg two or three times daily

Caution: **Methyldopa should be avoided** in patients with active liver disease, depression, or pheochromocytoma. Hemolytic anemia is a well-known complication, and myocarditis causing death has been reported (Seeverens et al. 1982, 47). The drug has a role mainly in pregnancy (see Chap. 20) and in special situations as combination therapy when other agents have failed or are contraindicated. Clonidine is not recommended because it causes significant depression and has variable antihypertensive effects.

Caution: Clonidine is contraindicated in patients with depression. Rebound hypertension can pose a major problem. **Newer agents have rendered centrally acting drugs obsolete.**

RESISTANT HYPERTENSION

Apart from increased salt intake, poor drug compliance or inappropriate drug combinations are common causes of so-called resistance. Some patients treated with triple therapy—ACE inhibitor, calcium antagonist, and beta-blocker—without an added diuretic may portray features of resistance. A diuretic, particularly chlorthalidone, is a necessity in the management of resistant hypertension. It is suggested that in patients with truly resistant hypertension, thiazide diuretics, particularly chlorthalidone, should be considered as one of the initial agents (Vongpatanasin 2014). An AHA scientific statement (Calhoun et al. 2008) and a review article cover this topic in depth (Sarafidis and Bakris 2008).

- If the GFR is 40–50 mL/min, chlorthalidone will be more effective than HCTZ.
- If the GFR is <40, metolazone is the only effective thiazide. Or, a loop diuretic becomes necessary but the short-acting furosemide does not cover 24 h blood-pressure control.
- Miscellaneous drugs that contribute to resistant hypertension include: corticosteroids, NSAIDS, decongestants, anorectics, amphetamines, cyclosporine, tacrolimus, cocaine and illicit drugs, oral contraceptive hormones, and erythropoietin. Other contributing substances include excess alcohol; herbal supplements such as ginseng, yohimbine, ma huang, bitter orange, and licorice stimulate mineralocorticoid production.
- Although rare, renal artery stenosis can cause accelerated resistant hypertension (Calhoun 2008).

Primary hyperaldosteronism

Studies have shown a prevalence of 6–20 % and appear similar in African American and white patients. In a study conducted in Seattle, Washington, primary aldosteronism was diagnosed in 17 % of patients with resistant hypertension (Gallay et al. 2001) and in Norway, this diagnosis was found in 23 %. In an evaluation of more than 600 patients with hypertension, the prevalence of primary hyperaldosteronism was found to be 6.1 % (Mosso et al. 2003).

Importantly, serum potassium levels were rarely low in patients confirmed to have primary aldosteronism. Thus, primary aldosteronism is not uncommon and physicians must not wait for the typical marked fall in serum potassium that occurs in Conn's syndrome. A serum potassium 3.1–3.5 mmol/L or a fall to <3 when diuretics are prescribed for a few weeks should raise suspicion.

- Amiloride antagonizes the epithelial sodium channel in the distal collecting duct of the kidney and thus functions as an indirect aldosterone antagonist (Eide et al. 2004). In a study of 38 patients with low-renin hypertension and resistant uncontrolled hypertension, despite multiple drugs, including a diuretic, substitution with the combination of amiloride 2.5/hydrochlorothiazide 25 mg daily for the prior diuretic lowered systolic and diastolic blood pressure by 31 and 15 mmHg, respectively (Eide et al. 2004).
- Amiloride 5 mg is more effective than spironolactone 25 mg.
- Also, spironolactone is a twice daily drug; amiloride is once a day and does not cause gynecomastia.

Caution is required, however, in prescribing these most beneficial aldosterone antagonists in patients with renal dysfunction to avoid hyperkalemia.

It is suggested that, in patients with truly resistant hypertension, thiazide diuretics, particularly chlorthalidone, should be considered as one of the initial agents (Vongpatanasin 2014).

CATHETER-BASED RADIOFREQUENCY RENAL DENERVATION

SYMPLICITY HTN-3 was a prospective, blinded, randomized, sham-controlled trial. The current analysis details the effect of renal denervation or a sham procedure on ABPM measurements 6 months post-randomization. Conclusions: This trial did not demonstrate a benefit of renal artery denervation on reduction in ambulatory BP in either the 24-h or day and night periods compared with sham (Bakris et al. 2014).

HYPERTENSIVE CRISIS

Hypertensive crisis is usually subclassified into either **hypertensive emergency or urgency**.

* *Hypertensive emergency* is defined as a severe sudden elevation in BP, generally diastolic >120–130 mmHg; some clinicians add: and/or systolic BP > 220 mmHg. The systolic pressures should reflect a knowledge of previous BPs, such as a rise within days from 160–170 to >220 mmHg systolic; the rate of rise of BP in relation to previous BP is more important than the absolute BP. Most important, the sudden excessive elevation in BP should be associated with **acute** organ damage or dysfunction, which confers an immediate threat to the integrity of the cardiovascular system and to life.

In aortic dissection or acute pulmonary edema, a BP of 200/110 mmHg must be reduced. Conditions associated with emergencies are given in Table 8-9.

Table 8-9
Types of hypertensive emergencies

* Accelerated malignant hypertension[a]
* Acute coronary insufficiency
* Acute pulmonary edema (LVF)
* Acute renal dysfunction
* Aortic dissection
* Catecholamine crisis
* Eclampsia
* Hypertensive encephalopathy
* Subarachnoid hemorrhage
* Perioperative hypertension

[a]Severe elevation of blood pressure with papilledema and/or microangiopathic hemolytic anemia, or encephalopathy, or renal dysfunction

Emergencies require reduction in BP within minutes by intravenous (IV) therapy.

For hypertensive emergencies, the goal is to produce an immediate but modest reduction in BP. The objective, in most patients, is to achieve no greater than a 20 % reduction from baseline of the mean arterial pressure or to reduce the diastolic BP to 110 mmHg and no less than 100 mmHg over a period of several minutes to several hours depending on the clinical situation. The BP is maintained at this level for a further 12–24 h, at which time oral therapy should be instituted and a decision made as to the necessity for further lowering of BP. These guidelines do not apply in patients with aortic dissection, in whom BP must be reduced to a much lower level along with the use of a beta-blocking agent to decrease the rate of rise of aortic pressure.

Caution is necessary: nitroprusside and labetalol have caused precipitous reductions in BP in some patients, resulting in cerebral and myocardial ischemia and/or MI.

Hypertensive urgencies refer to other situations in which it is advisable to reduce markedly elevated BP within a day or two, rather than within minutes using oral drugs. These situations include:

- Upper level of stage 3 hypertension: BP commonly systolic >220 mmHg, diastolic >120 mmHg; decrease to 180/100 mmHg.
- Presence of papilledema but without acute deterioration of specific organ systems.
- Progressive but not acute target organ damage, as outlined earlier for hypertensive emergencies.
- Rebound hypertension, for example, after withdrawal of methyldopa, clonidine, or DHPs. If stroke, decrease only to 180/105 mmHg.
- Refractory hypertension: patients in this category, with diastolic BP > 120 mmHg and no acute complications, should be tried first on oral antihypertensive therapy and sedation plus furosemide 40–80 mg IV initially; this is especially

necessary if the history suggests that volume expansion is present; with renal failure, volume overload is usually present.

Drug name:	**Sodium nitroprusside**
Trade name:	Nipride
Dosage:	See text

IV administration is given by infusion pump only. Take care to avoid extravasation. Wrap the infusion bottle in aluminum foil or other opaque material to protect it from light. The prepared solution must be used within 4 h.

One vial (50 mg) sodium nitroprusside in 500 mL 5 % dextrose = 100 µg/mL.

Dose/kg:	µg/kg/min	mL/kg/min
Average:	3	0.03
Range:	0.25–10	0.005–0.08
Dose for a 60-kg patient:	mg/60 kg/min	mL/60 kg/min
Average:	180	1.8
Range:	30–300	0.30–3.0

Start the infusion at the lower dose range (0.5–1 µg/kg/min) and adjust in increments of 0.2 µg/kg/min, usually every 5 min until the desired BP reduction is obtained. The average dose is 3 µg/kg/min (range, 0.5–8 µg/kg/min). A lower initial dose of 300 nanograms/kg/min has been used.

An alternative dosing schedule using less volume is given in Table 11-5.

Oral antihypertensive agents should be started immediately so that the patient can be weaned from nitroprusside as quickly as possible.

Action and Metabolism

Nitroprusside is a potent, rapidly acting, IV antihypertensive agent. The hypotensive effects are caused by peripheral vasodilation and reduction in peripheral resistance as a result of a direct action on vascular smooth muscle, partly through nitric oxide. There is also venous pooling. Because of vasodilation, variable reflex tachycardia occurs. There is a slight decrease in stroke volume and cardiac output. Myocardial oxygen consumption is reduced. The drug's effect on BP is almost immediate (within 0.5–2 min) and usually ends when the IV infusion has stopped. The brief duration of drug action is the result of its rapid biotransformation to thiocyanate. The ferrous ion in nitroprusside reacts with the sulfhydryl groups of red blood cells to produce cyanide ion, which is further reduced to thiocyanate in the liver, which, in turn, is excreted by the kidney.

Advice, Adverse Effects, and Interactions

Contraindications

- Hepatic failure.
- Compensatory hypertension, such as arteriovenous shunt or coarctation of the aorta, corrected hypovolemia or severe anemia.
- Abnormalities of cyanide metabolism: Leber's optic atrophy and tobacco amblyopia.
- Malnutrition, vitamin B_{12} deficiency, and hypothyroidism.
- Severe renal failure and inadequate cerebral circulation; caution is necessary in these patients.
- Pregnancy.
- Raised intracranial pressure.

Fatalities have resulted from cyanide poisoning. In the presence of liver disease, cyanide levels increase with evidence of metabolic acidosis, so it is necessary to measure cyanide levels. If kidney disease exists, thiocyanate levels must be monitored, especially if treatment is to be extended for more than 2 days. Acceleration of infusion from an accident or faulty equipment and failure to monitor the BP accurately have all been associated with hypotension and shock. Retrosternal chest pain and palpitations may also be experienced.

Methemoglobinemia has been reported. Hydroxocobalamin decreases cyanide levels and may be useful to increase the margin of safety. Rebound hypertension can be a problem.

Management of Adverse Effects. Amyl nitrite inhalations and IV sodium thiosulfate are used to treat acute cyanide poisoning. Nitrites form methemoglobin, which combines with cyanide ions to form relatively nontoxic cyanomethemoglobin.

Drug name:	**Labetalol**
Trade names:	Normodyne, Trandate
Dosage:	20–80-mg bolus over at least 1 min, repeat after 5 min, then every 10–15 min if needed to maximum 200 mg; IV infusion: 0.5–2 mg/min

Dosage (Further Advice). IV infusion of 20–160 mg/h (2 mg/min) under close and continuous supervision is given slowly to obtain the desired BP reduction. The onset of action is 5–10 min, and the duration is 3–6 h. The patient must be recumbent throughout the infusion and for at least 4 h afterward. The hypotensive effect may last 1–8 h after cessation of the infusion. Thus, labetalol is not as predictable as nitroprusside. Alternatively, bolus injections are used, starting with a 20-mg dose and gradually increasing the dosage every 10 min to a maximum of 80 mg bolus. Excessive bradycardia can be managed with IV atropine sulphate 0.6–2.4 mg in divided doses of 600 µg.

- Hypertension of pregnancy, 20 mg/h, doubled every 30 min; usual max. 160 mg/h.
- Hypertension complicating MI: 15 mg/h, gradually increased to max. 120 mg/h

Labetalol is a very useful drug for the management of hypertensive emergencies. The drug is especially useful for crises associated with dissecting aneurysm, renal failure, hypertensive encephalopathy, eclampsia, and clonidine withdrawal, as well as in malignant hypertension and in some patients with pheochromocytoma. It is useful perioperatively and postoperatively, such as during neurosurgery for clipping aneurysms and in ear surgery. Adverse effects include bronchospasm, nausea, vomiting, orthostatic hypotension, and, rarely, hepatic necrosis.

Drug name:	**Hydralazine**
Trade name:	Apresoline
Dosage:	10–20 mg; see text

Hydralazine intramuscularly, but preferably by IV infusion, is indicated for hypertensive emergencies, particularly if the condition is associated with renal failure or preeclampsia. The recommended test dose is 10 mg followed in 30 min by an IV infusion of 10–20 mg/h, depending on the response. A maintenance dose of 5–10 mg/h is recommended with continuous monitoring of heart rate and BP. Oral hydralazine is commenced within 24 h, 100–200 mg daily. If there is no contraindication to beta-blockers, propranolol is given IV 1–4 mg and then orally 120–240 mg daily in addition (or the equivalent dose of another beta-blocker). Furosemide 40 mg IV followed by oral HCTZ or furosemide greatly improves the control of BP.

Hydralazine is contraindicated in patients with IHD and aneurysms, in particular dissecting aneurysm, because the drug increases cardiac ejection velocity and the rate of rise of aortic pressure.

Other agents have relegated the use of hydralazine to a role in patients with renal failure and eclampsia.

Fenoldopam increases intraocular pressure and should be avoided in patients with glaucoma or high intraocular pressure; and many elderly may have glaucoma and this information may be missed during the panic to treat urgently. Decreases in serum potassium may occur and this is not desirable. Concomitant use of fenoldopam with beta-blockers should be avoided; but these agents may have been taken as usual therapy for hypertension. Also the drug is expensive.

Diazoxide: other agents have rendered *diazoxide obsolete for hypertensive emergencies.*

Nimodipine is indicated for hypertensive emergencies associated with subarachnoid hemorrhage.

REFERENCES

ACCOMPLISH, Jamerson K, Weber MA, Bakris GL, for the ACCOMPLISH Trial Investigators, et al. Benazepril plus amlodipine or hydrochlorothiazide for hypertension in high-risk patients. N Engl J Med. 2008;359:2417–28.

ALLHAT Officers and Coordinators for the ALLHAT Collaborative Research Group. Major cardiovascular events in hypertensive patients randomized to doxazosin vs chlorthalidone: the Antihypertensive and Lipid-Lowering Treatment to Prevent Heart Attack Trial (ALLHAT). JAMA. 2000;283:1967–75.

ALLHAT Officers and Coordinators for the ALLHAT Collaborative Research Group. Major outcomes in high-risk hypertensive patients randomized to angiotensin-converting enzyme inhibitor or calcium channel blocker vs. diuretic: the antihypertensive and lipid-lowering treatment to prevent heart attack trial (ALLHAT). JAMA. 2002;288:2981–97.

Bakris GL, Townsend RR, Liu M, et al. Impact of renal denervation on 24-hour ambulatory blood pressure: results from SYMPLICITY HTN-3. J Am Coll Cardiol. 2014. doi:10.1016/j.jacc.2014.05.012.

BHAT: β-Blocker Heart Attack Trial Research Group. A randomised trial of propranolol in patients with acute myocardial infarction, I: mortality results. JAMA. 1982;247:1707–14.

Binder EF, Cayabyab L, Ritchie DJ, et al. Diltiazem-induced psychosis and a possible diltiazem-lithium interaction. Arch Intern Med. 1991;151:373.

Biron P, Dessureault J, Napke E. Acute allergic interstitial pneumonitis induced by hydrochlorothiazide. Can Med Assoc J. 1991;145:28.

Boydak B, Nalbantgil S, Fici F, et al. A randomised comparison of the effects of nebivolol and atenolol with and without chlorthalidone on the sexual function of hypertensive men. Clin Drug Investig. 2005;25:409–16.

Brixius K, Middeke M, Lichtenthal A, et al. Nitric oxide, erectile dysfunction and beta-blocker treatment (MR NOED study): benefit of nebivolol versus metoprolol in hypertensive men. Clin Exp Pharmacol Physiol. 2007;34:327–31.

Bursztyn M, Tordjman K, Grossman E, et al. Hypertensive crisis associated with nifedipine withdrawal. Arch Intern Med. 1986;146:397.

Calhoun DA, Jones D, Textor S, et al. AHA scientific statement: resistant hypertension: diagnosis, evaluation, and treatment. Circulation. 2008;117:e510–26.

Calhoun DA, Nishizaka MK, Zaman MA, Thakkar RB, Weissmann P. Hyperaldosteronism among black and white subjects with resistant hypertension. Hypertension. 2002;40:892–6.

Calhoun DA, Jones D, Textor S, et al. AHA scientific statement: resistant hypertension: diagnosis, evaluation, and treatment. Circulation. 2008;117:e510–26.

CAPRICORN Investigators. Effect of carvedilol on outcome after myocardial infarction in patients with left-ventricular dysfunction: the CAPRICORN randomized trial. Lancet. 2001;357:1385.

CAPPP: Hansson L, Lindholm LH, Niskanen L, et al. Effect of angiotensin-converting-enzyme inhibition compared with conventional therapy on cardiovascular morbidity and mortality in hypertension: the Captopril prevention project randomised trial. Lancet. 1999;353(9153):611–16.

Casas JP, Chau W, Loukogeorgakis S, et al. Effect of inhibitors of the renin-angiotensin system and other antihypertensive drugs on renal outcomes: systematic review and meta-analysis. Lancet. 2005;366: 2026–33.

Caskey FJ, Thacker EJ, Johnston PA, et al. Failure of losartan to control blood pressure in scleroderma renal crisis. Lancet. 1997;349:620.

Chen TM, Chiou WL. Large differences in the biological half-life and volume of distribution of hydrochlorothiazide in normal subjects from eleven studies Correlation with their last blood sampling times. Int J Clin Pharmacol Ther Toxicol. 1992;30:34–7.

Clark JA, Zimmerman HF, Tanner LA. Labetalol hepatotoxicity. Ann Intern Med. 1990;113:210.

Cockcroft JR, Chowienczyk PJ, Brett SE, et al. Nebivolol vasodilates human forearm vasculature: evidence for a L-arginine/No-dependent mechanism. J Pharmacol Exp Ther. 1995;274:1067–71.

Cominacini L, Pasini AF, Garbin U, et al. Nebivolol and its 4-keto derivative increase nitric oxide in endothelial cells by reducing its oxidative inactivation. J Am Coll Cardiol. 2003;42:1838–44.

COPERNICUS, Packer M, Coats JS, Fowler MB, for the Carvedilol Prospective Randomized Cumulative Survival (COPERNICUS) Study Group, et al. Effect of carvedilol on survival in severe chronic heart failure. N Engl J Med. 2001;344:1651.

Dahlöf B, Devereux RB, Kjeldsen SE, LIFE Study Group, et al. Cardiovascular morbidity and mortality in the Losartan Intervention For Endpoint reduction in hypertension study (LIFE): a randomised trial against atenolol. Lancet. 2002;359(9311):995–1003.

Deary A, Schumann AL, Murfet H. Double-blind placebo-controlled crossover comparison of five classes of antihypertensive drugs. J Hypertens. 2002;20:771–7.

Devereux RB. Do antihypertensive drugs differ in their ability to regress left ventricular hypertrophy? Circulation. 1985;95:1983.

Dickerson JEC, Hingorani AD, Ashby MJ, et al. Randomisation of antihypertensive treatment by crossover rotation of four major classes. Lancet. 1999;353:2008–13.

Dunn FG, Venture HO, Messerli FH, et al. Time course of regression of left ventricular hypertrophy in hypertensive patients treated with atenolol. Circulation. 1987;76:243.

Eide IK, Torjesen PA, Drolsum A, Babovic A, Lilledahl NP. Lowrenin status in therapy-resistant hypertension: a clue to efficient treatment. J Hypertens. 2004;22:2217–26.

EPHESUS, Pitt B, Remme W, Zannad F, for the Eplerenone Post-Acute Myocardial Infarction Heart Failure Efficacy and Survival Study Investigators, et al. Eplerenone, a selective aldosterone blocker, in patients with left ventricular dysfunction after myocardial infarction. N Engl J Med. 2003;348:1309–21.

Ernst ME, Carter BL, Goerdt CJ, et al. Comparative antihypertensive effects of hydrochlorothiazide and chlorthalidone on ambulatory and office blood pressure. Hypertension. 2006;47:352–8.

Felson DT, Sloutskis D, Anderson J, et al. Thiaxide diuretics and the risk of hip fracture. JAMA. 1991;265:370.

Gallay BJ, Ahmad S, Xu L, Toivola B, Davidson RC. Screening for primary aldosteronism without discontinuing hypertensive medications: plasma aldosterone-renin ratio. Am J Kidney Dis. 2001;37:699–705.

Giles TD, Weber MA, Basile J, for the NAC-MD-01 Study Investigators, et al. Efficacy and safety of nebivolol and valsartan as fixed-dose combination in hypertension: a randomised, multicentre study. Lancet. 2014;383:1889–98.

Gillespie RL, Ferdinand KC, Fergus LV. Criticism of JNC-8P recommendations. J Am Coll Cardiol. 2014;64(4):394–402.

Gray CL, Ndefo UA. Nebivolol: a new antihypertensive agent. Am J Health Syst Pharm. 2008;65(12):1125–33.

HANE, Philipp T, Anlauf M, Distler A, on behalf of the HANE Trial Research Group, et al. Randomised double blind, multicentre comparison of hydrochlorothiazide, atenolol, nitrendipine, and enalapril in antihypertensive treatment: results of the HANE study. BMJ. 1997;315:154.

Hanley AJ, Zinman B, Sheridan P, et al. Effect of rosiglitazone and ramipril on b-cell function in people with impaired glucose tolerance or impaired fasting glucose. Diabetes Care. 2010;33:608–13.

HEAAL Investigators. Konstam MA, Neaton JD, Dickstein K, et al. Effects of high-dose versus low-dose losartan on clinical outcomes in patients with heart failure (HEAAL study): a randomised, double-blind trial. Lancet. 2009;374:1840–48.

Hoegholm A, Rasmussen SW, Kristensen KS. Pulmonary oedema with shock induced by hydrochlorothiazide: a rare side effect mimicking myocardial infarction. Br Heart J. 1990;63:186.

HYVET, Beckett NS, Peters R, Fletcher AE, for the HYVET Study Group, et al. Treatment of hypertension in patients 80 years of age or older. N Engl J Med. 2008;358:1887–98.

INSIGHT, Brown MJ, Christopher RP, Castaigne A. Morbidity and mortality in patients randomized to double blind treatment with a long acting calcium channel blocker or diuretic in the international nifedipine GITS study: Intervention as a Goal in Hypertension Treatment (INSIGHT). Lancet. 2000;356:366.

JNC8, James PA, Oparil S, Carter BL. Evidence-based guideline for the management of high blood pressure in adults report from the panel members appointed to the Eighth Joint National Committee (JNC 8). JAMA. 2014;311(5):507–20.

Kearney PM, Whelton M, Reynolds K. Global burden of hypertension: analysis of worldwide data. Lancet. 2005;365:217–23.

Khan MG. Clinical trials. In: Cardiac drug therapy. 6th ed. Philadelphia: WB Saunders/Elsevier; 2003. p. 502.

Khan MG. Angina. In: Heart disease diagnosis and therapy, a practical approach. 2nd ed. New York: Humana; 2005a p. 150–151.

Khan MG. Hypertension. In: Encyclopedia of heart diseases. 2nd ed. New York: Springer; 2011. p. 556.

Khan MG. Alpha-1 adrenergic blockers. In: Cardiac drug therapy. 4th ed. Philadelphia, PA: WB Saunders; 1995. p. 103.

Krakoff LR, Gillespie RL, Ferdinand KC, et al. Hypertension recommendations from the Eighth Joint National Committee Panel Members Raise Concerns for Elderly Black and Female Populations. J Am Coll Cardiol. 2014;64(4):394–402.

LaCroix AZ, Wienpahl J, White LR, et al. Thiazide diuretic agents and the incidence of hip fracture. N Engl J Med. 1990;322:288.

Maffei A, Lembo G. Nitric oxide mechanisms of nebivolol. Ther Adv Cardiovasc Dis. 2009;3(4):317–27.

Materson BJ, Reda D, Freiss ED, Henderson WG. Cigarette smoking interferes with treatment of hypertension. Arch Intern Med. 1988;148:2116.

Materson BJ, Reda DJ, Cushman WC, et al. Single-drug therapy for hypertension in men: a comparison of six antihypertensive agents with placebo. N Engl J Med. 1993;328:914.

Materson BJ, Reda DJ. Correction: single-drug therapy for hypertension in men. N Engl J Med. 1994;330:1689.

Morales-Salinas A, Coca A, Wyss FS. Guidelines for managing high blood pressure. JAMA. 2014;312(3):293–4.

Mosso L, Carvajal C, González A, Barraza A, Avila F, Montero J, Huete A, Gederlini A, Fardella CE. Primary aldosteronism and hypertensive disease. Hypertension. 2003;42:161–5.

Multicenter Diltiazem Postinfarction Trial Research Group. The effect of diltiazem on mortality and re-infarction after myocardial infarction. N Engl J Med. 1988;319:385.

Münzel T, Gori T. Nebivolol. The somewhat-different b-adrenergic receptor blocker. J Am Coll Cardiol. 2009;54:1491–9.

Murphy MB, Murray C, Shorten G. Fenoldopam: a selective peripheral dopamine-receptor agonist for the treatment of severe hypertension: Review article. N Engl J Med. 2001;345:1548.

Nissen SE. Angiotensin-receptor blockers and cancer: urgent regulatory review needed. Lancet Oncol. 2010. doi:10.1016/S1470-2045(10)70106-6. Early Online Publication.

NORDIL, Hansson L, Hedner T, Lund-Johansen P, et al. Randomized trial of effects of calcium antagonists compared with diuretics and beta-blockers on cardiovascular morbidity and mortality in hypertension: the Nordic Diltiazem study. Lancet. 2000;356:359.

Norwegian Multicentre Study Group. Timolol-induced reduction in mortality in reinfarction in patients surviving acute myocardial infarction. N Engl J Med. 1981;304:801.

PRAISE, Packer M, O'Connor CM, Ghali JK, for the Prospective Randomized Amlodipine Survival Evaluation (PRAISE), et al. Effect of amlodipine on morbidity and mortality in severe chronic heart failure. N Engl J Med. 1996;335:1107.

PRoFESS, Yusuf S, Diener HC, Sacco RL, for the PRoFESS Study Group, et al. Telmisartan to prevent recurrent stroke and cardiovascular events. N Engl J Med. 2008;359:1225–37.

PROGRESS Collaborative Group. Randomized trial of a perindopril-based blood pressure lowering regimen among, individuals with previous stroke or transient ischaemic attack. Lancet. 2001;358:1033.

Ray WA, Griffin MR, Downey W. Long-term use of thiazide diuretics and risk of hip fracture. Lancet. 1989;1:687.

Riess W, Dubach UC, Burckhardt D, et al. Pharmacokinetic studies with chlorthalidone (Hygroton) in man. Eur J Clin Pharmacol. 1977;12: 375–82.

Sarafidis PA, Bakris GL. Resistant hypertension an overview of evaluation and treatment. J Am Coll Cardiol. 2008;52(22):1749–57.

Seeverens H, de Bruin CD, Jordans JGM. Myocarditis and methyldopa. Acta Med Scand. 1982;211:233–5.

SENIORS, van Veldhuisen DJ, Cohen-Solal A, Bohm M, et al. Beta-blockade with nebivolol in elderly heart failure patients with impaired and preserved left ventricular ejection fraction: data from (Study of Effects of Nebivolol Intervention on Outcomes and Rehospitalization in Seniors with Heart Failure). J Am Coll Cardiol. 2009;53:2150–8.

SHEP Cooperative Study Group. Prevention of stroke by antihypertensive drug treatment in older persons with isolated systolic hypertension: final results of the Systolic Hypertension in Elderly Programs (SHEP). JAMA. 1991;265:3255.

Sipahi I, Debanne SM, Rowland DY. Angiotensin-receptor blockade and risk of cancer: meta-analysis of randomised controlled trials. Lancet Oncol. 2010;11(9):819–820.

Siscovick DS, Raghanathan TE, Psaty BM, et al. Diuretic therapy for hypertension and the risk of primary cardiac arrest. N Engl J Med. 1994;330:1852.

Staessen JA, Wang JG, Thijs L. Cardiovascular protection and blood pressure reduction: a meta-analysis. Lancet. 2001;358:1305.

STOP 2, Hansson L, Lindholm LH, Ekbom T, et al. Randomised trial of old and new antihypertensive drugs in elderly patients: cardiovascular mortality and morbidity, the Swedish Trial in Old Patients with Hyper-tension-2 study. Lancet. 1999;354:1751–6.

The seventh report of the Joint National Committee on Prevention, Detection, Evaluation, and Treatment of High Blood Pressure. JAMA. 2003;289:2560–72.

TRANSCEND, Yusuf S, Teo K, Anderson C, for the TRANSCEND Investigators, et al. Effects of the angiotensin-receptor blocker telmisartan on cardiovascular events in high-risk patients intolerant to angiotensin converting enzyme inhibitors: a randomised controlled trial. Lancet. 2008;372:1174–83.

Tuncer M, Fettser DV, Gunes Y, et al. Comparison of effects of nebivolol and atenolol on P-wave dispersion in patients with hypertension [in Russian]. Kardiologiia. 2008;48:42–5.

UKPDS: UK Prospective Diabetes Study Group. Efficacy of atenolol and captopril in reducing risk of macrovascular and microvascular complications in type 2 diabetes. BMJ. 1998;317:713.

Val-HeFT, Cohn JN, Tognoni G, for the Valsartan Heart Failure Trial Investigators. A randomized trial of the angiotensin-receptor blocker valsartan in chronic heart failure. N Engl J Med. 2001;345:1667–75.

VALIANT, Pfeffer MA, McMurray JJ, Velazquez EJ, et al. Valsartan, captopril, or both in myocardial infarction complicated by heart failure, left ventricular dysfunction, or both. N Engl J Med. 2003;349:1893–906.

Vongpatanasin W. Resistant hypertension: a review of diagnosis and management. JAMA. 2014;311(21):2216–24.

Zweifler AJ, Shahab ST. Pseudohypertension: a new assessment. J Hypertens. 1993;11:1–6.

9 Hypertension Controversies

BETA-BLOCKERS SHOULD NOT REMAIN FIRST CHOICE IN THE TREATMENT OF PRIMARY HYPERTENSION: TRUE OR FALSE?

A meta-analysis by Lindholm et al. (2005) concluded that beta-blockers should not remain as the first choice in the treatment of primary hypertension and should not be used as reference drugs in future randomized controlled trials (RCTs) of hypertension. Unfortunately, many experts in the field have endorsed the conclusions of this faulty meta-analysis produced by Lindholm et al. (2005).

Beta-blockers have been used for more than 40 years for the treatment of hypertension. The controversy regarding their continued use is of paramount importance, particularly because there are more than one billion hypertensive individuals who require treatment, and only four classes of antihypertensive agents are available: beta-blockers, diuretics, calcium antagonists, and angiotensin-converting enzyme (ACE) inhibitors or angiotensin receptor blockers (ARBs). The two other drug classes [alpha-blockers (doxazosin) and centrally acting agents (methyldopa, clonidine)] have been rendered relatively obsolete for the management of primary hypertension (see discussion and alpha-blocker section in Chap. 8). Methyldopa remains useful mainly for some patients with hypertension in pregnancy.

© Springer Science+Business Media New York 2015
M. Gabriel Khan, *Cardiac Drug Therapy*, Contemporary Cardiology,
DOI 10.1007/978-1-61779-962-4_9

Unfortunately, Lindholm and colleagues (2005), trialists, and physicians fail to realize that beta-blocking agents are not all alike and that the most prescribed beta-blocker, atenolol, has poor efficacy. Beta-blockers have subtle and important differences among them (Khan 2005) that have not been recognized by senior researchers and clinicians worldwide:

- In 14 studies analyzed by Lindholm et al., atenolol was the beta-blocker used; in four trials, mixtures of atenolol, metoprolol, and pindolol were used (see Table 9-1).
- In a Lancet letter, Cruickshank (2006) stated that by lumping together all randomized hypertension trials involving beta-blockers, Lars Lindholm and colleagues have arrived at misleading conclusions, but letters in journals are perused by few readers.
  - **Atenolol should not be used in hypertensive drug trials that compare it with other antihypertensive agents (Khan 2003). This widely prescribed beta-blocker should become obsolete** (Khan 2011). The author used atenolol from 1974 to 1984 and agrees that the drug probably causes less side effects than propranolol and metoprolol.
  - But less adverse effects equates with lower salutary effects because of poor brain concentration.
  - Unfortunately the majority of hypertensive RCTs done from 1985 to 2007 used atenolol. There are no sound RCTs in which propranolol, metoprolol or bisoprolol were used.

This discussion reviews trials selected by Lindholm and colleagues and emphasizes that the meta-analysis suggests that atenolol is not an effective choice for the management of hypertension but does not indicate that other beta-blockers are ineffective in decreasing cardiovascular disease (CVD) morbidity and mortality associated with hypertension.

Table 9-1

Clinical trials assessed in the meta-analysis by Lindholm et al. (2005) and relevant effects

Trial	No. of patients (year of follow-up)	Total mortality	Stroke	Myocardial infarction
MRC 1985	8,700			
Propranolol[a]				
vs. placebo		120 vs. 253 RR 0.93	42 vs. 109 RR 0.76	103 vs. 234 RR 0.87
vs. diuretic		120 vs. 128 RR 0.91	42 vs. 18 RR 2.28	103 vs. 119 RR 0.84
MRC[b] 1992	4,396 (5.8)			
Atenolol vs. diuretic		—[c]	—[c]	—[c]
IPPSH (1985)	6,357 (4)	108 vs. 114 RR 0.94	45 vs. 46 RR 0.97	96 vs. 104 RR 0.92
Oxprenolol[d] vs. placebo				
Berglund (1986)	106 (10)	5 vs. 4 NS	—	—
Propranolol vs. diuretic				
Yurenev (1992)	304 (4)	1 vs. 7 RR 0.15	6 vs. 11 RR 0.56	7 vs. 6 RR 1.2
Propranolol vs. non-beta-blocker				

(continued)

Table 9-1 (Continued)

Trial	No. of patients (year of follow-up)	Total mortality	Stroke	Myocardial infarction
Dutch TIA (1993)	1,473	64 vs. 58	52 vs. 62	45 vs. 40
Atenolol vs. placebo	(2.6)	RR 1.12	RR 0.85	RR 1.14
UKPDS (1998)	758	59 vs. 75	17 vs. 21	46 vs. 61
Atenolol vs. captopril	(9)[d]	RR 0.88	RR 0.90	RR 0.84[e]
LIFE (2002)	9,193	431 vs. 383	309 vs. 232	188 vs. 198
Atenolol vs. losartan	(4.8)	RR 1.13	RR 1.34	RR 0.95
ASCOT-BPLA (2005)	19,257	820 vs. 738	422 vs. 327	444 vs. 390
Atenolol + diuretic	(5.7)	RR 1.11	RR 1.29	RR 1.1[f]
Amlodipine + perindopril				
STOP-2 (Hansson et al. 1999a)	6,614	369 vs. 742	237 vs. 422	154 vs. 318
Atenolol		RR 0.99	RR 1.12	RR 0.96
Pindolol[d]				
Metoprolol	2,213			
vs. ACE inhibitor	(5)			
or	2,205			
calcium antagonist	2,196			

NORDIL (Hansson et al. 1999a) Any beta-blocker vs. diltiazem	10,881 (4.5)	228 vs. 221 RR 0.98	196 vs. 159 RR 1.22	157 vs. 183 RR 0.85[e]
CONVINCE (2003) Atenolol vs. verapamil	16,476 (3)	319 vs. 337 RR 0.93	118 vs. 133 NS	166 vs. 133 RR 1.23[g]
Not assessed by Lindholm et al.	10,985	82 vs. 95	193 vs. 149	163 vs. 164
CAPP (Hansson et al. 1999b) Captopril vs. atenolol or metoprolol	(6)	NS	RR 1.25[h]	NS

ACE angiotensin-converting enzyme, *NS* not significant, *RR* relative risk

[a]Not effective in smokers; *see* text

[b]Poorly run RCT; 25 % lost to follow-up; *see* text

[c]The only long-term RCT in diabetics, high-risk patients; beta-blocker = to captopril

[d]Has intrinsic sympathomimetic activity (ISA): destroys cardioprotection

[e]Marked significant reduction in fatal and nonfatal myocardial infarction (MI) in high-risk diabetic patients compared with captopril; surely a diuretic cannot outperform a beta-blocker in preventing coronary heart disease (CHD) events in any group of patients; trials that indicate this superior effect of diuretics are obscure; it is only observed in the poorly run MRC trials. In NORDIL, beta-blocker is better than diltiazem for CHD events

[f]Primary end point

[g]Verapamil caused a 30 % increase in congestive heart failure

[h]Captopril caused a 29.5 % increase in fatal and nonfatal strokes vs. beta-blocker; the opposite effect occurred in LIFE

- The reasons for the ineffectiveness of atenolol and the subtle differences that prevail among the available beta-blocking drugs are discussed.
- Trials selected for meta-analysis by Lindholm et al. include the following:
- The International Prospective Primary Prevention Study in Hypertension (IPPSH): Oxprenolol was used (IPPPSH collaborative group 1985). The drug has intrinsic sympathomimetic activity (ISA), which renders it noncardioprotective; thus, all beta-blockers cannot be blamed for a poor choice of oxprenolol.
- Berglund et al. (1986), Yurenev et al. (1992), and a Dutch trial (1993): These investigators studied only 106, 304, and 720 patients, respectively. Should clinicians accept this type of meta-analysis of apples and oranges?
- The Swedish Trial of Old Patients-2 (STOP-2) (Hansson et al. 1999a, b: 7): In 6,614 elderly hypertensive patients, a diuretic or beta-blocker (atenolol, metoprolol, and pindolol, an ISA beta-blocker) or both were compared with newer drugs – ACE inhibitors (enalapril, lisinopril) or calcium antagonists (felodipine or isradipine). The findings at 6 years were as follows: old and newer antihypertensive drugs were similar in the prevention of cardiovascular mortality or events. At the final visit, only 61–66 % of patients were still taking the agents allocated to them, and this was not a comparative beta-blocker trial. An unsound trial.
- Medical Research Council (MRC 1985) trial: For mild hypertension, propranolol was the beta-blocker used compared with diuretic therapy. Propranolol, but not diuretics, reduced the risk of myocardial infarction by 13 %, which increased to a significant 18 % when silent infarctions were included. In a subsequent subanalysis compared with placebo, the reduction in nonsmokers was 33 %. Nonsmokers given propranolol showed a trend toward reduction in coronary events and significant decrease in strokes; the diuretic bendrofluazide showed a reduction in strokes but not in coronary events. Another unsound trial. Methodology was poor.

- A Lancet editorial (1985) considered the possibility that beta-blockers were preferable in nonsmoking men. The expert author of the editorial did not know that the cardioprotective effects of beta-blockers other than propranolol are not decreased by cigarette smoking.

- Cigarette smoke increases the rate of metabolic degradation of propranolol, and a decrease in plasma propranolol levels has been shown in smokers. Timolol, a partially metabolized drug, was shown to be effective in significantly reducing total and cardiac deaths in smokers and nonsmokers (Norwegian trial 1981).

• MRC trial in the elderly (1992): The beta-blocker used was atenolol.

- **The MRC Working Party** (1992) **confirmed that 25 % of patients were lost to follow-up and more than half the patients were not taking the therapy assigned by the end of the study. A pathetic study used by Messerli et al. (1989) in an editorial condemning beta-blockers.**

- There was no difference in total mortality between atenolol and diuretic therapy, but, surprisingly, diuretics reduced coronary heart disease (CHD) events, and atenolol did not. This is a spurious finding; to this date, we do not use diuretics to effectively treat patients with CHD, but we do use beta-blockers.

- **This obscure and misleading finding nevertheless led Messerli et al. (1998) to publish an article in the *Journal of the American Medical Association* entitled "Are β-Blockers Efficacious as First-Line Therapy for Hypertension in the Elderly?"**

- These analysts concluded that beta-blockers should not be first-line therapy for elderly hypertensives.

- Unfortunately, this faulty opinion has gained access to notable textbooks and journals and the brains of medical teachers. **It appears that virtually all internists**

and guideline providers (UK and USA) share this faulty opinion, which has been spread worldwide.

- The Controlled Onset Verapamil Investigation of Cardiovascular End Points (CONVINCE 2003): 8,241 hypertensive patients received 180 mg of verapamil, and 8,361 received either 50 mg of atenolol or 12.5 mg of hydrochlorothiazide. The findings at 3 years were as follows: "There were 364 primary CVD-related events that occurred in the verapamil group vs. 365 in the atenolol or hydrochlorothiazide group [hazard ratio (HR), 1.02; 95 % confidence interval (CI), 0.88–1.18; $p = 0.77$]." Importantly, more cardiovascular disease (CVD)-related events occurred between 6 AM and noon in both the verapamil (99/277) and atenolol or hydrochlorothiazide (88/274) groups. A blunderbuss study.

- **It must be emphasized that atenolol does not provide a full 24-h action.** Neutel et al. (1993) indicated that bisoprolol reduced ambulatory systolic and diastolic pressures by 43 % and 49 %, respectively, more than atenolol during early morning hours. **The drug fails to quell early morning catecholamine surge, a time at which there is an increased risk of ischemia and sudden death. It is not surprising, therefore, that this beta-blocker is only partially CVD protective.**

Reasons for the poor cardiovascular protective effects of atenolol are given in Chaps. 1 and 2.

The JNC 8 (2014), the UK, and European guidelines have misled general physicians and clinicians worldwide by excluding beta-blockers as a first-line or second-line agent to treat selected patients with mild hypertension. There opinion is based on atenolol failures and not on the proven effectiveness of other beta-blockers: bisoprolol, carvedilol, metoprolol succinate (Toprol XL), and nebivolol.

Conclusion

- Clinicians are presented with the aforementioned facts and can draw their own conclusions.

- Beta-blockers, particularly bisoprolol, carvedilol, Toprol XL, nebivolol, and metoprolol succinate (extended release), should remain as the initial choice along with diuretics ACE inhibitors and calcium antagonists in the treatment of primary hypertension depending on age and ethnicity. Calcium antagonists and ACE inhibitors or ARBs are not superior.
- **It is now important for the physician to select an appropriate beta-blocker with the understanding that all beta-blockers are not alike.**

DIABETIC RISK WITH BETA-BLOCKERS AND DIURETICS

An Increased Risk: True or False?

An important area of concern is the so-called increased incidence of diabetes caused by beta-blockers and diuretics. The poor CVD outcomes in diabetic patients behoove us to be cautious in recommending agents that might increase the incidence of diabetes.

I have cited evidence from clinical trials to indicate that the increased incidence of type 2 diabetes mellitus reported in RCTs and editorials is unproved and is false.

- It is well established that diabetics have the same CVD risk as do patients with established CVD. Diabetes increases the risk of coronary artery disease (CAD) twofold in men and fourfold in women (Zanchetti et al. 2001). A proclaimed small increased risk for the development of type 2 diabetes caused by beta-blocker and diuretic therapy in hypertensive individuals has become a concern.
- Clinicians should ask whether this incidence is real or are there other explanations for the observed modest increase in fasting glucose concentrations observed in a few patients on long-term treatment with these agents.

Other explanations include:

- Incorrect diagnosis of type 2 diabetes mellitus. In virtually all clinical trials (randomized and nonrandomized), a definition of diabetes was an increase in glucose levels >126 mg/dL (7 mmol/L). This was the criterion used in several RCTs including ALLHAT, the largest RCT.
- A fasting glucose of 7–7.9 mmol/L, even if repeated twice, should qualify as glucose intolerance and is not diagnostic of diabetes mellitus in patients administered a beta-blocking drug and/or a diuretic.
- Mild reversible glucose intolerance is not necessarily diabetes mellitus. When diuretics and or beta-blocker therapy is discontinued, mild glucose intolerance reverts to normal in virtually all patients who are not genuinely diabetics, but glucose levels remain elevated in patients who are prediabetics.

Murphy et al. (1982) **reported on the results of a 14-year follow-up in hypertensive patients treated with a diuretic that showed a major increase in the incidence of glucose intolerance. This effect was promptly reversed on discontinuation of the diuretic in more than 60 % of individuals. The remaining patients were prediabetics.**

- It must be emphasized that based solely on the finding of glucose intolerance, the learned physicians (Murphy et al. 1982) did not classify these individuals as diabetics. Thus, current trialists and experts in the field should avoid putting a label of diabetes mellitus on individuals who might have reversible benign glucose intolerance, as did the subjects studied by Murphy and colleagues. Similar findings have been reported when beta-blocker therapy is discontinued.

In a few patients treated with a beta-blocking drug for more than 5 years, fasting glucose may increase to 6.5 or 7–7.5, but 2–3 months later revert to 5–5.9 even when on the same dose of the beta-blocking drug. This fluctuation may persist for several years without culminating in a true diabetic state.

HYPERTENSIVE AGENTS INCREASE HEART FAILURE RISK: TRUE OR FALSE?

Beta-blockers and diuretics are effective treatment for heart failure and in hypertensive individuals do not cause an increased risk for HF, but alpha-blockers, including doxazosin, and calcium antagonists have been shown to cause a significant increase in HF in hypertensive patients in long-term studies (ALLHAT 2000, 2002) (see Table 9-2).

1. In ALLHAT (2000), a significant 82 % higher rate for HF was observed for the alpha-blocker doxazosin. "HF risk was doubled (4-year rates, 8.13 % vs. 4.45 %; RR, 2.04; 95 % CI, 1.79–2.32; $p < 0.001$)." In the second edition of this book the author gave a warning, and in the fourth edition (1995), cautioned that the use of alpha-blockers should be curtailed.
2. In the INSIGHT trial (2000), a 46 % higher rate of HF was observed with calcium antagonist therapy vs. older drug regimens (Table 9-2).
   • There was no difference in RR for dihydropyridines compared with diltiazem and verapamil (Neal et al. 2000; Pahor et al. 2000).
   • The amlodipine group had a 32 % higher risk of HF ($p < 0.001$), with a 6-year absolute risk difference of 2.5 % and a 35 % higher risk of hospitalization for fatal

Table 9-2
Antihypertensive agents and risk for heart failure

Drugs	Trial	Risk for heart failure
Doxazosin	ALLHAT (2000)	82 % versus diuretic
Amlodipine	ALLHAT	32 % versus diuretic
Lisinopril	ALLHAT	19 % versus diuretic
Nifedipine	INSIGHT (2000)	46 % versus diuretic
Carvedilol	CAPRICORN (2001)	Significantly decreased risk

HF ($p<0.001$). Elderly blacks had the highest increase in HF. ACE inhibitor and lisinopril caused a 19 % higher risk of HF ($p<0.001$).

AGE AND ETHNICITY HOLD THE KEY FOR DRUG CHOICE

The choice of initial drug in patients without compelling reasons should be based on:

- Age younger or older than 60 years
- Ethnicity: nonblack or patients of African origin

It is well established that >60 % of hypertensive individuals require more than one drug to attain goal blood pressures. However, monotherapy is worth the effort because in patients with mild primary hypertension (stages I–II), if clinicians use the age and ethnicity formula, monotherapy is expected to obtain blood pressure (BP) goal in about 50 %.

- The advice to begin with a diuretic in most is logical and sound advice based on the results of numerous well-run RCTs including the hallmark ALLHAT (2002).
- Diuretics, however, are not very effective blood pressure-lowering agents in younger whites (Materson and Reda 1994; Deary 2002; Dickerson 1999) and, although effective in the elderly, may cause frequency of micturition and use should be individualized.
- ALLHAT (2002) and SHEP (1991) gave conclusive proof as to the salutary CVD effects of diuretics vs. newer agents in their study of patients with mean ages of 67 and 72 years, respectively.
  - For patients older than 80, HYVET (Beckett et al. 2008) proved the effectiveness of small dose diuretic: indapamide, 1.25 mg or chlorthalidone 25 mg alternate day; this should suffice in the majority; some may require a small dose of beta-blocker added, for example, bisoprolol 5 mg daily.

- The safety of a small dose of beta-blocker is assured because we do know that the majority of elderly patients (age 70–85) with atrial fibrillation are safely controlled with a small dose of bisoprolol 2.5–5 mg daily. The combination of small dose diuretic and very small dose of a beta-blocker is safer than the addition of an ACE inhibitor (ARB) or calcium antagonist because this addition may cause too excessive lowering of blood pressure and injury from falls. At this age, a systolic pressure of 145–155 does not require further lowering except in those with heart failure or renal failure in whom a pressure of 130–140 is advisable.

- ACE inhibitors or ARBs are as effective as beta-blockers in reducing CVD outcomes in nonblack individuals younger than age 60 years, and either agent may be chosen depending on the patient's characteristics.
- ACE inhibitors or ARBs, however, are not superior to beta-blocker therapy if atenolol is excluded.

The Perindopril Protection Against Recurrent Stroke Study (PROGRESS 2001) was a large, well-run RCT of 6,105 individuals with hypertension and previous stroke or transient ischemic attack.

- The ACE inhibitor perindopril attained blood pressure goal in only about 42 % of trial patients, and no discernible reduction in the primary outcome, reduction in the risk of stroke, was observed.
- Reduction in CVD events was observed only with the combination of captopril and diuretic.

In CAPP, fatal and nonfatal stroke was more common with the ACE inhibitor captopril (189 vs. 148) for the beta-blocker atenolol or metoprolol and diuretic therapy ($p=0.044$) (1999).

The British guidelines use age < or >55 years and ethnicity; this provides logical advice based on the renin hypothesis. However, their recommendation to use a calcium antagonist in the elderly black or nonblack individual should be reexamined because these agents increase HF risk, particularly so in black hypertensive individuals (see Table 9-1).

The following are suggested drug choices based on age and ethnicity:

1. Nonblack individuals aged < 60 years:
   - A hallmark randomized parallel group study in 1292 men by Materson et al. (1993) compared younger black patients, younger white patients, older black patients, and older white patients treated with a diuretic, a beta-blocker, an ACE inhibitor, or a calcium antagonist. The study indicated that in younger white patients, a beta-blocker or ACE inhibitor had equal BP-lowering effects and was superior to diuretic or calcium antagonist therapy.
   - Deary et al. (2002) completed a double-blind placebo-controlled crossover comparison of five antihypertensive drugs (amlodipine, doxazosin, lisinopril, bisoprolol. and bendrofluazide) and placebo in 34 young nonblack hypertensives and showed that bendrofluazide performed significantly worse ($p = 0.0016$) and a beta-blocker, bisoprolol, significantly better ($p = 0.004$).
   - Dickerson et al. (1999) undertook a crossover rotation of the four main classes of antihypertensive drugs in 40 untreated young white hypertensive patients aged < 55 years to assess the response rate with monotherapy achieved by a systematic rotation; 36 patients completed all four cycles. Success of monotherapy was achieved ($p = 0.0001$); in half the patients, BP on the best treatment was 135/85 mmHg or less. The responses to the ACE inhibitor or beta-blocker pair were, on average, at least 50 % higher than those to the calcium antagonist/diuretic pair. Both studies agree with the findings of Materson et al. that in younger white patients, a beta-blocker or ACE inhibitor is equally effective as monotherapy in approximately 45 % of nonblack patients with mild primary hypertension.

In this RCT, the ACCOMPLISH trial investigators assigned 11,506 patients with hypertension who were at high risk for cardiovascular events to receive treatment with either benazepril plus amlodipine or benazepril plus hydrochlorothiazide. The primary end point was the composite of death from cardiovascular causes, nonfatal MI, nonfatal stroke, hospitalization for angina, and coronary revascularization (ACCOMPLISH Trial Investigators, Jamerson et al. 2008).

– **After a mean follow-up of 36 months, the trial was halted. There were 552 primary-outcome events in the benazepril–amlodipine group (9.6 %) and 679 in the benazepril–hydrochloro-thiazide group (11.8 %), representing an absolute risk reduction with benazepril–amlodipine therapy of 2.2 % and a relative risk reduction of 19.6 % [hazard ratio, 0.80, 95 % confidence interval (CI), 0.72–0.90; $p < 0.001$].**

For the secondary end point of death from cardiovascular causes, nonfatal MI, and nonfatal stroke, the hazard ratio was 0.79; $p = 0.002$. The benazepril–amlodipine combination was superior to the benazepril–hydrochlorothiazide combination in reducing cardiovascular events (ACCOMPLISH Trial Investigators 2008).

The initial drug for nonblack individuals younger than 60 years should be an appropriate beta-blocker (carvedilol, bisoprolol, metoprolol succinate extended release (Toprol XL) carvedilol or nebivolol) or an ACE inhibitor or combination of amlodipine + ACE inhibitor as done in ACCOMPLISH (2008). An ACE inhibitor is an appropriate second choice for initial therapy, but physicians may appropriately choose these agents as first line. ACE inhibitors are fairly effective first-line agents in younger nonblack patients.

But they attain goal BP in only about 42 % of patients, a similar efficacy to monotherapy with beta-blocker or diuretic therapy. What is best for one is not as good for another; thus, monotherapy should be well tried in patients with mild essential hypertension.

2. Younger individuals of African origin aged < 60 years:
   - The Materson et al. study (1993) indicated that calcium antagonists were most effective followed by beta-blockers and then diuretics and a poor response to ACE inhibitors.

     Also, ACE inhibitors carry a grave risk for angioedema; to have loss of life or emergency visits is not acceptable when treating patients with mild to moderate hypertension at low risk. ACE inhibitors cause a higher risk for angioedema in black vs. white patients. Several studies have documented a lower efficacy of ACE inhibitors in blacks vs. nonblack patients. In two RCTs, greater differences were observed in black vs. nonblack patients for combined CVD along with a similar trend for HF and lesser BP reduction (Saunders et al. 1990; Cushman et al. 2000).

3. Older individuals of African origin aged > 60 years:
   - The initial agent advised is a diuretic because of safety.
   - If goal BP readings are not achieved, the diuretic should be discontinued and a beta-blocker given, preferably bisoprolol metoprolol succinate (Toprol XL), nebivolol, or carvedilol.

     If difficult to control on beta-blockers and diuretics, the combination of amlodipine and ARB is advisable: ARB (an ARB is chosen because of the risk of angioedema with ACE) (see ACCOMPLISH 2008).
   - The beta-blockers carvedilol, bisoprolol, and metoprolol are as effective as diuretics in achieving goal BP and in reducing CVD outcomes in the elderly nonblack patient. In the Materson et al. study, BP goal was achieved by 68 %, 64 %, and 52 % in older white patients treated with beta-blocker, diltiazem, and diuretic, respectively. However, in the MRC trial (1992) of hypertension in

elderly white patients, surprisingly, a reduction in CHD events was attained by diuretic therapy but not with atenolol. In this trial, more than 25 % of patients were lost to follow-up, and 63 % of patients in the atenolol group were either lost to follow-up or withdrawn for various reasons. This obscure trial finding nevertheless led Messerli and colleagues (1998: 13) to state incorrectly that diuretics and not beta-blockers are the treatment of choice in elderly hypertensives. Unfortunately, their advice was published in most textbooks and journals. A rebuttal with which I concur was made by Kendall and Cohen (1999) regarding the recommendation for treatment with beta-blockers in elderly hypertensives.

- Beta-blockers with proven cardioprotective properties, particularly carvedilol, bisoprolol, timolol, and metoprolol, have been shown to prevent fatal and nonfatal MI in the elderly with CHD with or without coexisting hypertension. Diuretics do not have a basis for a protective role in atheroma rupture and thus are not expected to prevent the occurrence of fatal and nonfatal MI.
- Failure to achieve target BP should result in a combination of diuretic and beta-blocker, each at small doses.
- Diltiazem or amlodipine should be tried next at a low dose plus low-dose diuretic; a low-dose combination decreases risk for HF. The British guideline recommends either a calcium antagonist or a diuretic. Caution is necessary because HF has reached epidemic proportions in the elderly population. Calcium antagonists are effective in achieving goal blood pressure in the elderly, but they carry a substantial risk for HF. In ALLHAT, participants were older than age 55 years (mean age 67 years), and amlodipine caused a 32 % increased risk for HF. Other RCTs have documented that calcium antagonists including the dihydropyridines verapamil and diltiazem increase the risk of HF in the elderly (see Table 9-2).

4. Patients of Non African origin aged > 60 years:
   - A diuretic is the drug of choice, as indicated in the Materson et al. study and proved in ALLHAT (2002), in

which CVD outcomes were significantly reduced by diuretics, with calcium antagonists showing no advantages.

- A calcium antagonist may be considered as second-line therapy in patients in whom diuretics cause adverse effects, and there is no suspicion of left ventricular dysfunction.
- An increased risk for HF was observed for verapamil in the CONVINCE study (2003), for amlodipine in ALLHAT (2002), and for the dihydropyridines in other RCTs. This risk is higher in patients older than age 60 years than in younger individuals.

REFERENCES

ACCOMPLISH, Jamerson K, Weber MA, Bakris GL et al. for the ACCOMPLISH Trial Investigators. Benazepril plus amlodipine or hydrochlorothiazide for hypertension in high-risk patients. N Engl J Med. 2008;359:2417–28.

ALLHAT Officers and Coordinators for the ALLHAT Collaborative Research Group. Major outcomes in high-risk hypertensive patients randomized to angiotensin-converting enzyme inhibitor or calcium channel blocker vs. diuretic: the antihypertensive and lipid-lowering treatment to prevent heart attack trial. JAMA 2002;288:2981–97.

ALLHAT Officers and Coordinators for the ALLHAT Collaborative Research Group. Major cardiovascular events in hypertensive patients randomized to doxazosin vs chlorthalidone: the antihypertensive and lipid-lowering treatment to prevent heart attack trial (ALLHAT). JAMA. 2000;283:1967–75.

ASCOT, Dahlof B, Sever PS, Poulter NR, et al. for the ASCOT investigators. Prevention of cardiovascular events with an antihypertensive regimen of amlodipine adding perindopril as required versus atenolol adding bendroflumethiazide as required, in the Anglo-Scandinavian cardiac outcomes trial-blood pressure lowering arm (ASCOT-BPLA): a multicenter randomised controlled trial. Lancet. 2005;366: 895–906.

Berglund G, Andersin O, Widgren B. Low-dose antihypertensive treatment with a thiazide diuretic is not diabetogenic. Acta Med Scand. 1986;220:419–24.

Beta-blocker Evaluation of Survival Trial Investigators. A trial of the beta-blocker bucindolol in patients with advanced chronic heart failure. N Engl J Med. 2001;362:1659–67.

CONVINCE, Black HR, Elliott WJ, Grandits G, et al. for the CONVINCE Research Group. Principal results of the controlled onset verapamil investigation of cardiovascular end points (CONVINCE) trial. JAMA 2003;289:2073–82.

Cruickshank JM. β blockers for the treatment of primary hypertension. Lancet 2006;367:209.

Cushman WC, Reda DJ, Perry HM, et al. Regional and racial differences in response to antihypertensive medication use in a randomized controlled trial of men with hypertension in the United States. Arch Intern Med. 2000;160:825–31.

Deary A, Schumann AL, Murfet H. Double-blind placebo-controlled crossover comparison of five classes of antihypertensive drugs. J Hypertens. 2002;20:771–7.

Dickerson JEC, Hingorani AD, Ashby MJ, et al. Randomisation of antihypertensive treatment by crossover rotation of four major classes. Lancet. 1999;353:2008–13.

Giles TD, Weber MA, Basile J, et al. for the NAC-MD-01 Study Investigators. Efficacy and safety of nebivolol and valsartan as fixed-dose combination in hypertension: a randomised, multicentre study. Lancet 2014;383:1889–98.

Hansson L, Lindholm LH, Niskanen L, et al. Effect of angiotensin-converting-enzyme inhibition compared with conventional therapy on cardiovascular morbidity and mortality in hypertension: the captopril prevention project (CAPPP). Lancet. 1999b;353:611–6.

HYVET, Beckett NS, Peters R, Fletcher AE et al. For the HYVET Study Group. Treatment of hypertension in patients 80 years of age or older. N Engl J Med. 2008;358:1887–98.

INSIGHT, Brown MJ, Palmer CR, Castaigne A, et al. Morbidity and mortality in patients randomised to double-blind treatment with a long-acting calcium-channel blocker or diuretic in the international nifedipine GITS study: intervention as a goal in hypertension treatment (INSIGHT). Lancet. 2000;356:366–72.

JNC8, James PA, Oparil, S Carter BL. Evidence-based guideline for the management of high blood pressure in adults report from the panel members appointed to the eighth joint national committee (JNC 8). JAMA 2014;311(5):507–20.

Kendall MJ, Cohen JD. β-Blockers as first-line agents for hypertension in the elderly. JAMA 1999;281:131–33.

Khan MG. Clinical trials. In: Cardiac drug therapy, 6th ed. Philadelphia, PA: WB Saunders Elsevier; 2003. p. 502

Khan MG. Hypertension. In: Encyclopedia of heart diseases, 2nd ed. New York: Springer; 2011. p. 556

LIFE, Dahlöf B, Devereux RB, Kjeldsen SE, et al. for the LIFE Study Group. Cardiovascular morbidity and mortality in the losartan intervention for endpoint reduction in hypertension study (LIFE): a randomised trial against atenolol. Lancet 2002;359:995–1003.

Lindholm LH, Carlberg B, Samuelsson O. Should β blockers remain first choice in the treatment of primary hypertension? A meta-analysis. Lancet. 2005;366:1545–53.

Materson BJ, Reda DJ. Correction: single-drug therapy for hypertension in men. N Engl J Med. 1994;330:1689.

Materson BJ, Reda DJ, Cushman WC, et al. Single-drug therapy for hypertension in men. A comparison of six antihypertensive agents with placebo: the department of veterans affairs cooperative study group on antihypertensive agents. N Engl J Med. 1993;328:914–21.

Messerli FH, Grossman E, Goldbourt U. Are β-blockers efficacious as first-line therapy for hypertension in the elderly? JAMA. 1998;279:1903–7.

MRC Working Party. MRC trial of treatment of mild hypertension: principal results. BMJ. 1985;291:97–104.

MRC Working Party. Medical research council trial of treatment of hypertension in older adults: principal results. BMJ. 1992;304:405–12.

Murphy MB, Lewis PJ, Kohner E, Schumer B, Dollery CT. Glucose intolerance in hypertensive patients treated with diuretics: a fourteen-year follow-up. Lancet. 1982;2:1293–5.

Neal B, MacMahon S, Chapman N. Effects of ACE inhibitors, calcium antagonists, and other blood-pressure-lowering drugs: results of prospectively designed overviews of randomised trials: blood pressure lowering treatment trialists' collaboration. Lancet. 2000;356:1955–64.

Neutel JM, Smith DHG, Ram CVS. Application of ambulatory blood pressure monitoring in differentiating between antihypertensive agents. Am J Med. 1993;94:181.

Norwegian Multicentre Group. Timolol induced reduction in mortality and reinfarction in patients surviving acute myocardial infarction. N Engl J Med. 1981;304:801–7.

Pahor M, Psaty BM, Alderman MH, et al. Health outcomes associated with calcium antagonists compared with other first-line antihypertensive therapies: a meta-analysis of randomised controlled trials. Lancet. 2000;356:1949–54.

PROGRESS Collaborative Group. Randomized trial of a perindopril-based blood pressure lowering regimen among, individuals with previous stroke or transient ischaemic attack. Lancet. 2001;358:1033–41.

Saunders E, Weir MR, Kong BW, et al. A comparison of the efficacy and safety of a beta-blocker, a calcium channel blocker, and a converting enzyme inhibitor in hypertensive blacks. Arch Intern Med. 1990;150:1707–13.

SHEP Cooperative Research Group. Prevention of stroke by antihypertensive drug treatment in older persons with isolated systolic hypertension: final results of the systolic hypertension in the elderly program
(SHEP). JAMA. 1991;265:3255–64.

The CAPRICORN Investigators. Effect of carvedilol on outcome after
myocardial infarction in patients with left-ventricular dysfunction:
the CAPRICORN randomised trial. Lancet. 2001;357:1385–90.

The Dutch TIA Trial Study Group. Trial of secondary prevention with
atenolol after transient ischemic attack or nondisabling ischemic
stroke. Stroke. 1993;24:543–8.

The IPPPSH Collaborative Group. Cardiovascular risk and risk factors in
a randomised trial of treatment based on the beta-blocker oxprenolol.
The international prospective primary prevention study in hypertension (IPPPSH). J Hypertens. 1985;3:379–92.

Treatment of hypertension: The 1985 results. Lancet 1985;2:645.

UKPDS, UK Prospective Diabetes Study Group. Efficacy of atenolol and
captopril in reducing risk of macrovascular and microvascular complications in type 2 diabetes: UKPDS. BMJ 1998;317:713–20.

Yurenev AP, Dyakonova HG, Novikov ID, et al. Management of essential
hypertension in patients with different degrees of left ventricular
hypertrophy. Multicenter trial. Am J Hypertens. 1992;(6 Pt 2):
182S–9S.

Zanchetti A et al. Effects of individual risk factors on the incidence of
cardiovascular events in the treated hypertensive patients in the
hypertension   optimal   treatment   study.   J   Hypertens.
2001;19:1149–59.

10 Angina

SALIENT CLINICAL FEATURES

Angina is a pain in the chest or adjacent areas caused by severe, but temporary, lack of blood (ischemia) to a segment of the heart muscle, hence the term myocardial ischemia. For stable angina, the most important feature is the causation of pain by a particular exertional activity and relief within minutes of cessation of the precipitating activity.

Angina may be classified as:

- Stable angina
- Unstable angina
- Variant angina (Prinzmetal's), coronary artery spasm (CAS), a rare disorder

The pain of angina must be differentiated from commonly occurring:

- Gastroesophageal reflux and motility disorders
- Musculoskeletal disorders, particularly costochondritis that causes tenderness without swelling of the second to fourth left costochondral junctions and may occur concomitantly with coronary artery disease

It is necessary to document the presence or absence of diabetes and cigarette smoking, which markedly increases risk and asthma, which contraindicates the use of beta-blocking drugs.

© Springer Science+Business Media New York 2015
M. Gabriel Khan, *Cardiac Drug Therapy*, Contemporary Cardiology,
DOI 10.1007/978-1-61779-962-4_10

Physical examination should exclude secondary factors that may precipitate angina:

- Anemia and hypertension
- Aortic stenosis, severe valvular disease, and hypertrophic cardiomyopathy
- Arrhythmias

Relevant baseline investigations include resting and stress electrocardiogram (ECG), total cholesterol, high-density lipoprotein (HDL) cholesterol, low-density lipoprotein (LDL) cholesterol, and triglycerides, as well as hemoglobin, glucose serum creatinine, and estimated glomerular filtration rate (eGFR).

Pathophysiologic Implications

Three determinants play major roles in the pathogenesis of myocardial ischemia to cause stable or unstable angina:

- Atheromatous lesions are mainly concentric with stable angina and eccentric with unstable angina and cause >70 % coronary stenosis.
- Myocardial oxygen demand is increased.
- Catecholamines are released in response to exertional and emotional stress or other activity. Catecholamines cause an increase in heart rate, velocity, and force of myocardial contraction that increase oxygen demand and ischemia. Increased heart rate decreases the diastolic interval during which coronary artery perfusion occurs. Ischemia further stimulates catecholamine release, thereby perpetuating the vicious circle.

Catecholamine release initiates and perpetuates a dynamic process. Thus, beta-blocking agents play a key role in the management of patients with myocardial ischemia manifested by anginal pain or silent ischemia. The pathophysiology of unstable angina is more complex and is dealt with later in this chapter.

TREATMENT OF STABLE ANGINA

The ACC/AHA provided guidelines in 2014. It is crucial to control known risk factors for coronary artery disease strictly:

- Cigarette smoking must be curtailed; weight and stress must be addressed.
- Hypertension must be controlled with an appropriate drug; goal blood pressure (BP): systolic < 135 mmHg.
- Hyperlipidemia must be brought to goal levels: LDL < 2.0 mmol/L (70 mg/dL) and for high-risk patients, example unstable angina < 60 mg/dL (1.6 mmol/L).
- Diabetes must be treated aggressively.

The Clinical Outcomes Utilizing Revascularization and Aggressive Drug Evaluation (COURAGE Boden et al. 2007) trial compared an initial strategy of PCI plus optimal medical therapy with optimal medical therapy alone for patients with stable angina. This RCT studied 2,287 patients who had objective evidence of myocardial ischemia, 1,149 patients to undergo PCI with optimal medical therapy (PCI group), and 1,138 to receive optimal medical therapy alone (medical-therapy group). The primary outcome was death from any cause and nonfatal MI during a median follow-up of 4.6 years.

There were 211 primary events in the PCI group and 202 events in the medical-therapy group. The 4.6-year cumulative primary-event rates were 19 % in the PCI group and 18.5 % in the medical-therapy group.

In patients with stable angina, PCI did not reduce the risk of death, MI, or other major cardiovascular events when added to optimal medical therapy COURAGE Trial (Boden et al. 2007). During the trial period, 21 % crossed over and received PCI. There was rapidity of improvement in health status in both treatment groups; the majority of patients who received optimal medical therapy alone had improved symptoms within 3 months. This suggests that optimal antianginal medications are underused in practice.

The "take-home" message from the COURAGE trial is to pursue optimal medical therapy initially as it is effective in 75 % and if this is ineffective in 25 % resort to PCI (Peterson and Rumsfeld 2008).

Schomig et al. (2008) pooled together the results of 17 randomized trials comparing PCI and medical treatment as strategies in patients with stable angina and no acute coronary syndromes. Their meta-analysis concluded that a PCI-based invasive strategy may improve long-term survival in patients with stable coronary artery disease (CAD) and that this justifies a new clinical trial sufficiently powered to evaluate the impact of PCI on long-term mortality.

• Based on the strength of available evidence, O'Rourke recommends "more aggressive medical therapy for patients with moderate to severe angina, and PCI or CABG for patients whose symptoms are bothersome. Optimal medical therapy is a proven option for chronic stable angina" (O'Rourke 2008). But there is little doubt that most post-PCI patients can engage in many more activities including golfing, swimming, and traveling, whereas medically treated patients do have to be cautious, and many cannot engage in activities that they like.

Usually PCI is done to relieve bothersome angina, but data are emerging to suggest that there may also be functional and a mortality benefit. Successful PCI for chronic total coronary occlusion was associated with improved long-term survival. The improvement was greatest in patients when complete revascularization was achieved (George et al. 2014).

Beta-Adrenoceptor Blocking Agents

All cardiologists now agree that beta-blockers are standard first-line therapy for stable and unstable angina. A table that compared beta-blockers, nitrates, and calcium

Table 10-1
Beta-blocker: first-line oral drug treatment in angina pectoris

Effect on	Beta-blocker	Calcium antagonist	Oral nitrate
Heart rate	↓	↑↓	—
Drastolic filling of coronary arteries	↑	—	—
Blood pressure	↓↓	↓↓	—
Rate pressure product (RPP)	↓	—[a]	—
Relief of angina	Yes	Yes	Variable
Blood flow (subendocardial ischemic area)[b]	↑	↓	Variable
First-line treatment for angina pectoris	Yes	No	No
Prevention of recurrent ventricular fibrillation	Proven	No	No
Prevention of cardiac death	Proven	No	No
Prevention of pain from coronary artery spasm	No	Yes	Variable
Prevention of death in patient with coronary artery spasm	No	No	No

↓, decrease; ↑, increase: —, no significant change

[a]RPP variable decrease on exercise, but no significant at rest or on maximal exercise.

[b]Distal to organic obstruction

antagonists and indicated the rationale for beta-blockers as first-line treatment has remained unaltered since the first edition in 1984 (Table 10-1).

Many patients with left ventricular (LV) dysfunction and borderline and class II–III heart failure (HF) were deprived of beta-blocker therapy from 1970 to 1999. These drugs were believed to be contraindicated in HF. However, beta-blockers continue to surprise us (Cruickshank 2000).

Randomized controlled trials (RCTs) have proved solidly that these drugs decrease mortality and morbidity in patients with all grades of HF (see Chap. 12), and at present they are strongly recommended in patients with angina and HF or LV dysfunction. Calcium antagonists and nitrates cannot reduce mortality or morbidity in these patients and are relegated to second-line therapy.

- **Virtually all patients with angina should receive a beta-blocker, preferably bisoprolol, carvedilol, metoprolol, propranolol, or timolol at a cardioprotective dosage** (see the later discussion of cardioprotective dose); the widely used atenolol is not advisable; it is a poorly effective beta-blocker because it is non-lipophilic and attains poor brain concentration.

  "Use should be limited to bisoprolol, carvedilol, metoprolol succinate (Toprol XL), or timolol which have been shown to reduce risk of death" (*Level of Evidence: A*).

  These beta-blockers are chosen because they have been shown to decrease mortality in patients with coronary heart disease (see Chap. 1). *Atenolol, a water-soluble* drug, is frequently used worldwide for angina and hypertension. The water-soluble, non-lipid-soluble beta-blockers atenolol and nadolol, also pindolol and acebutolol, are not recommended (see Chaps. 1 and 2).

- It is important to reemphasize that only the cardioselective, lipid-soluble beta-blockers metoprolol, timolol (Norwegian Multicenter Study Group 2001), propranolol (in nonsmokers), and carvedilol (CAPRICORN 2001) have been shown in RCTs to decrease mortality in post-MI patients. Beta-blockers have important subtle clinical differences (Khan 2005).
- It remains probable that beta 1 and beta 2 effects are needed to render further cardioprotection (see Chap. 1). Timolol caused an outstanding unmatched 67 % reduction in sudden deaths in post-infarct patients (Norwegian Multicenter

Study Group 1981), a result that has been lost to the cardiology world. The drug is rarely if ever used in the USA and Canada.

Beta-blockers significantly reduce the number of episodes of angina in more than 75 % of patients. Beta-blockers may prevent deaths in patients with angina, but reduction in mortality has not been documented in RCTs of patients with angina. Only a few small trials have been conducted and with poor methodology. Patients receiving a beta-blocking agent have the advantage of pretreatment before a subsequent severe ischemic episode (Norwegian Multicenter Study Group 1981; CAPRICORN 2001).

Observations have established that silent ischemia is common and is easily provoked by daily stressful activities (Deanfield et al. 1983, 1984). Patients with angina may have more silent than painful episodes. Beta-blockers and calcium antagonists have been shown to ameliorate silent ischemic episodes, but beta-blockers are superior. The salutary effects of beta-adrenoceptor blockade are illustrated in Fig. 1-1. These beneficial effects in myocardial ischemia result from:

- A decrease in myocardial oxygen demand as a result of a decrease in heart rate.
- A decrease in the velocity and force of myocardial contraction.
- A fall in cardiac output and blood pressure; thus the rate pressure product (heart rate × systolic blood pressure) is reduced.
- Improvement in blood supply caused by a decrease in heart rate, which lengthens the diastolic interval. Because the coronary arteries fill during diastole, coronary perfusion improves.
- Blocking of exercise-induced catecholamine vasoconstriction at sites of coronary stenosis where atheroma could impair the relaxing effects of the endothelium.
- Decreased conduction through the atrioventricular (AV) node resulting in the slowing of the ventricular response in

atrial fibrillation or other supraventricular arrhythmias that may occur in patients with myocardial ischemia.

- Decrease in phase four diastolic depolarization producing suppression of ventricular arrhythmias, especially those induced by catecholamines and/or ischemia.
- Increase in ventricular fibrillation (VF) threshold reduces the incidence of VF and sudden deaths that could, at some stage, occur in patients with angina (see Chap. 1 for other mechanisms).

Cardioprotection and Dosage of Beta-Blocker

Table 1-4 gives dosages of beta-blockers. The dose of metoprolol is 100–200 mg, that of propranolol in nonsmokers is 160–240 mg, and that of timolol is 10–20 mg daily, because these doses have been shown to be effective in preventing sudden death and decreasing total cardiac deaths in well-designed clinical trials albeit in patients after MI. The salutary effect of smaller doses is unknown, and larger doses are likely to be nonprotective (*see* Chap. 1).

The dose of beta-blocker is kept within the cardioprotective range, to maintain a resting heart rate of 52–60 beats/min bearing in mind that no patient should be allowed to have significant adverse effects from medication. If side effects occur, the dose is reduced, and a nitrate or calcium antagonist is added. If the maximum cardioprotective dose is used and angina is not controlled, the dose of beta-blocker can be increased, but adverse effects may limit the increase. Some patients do better on an average dose of beta-blocker plus a nitrate or calcium antagonist. Trial and error is necessary in many patients.

Contraindications to Beta-Blockers

Contraindications to the use of a beta-blocking drug are the following:

- Asthma.
- Severe chronic obstructive pulmonary disease. Mild stable disease is not a contraindication.

- Severe HF (decompensated class IV). These agents have been approved for cautious use in patients with compensated class IV HF.
- Bradyarrhythmias (second- or third-degree AV block).
- Brittle insulin-dependent diabetes and patients prone to hypoglycemia.
- Raynaud's phenomenon.

Calcium Antagonists

These agents are used as second-line therapy when beta-blockers are genuinely contraindicated. Several trials have shown that verapamil is as effective as beta-blockers in the control of angina, but this agent does not prolong life. Verapamil is a more effective antianginal agent than diltiazem or dihydropyridines (DHPs) and is considered a first choice, but the drug must be used with caution and must not be combined with a beta-blocker.

Contraindications to the use of verapamil and diltiazem include:

- Heart failure, suspected LV dysfunction, and ejection fraction (EF) <40 %, because verapamil has a strongly negative inotropic action and diltiazem is moderately so.
- Sinus or AV node disease.
- Bradycardia.

Amlodipine (Norvasc) has a less negative inotropic effect than other DHPs, but in the Prospective Randomized Amlodipine Survival Evaluation (PRAISE 1996) study, although amlodipine use was generally safe in patients with HF, it caused an increased incidence of pulmonary edema in patients with EF< 30 %. The drug is not recommended if the EF is <35 % and should not be combined with a beta-blocker if the EF is <40 %.

Combination of Beta-Blockers and Calcium Antagonists

Amlodipine has minimal negative inotropic effects and can be combined with a beta-blocker in patients with EF > 35 %. Although beta-blockers may be used in patients with EF < 30 %, the combination of a beta-blocker with diltiazem or dihydropyridine should be avoided in patients with EF < 40 %. Verapamil is contraindicated in patients with an EF < 40 %.

Verapamil and, to a lesser extent, diltiazem, when added to a beta-blocker, may cause conduction disturbances or HF, and the verapamil combination is considered unsafe. The hemodynamic, electrophysiologic, and pharmacokinetic effects, adverse effects, and relative effectiveness of calcium antagonists are given in Tables 5-2 and 5-3 and are discussed in Chap. 5.

Nitrates

Drug name:	Nitroglycerin: glyceryl trinitrate
Supplied:	Sublingual nitroglycerin: 0.15, 0.3, 0.4 mg
Sublingual glyceryl trinitrate:	300, 500, 600 µg (UK)
Spray (Nitrolingual):	0.4 mg metered dose, 200 doses/vial

Dosage: Start with nitroglycerin 0.15 or 0.3 mg or glyceryl trinitrate 300 µg as a test dose with the patient sitting. The drug will not be as effective if the patient is lying down; if the patient is standing, dizziness or presyncope may occur. Thereafter, prescribe 0.3 mg nitroglycerin or 300 µg glyceryl trinitrate or 0.4 mg nitrolingual spray. If the systolic blood pressure in routine follow-up is more than 130 mmHg, then it is safe to give 0.4 mg sublingual tablets depending on patient choice.

The patient must be instructed that nitroglycerin tablets are to be kept in their dark, light-protected bottles; they may be rendered useless after 6 months, or even earlier, if they are not protected from light. Patients should be advised to have at least two bottles available. These two bottles must contain approximately 1-month supply and no cotton wool, to ensure rapid availability in emergencies. At the end of each month, the containers should be emptied and the supply replenished from a third-stock bottle. If pain occurs and is not relieved by two tablets, three 80–81 mg soft chewable aspirins should be taken; obtain ambulance assistance to a coronary intervention center or an emergency department.

Oral Nitroglycerin Tablets: For Nitrong SR 2.6 mg, the dosage is 1 tablet at 7 AM and 2 PM daily (Table 10-2). This will allow a 12-h nitrate-free interval to maintain the efficacy of the drug. The maximum dose 6.25-mg tab may cause bothersome headaches.

Action: Nitrates bind to "nitrate receptors" in the vascular smooth muscle wall that activate guanylate cyclase and thereby stimulate the generation of cyclic guanosine monophosphate, which causes relaxation of the vascular smooth muscle and thus dilation of the veins and, to a lesser extent, arteries. The reason that venous dilation is greater than arterial is unknown. The result is marked dilation of the venous bed and therefore reduction in preload and a minimal decrease in afterload. A modest variable dilation of coronary arteries occurs. Nitrates have a direct effect on the compliance of the left ventricle and cause a downward shift in pressure–volume relationship.

The nonmononitrates are rapidly metabolized in the liver. The large first-pass inactivation of orally administered nitrates causes poor bioavailability to vascular receptors. Transdermal, buccal mononitrates, or intravenous (IV) preparations partially overcome this problem.

Cutaneous Nitroglycerins

Long-acting or slow-release cutaneous nitroglycerin preparations are available.

Transderm-Nitro: 0.2, 0.4, 0.6 mg released/h.

Table 10-2
Nitrates

Generic	Trade name or available as[a]	Supplied and dosage[b]
Sublingual		
Nitroglycerin	Nitroglycerin	0.15, 0.3, 0.4, 0.6 mg (USA)
	Nitrostat	0.3, 0.6 mg (C)[c]
	Nitrostabiin	600 µg (C)
	Nitrolingual spray	Metered dose of 0.4 mg
Glyceryl trinitrate (UK)	Giyceryl trinitrate (GTN)	300, 500, 600 µg
	Coro-nitro spray	400 µg/metered dose
	Nitrolingual spray oral	400 µg/metered dose
Nitroglycerin oral tablets	Nitrong SR	2.6 mg (USA, C)
	Nitrostat SR, Nitrobid	7 AM, 2 PM
Buccal tablets	Nitrogard (USA)	1, 2, 3 mg
	Susadrin (USA)	1, 2, 3 mg
	Nitrogard SR (C)	1, 2, 3 mg
	Suscard (UK)	1, 2, 3, 5 mg
Isosorbide dinitrate oral, tablets	Isosorbide dinitrate	10, 20, 30, 40 mg (USA)
		10, 20, 30 mg (UK)
		10, 30 mg (C)
	Isordil	10, 20, 30, 40 mg (USA)
		10, 30 mg (UK)
		10, 30 mg (C)
	Cedocard 10, Cedocard 20	10, 20 mg (UK)
	Cedocard Retard	20 mg
	Isordil Tembids	40 mg capsules
	Sorbitrate	10, 20 mg (USA, UK)

(continued)

Table 10-2 (continued)

Generic	Trade name or available as[a]	Supplied and dosage[b]
Isosorbide mononitrate	Isosorbide mononitrate	20 mg
	Elantan 20	20 mg
	Elantan 40	40 mg
	Ismo	20 mg b.i.d., 7 h apart
	Imdur	60–120 mg once daily

[a]Several other trade names are available
[b]For dosage see text
[c]C, Canada

Cutaneous Nitrates

Transderm-Nitro: 0.2, 0.4, 0.6 mg released/h.

Nitro-Dur II: 0.2, 0.4, 0.6 mg released/h.

The advantage of a cutaneous preparation is that the active drug reaches the target organs before it is inactivated by the liver. A therapeutic effect can be anticipated in 30–60 min and will last 4–6 h with the paste and about 20 h with long-acting preparations. Transdermal preparations should not be applied to the distal parts of the extremities or to the precordium where defibrillator paddles or chest leads may be placed. (Rare explosive events have been reported when contact was made with defibrillator paddles.) Cutaneous preparations are useful during dental work or minor or major surgery in patients with ischemic heart disease or hypertension. It is important, however, to ensure that such patients have tried the preparation and that the systolic blood pressure does not fall to <110 mmHg, because premedication and anesthetics can cause a further decrease in blood pressure. An attempt should be made by the physician to restrict the continuous use of transdermal preparations to up to 3 days and then 12 h daily, allowing at least a 10-h nitrate-free interval. The patient should be weaned from the drug slowly, to avoid rebound.

Nitrate Tolerance

- It is well established that nitrate tolerance commonly occurs after several weeks of continuous nitrate use. Continuous infusion of nitroglycerin can result in tolerance within 24 h (Elkayam 1991; Packer et al. 1986).

- All long-acting nitrate preparations—transdermal, isosorbide dinitrate (ISDN) regular strength, or sustained-release isosorbide-5-mononitrate (ISDN 5. MN)—have shown complete attenuation of antianginal effects after 1–2 weeks of continuous daily use (Abrams 1989).

- A nitrate-free interval limits the development of nitrate tolerance. When 20 mg ISDN was given at 8 AM and 1 PM for 8 days, leaving a nitrate-free interval during the night, no alteration of the anti-ischemic effect of the drug occurred (Rudolph 1983: 22). However, 15 days of continuous therapy with long-acting ISDN caused a 35–60 % alteration of both the ST segment and the EF response to exercise (Sharpe et al. 1987). The vasodilator effect of transdermal nitroglycerin in HF is maintained with intermittent treatment, whereas tolerance develops with continuous therapy (Juul Moller et al. 1992).

- Veins and arteries are important sites of nitrate biotransformation. Organic nitrates are converted by intracellular sulfhydryl (SH) groups to nitric oxide and sulfhydryl-containing compounds. Vascular tolerance to nitrates is believed to result from a relative depletion of SH groups in vascular smooth muscle cells. A nitrate-free interval is necessary to allow intracellular generation of an adequate supply of SH groups and to restore vascular responsiveness.

- A nitrate-free interval of 10–12 h is necessary to prevent nitrate tolerance. Suggested steps include the following: ISDN 15–40 mg given at 7 AM, 12 noon, and 5 PM daily or sustained release one tablet 8 AM daily; Nitrong SR 7 AM and 2 PM daily; Ismo 20 mg twice daily 7 h apart; Imdur 30–120 mg once daily. Transdermal preparations should be used for about 12 h daily.

Drug name:	**Isosorbide dinitrate**
Trade names:	Coronex, Isordil, Iso-Bid, Sorbitrate (UK)
Supplied:	Isordil: 5-, 10-, 20-, and 30-mg tablets; 40-mg capsules; 10-mL ampules for IV use (1 mg/mL)
Dosage:	30 mg 7 AM and 2 PM daily; *see* text

IV: 2–7 mg/h (polyethylene apparatus)
Oral: 10–30 mg three times daily; if possible ½–1 h before meals or on an empty stomach. Maintenance: 30 mg at 7 and 11 AM and 4 PM; allow a 12-h nitrate-free interval to prevent tolerance. The 10-mg dose is ineffective.

Drug name:	**Isosorbide mononitrate**
Trade names:	Imdur, Elantan, Ismo (UK)
Dosage:	Initial 30 mg, then 60–120 mg once each AM; max. 240 mg if tolerated
Dosage advice:	Half the dose for 1 week if headache occurs with oral nitrate

The 5-mononitrate of isosorbide achieves consistent plasma nitrate levels, but tolerance quickly develops. The drug does not undergo hepatic degradation. It is excreted by the kidneys, unchanged and partially as an inactive compound. Activity lasts for 12 h and thus with once daily use nitrate tolerance is avoided.

Caution: gradually discontinue long-term nitrate therapy to avoid the rare occurrence of rebound increase in angina. Cover the nitrate-free interval with a beta-blocker or, if these drugs are contraindicated, administer a calcium antagonist.

Intravenous nitroglycerin is of proven value in the management of unstable angina. Onset of action is within 1.5 min, with a duration of about 9 min.

• Low doses predominantly dilate the venous capacitance vessels and therefore decrease preload. The drug reduces LV dimensions and LV wall tension, thereby reducing myocardial oxygen consumption. The drug can also cause an increased myocardial oxygen consumption because of a reflex increase in the heart rate.

- Higher doses cause systemic arteriolar dilation and reduction in afterload.
- In rare instances when the patient does not respond and seems to be doing worse, the physician should entertain the possibility that the nitroglycerin has caused a shunting of blood from the ischemic to the nonischemic zone.

Indications

- Refractory or unstable angina, chest pain, or acute coronary insufficiency. In this setting, continuous IV nitroglycerin is necessary without consideration of tolerance. The dose is titrated to control pain but with careful monitoring of BP.
- CAS.
- Pulmonary edema resulting from LV failure.
- Intraoperative arterial hypertension, especially during cardiac surgery (not routine) and in patients with Prinzmetal's angina and organic obstruction who are undergoing bypass surgery.
- To reduce the size of MI (not proved to be effective). A modest decrease in mortality rate was observed in one study of patients with acute MI.

Contraindications to intravenous nitrate or high-dose therapy:

- Hypovolemia
- Increased intracranial pressure
- Cardiac tamponade and constructive pericarditis
- Obstructive cardiomyopathy, severe aortic stenosis, or mitral stenosis
- Right ventricular infarction (decrease in preload may cause clinical and hemodynamic deterioration in categories 3, 4, and 5)
- Glaucoma: closed-angle glaucoma or severe uncontrolled glaucoma

Warnings: IV nitroglycerin is a potent vasodilator, and hemodynamic monitoring is usually necessary. The systolic blood pressure should not drop by >20 mmHg; reduce the dose if the systolic blood pressure is <100 mmHg. A diastolic blood pressure of >60 mmHg is necessary for adequate coronary artery perfusion.

- The pulmonary wedge pressure should be maintained at 15–18 mmHg in patients with acute MI.
- As much as 80 % of the nitroglycerin may bind to the polyvinyl chloride infusion set. If such an apparatus is used, the infusion should be slowed down after 2 h because the binding sites in the tubing become saturated. Special polyethylene tubing sets should therefore be used.
- Use an infusion pump to ensure titrated dose response (Table 10-3). IMED infusion pumps are not compatible with the new non-polyvinyl chloride administration sets; however, new pump systems are being developed.
- Wean the patient from the drug slowly.
- Methemoglobinemia may occur after extended, continuous, high doses at levels greater than 7 µg/kg/min; cyanosis with normal arterial blood gases and methemoglobin levels >1.5 g/dL confirms the diagnosis. Hypoxemia may result from increased venous admixture.
- Interactions with heparin or tissue plasminogen activator may occur.

Aspirin

All patients with stable angina should be administered a soft chewable aspirin 75–81 mg once daily after a meal; if gastritis or stomach problem exists, then the enteric coated, 75–81 mg daily, is advisable. Aspirin is a potent antiplatelet agent and has been shown to improve survival and to prevent infarction in patients with unstable angina or at onset of MI. Enteric-coated ASA is not advisable because the formulation is not adequately absorbed.

Table 10-3
Nitroglycerin infusion pump chart
(50 mg in 500 mL 5 % dextrose/water = 100 μg/
mL)[a]

Dose (µg/min)	Infusion rate (mL/h)
5	3
10	6
15	9
20	12
25	15
30	18
35	21
40	24
45	27
50	30
60	36
70	42
80	48
90	54
100	60
120	72
140	84
160	96
200	120
250	150

[a]Increase by 5 μg/min every 5 min until relief of chest pain; decrease rate if systolic blood pressure < 100 mmHg or falls to 20 mmHg below the baseline, or diastolic blood pressure < 65 mmHg

Grosser et al. (2013) assessed aspirin resistance and identified a high occurrence of pseudoresistance that is clinically meaningful. Healthy volunteers ($n=400$) were screened for their response to a single dose of 325-mg immediate-release or enteric-coated aspirin. Response parameters reflected the activity of the molecular target of aspirin, cyclooxygenase-1. Absorption proved very variable and caused up to 49 % apparent resistance to a single dose of enteric-coated aspirin but not to immediate-release aspirin (0 %). Genuine pharmacologic resistance to aspirin is rare; the study failed to identify a single case of true aspirin resistance. Pseudoresistance, reflecting delayed and reduced drug absorption, complicates enteric coated but not immediate-release aspirin administration (Grosser et al. 2013).

The author abandoned the use of enteric-coated aspirin since 2009 and instead prescribes soft chewable aspirin 81 mg for CVD prevention:

* The non-coated, soft chewable aspirin 80–81 mg is highly recommended taken once daily after a meal. **This soft aspirin is thus available to be taken 240–320 mg chewed immediately when an ambulance is called, if chest pain suggestive of a heart attack occurs**.

Aspirin inhibits cyclooxygenase and the subsequent suppression of thromboxane A2, the key moderator of irreversible platelet aggregation. A prospective study (Juul Moller 1992) of 2,035 patients with stable angina showed that 75 mg aspirin added to sotalol produced a 34 % decrease in primary outcome events of MI and sudden death ($p = 0.003$). If aspirin use is contraindicated, 75 mg clopidogrel is advisable.

Ranolazine

Ranolazine is a second-line antianginal agent. The drug acts as a selective inhibitor of the late sodium current, which acts to reduce intracellular calcium in myocytes, thereby reducing the tension or stiffness of the myocardium that occurs during ischemia or HF. The drug may be combined with beta-blockers and ACE inhibitors because the drug does not cause a reduction in heart rate or BP:

* In small RCTs the drug reportedly reduced the number of anginal attacks per week and caused a modest improvement in treadmill exercise duration.

- Large-scale RCTs are required to establish this agent as an effective and safe antianginal agent. The drug causes a prolongation of the QT interval, and syncope has been reported.
- Significant interaction occurs with potent CYP3A inhibitors including the antianginal agent diltiazem.
- **The drug is contraindicated in patients with heart failure of all grades;** the drug causes QT interval prolongation, and caution is required.
- Avoid if elderly, body weight less than 60 kg. Use with caution if eGFR 40–60 mL/min; avoid if eGFR < 40 ml/min.

Dosage: Initially 375 mg twice daily, increased after 2–4 weeks to 500 mg twice daily. Several side effects have been reported. The drug should not replace beta-blocker use. **If a combination of a beta-blocker and nitrate or calcium antagonist fails to prevent bothersome chest discomfort, PCI is more logical therapy than a trial of ranolazine or nicorandil**.

NICORANDIL

This nicotinamide nitrate acts as a potassium channel activator but also has a nitrate-like action. The drug reportedly causes modest dilation of large coronary arteries and reduces preload and afterload. Indications include prophylaxis and treatment of angina. The drug is used sparingly in the United Kingdom but extensively in Japan. The drug has shown low efficacy in small RCTs and is not used in the United States and Canada:

- May be tried in patients with stable angina inadequately controlled or intolerant of first-line antianginal therapies. It has a small role in the management of stable angina (including risk reduction of acute coronary syndromes in patients at high risk).
- Cautions: Hypovolemia, low systolic blood pressure, acute pulmonary edema, acute myocardial infarction, left ventricular failure, and low filling pressures. Several side effects have been reported and hypotension may occur, a detrimental effect in coronary disease.

Dosage: Initially 10 mg twice daily (if susceptible to headache, 5 mg twice daily), usual dose 10–20 mg twice daily.

The author does not advise the use of verapamil or other calcium antagonist as initial therapy instead of beta-blocker. These agents are tried judiciously only if beta-blocker therapy is contraindicated or adverse effects are unacceptable. They have not proven cardio-protective in post-MI patients, and verapamil is contra-indicated in patients with acute MI. The patient with angina is at risk for development of acute MI.

CONSIDER INTERVENTIONAL THERAPY

If symptoms are not controlled with beta-blocker and nitrate administration instead of a trial of calcium antagonists or ranolazine, interventional therapy (PCI) should be considered.

MANAGEMENT OF UNSTABLE ANGINA

The pathophysiology of unstable angina has been clarified. In most cases, plaques are asymmetric, with irregular borders and a narrow neck. Rupture of the plaque with over-lying thrombus is a common finding on angioscopy. Lipid-rich plaques have a predilection for rupture. Silent ischemia is frequently observed in patients with unstable angina (Gottlieb et al. 1986; Nademanee et al. 1987).

Investigations

- Serial ECGs.
- Troponin T or troponin I, to exclude non-ST elevation MI (NSTEMI) assist with risk stratification; measurement of creatine kinase, myocardial bound (CK-MB) isoenzyme levels, if troponin is not available.
- Serum cholesterol, HDL, LDL cholesterol, and triglycerides.

- Hb for anemia is relevant to angina occurrence.
- Creatinine clearance (eGFR) for adjustment of drug doses particularly low-molecular-weight heparin (LMWH) in patients older than age 70.
- Coronary angiograms with a view to PCI, in virtually all patients without serious comorbidities. Bypass surgery is considered for a selected few.
- Unstable angina, unlike NSTEMI, is a heterogeneous entity and exhibits marked variations in risk for coronary events.

Medications

- IV nitrates (if unavailable, use transdermal nitrate plus oral nitrates in high doses). Reduce the dose if the systolic blood pressure is <100 mmHg. A nitrate-free interval may place the patient at risk. It is advisable to continue IV nitroglycerin and titrate the dose upward to pain relief. Failure to gain complete pain relief with IV nitroglycerin, a beta-blocker, and diltiazem, if there is no contraindication to the last combination, should prompt consideration of coronary angiography and interventional therapy.
- Morphine should be avoided if PCI is an option because the drug decreases the effectiveness of clopidogrel (Hobl et al. 2014).
- A beta-blocker in sufficient doses (metoprolol, bisoprolol, carvedilol, timolol or propranolol, **not atenolol**). Hold the dose if the systolic blood pressure is <100 mmHg or the heart rate is <48 per min.
- If pain is not completely controlled, add calcium antagonist: preferably amlodipine 5 mg, if no contraindication to the combination with beta-blocker (LV dysfunction, EF < 35 %, systolic BP < 120 mmHg). Monitor the BP carefully, because calcium antagonists may cause severe hypotension, especially if used concomitantly with IV nitroglycerin, and diltiazem may cause severe bradycardia or sinus arrest in patients with sick sinus syndrome, and a combination with a beta-blocker may be hazardous. Diltiazem plus nitrates should be started at the time of admission if beta-blockers are contraindicated because of asthma. Chronic obstructive pulmonary disease is not a contraindication.

Aspirin: A timely Veterans Administration study using 324 mg aspirin in patients with unstable angina resulted in a 50 % reduction in mortality rate and nonfatal MIs (Lewis et al. 1983):

- In another randomized study, aspirin was shown to reduce the cardiac mortality rate by 50 % in patients with unstable angina (Cairns et al. 1985).
- A Swedish study using 75 mg aspirin in patients with stable angina showed a 34 % reduction in MI and death.

All patients should receive chewable aspirin 3×75 mg tab or 3×81 mg immediately on presentation if not given by paramedics, then 75–81-mg soft chewable aspirin daily after a meal. Enteric-coated aspirin is not recommended because absorption is incomplete (see aspirin in Chap. 19).

Clopidogrel: 600 mg loading dose is given on presentation as soon as the diagnosis of probable NSTEMI/unstable angina is made and is given at the same time as chewable aspirin. In some centers clopidogrel is given 600 mg <2 h before percutaneous coronary intervention (PCI).

Morphine decreases salutary effects of clopidogrel. (See Chaps. 11, 19, and 22 for further discussion regarding clopidogrel administration.)

An early invasive strategy (i.e., diagnostic angiography with intent to perform revascularization) is indicated in initially stabilized UA/NSTEMI patients who have an elevated risk for clinical events (GRACE score > 140):

- An early invasive strategy (angiography with intent to perform revascularization within the first 24 h of presentation) is indicated in UA/NSTEMI patients who have refractory angina or hemodynamic or electrical instability. A delayed invasive strategy is advisable in low- to intermediate-risk patients. (See Chap. 22, hallmark clinical trials.) But virtually all patients should have coronary angiograms with view to PCI (See focused update Fihn et al. 2014).

STATINS

- It is imperative to maintain the LDL cholesterol level at <60 mg/dL (1.6 mmol/L) in patients with unstable angina.
- A level of 60 mg (1.6 mmol/L) or less is now preferred (see ASTEROID and SATURN trial in Chap. 22).

Thus, the use of a high-dose statin (e.g., rosuvastatin 20–40 mg daily or atorvastatin 60–80 mg) should be commenced in virtually all patients (Cannon et al. 2004). Statins decrease elevated CRP levels; it is advisable to initiate potent statin therapy when the patient is admitted for ACS (Chaps. 17 and 22).

The course of patients with unstable angina and NSTEMI after hospital discharge is improved by an intensive reduction in LDL cholesterol levels (Cannon et al. 2004) and administration of a new anticoagulant, rivaroxaban (Mega et al. 2012) (see Chap. 22). Clopidogrel is given for 1–2 years, but omeprazole use must be avoided. A study indicated that pantoprazole was not associated with recurrent MI among patients receiving clopidogrel, possibly due to pantoprazole's lack of inhibition of CYP450 2C19 (Juurlink et al. 2009).

The use of a PPI that inhibits CYP450 2C19, including omeprazole, lansoprazole, or rabeprazole, should be avoided. Evidence is certain for omeprazole.

VARIANT ANGINA (PRINZMETAL'S)

Clues to Diagnosis

- Pain usually occurs at rest (often during sleep between midnight and 8 AM).
- The ECG shows ST segment elevation during pain.
- Patients have a poor response to beta-blockers alone or a worsening of pain.
- CAS can be provoked by the use of IV ergonovine (with IV nitroglycerin drip on standby; nifedipine may be necessary

to reverse spasm, which should be precipitated only in the cardiac laboratory). The test is not necessary, however, to initiate therapy.

- A few patients have ST segment depression, and it is impossible to separate them from patients with angina from ischemic heart disease with fixed obstruction, except by a history of variable threshold or by an ergonovine test.
- Variable threshold angina may exist.

A subset of patients with variant angina may have significant obstructive coronary artery disease with spasm at the site of the plaque (Prinzmetal's) and may demonstrate any or all of the aforementioned features:

- Coronary arteriography should be considered in most patients.
- Patients should stop smoking.
- Nitroglycerin tablets are taken sublingually.
- Among calcium antagonists, DHPs, verapamil, and diltiazem are equally effective.
- It may be necessary to combine both a calcium antagonist and ISDN or isosorbide-5-mononitrate. Occasionally, the patient may respond to nitrates only, but at high doses.
- Avoid aspirin because the drug can precipitate spasm in patients with variant angina (Miwa et al. 1983).

Unfortunately, patients with variant angina, even when the syndrome is completely controlled by calcium antagonists, have died or have had MIs. Although calcium antagonists are efficient in controlling the pain of variant angina, they do not prevent death. Nitrates are much less effective and also do not appear to improve survival.

REFERENCES

Abrams J. Interval therapy to avoid nitrate tolerance: paradise regained. Am J Cardiol. 1989;64:931.

Cairns JA, Gent M, Singer J, et al. Aspirin, sulfinpyrazone or both in unstable angina. N Engl J Med. 1985;313:1369.

Cannon CP, Braunwald E, McCabe CH, et al. Intensive versus moderate lipid lowering with statins after acute coronary syndromes. N Engl J Med. 2004;350:1495–504 [Erratum, N Engl J Med 2006;354:778.].

CAPRICORN investigators. Effect of carvedilol on outcome after myocardial infarction in patients with LV dysfunction. Lancet. 2001; 357:1385.

Cohn PF. Total ischemic burden: pathophysiology and prognosis. Am J Cardiol. 1987;59:3C.

COURAGE Boden WE, O'Rourke RA, Teo KK, et al. for the COURAGE trial research. Optimal medical therapy with or without PCI for stable coronary disease. N Engl J Med. 2007;356:1503–1516.

Cruickshank JM. Beta-blockers continue to surprise us. Eur Heart J. 2000;21:354.

Elkayam U. Tolerance to organic nitrates: evidence, mechanisms, clinical relevance and strategies for prevention. Ann Intern Med. 1991;114:667.

Fihn SD, Blankenship JC, Alexander KP, et al. ACC/AHA/AATS/PCNA/ SCAI/STS focused update of the guideline for the diagnosis and management of patients with stable ischemic heart disease: a report of the American College of Cardiology/American Heart Association Task Force on Practice Guidelines, and the American Association for Thoracic Surgery, Preventive Cardiovascular Nurses Association, Society for Cardiovascular Angiography and Interventions, and Society of Thoracic Surgeons. J Am Coll Cardiol. 2014;28:2014. doi:10.1016/j.jacc.2014.07.017.

George S, Cockburn J, Clayton TC. Long-term follow-up of elective chronic total coronary occlusion angioplasty analysis from the U.K. Central Cardiac Audit Database. J Am Coll Cardiol. 2014;64:235–43.

Gottlieb SO, Weisfeldt ML, Ouyang P, et al. Silent ischemia as a marker for early unfavorable outcomes in patients with unstable angina. N Engl J Med. 1986;314:1214.

Grosser T, Fries S, Lawson JA, et al. Drug resistance and pseudoresistance an unintended consequence of enteric coating Aspirin. Circulation. 2013;127:377–85.

Hobl E, Stimlfl T, Ebner J, et al. Morphine decreases clopidogrel concentrations and effects. A randomized double—blind placebo-controlled trial. J Am Coll Cardiol. 2014;63(7):630–5.

Juul Moller S, Edvardsson N, Jhnmatz B, et al. Double blind trial of aspirin in primary prevention of myocardial infarction in patients with stable angina pectoris. Lancet. 1992;340:1421.

Juurlink DN, Gomes T, Ko DT, et al. A population-based study of the drug interaction between proton pump inhibitors and clopidogrel. CMAJ. 2009;180:713–8.

Khan MG. Angina. In: Heart disease, diagnosis and therapy. Totowa, NJ: Humana Press, 2005, p. 55.

Lewis HD, Davis JW, Archibald DG, et al. Protective effects of aspirin against acute myocardial infarction and death in men with unstable angina: results of a Veterans Administration Cooperative Study. N Engl J Med. 1983;309:396.

Mega JL, Braunwald E, Wiviott SD, et al. Rivaroxaban in patients with a recent acute coronary syndrome. N Engl J Med. 2012;366:9–19.

Miwa K, Kambara H, Kawai C. Effect of aspirin in large doses on attacks of variant angina. Am Heart J. 1983;105:351.

Nademanee K, Intarachot V, Josephson MA, et al. Prognostic significance of silent myocardial ischemia in patients with unstable angina. J Am Coll Cardiol. 1987;10:1.

Norwegian MultiCenter Study Group. Timolol-induced reduction in mortality and reinfarction in patients surviving acute myocardial infarction. N Engl J Med. 1981;304:801.

O'Rourke RA. Optimal medical therapy is a proven option for chronic stable angina. J Am Coll Cardiol. 2008a;52:905–7.

Packer M, Le WH, Kessler P, et al. Induction of nitrate tolerance in heart failure by continuous infusion of nitroglycerin and reversal of tolerance by N-acetylcysteine, a sulfhydryl donor (abstract). J Am Coll Cardiol. 1986;7:27A.

Peterson ED, Rumsfeld JS. Finding the courage to reconsider medical therapy for stable angina. N Engl J Med. 2008;359:751–3.

PRAISE, Packer M, O'Connor CM, Ghoul JK, et al. Effect of amlodipine on morbidity and mortality in severe chronic heart failure. Prospective Randomized Amlodipine Survival Evaluation study group. N Engl J Med. 1996;335:1107.

Rudolph W. Tolerance development during isosorbide dinitrate treatment: can it be circumvented? Z Kardiol. 1983;72:195.

Schömig A, Mehilli J, de Waha A, et al. A meta-analysis of 17 randomized trials of a percutaneous coronary intervention-based strategy in patients with stable coronary artery disease. J Am Coll Cardiol. 2008;52:894–904.

Sharpe N, Coxon R, Webster M, et al. Hemodynamic effects of intermittent transdermal nitroglycerin in chronic congestive heart failure. Am J Cardiol. 1987;59:895.

11 Myocardial Infarction

OVERVIEW

- Acute coronary syndrome [ACS = ST-segment elevation myocardial infarction (STEMI) or non-ST-elevation myocardial infarction (NSTEMI) and unstable angina] is a life-threatening condition (see Fig. 11-1).
- Patients presenting with ACS are at high risk for cardiac events: death which may be sudden, recurrence of Myocardial Infarction (MI), or ischemia.
- Events can be significantly reduced by percutaneous coronary intervention [PCI] or thrombolytic therapy accomplished within 2–3 h of onset of MI. Ways to reduce delays in doing percutaneous coronary intervention soon after STEMI onset include early recognition of symptoms by patients and prehospital diagnosis by paramedics so that the emergency room can be bypassed in favor of direct admission to the catheterization laboratory (Windecker et al. 2013). The late Dr JF Pantridge, founder of coronary care units (1967), uttered the statement: "He advocated that a cardiac defibrillator should be considered in the same light as a *fire extinguisher* and thus should be available *in most homes*, place of work and sports arenas" (Pantridge 1974, personal conversation).
- An acute MI remains a fatal event in >33 % of patients. Approximately 50 % of deaths occur within 1 h of onset of symptoms, mainly because of ventricular fibrillation (VF).

Of 55 million deaths globally every year, about 30 % are from cardiovascular diseases. Of these, 40–50 % are likely to be due to acute MI (Yusuf et al. 2001).

© Springer Science+Business Media New York 2015
M. Gabriel Khan, *Cardiac Drug Therapy*, Contemporary Cardiology,
DOI 10.1007/978-1-61779-962-4_11

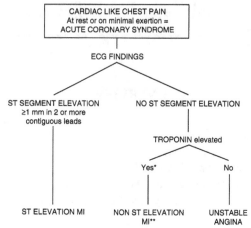

*Exclude false +ve. If troponins unavailable, creatine kinase, myocardial bound (CK-MB) + ve also confirms diagnosis; CK-MB –ve with the associated ECG changes = unstable angina high risk.

**ACC/AHA guideline: associated with ST depression ≥ 0.05 mV, 0.5 mm. European Society of Cardiology ≥ 0.1 mV, 1 mm.

Fig. 11-1. Diagnosis of ST-segment elevation MI (STEMI) and non-ST-segment elevation MI (NSTEMI) Acute coronary syndrome. *Exclude false +ve. If troponins are unavailable, creatine kinase, myocardial bound (CK-MB) +ve also confirms diagnosis; CK-MB –ve with the associated ECG changes = unstable angina high risk. **ACC/AHA guideline: associated with ST depression ≥0.05 mV, 0.5 mm in two or more contiguous leads. European Society of Cardiology ≥0.1 mV, 1 mm.

- About 15 % of patients will either have died or had another MI or significant ischemia within 6 months following acute STEMI or NSTEMI.
- The incidence of AMI is similar in Europe; unfortunately, the incidence is increasing in Asia and Latin America.
- Although more than 50 million American adults have some atheromatous coronary artery disease (CAD), only a small fraction will ever develop erosion, fissuring, or plaque rupture that culminates in AMI (Topol 2005)

LIFESTYLE: Willett (2002) estimated that more than 80 % of coronary artery disease (CAD) may be accountable for by lifestyle issues: weight, diet, exercise, and control of risk factors such as blood pressure and smoking. There is evidence that a small consumption of alcohol, 1 drink for women and 2 for men, confers some cardiovascular protection. But a Prospective Study and Dose-Response Meta-Analysis indicated that alcohol consumption, even at moderate intakes, is a risk factor for atrial **fibrillati**on. All studies reported a positive association, with an overall 8 % (6–10 %) increase in AF risk per 1 drink/day increment in alcohol consumption. In this large prospective study, both moderate (1–3 drinks/day) and high (>3 drinks/day) alcohol consumption was associated with increased AF risk. With regard to specific alcoholic beverages, **consumption of liquor and wine but not beer was significantly positively associated with AF risk** (Larsson et al. 2014).

FAMILY HISTORY: Nevertheless the evidence for heritability of AMI is striking, with a positive family history being one of the most important risk factors for this complex trait (Wang et al. 2004). Genetic studies indicate that the heritability of AMI is much more impressive than that of atherosclerotic CAD (Willett 2002; Topol et al. 2001), which in the majority remains stable and without plaque erosion or rupture.

TRIGGERS FOR ACS

- **Cocaine** is the most likely to trigger an event in an individual, although only 0.9 % of MI cases were estimated to be triggered by cocaine.
- **Traffic**, has the greatest population effect as more people are exposed to the trigger (Nawrot et al. 2011). Most city dwellers are exposed to traffic pollution which is now believed to be a major trigger for heart attacks and supersedes other triggers such as physical exertion in relatively sedentary individuals, air pollution, and anger.

  Importantly, drivers of vehicles in heavy city traffic are exposed to exhaust fumes which circulate within their vehicles. It is not surprising therefore that in China, India, and other countries there is a rise in the occurrence of ACS as large population groups move from country living and become city dwellers.

- **LDL-C**: The importance of maintaining LDL-C at goal levels in patients at intermediate and high risk cannot be overemphasized. Low HDL-C is a novel lipid phenotype that appears to be more prevalent among Asian populations, in whom it is associated with increased coronary risk (Huxley et al. 2011). Some genetic mechanisms that raise plasma HDL cholesterol, however, do not lower risk of MI. These data challenge the concept that raising of plasma HDL cholesterol will uniformly translate into reductions in risk of MI (Voight et al. 2012).

- **Serum Potassium stability is most important**. Among inpatients with AMI, the lowest mortality was observed in those with post-admission serum potassium levels 3.5–4.4 mEq/L compared with those who had higher or lower potassium levels. Rates of ventricular fibrillation (VF) or cardiac arrest were higher only among patients with potassium levels of less than 3.0 mEq/L and at levels of 5.0 mEq/L or greater (Goyal et al. 2012).

DIAGNOSIS

- Patients with symptoms of STEMI (chest discomfort with or without radiation to the arms, neck, jaw, epigastrium, or back; shortness of breath; weakness; diaphoresis; nausea; light-headedness) should be transported to the hospital by ambulance rather than by relatives. If nitroglycerin is available, one tablet or two puffs sublingual should be used and three chewable aspirins (total 240 mg) are taken while awaiting the ambulance.

- Thuresson et al. (2005) point out that the typical symptom onset of AMI is observed in less than 50 % of patients with STEMI; only one in five fulfill all the criteria usually associated with an acute MI.

- Symptoms of AMI in women may differ from those in men but not markedly. Most important, women more frequently report pain/discomfort in the neck or jaw and back, as well as nausea; they score their pain/discomfort slightly higher than men (Thuresson et al. 2005).

- In younger women aged 35–55 presenting with severe but somewhat atypical chest pain precipitated by an acute stressful event, stress cardiomyopathy (Takotsubo cardiomyopathy) should be excluded by an urgent echocardiographic assessment (see Fig. 11-2).
- Astute observation of the electrocardiographic (ECG) changes of STEMI remains crucial for diagnosis and must be mastered to command rapid commencement of PCI or thrombolytic therapy.
- STEMI can be diagnosed within 10–30 min by observation of ST-segment changes in two or three serial ECGs. The ECG is the crucial test needed for diagnosis. Troponins or MRI are second runners because time is of the essence.

Troponin levels are important in defining high-risk NSTEMI, but have no role to play in diagnosis of STEMI prior to PCI done within 90 min of arrival at a PCI facility. It is also of no value in areas where only thrombolytic therapy is available and can be given during ambulance transport or within 20 min of arrival at an emergency room.

- Serial changes in highly sensitive troponin I assay and earlier diagnosis of MI may evolve (Keller et al. 2011). But there are many other conditions that can cause troponin elevation: Causes of elevated troponin values in clinical settings other than acute MI (White and Chew 2008) include: tachyarrhythmia, bradyarrhythmia, heart block, severe hypertension, cardiogenic shock, hypotension, heart failure, aortic dissection, hypertrophic cardiomyopathy, rhabdomyolysis with cardiac myocyte necrosis, Takotsubo cardiomyopathy, transplant vasculopathy, myopericarditis, rheumatoid arthritis, systemic vasculitis, post-viral infiltrative diseases of the myocardium, amyloidosis, sarcoidosis, hemochromatosis, scleroderma, atrioventricular ablation, defibrillation, chest wall trauma, cardiac surgery renal failure, transient ischaemic attack, stroke, or subarachnoid hemorrhage, drug

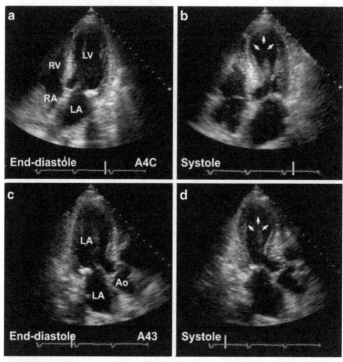

Fig. 11-2. Transient myocardial stunning: stress-related Takotsubo: transient left apical ballooning. Apical four-chamber views in this 62-year-old female who presented with chest pains show (**a, b**) akinetic apical segments, markedly hypokinetic mid-ventricular segments, with preserved basal segments—a pattern not consistent with coronary artery anatomy. Work-up for acute myocardial infarct—enzymes, electrocardiogram, and cardiac catheterization—was nondiagnostic. Follow-up echocardiogram 6 weeks later (**c, d**) showed normal cardiac function (Reproduced with permission from Bulwer BE, Solomon SD (2007) Cardiomyopathies. In: Solomon SD, Bulwer BE, editors. *Essential Echocardiography: A Practical Handbook.* Totowa, NJ: Humana Press, 2007; p. 187. With kind permission from Springer Science + Business Media.)

toxicity (e.g., adriamycin, 5-fluorouracil, daunorubicin, herceptin, etc.), hypothyroidism pulmonary embolism, severe asthma, pulmonary hypertension, sepsis (including sepsis occurring with shock), critically ill patients, pheochromocytoma, severe burns, kawasaki disease, extreme exertion, and snake venom.

CK-MB still has a role for the diagnosis of NSTEMI where troponin estimation is not available.

- The ECG remains unchallenged, therefore, for the diagnosis of STEMI which by definition engages abnormal elevation of the ST segment.

ELECTROCARDIOGRAPHIC FEATURES

Although sophisticated tests have evolved to improve diagnostic accuracy, they are of limited value in the era of aggressive PCI and thrombolysis. Thus, a rapid relevant history and correct interpretation of the ECG repeated within minutes are of paramount importance in the implementation of early PCI, or thrombolytic therapy, either of which will be of greatest benefit if instituted within 2 h of symptom onset.

Inferior MI Diagnosis

Abnormal contour ST-segment elevation of more than 1 mm (0.1 mV) in two or more contiguous inferior leads II, III, and aVF. Figures 11-3 and 11-4 reveal abnormally coved ST-segment elevation in inferior leads with reciprocal depression in leads I and AVL diagnostic of inferior STEMI. Note the reciprocal depression in 1, AVL, V1–V3

Anterior MI Diagnosis

Greater than 1 mm (0.1 mV) abnormal contour ST-segment elevation in two or more contiguous precordial leads. But leads V2 and V3 often show some ST elevation in normal men and the following adjustment is advisable: V2 and V3 should be >2 mm in men; >1.5 mm in women to be considered

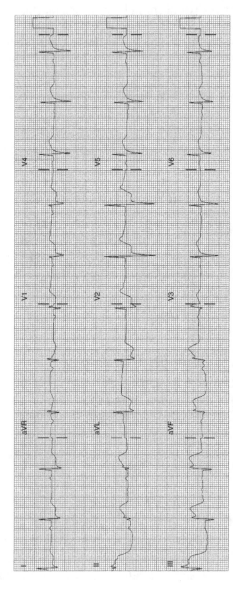

Fig. 11-3. Acute inferior MI (STEMI); abnormally shaped high ST-segment elevation in inferior leads. Note the reciprocal ST-segment depression in leads I, aVL, V1, V2. Reciprocal ST-segment depression strengthens the diagnosis of acute MI (Reproduced with permission from Khan M Gabriel, *Encyclopedia of Heart Diseases*, 2nd edition. New York: Springer; 2011. With kind permission from Springer.)

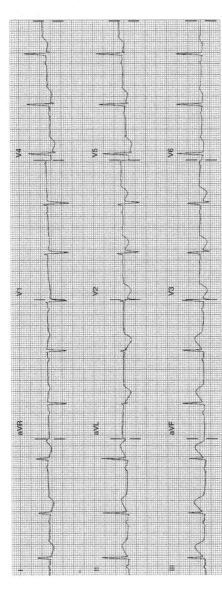

Fig. 11-4. ST elevation is less than that shown in Fig. 11.3, but the ST contour is frankly abnormal in inferior leads; note in both Figs. 4 and 5 the ST elevation in lead III is greater than that seen in lead 2, a typical feature of inferior MI. ST-segment reciprocal depression in 1, aVL, V2 V3 (Reproduced with permission from Khan M Gabriel, *Encyclopedia of Heart Diseases*, 2nd edn. New York: Springer; 2011. With kind permission from Springer.)

significant; note ST elevation should be preferably in three contiguous precordial leads: thus, elevation in V1–V3; or V2–V4. This caution may avoid administration of thrombolytic agents or coronary angiograms to individuals without MI.

Figure 11-5a shows anteroseptal MI; Fig. 11-5b shows marked ST elevation V2–V5, lead I aVL, and Q-waves, diagnostic of acute anterior MI.

- Where symptoms are not typical, the response to nitroglycerin must be ascertained. Also, minimal ST-segment elevation in black patients, other ethnic groups, and athletes must be reassessed to exclude the occasional normal variant.

ECG Mimics of Acute Myocardial Infarction

- Normal Variants: see Figs. 11-6 and 11-7 which show so-called early repolarization pattern
- Acute Pericarditis; see Fig. 11-8
- MI in recent past, age indeterminate; see Fig. 11-9
- Left bundle branch block: see Fig. 11-10. The V leads commonly show small r-waves in V1, V2, or QS complexes; poor R-wave progression with ST elevation V 1–V 3 that can be misinterpreted as an anteroseptal infarct if the interpreter fails to note the QRS duration greater than 0.12 s. LBBB caused by acute MI is a diagnostic problem
- Stress cardiomyopathy (Takotsubo cardiomyopathy, Fig. 11-2)
- Brugada syndrome; see Fig. 11-11

Other causes of ST-segment elevation include:

- Prinzmetal's (Variant) Angina

  This disorder is caused by coronary artery spasm. In this uncommon condition, transient ST elevation occurs during pain and resolves with relief of pain or with the administration of nitroglycerin.

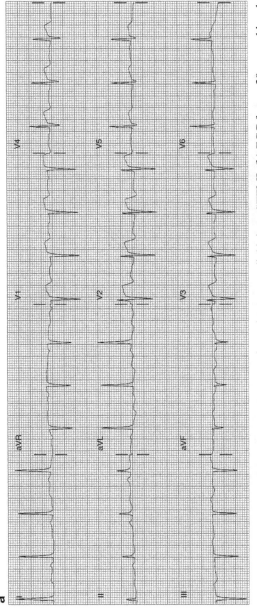

Fig. 11-5. (a) Abnormal coving, typical features of anterior myocardial injury, STEMI. **(b)** ECG from a 39-year-old male with ST-segment elevation V2–V5: acute anterior MI (Reproduced with permission from Khan M Gabriel, *Encyclopedia of Heart Diseases*, 2nd edition. New York: Springer; 2011. With kind permission from Springer.)

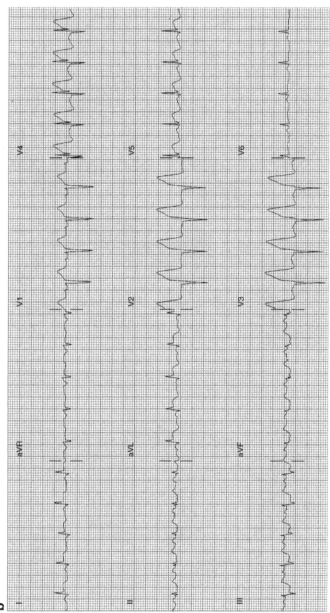

Fig. 11-5. *Continued.* ECG minutes later show further ST elevation and Q waves V2 -V5.1, aVL

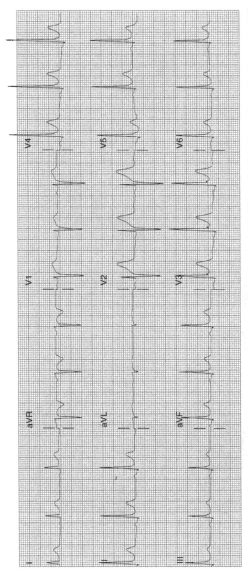

Fig. 11-6. ECG from a 25-year-old male: ST elevation 1.5 mm in leads II, III, and aVF; also, elevation 2 mm in V2–V4, but normal curve, and fishhook in V3: typical normal variant (Reproduced with permission from Khan M Gabriel, *Encyclopedia of Heart Diseases*, 2nd edition. New York: Springer; 2011. With kind permission from Springer.)

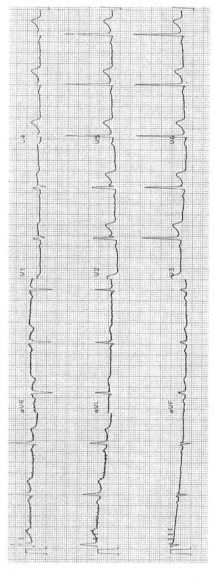

Fig. 11-7. ECG from a 45-year-old male: ST elevation 2 mm in V2, V3; fishhook in V2 (Reproduced with permission from Khan M Gabriel, *Encyclopedia of Heart Diseases*, 2nd edition. New York: Springer; 2011. With kind permission from Springer.)

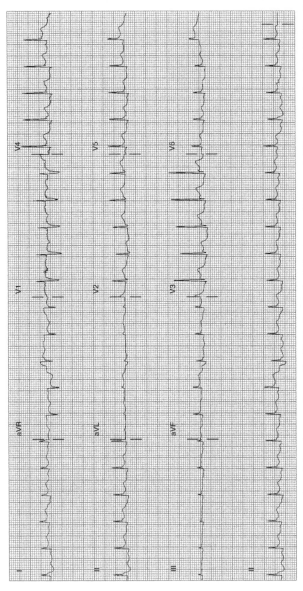

Fig. 11-8. Acute pericarditis: sinus tachycardia 126/min; typical features: widespread ST-elevation leads I, II, III, aVF, V3–V6. Note aVR shows ST-segment depression and PR-segment elevation. In addition, the J-point level almost equals the height of the T-wave in V6 (Reproduced with permission from Khan M Gabriel, *Encyclopedia of Heart Diseases*, 2nd edition. New York: Springer; 2011. With kind permission from Springer.)

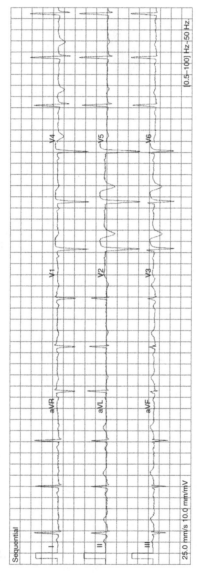

Fig. 11-9. QS in V1 V2; abnormal ST elevation V1–V3, with T inversion: anteroseptal MI age indeterminate; comparison with old ECG and clinical correlation needed; note absence of reciprocal depression as not acute MI (Reproduced with permission from Khan M Gabriel, *Encyclopedia of Heart Diseases*, 2nd edition. New York: Springer; 2011. With kind permission from Springer.)

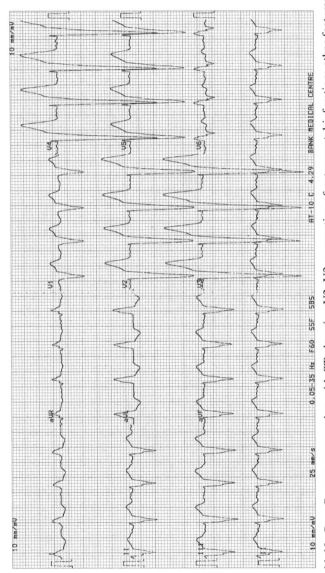

Fig. 11-10. Poor R-wave progression with ST elevation V2, V3, suggestive of anteroseptal infarction; other features of left bundle branch block (Reproduced with permission from Khan M Gabriel, *Rapid ECG Interpretation*, 3rd edition. New York: Humana Press/Springer; 2008, p. 347. With kind permission from Springer.)

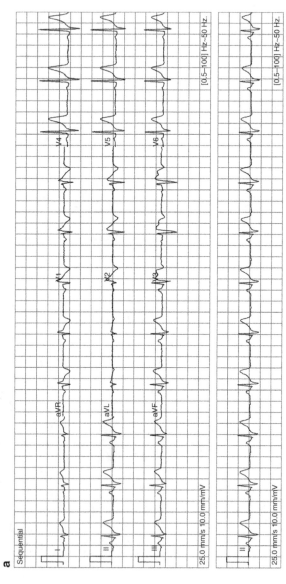

Fig. 11-11. (a) Typical features of Brugada syndrome. Atypical, incomplete right bundle-branch block (RBBB) with a curious (*odd shape*) ST-segment elevation/deformity in V1–V3, described as the coved (in V1, V2) and saddle-back patterns (V3). Note there is no widened S-wave in lead 1 V5 or in V6, as seen in true incomplete or complete RBBB. Thus, if you recognize an atypical RBBB think of Brugada syndrome and reassess for the characteristic features of this rare but important diagnosis. ECG from a 40-year-old man with episodes of syncope/collapse. No recurrence of syncope over

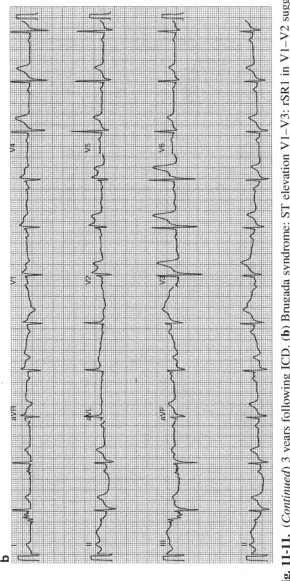

Fig. 11-11. (*Continued*) 3 years following ICD. (**b**) Brugada syndrome: ST elevation V1–V3: rSR1 in V1–V2 suggests incomplete RBBB, but there is no slurred or widened S-wave (the S-wave is not of prolonged duration) in lead I, V5, or V6 to indicate true RBBB or IRBBB. This should alert the interpreter to assess for atypical RBBB, a feature of Brugada syndrome. Scrutiny of the ST segment in V1 and V2 reveals a coved and saddle-back deformity, characteristic features of the syndrome (Reproduced with permission from Khan M Gabriel, *Encyclopedia of Heart Diseases*, 2nd edition. New York: Springer; 2011. With kind permission from Springer.)

Hyperkalemia can cause ST elevation and, rarely, transient Q-waves.

- Hypothermia with rectal temperatures below 93 °F (34 °C) may cause distortion of the earliest stage of repolarization; the ST segment becomes elevated in a curious "hitched up" pattern
- Primary or secondary tumors may cause ST elevation and Q-waves
- Acute myocarditis may present with ST elevation with or without Q-waves (Myocarditis)
- Chagasic myocarditis can cause ST and Q-wave changes (Chagas Disease)
- Subarachnoid hemorrhage or intracranial hemorrhage may cause ST-segment shifts or alteration of the QT

THERAPY

- Aspirin: 240–324 mg (3–4 tabs, 75–81 mg) chewed and swallowed at onset of pain caused by a probable heart attack. UK: Aspirin 300 mg (chewed or dispersed in water) is recommended
- Prophylaxis: 75–81 mg (non enteric coated) daily after a meal for post-MI, ischemic heart disease, or for others with atherosclerotic disease. See Chaps. 10 and 19 for aspirin pseudoresistance and reason for using soft/chewable aspirin
- Clopidogrel 600 mg loading dose; note: morphine decreases effectiveness (Hobl et al. 2014)
- Beta-blockers: metoprolol; if LV dysfunction advise carvedilol, bisoprolol, or metoprolol succinate sustained release). Avoid atenolol (see Chaps. 1 and 2)
- PCI, which if readily available, is the first choice for reperfusion
- Statins at high dose; rosuvastatin 20–40 mg or atorvastatin 60–80 mg daily to maintain LDL-C levels<1.8 (70 mg/dL mmol/L)
- Nitrates should not be used by patients who have received a phosphodiesterase inhibitor for erectile dysfunction within the last 24 h (48 h for tadalafil)

Acute MI is usually caused by occlusion of a coronary artery by thrombosis (DeWood et al. 1980) overlying a fissured or ruptured atheromatous plaque. The contents of a ruptured plaque are highly thrombogenic, and exposed collagen provokes platelet aggregation. Thus, the efficacy of aspirin should not be underestimated. Aspirin administered at the onset of symptoms markedly improves survival. In the Second International Study of Infarct Survival (ISIS-2 1988), aspirin caused a 32 % reduction in the 35-days vascular mortality rate. Thus, all patients with known coronary heart disease must be strongly advised to chew and swallow this life-saving agent if chest discomfort exceeds 10 min or if chest pain is not relieved by nitroglycerin (glyceryl trinitrate).

- Patients and the public must be informed that the use of 160–325 mg chewable tablets (not enteric coated) taken at the onset of a heart attack can cause a 20 % decrease in the incidence of heart attack or death. Aspirin should be taken once the decision has been made to proceed to the nearest emergency room. Individuals over age 40 (the MI age) should be warned that chewable aspirin acts rapidly and prevents fatal and nonfatal MI, but that nitroglycerin does neither. Nitroglycerin is effective mainly for coronary artery spasm, which is indeed a rare cause of acute MI
- In the United Kingdom advice for aspirin is as follows: chewed or dispersed in water at a dose of 150–300 mg. If aspirin is given before arrival at hospital, a note saying that it has been given should be sent with the patient
- Patients may be motivated to use this strategy if they are informed that aspirin is more important than the use of nitroglycerin because nitroglycerin may relieve pain of mild angina but does not prevent a heart attack or save lives. If chewable aspirin has not been used, then the dose should be given immediately on arrival at an emergency room

Aspirin does not block catecholamine-induced platelet aggregation and does not decrease the incidence of sudden cardiac death or the occurrence of early-morning AMI. Beta-blocking drugs have good effects here. The combination of aspirin and beta-blockers is life-saving and has proved to be effective.

Pain Relief

Pain relief must be achieved immediately and completely. Pain precipitates and aggravates autonomic disturbances, which may cause arrhythmias, hypotension, or hypertension, thus increasing the size of infarction.

1. **Morphine** Dosage: Initial dose of 4–8 mg IV at a rate of 1 mg/min repeated if necessary at a dose of 2–4 mg at intervals of 5–15 min until pain is relieved. The dose is reduced or morphine is discontinued if toxicity is observed, that is, depression of respiration, hypotension, or severe vomiting. The drug allays anxiety, relieves pain, causes venodilation, and therefore reduces preload. In addition, the drug has a favorable effect on VF threshold.

   Caution: Morphine has been shown to decrease clopidogrel absorption, decrease concentrations of clopidogrel active metabolite, and diminish its salutary effects. This can cause treatment failure in susceptible patients (Hobl et al. 2014). The drug is avoided or is used under close supervision if severe respiratory insufficiency is present. Severe vomiting and occasionally aspiration may increase cardiac work. Bradycardia is occasionally made worse, so care is required in patients with inferior MI in whom intense vagotonia already exists. Respiratory depression can be treated with the narcotic antagonist naloxone (Narcan) at a dose of 0.4–0.8 mg every 10–15 min as necessary to a maximum of 1.2 mg. Nausea and vomiting can be suppressed by IV metoclopramide 5–10 mg. The antiemetic should be given 5–15 min before the second injection of morphine.

   The dose of the antiemetic is titrated to avoid sinus tachycardia.

Diamorphine: In the UK the pain and anxiety of AMI are managed with slow IV injection of diamorphine: 2–5 mg (over 1–2 mg/min), followed by a further 2.5–5 mg if necessary every 4 h. Reduce dose by half for elderly or frail patients.

The drug appears to have a more euphoriant effect than morphine and is preferred physicians in the United Kingdom. An antiemetic such as metoclopramide (if LV function is not compromised) or cyclizine by intravenous injection.

2. **Beta-blockers** must be given a more important place in the management of chest pain resulting from MI. Beta-blockers can be considered important second-line agents for the control of ischemic pain. This is of particular importance in patients with anterior infarction accompanied by sinus tachycardia and systolic blood pressure (BP)>110 mmHg. Dramatic pain relief and reduction of ST-segment elevation can be obtained by the administration of a beta-blocking agent. The requirement for opiates is thus reduced. In some patients, pain has been documented to be relieved by the administration of beta-blockers without concomitant use of opiates. Pain may be relieved even in the absence of sympathetic overactivity. Beta-blocking agents. Administer a beta-blocker as soon as possible if it is not contraindicated. Beta-blockers (metoprolol, bisoprolol, carvedilol) given within the first 3 h of onset of chest pain improve survival provided they are used orally in patients with stable BP (systolic >105 mmHg) and there is no evidence of heart failure (HF).

Caution is needed because beta-blockers may increase cardiac mortality when used indiscriminately in patients in whom the drugs are contraindicated, particularly IV use in patients who are hemodynamically unstable, with impending cardiogenic shock, pulmonary edema, or acute MI with HF as was done in COMMIT/Second Chinese Cardiac Study (CCS–2; 2005).

In patients with anterior Killip class less than or equal to 11 ST elevation MI undergoing PCI, early IV metoprolol before reperfusion resulted in higher long-tem left ventricular ejection fraction. This administration reduced the incidence of severe left ventricular dysfunction and implantable cardioverter defibrillator indications and fewer admissions for heart failure (Pizarro et al. 2014). Carvedilol proved beneficial in the Carvedilol Postinfarct Survival Controlled Evaluation (CAPRICORN) study (2001) in patients with ejection fraction (EF) <40 %.

PERCUTANEOUS CORONARY INTERVENTION

Policies are being mustered at all levels to ensure a door-to-balloon time of <90 min. Unfortunately, despite active public education, triage in the United States, and in many countries, remains difficult, particularly because only approx. 50 % of patients with STEMI reach emergency rooms by ambulance.

PCI performed within the first 2 h of onset of symptoms markedly improves survival and morbidity. Although improvement in survival has been shown in clinical trials to occur with thrombolytic therapy given up to 4 h after the onset of symptoms, the gain is greatest within the first 2 h and then falls off dramatically after the fourth hour. For those who cannot reach a coronary intervention within 2 h or facilities are not available, thrombolytic therapy administered at the earliest moment (<2 h) is of the utmost importance. The delay in the emergency room from the arrival of the patient to the administration of thrombolytic therapy varies from 30 to 90 min. The door-to-needle time is stated to vary widely among hospitals. A delay beyond 20 min is inexcusable.

Extensive public education is essential. This is especially important in patients with known CAD. The patient and relatives must be aware of the early symptoms and signs of

AMI. The patient may therefore quickly summon transport by a mobile emergency service that should be equipped with semiautomated defibrillators and provide the use of life-saving thrombolytic therapy; in the absence of such facilities, the patient should present without delay to the nearest emergency room for early therapy which should be given within the golden 1 h

Clopidogrel

Antiplatelet therapy should be initiated before diagnostic angiography with clopidogrel (loading dose 600 mg followed by daily maintenance dose 75 mg).

Morphine has been shown to decrease clopidogrel absorption, decrease concentrations of clopidogrel active metabolite, and diminish its salutary effects. This can cause treatment failure in susceptible patients (Hobl et al. 2014).

Studies have suggested that adverse cardiovascular outcomes with the combination of clopidogrel and a proton pump inhibitor (PPI) are explained by the individual PPI. The use of a PPI inhibits CYP450 2C19, including omeprazole, lansoprazole, or rabeprazole. In particular, omeprazole has been reported to significantly decrease the inhibitory effect of clopidogrel on platelet aggregation. A study reported that the PPI pantoprazole was not associated with recurrent MI among patients receiving clopidogrel, possibly due to pantoprazole's lack of inhibition of CYP450 2C19 (Juurlink 2009)

Prasugrel

The pharmacokinetic and pharmacodynamic advantages of prasugrel over clopidogrel is clinically important when pretreatment is not possible, and fast inhibition of platelet aggregation is desirable for primary PCI for STEMI (Montalescot et al. 2009). "A loading dose of 60 mg prasugrel achieves faster, more consistent, and greater inhibition of ADP-induced platelet aggregation than does 600 mg of clopidogrel, with a significant effect seen 30 min after administration of prasugrel when no effect is detectable with clopidogrel" (Wiviott et al. 2007; Wallentin et al. 2008).

TRITON-TIMI 38 (2009), a double-blind, randomized controlled trial, compared prasugrel with clopidogrel in patients undergoing PCI for STEMI (Montalescot et al. 2009). See Chaps. 19 and 24.

Prasugrel must not be administered to patients with a history of TIA or stroke. Patients <60 kg have an increased exposure to the active metabolite and an increased risk of bleeding on a 10-mg once-daily dose. It is advisable to lower the maintenance dose to 5 mg in patients who weigh <60 kg, although the effectiveness and safety of the 5-mg dose have not been studied prospectively (Wright et al. 2011).

In the UK: Indications in combination with aspirin for the prevention of atherothrombotic events in patients with ACS undergoing PCI (with aspirin—initially 60 mg as a single dose and then body weight over 60 kg, 10 mg once daily, or body weight under 60 kg or elderly, 5 mg once daily).

Ticagrelor (BRILINTA; Brilique in UK)

Ticagrelor is an oral non-thienopyridine cyclo-pentyl triazolo-pyrimidine ADP-receptor (P2Y12) antagonist, which like prasugrel is more potent and rapid acting than clopidogrel.

Cannon and colleagues for the Platelet Inhibition and Patient Outcomes (PLATO) investigators compared ticagrelor with clopidogrel. Subjects were 13,408 (72 %) of 18,624 patients hospitalized for STEMI and NSTEMI. At 1 year, the primary composite end point occurred in fewer patients in the 6,732 ticagrelor-treated group than in the 6,676 clopidogrel group: $p = 0.0025$. Ticagrelor compared with clopidogrel significantly *reduced all-cause mortality* at 12 months in all patients (4.5 % vs. 5.9 %, hazard ratio 0.78, $p < 0.001$).

- Unlike clopidogrel and prasugrel, which bind irreversibly to the platelet surface-membrane (P2Y12) receptor, ticagrelor is a reversible P2Y12 receptor blocker, with platelet function returning to normal, 2–3 days after discontinuation (Gurbel et al. 2009) compared with 5–10 days after discontinuation of clopidogrel and prasugrel. Within 30 min, a ticagrelor loading dose of 180 mg results in roughly the same level of inhibition of platelet aggregation as that achieved 8 h after a clopidogrel loading dose of 600 mg (Gurbel et al. 2009).
- Ticagrelor, compared with clopidogrel, reduced the composite of cardiovascular death, MI, and stroke in patients with extensive coronary heart disease (14.9 % vs. 17.6 %) similar to its reduction in those without extensive CAD (6.8 % vs. 8.0 %) (Kotsia et al. 2014).

Bivalirudin: Gregg et al. (2011) was a prospective, open-label, randomized trial in patients with acute STEMI, within 12 h after the onset of symptoms, and who were undergoing PCI (Stone et al. 2011).

Results at 3 years: Compared with 1,802 patients allocated to receive heparin plus a GPI, 1,800 patients allocated to bivalirudin monotherapy had lower rates of all-cause mortality (5.9 % vs. 7.7 %, $p=0.03$), cardiac mortality (2.9 % vs. 5.1 %, $p=0.001$), and reinfarction (6.2 % vs. 8.2 %, $p=0.04$). Major bleeding not related to bypass graft surgery was significantly reduced (6.9 % vs. 10.5 %, $p=0.0001$) (Stone et al. 2011).

Bivalirudin in ISAR-REACT 4 Trial: Abciximab and Heparin vs. Bivalirudin for Non-ST-Elevation Myocardial Infarction. Bivalirudin was administered to 860 and abciximab to 861 patients. A strategy of early invasive intervention (within 24 h after admission) was the standard of care at all centers for patients presenting with an ACS and elevated biomarker levels. All the patients in the trial were given 325–500 mg of aspirin and 600 mg of clopidogrel before they received a study drug. There were no significant differences in deaths or recurrent MI.

- But major bleeding was ~ 84 % increased by abciximab (4.6 %) compared with bivalirudin (2.6 %) Kastrati et al. 2011). Bivalirudin should be the preferred anticoagulant agent for all PCIs. See Chap. 22 for other anticoagulant RCTs.

A deferred angioplasty strategy of nonculprit lesions should remain the standard approach in patients with STEMI undergoing primary PCI, as multivessel PCI may be associated with a greater hazard for mortality and stent thrombosis (Kornowski et al. 2006).

Rivaroxaban: In ATLAS ACS 2–TIMI 51 patients received the first dose of rivaroxaban no sooner than 4 h after the final dose of IV heparin, 2 h after the final dose of bivalirudin, and 12 h after the final dose of other intravenous or subcutaneous enoxaparin or fondaparinux. Patients were randomly assigned to twice-daily administration of either 2.5 or 5.0 mg of rivaroxaban or placebo, with a maximum follow-up of 31 months. Rivaroxaban significantly reduced the primary efficacy end point of death from cardiovascular causes, MI, or stroke, as compared with placebo. The 2.5 mg twice daily achieved efficacy without increased life-threatening bleeding (Mega et al. 2012). There was no significant difference in the rates of fatal bleeding associated with rivaroxaban as compared with placebo (0.3 % vs. 0.2 %, $P = 0.66$). Rivaroxaban significantly increased the rate of TIMI major bleeding that was not related to CABG, as compared with placebo, with rates of 2.1 and 0.6 %, respectively (hazard ratio, 3.96; 95 % CI, 2.46–6.38; $P < 0.001$), TIMI bleeding requiring medical attention (14.5 % vs. 7.5 %, $P = <0.001$), and intracranial hemorrhage (0.6 % vs. 0.2 %, $P = 0.009$).

The Role of Residual Thrombus was emphasized by Applegate (2011). Rivaroxaban should have a role in the prevention of residual thrombus post-PCI or following thrombolytic therapy or fondaparinux administration.

THROMBOLYTIC THERAPY

Although improvement in survival has been shown in clinical trials to occur with thrombolytic therapy given up to 6 h after the onset of symptoms, the gain is greatest within the first 2 h and then falls off dramatically after the fourth hour. Thrombolytic therapy administered at the earliest moment (<2 h) is of the utmost importance. Lives saved / 1000 treated: within 1, 3 and 7 hours respectively: 65 %, 27 %, 8 %.

The delay in the emergency room from the arrival of the patient to the administration of thrombolytic therapy varies from 30 to 90 min. The door-to-needle time is stated to vary widely among hospitals. A delay beyond 20 min is inexcusable. Delays may result from duplication of assessments by different teams of clinicians. Thrombolytic therapy should be administered in the emergency room. The emergency room physician and assistants should have the training and authority necessary to administer a thrombolytic agent.

Thrombolytic therapy is the mainstay of therapy in many countries worldwide where PCI is not immediately available.

Approximately 90 % of patients with AMI are observed on coronary arteriography to have a thrombus completely occluding the infarct-related artery (DeWood et al. 1980). There is little doubt that coronary thrombosis is the major cause of MI and that prevention of plaque rupture and thrombosis or its immediate lysis with maintenance of a patent infarct-related artery improves short- and long-term survival.

The Italian trial of IV streptokinase (SK) the GISSI trial (1986) and others have demonstrated that IV SK produces adequate reperfusion if it is given within the first 2 h of the onset of the ischemic event (ISIS 1987).

The GISSI study and ISIS-2 indicate that an IV infusion of 1.5 million U of SK over about 1 h is not particularly expensive or troublesome to give routinely, and heparin is not required.

The randomization of over 6,000 patients in ISIS-3 and GISSI-2 indicated no real difference in early mortality between SK and t-PA, and, although there was a small trend suggestive of a slightly higher incidence of intracranial bleeding resulting from t-PA plus heparin, the total death or stroke rate with SK was approximately 11.1 and 11.1 %, respectively, for tPA in ISIS-3, i.e., no difference in "net clinical outcome."

IV heparin is essential to maintain patency of the infarct-related artery after the administration of tPA or tenecteplase because the raw surface of a fissured plaque is highly thrombogenic and continuous heparinization is required to prevent reocclusion.

The Global Utilization of Streptokinase and Tissue Plasminogen Activator for Occluded Coronary Arteries (GUSTO 1993) trial studied 41,021 patients with acute infarction. The primary end point, 30-day mortality, was modestly but significantly lowered with accelerated t-PA (6.3 %) vs. SK (7.3 %) a 14 % risk reduction (p=0.006). Not surprisingly, SK outcomes did not differ by heparin regimen.

The Assessment of the Safety and Efficacy of a New Thrombolytic (ASSENT)-2 (1999) trial compared single-bolus tenecteplase (TNKase) with front-loaded t-PA in 16,949 patients (20). At 30 days, mortality rates were almost identical, but in patients treated after 4 h, the mortality rate was 7 % for TNKase and 9.2 % for t-PA (p=0.018).

In patients presenting within 4 h of symptom onset, speed of reperfusion is important, and TNKase is preferred, particularly in patients at high risk: with anterior MI, new left bundle branch block, diabetes, and HF. The patient of advanced age is at high risk, but there is also a higher risk of intracranial hemorrhage (ICH), and the choice of TNKase or SK should be individualized.

It is not logical to administer TNKase to all patients with AMI, based on the net clinical benefit and cost-effectiveness; the choice of TNKase or SK is of little consequence to public health worldwide (Collins et al. 1997), particularly when the real problem is the emergency room door-to-needle time, which is still inexcusably high, in excess of 30 min.

The incidence of ICH in RCTs was reported as follows

GUSTO III (1997): SK 0.37, t-PA 0.72, ASSENT-2: t-PA 0.93, TNK/t-PA, 0.94

- Analysis of the Medicare database suggests that thrombolytic therapy is harmful in patients >75 years old (Thiemann et al. 2000). Reportedly, the incidence of stroke is >4 % for t-PA and approx 2.85 % for SK in patients older than age 75.
- There appears to be a four- to fivefold greater incidence of ICH in patients >75 years who are treated with t-PA vs. SK.

Contraindications

- Existing or very recent hemorrhage; known or suspected bleeding diathesis; local tendency to bleeding (gastrointestinal disease with existing hemorrhages, translumbar aortography within the last 2 months, recent punctures of large arteries).
- History of cerebrovascular accident with any residual disability, intracranial or intraspinal aneurysm, brain tumor, or arteriovenous malformation.
- Major surgery or serious trauma within the last 2 months; eye surgery up to 3 months previously; severe, poorly controlled hypertension with systolic values >200 mmHg and/or diastolic values >110 mmHg, but in the elderly aged >75 years, systolic BP >200 mmHg or diastolic > 100 mmHg without therapy.
- Severe liver or kidney disease.
- Severe anemia.
- Disease of the urogenital tract with existing sources of bleeding.
- Diabetic proliferative retinopathy.
- Acute pancreatitis.
- Age over 75 years with suspicion of cerebral arteriosclerotic vascular degeneration, agitation, or confusion.

- Mitral valve disease with atrial fibrillation because of a danger of embolism from the left side of the heart.
- Suspected aortic dissection.
- Allergy to SK or anistreplase or therapy with either drug from 5 days to 1 year previously, but not contraindicated for t-PA or TNKase.
- Recent prolonged or traumatic cardiopulmonary resuscitation.
- Infective endocarditis.
- Pregnancy.

Patients older than age 65 years presenting after 12 h should not be given a thrombolytic drug; there is a high risk of cardiac rupture, particularly in women.

Streptokinase [Kabikinase, Streptase]

Dosage: 1.5 million IU in 100 mL 0.9 % saline IV over 30–60 min.

SK is an enzyme derived from cultures of beta-hemolytic streptococci. SK forms an activator complex with plasminogen, converting circulating plasminogen to plasmin, which causes lysis of fibrin. Also, SK causes activation of fibrin-bound plasminogen. A patency rate of approximately 65 % is expected if the usual dose of 1.5 million U is given within 3 h of onset of symptoms.

Advice and Adverse Effects: Anaphylaxis occurs in fewer than 0.5 % of patients; angioneurotic edema, periorbital edema, and bronchospasm may occur. A skin test is available and can be done in the emergency room and read in 15 min.

Hydrocortisone or methylprednisolone is rarely used, because fatalities have not been reported, and reactions are easy to control with epinephrine and antihistamines. Hypotension is seen in fewer than 5 % of patients and, fortunately, does not worsen with the administration of SK. The most common reaction is mild fever in 5–25 % of patients, rigors, rash, flushing, and dyspnea. Hemorrhage is often confined to puncture sites and responds to pressure. Serious hemorrhage calls for discontinuation of SK and, if needed, blood products; clotting factors as well as a protein-ase inhibitor such as Antagosan should be given: initially 200,000–1 million KIU, followed by 50,000 KIU/h IV until the bleeding stops.

There is an increased risk of hemorrhage in patients who are receiving or who have been recently treated (past 5 days) with anticoagulants, indomethacin, and similar antiinflammatory agents, sulfinpyrazone, allopurinol, and sulfonamides.

Tenecteplase

Dosage: 0.5-mg/kg bolus

TNKase is a genetically engineered triple-combination mutant of native t-PA. The major advantage is the ease of single-bolus injection.

UK: IV bolus over 10 s (initiated within 6 h of symptom onset), 30–50 mg according to body weight—max. 50 mg

Reteplase is a deletion mutant of alteplase. Reteplase can be administered as a bolus injection; this is an advantage over t-PA and SK. Reteplase, however, showed only a small benefit over SK in the INJECT trial (1995), but it had mortality, ICH, and stroke rates similar to those of t-PA in the GUSTO-III trial. Heparin must not be given through the same IV line. Dosage: 10 U over 10 min; the same dose is repeated 30 min later.

UK: Reteplase Rapilysin® (Actavis) (initiated within 12 h of symptom onset), IV 10 units over not more than 2 min, followed after 30 min by a further 10 units.

ENOXAPARIN

Enoxaparin SC is as effective as IV heparin for the prevention of adverse outcomes in patients with ACS. Major bleeding is still a concern, however. The risk for major bleeding can be reduced by decreasing the enoxaparin dose to 0.75 mg/kg once daily in patients aged 75 and over and halving the dose administered once daily if the estimated glomerular filtration rate (GFR) is <50 mL/min, as shown in the Enoxaparin and Thrombolysis Reperfusion for Acute Myocardial Infarction Treatment—Thrombolysis in Myocardial Infarction EXTRACT-TIMI 25 trial (2006, 25). Importantly, the estimated GFR formula is inaccurate in patients older than 70 years, and an adjustment must be made in patients of African origin (multiply the estimated GFR by a factor of 1.21; see Chap. 22 for advice on LMWH dosage).

The EXTRACT-TIMI 25 (2006) results for enoxaparin vs. heparin were as follows:

- At 30 days of follow-up: The primary end point occurred in 12.0 % of patients in the UF heparin group vs. 9.0 % in the enoxaparin group (17 % reduction in relative risk; $p < 0.001$). There was no difference in total mortality (25). Major bleeding occurred in 1.4 % with UF heparin vs. 2.1 % with enoxaparin ($p < 0.001$). The exclusion of men with a creatinine level >2.5 mg/dL (220 μmol/L) and women with a creatinine level >2.0 mg/dL (177 μmol/L) was an important adjustment to prevent bleeding.
- This curtailment could have been adjusted further, however, using the suggested cutoff: for estimated GFR of 30–50 mL/min, give the 0.75-mg/kg dose once daily. If the GFR is <30 mL/min, the latter reflects poor renal function and enoxaparin should be avoided to prevent a high risk of bleeding with LMWH or fondaparinux (see Chap. 22 for enoxaparin RCTs).

FONDAPARINUX

Fondaparinux, a synthetic pentasaccharide, is a factor Xa inhibitor that selectively binds antithrombin and rapidly inhibits factor Xa and, thus, is an indirect inhibitor of activated factor X (Xa).

In OASIS-6, fondaparinux reduced death and reinfarction in those receiving thrombolytic therapy by 21 % and death by 19 % at 30 days and those not receiving reperfusion therapy. OASIS 6 (2006) explored the effects of fondaparinux on mortality and reinfarction in patients with acute STEMI through an RCT of fondaparinux vs. usual care in 12,092 STEMI patients [AGE 61±12]. A 7–8-day course of fondaparinux was compared with either no anticoagulation or UF heparin (75 % received UF heparin for less than 48 h). Sreptokinase was the main fibrinolytic used (given to 73 % of those who received lytics). The primary outcome was a composite of death or reinfarction at 30 days.

- A conclusion from this trial is that fondaparinux is highly beneficial in patients in whom PCI is not available or feasible. The most common thrombolytic agent used was streptokinase. There is no pharmacological reason why the benefits of fondaparinux should differ with different thrombolytic agents.
- Advantages over UF heparin include the lack of monitoring, the once-daily dose, much lower major bleeding and ICH, and absence of heparin-induced thrombocytopenia (HIT), although thrombocytopenia can occur and platelet counts should be monitored. The half-life is approx 15 h.
- Dosage: 2.5 mg SC once daily. Risk of hemorrhage is increased in patients with severe renal dysfunction, and the dose must be reduced if the estimated GFR is <50 mL/min. As advised for LMWH, the drug should be avoided if the GFR is <40 mL/min to avoid major bleeding (see warning for estimated GFR in patients over age 70. Rivaroxaban can be commenced 12 h after the final dose of fondaparinux (Mega et al. 2012).

BETA-BLOCKERS

The salutary effects of beta-blockers are depicted in Fig. 1-1. Beta-blockers cause a decrease in heart rate, BP, rate pressure product, and myocardial contractility, and they improve ventricular diastolic relaxation, thus producing a reduction in myocardial oxygen consumption. Additional benefits include the following:

- Myocardial oxygen consumption is increased by raised levels of fatty acids. Beta-blockers decrease levels of circulating free fatty acids. Improvement of coronary diastolic filling is achieved at a lower heart rate (see Chap. 1)
- Arrhythmias, including VF, which are probably induced by increased levels of catecholamine commonly present during the early phase of infarction, are prevented

Theoretically, to achieve a favorable effect on infarct size, beta-blockers must be initiated before or within the first 3 h of infarction and certainly not later than 4 h from the onset of symptoms.

MIAMI: The Metoprolol in Acute MI trial (1985) is often quoted as showing no reduction in mortality, but the mean time to treatment was 11 h.

In ISIS-1 (1986), 80 % of patients were treated with atenolol for up to 8 h and <30 % within 4 h; this approach resulted in a 15 % decrease in mortality and significant prevention of myocardial rupture. Although atenolol has weak cardioprotective properties and is expected to confer less cardioprotection than carvedilol and metoprolol, the drug showed a positive result (see Chap. 2, Beta-Blocker Controversies, and discussion of atenolol's poor efficacy). The use of atenolol in clinical trials should be curtailed (Khan 2003).

Pooled trial results covering mainly 4–8 h indicated a 23 % decrease in mortality occurring on days 1–2. Reduction of infarct size has been documented in an RCT (International Collaborative Study Group 1984).

- The ACC/American Heart Association (AHA) recommends beta-blocker therapy given at the same time as aspirin, as soon as the diagnosis of AMI is entertained; thus, treatment should be given within 15 min after arrival at the emergency room, at which time an ECG should have been scrutinized and preparations made for PCI or administration of a thrombolytic drug

These agents are indicated in all patients with AMI unless they are contraindicated by HF, heart block, bradycardia<55 per min, systolic BP<100 mmHg, or asthma. They are strongly indicated for anterior MI, with sinus tachycardia>110 and BP>110 mmHg. Sinus tachycardia, which is commonly present with anterior wall STEMI in the absence of HF, stimulates sensory nerves in the myocardium that initiate sympathetic overactivity and thus tachycardia and hypertension. Tachycardia lowers the VF threshold and predisposes to VF. The use of beta-blockers in this clinical situation often results in relief of chest pain and a decrease in the current of injury observed on the ECG. Beta-blockers are contraindicated, however, in patients in whom sinus tachycardia is a manifestation of HF. They are strongly indicated in AMI for

- Recurrent ischemic pain.
- LV dysfunction.
- Atrial fibrillation, rate control.
- Frequent or complex ventricular ectopy, particularly within days after MI.
- Virtually all patients from day 1 for several years, which has been proved to reduce mortality, recurrent MI, and HF.

Therapy is expected to save 4 lives annually of 100 treated, as indicated by the Norwegian timolol trial (1981) and the Beta-Blocker Heart Attack Trial (BHAT 1982) propranolol study. Data from the Survival and Ventricular Enlargement (SAVE) trial (1997) and CAPRICORN (2001) indicate that beta-blockers given during acute-phase MI decrease 1-year post-MI mortality in patients with low EF independent of the use of ACE inhibitors; the benefit from the use of both agents was additive.

Beta-blockers (not atenolol) should be administered to all patients initially if there are no contraindications. Beta-blockade should be continued indefinitely for all patients who have residual LV dysfunction and who are at risk of ischemia.

ACE INHIBITORS

On the day of admission, after routinely recommended AMI therapies have been instituted, including aspirin, and, when appropriate, beta-blockers, and the patient has been stabilized, all patients with AMI should be considered for ACE inhibitor therapy. There is a general agreement that high-risk patients—those with anterior MI, previous infarction, congestive HF, or, in the absence of HF, an EF<40 %—should be administered an ACE inhibitor.

An RCT by Ambrosioni and colleagues, the Survival of Myocardial Infarction Long-Term Evaluation (SMILE 1995) study, showed that zofenopril, an analogue of captopril, commenced at approximately 15 h after the onset of anterior MI and continued for 6 weeks, caused a significant reduction in mortality and occurrence of severe HF at 6 weeks and at 1 year follow-up.

Patients with anterior infarcts, particularly those with previous infarction, should be commenced soon after admission on captopril 6.25 mg, increasing to 25 mg twice daily, or zofenopril 7.5 mg, increasing to 15 mg twice daily, or ramipril 2.5, increasing to 5–10 mg, provided the systolic BP remains >110 mmHg. ACE inhibitors are recommended in the first 24 h of an anterior MI or MI complicated by congestive HF or EF<40 % or both. The dose must be titrated to avoid hypotension. The first dose may be administered on the first hospital day if the BP is stable.

ACE inhibitors improve LV remodeling, prevent LV dilation, and preserve EF (1992 13). Systemic and coronary vasodilation has been suggested to limit infarct expansion and to prevent early remodeling. Patients with uncomplicated inferior MI, with EF>40 %, are unlikely to benefit significantly. Patients at high risk should receive lifelong treatment.

ACE inhibitors are contraindicated in patients with systolic BP<100 mmHg, renal failure, aortic stenosis, bilateral renal artery stenosis, a solitary kidney, and known allergy to

ACE inhibitors. If ACE inhibitors are not tolerated, an angiotensin receptor blocker (ARB) is advisable (candesartan or irbesartan; avoid telmisartan, olmesartan, and valsartan; see Chap. 3).

In the VALIANT (2003) RCT Patients receiving conventional therapy were randomly assigned, 0.5–10 days after acute myocardial infarction, to additional therapy with valsartan (4,909 patients), valsartan plus captopril (4,885 patients), or captopril (4,909 patients). The primary end point was death from any cause.

During a median follow-up of 24.7 months, 979 patients in the valsartan group died, as did 941 patients in the valsartan-and-captopril group and 958 patients in the captopril group.

The investigators concluded: valsartan is as effective as captopril in patients who are at high risk for cardiovascular events after MI, but there was no control group; ~70 % received a beta-blocker.

But caution is needed: valsartan should not be combined with a beta-blocker as shown in Val-HeFT; **the post hoc observation of an adverse effect on mortality and morbidity in the subgroup receiving valsartan, an ACE inhibitor, and a beta-blocker raises concern about the potential safety of this specific combination** (Cohn and Tognoni 2001).

NITRATES

IV nitrate is indicated for the relief of chest pain if more than the usual dose of an opiate is required and for the management of HF. ISIS-4 and GISSI-3 indicate that nitrates do not significantly influence survival in patients with AMI. The ISIS-4 trial (1995) yielded an insignificant mortality reduction in patients randomized to nitrates. When data from randomized AMI trials are pooled, there is only a modest a 5.5 % reduction in mortality rate with nitrate administration ($p = 0.03$). These agents are, therefore, not recommended for the routine management of acute infarction. There is an unjustifiable overuse of these agents for the management of pain during AMI.

The administration of IV nitrate requires careful monitoring to prevent harmful hypotension, reflex tachycardia, and hypoxemia. Hypotension is more common in patients who are volume depleted by diuretics or in those with inferior and right ventricular infarction. In the latter subset, bradycardia is not uncommon. Prolonged use of IV nitrates at high infusion rates may produce significant methemoglobinemia. Avoid the use of nitrates in patients with right ventricular infarction, inferior MI with suspected posterior or right ventricular infarction, hypotension, bradycardia, and aortic stenosis.

STATINS

High-dose statins have proved to be effective in reducing morbidity and mortality rates in patients with ACS (Cannon et al. 2004; Murphy et al. 2009) (see Chaps. 17 and 22).

MANAGEMENT OF COMPLICATIONS OF INFARCTION

Arrhythmias

1. Bradycardia is common and is usually not harmful. The cautious use of atropine to correct severe bradycardia that is causing hypotension or ventricular ectopy is helpful. Atropine is given judiciously to increase the heart rate to a maximum of 60 beats/min. A slow rate is probably protective because the myocardium requires less oxygen. Overzealous use of atropine can cause sinus tachycardia and, very rarely, ventricular tachycardia (VT) or VF. Bradycardia associated with second-degree type II AV block and complete AV block unresponsive to atropine usually requires temporary pacing.

2. Tachyarrhythmias: sinus tachycardia has been adequately discussed.

VF is most common during the first 4 h of infarction and is observed in about 5.5 % of patients in the first 4 h and in 0.4 % of those admitted subsequently (Lawrie et al. 1968, p. 40). It is now clear that

- VF cannot be predicted accurately.
- Warning arrhythmias are misleading.
- VF can occur without warning arrhythmias and in the absence of HF or cardiogenic shock.
- VF may occur despite the adequate suppression of premature ventricular contractions (PVCs).
- Warning arrhythmias are seen frequently in those who have VF or do not go into VF.

Clearly, there is a relationship between the R-on-T phenomenon and VF, but the R-on-T phenomenon often occurs without precipitating VF. It is possible that when VF is precipitated by the R-on-T phenomenon, the VF threshold at that time has been decreased by factors such as

- Ischemia.
- Catecholamine release in the area of infarction (catecholamines increase cyclic adenosine monophosphate activity, which is believed to be important in facilitating the development of VF).
- Tachycardia (increases VF threshold).
- Hypoxemia.
- Alkalosis or acidosis.
- Hypokalemia, which lowers VF threshold (catecholamines may produce transient acute depressions in serum K+ levels).

Lidocaine suppresses PVCs but does not sufficiently raise the VF threshold.

Management of PVCs in AMI: Most cardiologists have abandoned prophylactic lidocaine. PVCs, nonsustained VT (runs of three or more PVCs <30 s) as warning arrhythmias, are generally ignored. Beta-blockers administered promptly to patients with MI should suffice for most of those with PVCs. This therapy has been shown to reduce the incidence of VF and death from AMI.

Prophylactic lidocaine may be important where facilities for monitoring cardiac rhythm are poor, but with heavy monitoring lidocaine is unnecessary and potentially toxic.

Dosage: For sustained VT, hemodynamically stable rate <150 min: lidocaine IV initial bolus 1.0–1.5 mg/kg (75–100 mg). After 5–10 min, administer a second bolus, 1 mg/kg. Halve the dose in the presence of severe hepatic disease or reduced hepatic blood flow or a hepatically metabolized beta-blocker and in patients over the age 65 years.

The initial bolus is given simultaneously with the commencement of the IV infusion of lidocaine, so a lag between the bolus and the infusion does not occur. Commence the infusion at 2 mg/min; if arrhythmias recur, administer a bolus of 50 mg and increase the infusion rate to 3 mg/min. Carefully reevaluate the clinical situation and rationale before increasing the rate to the maximum of 4 mg/min. The maximum dose in 1 h equals 300 mg. Patients should be observed for signs of lidocaine toxicity and the dose reduced appropriately. Seizures may be controlled with diazepam.

VT: Electrical cardioversion is used if there is any hemodynamic deterioration. If the patient remains stable and VT persists, a further bolus of lidocaine is tried, followed by procainamide given as an IV 100-mg bolus: 25 mg/min; then 10–20 mg/min to 1 g in the first hour; and then 1–4 mg/min.

Other arrhythmias: Atrial flutter or atrial fibrillation causing hemodynamic deterioration is converted electrically using low energy levels. If there is no hemodynamic disturbance, digoxin is administered. Esmolol may be used to control the ventricular rate.

Supraventricular tachycardia may require electrical conversion, but if there is no hemodynamic disturbance and HF is absent, esmolol or another beta-blocker is advisable.

Sinus bradycardia: Inferior and posterior MI initiates mainly vagal overactivity, which commonly causes sinus bradycardia and occasionally a nodal escape rhythm or AV block. Hypotension is often observed in this subset of patients. Bradycardia is commonly observed during the first hour of infarction (Adgey et al. 1968). Bradycardia may predispose to VF, especially if hypotension is present. Symptomatic bradycardia accompanied by hypotension or PVCs is managed effectively by the administration of atropine. The drug should be used judiciously.

Atropine dosage: Titrated aliquots of 0.5 or 0.6 mg are given slowly IV every 3–10 min to increase the heart rate to approximately 60 per min. Maximum atropine dose is 2.0 mg.

- Caution: Atropine in too large a dose (even 1.2 mg) or too rapid an administration may precipitate sinus tachycardia, and this is observed in about one-fifth of such patients despite careful titration. Rarely, VF may be precipitated (Massumi et al. 1972). Severe bradyarrhythmias (AV block not responsive to atropine) are managed with pacing.

Heart Failure

Mild LVF is not uncommon and may resolve spontaneously.

- Furosemide is given IV 20–40 mg followed by 20–40 mg every 3–4 h if absolutely necessary. Serum K+ must be maintained at a level 3.5–4.5 mEq (mmol)/L.
- Sublingual, transdermal, or IV nitrate: Nitrates are useful to reduce preload when pulmonary congestion is present with a high pulmonary capillary wedge (PCW) pressure. They are contraindicated in patients with low cardiac output in the absence of a raised PCW pressure, right ventricular infarction, and cardiac tamponade and when nitroprusside is given.

Right Ventricular Infarction

Approximately 42 % of acute inferior infarcts are accompanied by right ventricular infarction (Wellens 1993). Patients with inferior MI and ST elevation in V4R indicating right ventricular infarction were observed to have a 31 % mortality rate and 64 % in-hospital complications, versus 6 and 28 %, respectively, for those with inferior infarction (Zehender et al. 1993). The hypotension of right ventricular infarction may be confused with hypovolemic hypotension because both are associated with a low or normal PCW pressure. The markedly raised jugular venous pressure, Kussmaul's sign, absence of crepitations on examination and clear lung fields on chest radiography, a normal PCW, right atrial pressure >10 mmHg, or a ratio of right atrial pressure to PCW pressure >0.8, in association with ECG findings of an inferoposterior MI and ST elevation in V4R.

Cardiogenic Shock

Cardiogenic shock usually results from extensive MI or development of mechanical defects such as rupture of a papillary muscle or ventricular septum. Cardiogenic shock occurs in approximately 5–8 % of patients hospitalized with STEMI (Reynolds and Hochman 2008) and in <3 % of patients with NSTEMI. Mortality rates have been reported to range from 65 to 80 % (Rosamond et al. 2008).

Characteristic features are marked hypotension, systolic BP <80 mmHg, marked reduction in cardiac index <1.8 L/min/m², and raised PCW pressure >18 mmHg. BP should be measured by a direct intraarterial method. Systemic vascular resistance should be calculated. Accurate determination of urinary volume output is essential. Guidelines to hemodynamic parameters include the following:

- The central venous pressure is inaccurate in the critically ill and in particular in a patient with cardiogenic shock.
- The pulmonary artery occlusive pressure (=PCW) is a reliable indicator of LVFP and is the preferred method of

monitoring volume status. Normal LVFP is 8–12 mmHg. In AMI, because of reduction in LV compliance, allow a normal value of 13–18 mmHg; an LVFP of 16–20 mmHg may be necessary for optimal cardiac output.

Management

1. Hypovolemic hypotension, right ventricular infarction, cardiac tamponade, and pulmonary embolism are excluded or treated. Hypovolemic hypotension is a correctable condition and should be given first priority in the diagnostic checklist. Hypotension and reduced cardiac output are present with a PCW <9 mmHg; this measurement can range from 9 to 12 mmHg and occasionally from 13 to 17 mmHg (Right ventricular infarction is excluded by the presence of a markedly raised jugular venous pressure with a normal PCW.) If hypotension is present with a PCW <17 mmHg, 50-mL IV bolus infusions of crystalloid or colloid are given with serial estimation of PCW and cardiac output.
2. Mechanical defects such as ruptured papillary muscle or ventricular septum require consultation with the cardiac surgeon. Temporary support is often attained with the combined use of nitroprusside and intraaortic balloon counterpulsation to allow catheterization.
3. Dopamine or dobutamine used alone or in combination improves hemodynamics. Overgaard and Džavík emphasized in a review that the use of vasopressin at low-to-moderate doses may allow catecholamine sparing. In cardiogenic shock complicating STEMI, guidelines based on expert opinion recommend dopamine or dobutamine as first-line agents with moderate hypotension (systolic blood pressure 70–100 mmHg) and norepinephrine as the preferred therapy for severe hypotension (systolic blood pressure <70 mmHg) (Overgaard and Džavík 2008).

When the extent of myocardial damage is severe and systemic diastolic pressure remains <60 mmHg, mortality is not significantly reduced by dopamine, dobutamine, other cardiotonic agents, or vasodilators. A State-of-The-Art Paper on Inotropes gives a needed update (Francis et al. 2014).

4. Norepinephrine in doses of 2–10 mg/min may be given a trial when the systemic vascular resistance is not raised, but it does not significantly affect mortality. Norepinephrine in general is recommended only if all measures including balloon counterpulsation fail to maintain systemic arterial diastolic BP>60 mmHg. Intraaortic balloon counterpulsation reduces afterload and increases diastolic pressure, thus improving coronary perfusion pressure.
5. Isoproterenol, methoxamine, and phenylephrine are contraindicated. The overall mortality rate is not improved by any of the suggested steps outlined.
6. Intraaortic balloon counterpulsation is needed to stabilize patients selected for angiography and revascularization.

Early Reperfusion

There is little doubt that early reperfusion therapy significantly prevents shock. Thrombolytic therapy administered in-ambulance vs. PCI found no cardiogenic shock among patients assigned to prehospital thrombolysis (Steg et al. 2003). It must be reemphasized that in the APSAC trial, the early administration of thrombolytic therapy caused a significantly lower incidence of shock (3.2 vs. 9.5 %, $p=0.03$). The early recognition and reopening of the culprit coronary is crucial and if done within 2 h of onset of symptoms would dramatically reduce the occurrence of cardiogenic shock and should be a major focus of public health campaigns.

PCI has a role in these critically ill patients and has resulted in an improvement in survival in this group. The randomized SHOCK trial found a 13 % absolute increase in 1-year survival in patients assigned to early revascularization (Hochman et al. 1999, 2006). Among PCI-assigned patients, just 0.5 % developed CS in the group randomized <2 h from symptom onset. Many older adults are, however, "subjected to unwanted, costly, painful, and futile life-prolonging efforts." When appropriate, we should strive for comfortable death with dignity, for older adults with cardiogenic shock (Hochman and Skolnick 2009).

As in MI without shock, earlier revascularization is better in patients with cardiogenic shock. Prevention of cardiogenic shock is crucial and can be successful if PCI or thrombolysis is employed within 2 h of onset of symptoms.

Rapid thrombolysis commenced in ambulances deserves further clinical trials.

MANAGEMENT OF NON-ST-ELEVATION MYOCARDIAL INFARCTION

It is necessary to risk stratify patients with NSTEMI. High-risk factors include:

1. ST-segment changes in keeping with ischemia: If the ST-segment burden is high the risk is increased.
2. Positive biomarkers (troponin or CK-MB).
3. Recurrent ischemia: chest pain with further ECG changes of ischemia.
4. LV dysfunction: EF<45 % or manifest HF.

These patients should preferably have coronary angiograms to define coronary obstructive lesions within 12 h of admission to an emergency room, with a maximum delay of 24 h.

Atorvastatin 80 mg is advisable to maintain LDL-C<1.8 mmol/L (70 mg/dL). A beta-blocker [often metoprolol or bisoprolol but if LV dysfunction or EF<45 % is present carvedilol] is advisable.

Clopidogrel 300–600 mg should be given as early as possible before or at the time of PCI or prasugrel 60 mg may be used. Prasugrel is not recommended for patients with prior stroke or TIA, or over age 74 or weight<60 kg.

In **ISAR-REACT 4 Trial**, there were no significant differences in deaths, or recurrent MI, but major bleeding was ~84 % increased by abciximab [4.6 %] compared with bivalirudin [2.6 %]. Kastrati et al. 2011) Bivalirudin is now the preferred anticoagulant agent for all PCIs.

TACTICS-TIMI 18 (2001): Only patients with NSTEMI (as defined by positive troponin levels) achieved the greatest benefit from an early invasive strategy (14.3 % vs. 24.2 %; $p<0.001$. Coronary angiography was completed within 4–48 h, and PCI was accomplished in the invasive arm.

- The cumulative incidence of the primary end point of death, nonfatal MI, or rehospitalization for an ACS during the 6-month follow-up period was lower in the invasive-strategy group than in the conservative-strategy group (15.9 % vs. 19.4 %; OR, 0.78; $p=0.025$).

TIMACS (2009) randomly assigned 3,031 patients with ACS to undergo either routine early intervention (coronary angiography ≤24 h after randomization) or delayed intervention (coronary angiography ≥36 h after randomization).

About 80 % had ECG changes in keeping with ischemia (ST of equal to or >1 mm or transient ST-segment elevation or T-wave inversion of >3 mm). About 77 % of the patients had elevated biomarkers (NSTEMI) (Mehta et al. 2009). Thus, about 77 % were NSTEMI and 23 % were unstable angina. Unfortunately, the presence of these 23 % lower-risk patients dilutes the treatment effects.

Coronary angiography was performed in 97.6 % of patients in the early-intervention group (median time, 14 h) and in 95.7 % of patients in the delayed-intervention group (median time, 50 h). At 6 months, the primary outcome occurred in 9.6 % of patients in the early-intervention group, as compared with 11.3 % in the delayed-intervention group (hazard ratio in the early-intervention group, 0.85; $P=0.15$). There was a relative reduction of 28 % in the secondary outcome of death, MI, or refractory ischemia in the early-intervention group (9.5 %), as compared with the delayed-intervention group (12.9 %) (hazard ratio, 0.72; $P=0.003$).

In patients with a **GRACE risk score of more than 140** (the third with the highest risk), the primary outcome occurred in 13.9 % of patients in the early-intervention group, as compared with 21.0 % in the delayed-intervention group, a reduction of 35.0 % in the early-intervention group (hazard ratio, 0.65; 95 % CI, 0.48–0.89; $P=0.006$).

Among patients with a score of 140 or less (a combination of the low-risk and intermediate-risk thirds), there was no significant difference between groups (7.6 % vs. 6.7 %)

Angioplasty to Blunt the Rise of Troponin in Acute Coronary Syndromes (ABOARD) study investigators (2009) compared angiography and intervention performed immediately on presentation with intervention carried out on the next working day.

A total of 352 patients with unstable ischemic symptoms, ECG changes, or troponin elevation were randomized to immediate (at a median 70 min after enrollment) vs. delayed (at a median 21 h) angiography and revascularization.

These RCTs provide support for a strategy of early PCI [within the first 24 h after hospital presentation], among those at high risk (defined by a GRACE score >140). The GRACE risk calculator available at www.outcomes.org/grace can be used to derive a prognostic score (Fox et al. 2006).

- **A delayed approach [36–48 h] is reasonable in low- to intermediate-risk patients**. There is no evidence that incremental benefit is derived by angiography and intervention performed within the first few hours of hospital admission even in high-risk patients
- In high-risk patients, **intervention within 12–24 h is superior to a strategy of delaying intervention to more than 36 h**. For all other patients with ACS, either an early or a delayed approach is safe and acceptable

Fox and colleagues assessed a meta-analysis ($n=5,467$ patients) designed to determine whether outcomes are improved despite trial differences: "a routine invasive strategy reduces long-term rates of cardiovascular death or MI and the largest absolute effect is seen in higher-risk patients" (Fox et al. 2010).

Invasive generally preferred within 12–24 h.

- Recurrent angina or ischemia at rest or with low-level activities despite intensive medical therapy.
- Elevated cardiac biomarkers (TnI, troponin I; TnT, troponin T; or CK-MB)
- New or presumably new ST-segment depression.
- Signs or symptoms of HF or new or worsening mitral regurgitation.
- High-risk findings from noninvasive testing. Hemodynamic instability.
- Sustained ventricular tachycardia.
- PCI within 6 months.
- Prior CABG.
- High-risk score, e.g., TIMI (Antman et al. 2000) or GRACE>140).
- Mild-to-moderate renal dysfunction.
- Diabetes mellitus.
- Reduced left ventricular function (LVEF <40 %)

Conservative Generally Preferred [angiogram 24–36 h]

- Low-risk score, e.g., TIMI or GRACE (Fox et al. 2006).
- Patient/physician preference in the absence of high-risk features

MEDICATIONS ON DISCHARGE

The course of post-MI patients STEMI and NSTEMI after hospital discharge and in the ensuing years is improved by an intensive reduction in LDL-C cholesterol levels (Cannon et al. 2004) and administration of an anticoagulant (Mega 2012).

1. Clopidogrel 75 mg daily for 1 year if drug eluting stent. Controversies will continue. In the large Clopidogrel for High Atherothrombotic Risk and Ischemic Stabilization, Management and Avoidance (CHARISMA) trial, dual anti-

platelet therapy [DAPT] was not superior to aspirin monotherapy (Bhatt et al. 2006). The 2010 European guidelines
on myocardial revascularization (Wijns et al. 2010) state that
convincing evidence for the duration of DAPT after DES
implantation exists only up to 6 months, keeping in mind
that the 12-month time period was suggested primarily for
safety reasons. Main concerns against a DAPT duration
≥6 months after DES are the following: increased bleeding
rates and costs; occurrence of ST irrespective of DAPT
beyond 6 months (Wijns et al. 2010)

2. A beta-blocker (carvedilol, metoprolol, timolol, or bisoprolol) should be taken daily for at least 2 years and several
years if LV dysfunction, EF<40 %, or probable ischemia
persists; avoid atenolol the drug should be rendered obsolete
(see chapter 1) (Khan, 2011)

3. Aspirin soft chewable 75–81 mg once daily after a meal.

4. A statin to maintain LDL<1.8 mmol/L

5. An ACE inhibitor: lisinopril, enalapril, or ramipril for anterior MI or LV dysfunction or EF<40 %; an ARB is used only
if cough or other adverse effects occur; avoid telmisartan
and olmesartan; valsartan interacts unfavorably with beta-
blocking agents.

6. Current clinical guidelines give Class I recommendations to
long-term aldosterone receptor blockade [eplerenone] for
MI patients without significant renal dysfunction or hyperkalemia who are already receiving therapeutic doses of an
ACE inhibitor, have an EF<0.40, and have either symptomatic heart failure or diabetes mellitus.

REFERENCES

Adgey AAJ, Geddes JS, Mulholland HC, et al. Incidence, significance,
and management of early brady-arrhythmia complicating acute myocardial infarction. Lancet. 1968;2:1097.

Ambrosioni E, Borghi C, Magnani B, for the Survival of Myocardial
Infarction Long-Term Evaluation (SMILE) Study Investigators, et al.
The effect of the angiotensin-converting enzyme inhibitor zofen-opril
on mortality and morbidity after anterior myocardial infarction. N
Engl J Med. 1995;332:80.

Antman M, Cohen M, Bernink P, et al. The TIMI risk score for unstable angina/non–ST elevation MIA method for prognostication and therapeutic decision making. JAMA. 2000;284(7):835–42.

ASSENT-2 Investigators. Assessment of the safety and efficacy of a new thrombolytic: single-bolus tenecteplase compared with front-loaded alteplase in acute myocardial infarction: The ASSENT-2 double-blind randomized trial. Lancet. 1999;354:716.

Beta-blocker heart attack study group (BHAT). The beta blocker heart attack trial. JAMA. 1981;246:2073.

BHAT: β-Blocker Heart Attack Trial Research Group. A randomised trial of propranolol in patients with acute myocardial infarction. I: mortality results. JAMA. 1982;247:1707–14.

Bhatt DL, Fox KA, Hacke W, CHARISMA, et al. Clopidogrel and aspirin versus aspirin alone for the prevention of atherotrombotic events. N Engl J Med. 2006;354:1706–17.

Cannon CP, Braunwald E, McCabe CH, et al. Intensive versus moderate lipid lowering with statins after acute coronary syndromes. N Engl J Med. 2004;350:1495–504.

Collins R, Peto R, Baigent C, et al. Aspirin, heparin and fibrinolytic therapy in suspected acute myocar-dial infarction. N Engl J Med. 1997;336:847.

COMMIT/CCS-2 (Clopidogrel and Metoprolol in Myocardial Infarction Trial) Collaborative Group. Early intravenous then oral metoprolol in 45,852 patients with acute myocardial infarction: randomised placebo-controlled trial. Lancet. 2005;366:1622–32.

DeWood MA, Spores J, Notske R, et al. Prevalence of total coronary occlusion during the early hours of transmural myocardial infarction. N Engl J Med. 1980;303:897.

EXTRACT-TIMI 25, Antman EM, Morrow DA, McCabe CH, et al. Enoxaparin versus unfractionated heparin with fibrinoly-sis for ST-elevation myocardial infarction for the ExTRACT-TIMI 25 investigators. N Engl J Med. 2006;354:1477–88.

Fox KA, Dabbous OH, Goldberg RJ, et al. Prediction of risk of death and myocardial infarction in the six months following presentation with acute coronary syndrome: a prospective, multinational, observational study (GRACE). BMJ. 2006;333:1091.

Fox KAA, Clayton TC, Damman P, for the FIR Collaboration, et al. Long-term outcome of a routine versus selective invasive strategy in patients with Non–ST-segment elevation acute coronary syndrome. A meta-analysis of individual patient data. J Am Coll Cardiol. 2010;55:2435–45.

Francis GS, Bartos JA, Adatya S, et al. Inotropes. J Am Coll Cardiol. 2014;63:2069–78.

GISSI: Italian Group. Effectiveness of intravenous thrombolytic treatment in acute myocardial infarction. Lancet. 1986;1:397.

Goyal A, Spertus JA, Gosch K, et al. Serum potassium levels and mortality in acute myocardial infarction. JAMA. 2012;307(2):157–64.

Gregg W Stone, Bernhard Witzenbichler, Giulio Guagliumi et al. Heparin plus a glycoprotein IIb/IIIa inhibitor versus bivalirudin monotherapy and paclitaxel-eluting stents versus bare-metal stents in acute myocardial infarction (HORIZONS-AMI): final 3-year results from a multicentre, randomised controlled trial The Lancet, 2011;377: 2193–2204.

Gurbel PA, Bliden KP, Butler K, et al. Randomized double-blind assessment of the ONSET and OFFSET of the antiplatelet effects of ticagrelor versus clopidogrel in patients with stable coronary artery disease: the ONSET/OFFSET study. Circulation. 2009;120:2577–85.

GUSTO Investigators. An international randomized trial comparing four thrombolytic strategies for acute myocardial infarction. N Engl J Med. 1993;329:673.

GUSTO III: Global Use of Strategies to Open Occluded Coronary Arteries (GUSTO-III) Investigators. A comparison of reteplase with alteplase for acute myocardial infarction. N Engl J Med. 1997;337:1118.

Hobl E, Stimlfl T, Ebner J, et al. Morphine decreases clopidogrel concentrations and effects. A randomized double - blind placebo-controlled trial. J Am Coll Cardiol. 2014;63(7):630–5.

Hochman JS, Skolnick AH. Contemporary management of cardiogenic shock: age is opportunity. J Am Coll Cardiol Intv. 2009;2(2):153–5.

Hochman JS, Sleeper LA, Webb JG, for the SHOCK investigators, et al. Early revascularization in acute MI complicated by cardiogenic shock: should we emergently revascularize occluded coronaries for cardiogenic shock? N Engl J Med. 1999;341:625.

Hochman JS, Sleeper LA, Webb JG, et al. Early revascularization and long-term survival in cardiogenic shock complicating acute myocardial infarction. JAMA. 2006;295:2511–5.

Huxley RR, Barzi F, Lam TH, Czernichow S, Fang X, Welborn T, Shaw J, Ueshima H, Zimmet P, Jee SH, Patel JV, Caterson I, Perkovic V, Woodward M. Isolated low levels of high-density lipoprotein cholesterol are associated with an increased risk of coronary heart disease: an individual participant data meta-analysis of 23 studies in the Asia-Pacific region. Circulation. 2011;124:2056–64.

INJECT: International Joint Efficacy Comparison of Thrombolytics. Randomized, double blind comparison of reteplase-double bolus administration with streptokinase in acute myocardial infarction (INJECT): trial to investigate equivalence. Lancet. 1995;46:329.

International Collaborative Study Group. Reduction of infarct size with the early use of timolol in acute myocardial infarction. N Engl J Med. 1984;310:9.

Investigators CAPRICORN. Effect of carvedilol on outcome after MI in patients with left ventricular dysfunction; the CAPRICORN randomized trial. Lancet. 2001;357:1385–90.

ISIS Steering Committee. Intravenous streptokinase given within 0–4 h of onset of myocardial infarction reduced mortality in ISIS-2. Lancet. 1987;1:501.

ISIS-1 Group. Randomized trial of intravenous atenolol among 16,027 cases of suspected acute myocar-dial infarction: ISIS-1. Lancet. 1986;2:57.

ISIS-2 (Second International Study of Infarct Survival) Collaborative Group. Randomised trial of intravenous streptokinase, oral aspirin, both, or neither, among 17,187 cases of suspected acute myocardial infarction: ISIS-2. Lancet. 1988;2:350.

Juurlink DN, Gomes T, Ko DT, et al. A population-based study of the drug interaction between proton pump inhibitors and clopidogrel. CMAJ. 2009;180:713–8.

Kastrati A, Neumann F-J, Schulz S, for the ISAR-REACT 4 Trial Investigators, et al. Abciximab and heparin versus bivalirudin for non-ST-elevation myocardial infarction. N Engl J Med. 2011;365: 1980–9.

Keller T, et al. Serial changes in highly sensitive troponin I assay and early diagnosis of myocardial infarction. JAMA. 2011;306:2684–93.

Khan MG. Clinical trials. In: Cardiac drug therapy. 6th ed. Philadelphia, PA: WB Saunders/Elsevier; 2003. p. 502.

Khan MG. Hypertension. In: Encyclopedia of heart diseases. 2nd ed. New York: Springer; 2011. p. 556

Kornowski R, Mehran R, Dangas G, et al. Randomized trial. The OASIS-6 trial group. JAMA. 2006;295:1519–30.

Kotsia A, Brilakis ES, Held C, et al. Extent of coronary artery disease and outcomes after ticagrelor administration in patients with an acute coronary syndrome: insights from the PLATelet inhibition and patient Outcomes (PLATO) trial. Am Heart J. 2014;168(1):68–75.e2.

Larsson SC, Drca N, Wolk A. Alcohol consumption and risk of atrial fibrillation: a prospective study and dose-response meta-analysis. J Am Coll Cardiol. 2014;64(3):281–9.

Lawrie DM, Higgins MR, Godman MJ, et al. Ventricular fibrillation complicating acute myocardial infarction. Lancet. 1968;2:523.

Massumi RA, Mason DT, Amsterdam EA, et al. Ventricular fibrillation and tachycardia after intravenous atropine for treatment of bradycardias. N Engl J Med. 1972;287:336.

Mega JL, Braunwald E, Wiviott SD, et al. Rivaroxaban in patients with a recent acute coronary syndrome. N Engl J Med. 2012;366:9–19.

MIAMI Trial Research Group. Metoprolol in acute MI (MIAMI): a randomized placebo-controlled international trial. Eur Heart J. 1985;6:199.

Montalescot G, Cayla G, Collet JP, et al. Immediate vs. delayed intervention for acute coronary syndromes: a randomized clinical trial. JAMA. 2009;302:947–54.

Murphy SA, Cannon CP, Wiviott SD, et al. Reduction in recurrent cardiovascular events with intensive lipid-lowering statin therapy compared with moderate lipid-lowering statin therapy after acute coronary syndromes: from the PROVE IT–TIMI 22 (Pravastatin or Atorvastatin Evaluation and Infection Therapy – Thrombolysis in Myocardial Infarction 22) trial. J Am Coll Cardiol. 2009a;54:2358–62.

Nawrot TS, Perez L, Künzli N, Munters E, Nemery B. Public health importance of triggers of myocardial infarction: a comparative risk assessment. Lancet. 2011;377:732–40.

Norwegian Multicenter Study Group. Timolol-induced reduction in mortality and reinfarction in patients surviving acute MI. N Engl J Med. 1981;304:801.

Overgaard CB, Džavík V. Inotropes and vasopressors: review of physiology and clinical use in cardiovascular disease. Circulation. 2008;118: 1047–56.

Pantridge JF, Geddes JS. A mobile intensive-care unit in the management of myocardial infarction. Lancet. 1967;2:270–3.

Pizarro G, Fernandez-Friera L, Fuster V, et al. Long-term benefit of early pre-reperfusion metoprolol administration in patients with acute MI: results from the METOCARD-CNTC trial (effect of metoprolol in cardioprotection during an acute myocardial infarction. J Am Coll Cardiol. 2014;63(22):2356–62.

Reynolds HR, Hochman JS. Cardiogenic shock: current concepts and improving outcomes. Circulation. 2008;117:686–97.

Rosamond W, Flegal K, Furie K, For the American Heart Association Statistics Committee and Stroke Statistics Subcommittee, et al. Heart disease and stroke statistics—2008 Update: a report from the American Heart Association Statistics Committee and Stroke Statistics Subcommittee. Circulation. 2008;117:e25–146.

SAVE, Vantrimpont P, Roleau JL, Chaun-Chaun W, et al. Additive beneficial effects of beta-blockers to angio-tensin converting enzyme inhibitors in Survival and Ventricular Enlargement (SAVE) study. J Am Coll Cardiol. 1997;29:229.

Steg PG, Bonnefoy E, Chabaud S, et al. Impact of time to treatment on mortality after prehospital fibrinolysis or primary angioplasty: data from the CAPTIM randomized clinical trial. Circulation. 2003;108: 2851–6.

Stone GW, Witzenbichler B, Guagliumi G, et al. Heparin plus a glycoprotein IIb/IIIa inhibitor versus bivalirudin monotherapy and paclitaxel-eluting stents versus bare-metal stents in acute myocardial infarction

(HORIZONS-AMI): final 3-year results from a multicentre, randomised controlled trial. Lancet. 2011;377:2193–204.

Thiemann DR, Coresh J, Schulman SP, et al. Lack of benefit for IV thrombolysis in patients with MI who are older than 75 years. Circulation. 2000;101:2239.

Thuresson M, Jarlov MB, Lindahl B, et al. Symptoms and type of symptom onset in acute coronary syndrome in relation to ST elevation, sex, age, and a history of diabetes. Am Heart J. 2005;150:234–42.

TIMACS, Mehta SR, Granger CB. Boden WE et al for the TIMACS Investigators Early versus delayed invasive intervention in acute coronary syndromes. N Engl J Med. 2009;360:2165–75.

Topol EJ. The genomic basis of myocardial infarction. J Am Coll Cardiol. 2005;46:1456–65.

Topol EJ, McCarthy J, Gabriel S, GeneQuest Investigators, et al. Single nucleotide polymorphisms in multiple novel thrombospondin genes may be associated with familial premature myocardial infarction. Circulation. 2001;104:2641–4.

TRITON-TIMI 38 Investigators, Montalescot G, Wiviott SD, Braunwald E, et al. Prasugrel compared with clopidogrel in patients undergoing percutaneous coronary intervention for ST-elevation myocardial infarction double-blind, randomised controlled trial. Lancet. 2009;73: 723–31.

Val-HeFT, Cohn JN, Tognoni G. For the Valsartan Heart failure trial investigators. N Engl J Med 2001;345:1667–675.

VALIANT, Pfeffer MA, McMurray JJ, Velazquez EJ, et al. Valsartan, captopril, or both in myocardial infarction complicated by heart failure, left ventricular dysfunction, or both. N Engl J Med. 2003;349: 1893–906.

Voight BF, Peloso GM, Orho-Melander M. Plasma HDL cholesterol and risk of myocardial infarction: a mendelian randomisation study. Lancet. 2012;380(9841):572–80. http://www.lancet.com/journals/lancet/issue/vol380no9841/PIIS0140-6736(12)X6033-1. Accessed 11 Aug 2012.

Wallentin L, Varenhorst C, James S, et al. Prasugrel achieves greater and faster P2Y12receptor-mediated platelet inhibition than clopidogrel due to more efficient generation of its active metabolite in aspirin-treated patients with coronary artery disease. Eur Heart J. 2008; 29:21–30.

Wang Q, Rao S, Shen G-Q, et al. Premature myocardial infarction novel susceptibility locus on chromosome 1p34-36 identified by genome-wide linkage analysis. Am J Hum Genet. 2004;74:262–71.

Wellens HJJ. Right ventricular infarction. N Engl J Med. 1993;328:1036.

White HD, Chew DP. Acute myocardial infarction. Lancet. 2008; 372(9638):570–84.

Wijns W, Kolh P, Danchin N, et al. Guidelines on myocardial revascularization. Eur Heart J. 2010;31:2501–55.

Willett WC. Balancing life-style and genomics research for disease prevention. Science. 2002;296:695–8.

Windecker S, Bax JJ, Myat A. Future treatment strategies in ST-segment elevation myocardial infarction. Lancet. 2013;382(9892):644–57.

Wiviott SD, Trenk D, Frelinger AL, et al. Prasugrel compared with high loading- and maintenance-dose clopidogrel in patients with planned percutaneous coronary intervention: the Prasugrel in Comparison to Clopidogrel for Inhibition of Platelet Activation and Aggregation-Thrombolysis in Myocardial Infarction 44 trial. Circulation. 2007;116:2923–32.

Wright RS, Anderson JL, Adams CD. ACCF/AHA focused update of the guidelines for the management of patients with unstable Angina/ Non-ST-elevation myocardial infarction (Updating the 2007 Guideline): a report of the American College of Cardiology Foundation/American Heart Association Task Force on Practice Guidelines American Academy of Family Physicians, American College of Emergency Physicians, Society for Cardiovascular Angiography and Interventions, and Society of Thoracic Surgeons. J Am Coll Cardiol. doi:10.1016/j.jacc.2011.02.009. http://content. onlinejacc.org/cgi/content/full/j.jacc.2011.02.009v1. Accessed 28 Mar 2011.

Yusuf S, Reddy S, Ôunpuu S, Anand S. Global burden of cardiovascular diseases, Part I: general considerations, the epidemiologic transition, risk factors, and impact of urbanization. Circulation. 2001;104: 2746–53.

Zehender M, Casper W, Kauder E, et al. Right ventricular infarction as an independent predictor of prognosis after acute inferior myocardial infarction. N Engl J Med. 1993;328:981.

12 Heart Failure

THE SIZE OF THE PROBLEM

The world faces an epidemic of heart failure (HF). The plague of HF is common in developed and in developing countries.

Although treatment strategies have improved considerably over the past two decades, improvement in outcomes remains modest and the incidence of HF is increasing. Some of this increase is owing to an aging population in all countries and poor choice of optimal medications, particularly a reliance on angiotensin-receptor blockers (ARBs). In **Val-HeFT**, "valsartan when combined with a beta blocker caused significantly more cardiac events" (Val-HeFT, Cohn, and Tognoni 2001).

In patients with HF, a beta-blocker is needed as proven therapy. Thus an ACE inhibitor must be used, not an ARB; importantly, telmisartan failed in the HF trial. Telmisartan therapy for 56 months, although shown in ONTARGET to be equivalent to ramipril surprisingly, **failed to decrease total mortality and had no significant effect on the primary outcome, hospitalizations for HF (TRANSCEND). See further discussion of ARB failures in HF randomized control trials (RCTs).**

Caution: valsartan must not be combined with a beta-blocker.

© Springer Science+Business Media New York 2015
M. Gabriel Khan, *Cardiac Drug Therapy*, Contemporary Cardiology,
DOI 10.1007/978-1-61779-962-4_12

In **VALIANT** (Pfeffer et al. 2003): a clinical trial of valsartan, captopril, or both in MI complicated by HF, left ventricular dysfunction, or both, during a median follow-up of 24.7 months, **total mortality was not reduced by valsartan**: 979 patients in the valsartan group died, as did 941 patients in the valsartan-and-captopril group and 958 patients in the captopril group. There was no placebo group.

Caution: Valsartan is not advisable in HF patients because in this large number of patients a beta-blocker is needed therapy.

Although medical therapy for acute HF has improved dramatically from 1990, **unfortunately, more than 45 % of patients require readmission within 6 months of discharge**.

A major advance may be on its way: a novel drug, LCZ696, a dual inhibitor of angiotensin II receptor and neprilysin proved to be more effective than enalapril, (Jessup 2014). **Our current drugs are not used adequately. For example:**

1. **Digoxin** has been shown to significantly reduce readmissions and decreases mortality in patients with cardiomegaly or $EF < 35$ %, and is useful in most HF patients with atrial fibrillation, yet the drug is rarely used because of fear of digoxin toxicity, a complication that can be completely avoided by a watchful physician (see discussion under digoxin).

   – About 20 % of patients would not be able to use digoxin because of renal failure ($GFR < 40$ ml/min). More than 70 % of patients, however, can be given digoxin, but worldwide <15 % receive a useful inexpensive drug because of poor logic amongst those experts who formulate guidelines or prepare editorials.

   – Only those who had the pleasure of carefully dissecting the digoxin trial results and hearing an S3 gallop disappear after 3–4 days of digoxin administration would understand the salutary myocardial effects of this simple drug. Deaths and rehospitalizations continue with much outcry about health cost of HF.

- Digoxin is best suited for the multitude of hearts that are genuinely failing with an ejection fraction (EF)<40 % or with manifested mild or moderate cardiomegaly. In this large subset of patients worldwide, digoxin can be an asset to prevent some deaths but definitely prevent rehospitalization if used along with a beta-blocker and ACE inhibitor. Rosuvastatin in CORONA did not alter mortality and had a small significant effect in preventing rehospitalization; this is considered a breakthrough (Rogers et al. 2014).

   Since the downfall of digoxin during the past 20 years inotropes have been developed and much research is presently under way. Yet none has emerged to save more than a few lives (see section entitled "New Developments".) A new novel intravenous inotropic agent would have little impact on lives saved because that subset of nearly terminally ill patients require compassionate care and a transplant in some.

2. **Spironolactone and eplerenone** are proven effective for selected patients, but the agents are rarely prescribed because of the fear of hyperkalemia. This complication can be prevented by a watchful clinician. More than 40 % of patients can be treated with these agents but <20 % receive them. If the patient is stable and free from pulmonary congestion, ACE inhibitor or ARB dose should be slightly reduced prior to discharge to allow the maintenance of an aldosterone antagonist.

   - Spironolactone and ACE inhibitors or ARBs, however, have been shown to be noneffective for HF with preserved EF (HFPEF), a large subset of HF patients in whom no decisive therapy is available.
   - Digoxin and nebivolol are the two agents that have shown some salutary effects, but this information remains hidden

3. **ACE inhibitors** must be used as they are effective but with aid from other agents. They are more effective than angiotensin-receptor blockers (ARBs), yet their use is declining because ARBs are prescribed. **See discussion of the poor effects on total mortality of ARBS given in Chaps. 3 and 4.**

4. **Beta-blockers** are proven to be most effective and equal to ACE inhibitor therapy, yet many patients are denied for various reasons, particularly a fear for beta-blocker use in the elderly. But HF is a disease of the elderly age over 65.

   - In addition the correct choice of a beta-blocking drug is crucial: carvedilol, bisoprolol, and nebivolol are the beta-blockers to choose; also (metoprolol succinate (Toprol XL) if available).
   - **Atenolol is commonly used worldwide but is not recommended by the author** (see Chap. 1 for reasons).

5. **Furosemide** dosing is often inadequate: a single dose of 160 mg on an empty stomach is more effective than 80 mg twice daily (see Chap. 7). Salutary effects are much enhanced with the addition of spironolactone, eplerenone, or amiloride and in selected cases metolazone. **The combination of furosemide and metolazone decreases hyperkalemia when an aldosterone antagonist is added to the HF regimen. See later section under Diuretics.**

6. **Metolazone** has a role in patients with a GFR < 50, and is underused.

7. Acetazolamide is rarely indicated and proved useful in patients with refractory HF complicated by diuretic-induced normokalemic hypochloremic metabolic alkalosis (Khan 1980).

Prevention of HF is crucial, and physician education concerning the most appropriate drug cocktail to prescribe is vital.

CAUSES OF HEART FAILURE

The many diseases causing HF must be sought (see Table 12-1) and treated aggressively prior to symptomatic HF.

Basic Cause

Determine the basic cause of the heart disease. If the specific cause is present but is not recognized (e.g., surgically correctable causes: significant mitral regurgitation may be missed clinically; atrial-septal defect, arteriovenous fistula,

Table 12-1
Causes of systolic heart failure and diastolic heart failure

Systolic heart failure
  Coronary heart disease   ~40 %[a]
  Hypertensive heart disease   ~40 %
  Valvular heart disease   ~15 %
  Other causes   ~5 %
    Diabetes
    Dilated cardiomyopathy
    Myocarditis
    Cardiotoxins
Diastolic heart failure: HFPEF
  Left ventricular hypertrophy
  Hypertensive heart disease (systolic and diastolic HF)
  Chronic CHD
  Diabetes
  Myocardial fibrosis
  Cardiomyopathy
    Hypertrophic and restrictive
    Amyloid heart disease
    Sarcoidosis, Hemochromatosis, metabolic storage disease
    Hypertensive hypertrophic "Cardiomyopathy" of the
    elderly: aging heart (particularly woman)
    Arrhythmogenic right ventricular dysplasia
    Constrictive pericarditis, pericardial effusion, and
    tamponade
    Atrial myxoma
Systolic dysfunction is a principal cause of diastolic dysfunction

[a]CHD is approx 60 % in the United States, but worldwide hypertension is more common, particularly in blacks and Asians

constrictive pericarditis, and cardiac tamponade are important considerations), the possibility of achieving a complete cure, although rare, may be missed or the HF may become refractory.

Note: Pulmonary edema and HF are not complete diagnoses; the basic cause and precipitating factors should be stated.

The search for the etiology must be systematic, and the following routine check is suggested:

1. Myocardial damage:
   - Ischemic heart disease and its complications
   - Myocarditis
   - Cardiomyopathy
2. Ventricular overload:
   - Pressure overload.
     - (a) Systemic hypertension
     - (b) Coarctation of the aorta
     - (c) Aortic stenosis
     - (d) Pulmonary stenosis
   - Volume overload
     - (a) Mitral regurgitation
     - (b) Aortic regurgitation
     - (c) Ventricular septal defect
     - (d) Atrial-septal defect
     - (e) Patent ductus arteriosus
3. Restriction and obstruction to ventricular filling:
   - Mitral stenosis
   - Cardiac tamponade
   - Constrictive pericarditis
   - Restrictive cardiomyopathies
   - Atrial myxoma
4. Cor pulmonale
5. Others:
   - Arteriovenous fistula
   - Thyrotoxicosis
   - Myxedema

Factors precipitating heart failure:

1. Patient–physician problems:
   - Reduction or discontinuation of medications
   - Salt binge
   - Increased physical or mental stress
   - Obesity

2. Increased cardiac work precipitated by:
   - Increasing hypertension (systemic or pulmonary)
   - Arrhythmia; digoxin toxicity
   - Pulmonary embolism
   - Infection, e.g., bacterial endocarditis, chest, urinary, or others
   - Thyrotoxicosis or myxedema
3. Progression or complications of the basic underlying heart disease:
   - Ischemic heart disease—acute MI, left ventricular aneurysm, papillary muscle dysfunction causing mitral regurgitation
   - Valvular heart disease—increased stenosis or regurgitation
4. Blood problems:
   - Increased volume—transfusions of saline or blood
   - Decreased volume—overzealous use of diuretics
   - Anemia: hemoglobin in cardiacs <10 g/100 mL (100 g/L)
   - Electrolytes and acid–base problems (potassium, chloride, magnesium)
5. Drugs that affect cardiac performance and may precipitate HF:
   - Nonsteroidal anti-inflammatory drugs (NSAIDs):
   - Alpha-blockers are contraindicated all patients at risk for heart failure
   - Beta-blockers: uncommon if used appropriately
   - Corticosteroids
   - Disopyramide, procainamide
   - Calcium antagonists: verapamil, diltiazem, nifedipine, and amlodipine commonly used to treat hypertension (see Table 9-2)
   - Digitalis toxicity
   - Vasodilators and antihypertensive agents that cause sodium and water retention. These agents are further likely to precipitate HF if they cause an inhibition of increase in heart rate, which is especially important in patients with severe bradycardia or sick sinus syndrome.
   - Drugs that increase afterload and increase blood pressure

- Adriamycin, daunorubicin, and mithramycin
- Alcohol, acute excess (e.g., 8 oz of gin in a period of less than 2 h causes cardiac depression and a fall in the ejection fraction [EF]).
- Antidepressants: tricyclic compounds
- Ephedra can cause HF

DIAGNOSIS

1. Ensure that the diagnosis is correct by critically reviewing the history, physical exam, and posteroanterior (PA) and lateral chest radiographs. Many patients are incorrectly treated for HF on the basis of the presence of crepitations at the lung bases or peripheral edema. Crepitations may be present in the absence of HF and may be absent with definite LV failure. Edema is commonly owing to causes other than cardiac. The chest radiograph may be positive before the appearance of crepitations. Edema or raised jugular venous pressure (JVP) may be absent or incorrectly assessed.
2. Chest radiograph confirms the clinical diagnosis. It is most important to recognize the radiologic findings of HF, listed as follows:
   - Obvious constriction of the lower lobe vessels and dilation of the upper vessels related to pulmonary venous hypertension are commonly seen in left HF, in mitral stenosis, and occasionally with severe chronic obstructive pulmonary disease (COPD).
   - Interstitial pulmonary edema: pulmonary clouding; perihilar haze; perivascular or peribronchiolar cuffing; septal Kerley A lines and more commonly B lines.
   - Effusions, subpleural or free pleural; blunting of the costophrenic angle, right greater than left.
   - Alveolar pulmonary edema (butterfly pattern).
   - Interlobar fissure thickening related to accumulation of fluid (best seen in the lateral film).
   - Dilation of the central right and left pulmonary arteries. A right descending pulmonary artery diameter >17 mm (normal 9–16 mm) indicates an increase in pulmonary artery pressure.

- Cardiac size: cardiomegaly is common; however, a normal heart size can be found in several conditions causing definite HF:
  (a) Acute myocardial infarction (MI).
  (b) Mitral stenosis.
  (c) Aortic stenosis.
  (d) Acute aortic regurgitation.
  (e) Cor pulmonale.
- Cardiomegaly lends support to the diagnosis, severity, and etiology of HF but has been overrated in the past. Such phrases as "no HF if the heart size on PA film is normal" are to be discarded. The heart size may be normal in the presence of severe cardiac pathology, that is, an LV aneurysm or repeated MIs that can cause hypokinetic, akinetic, or dyskinetic areas that may be observed on inspection of the chest wall but may not be detectable on PA chest radiographs. Echocardiography is often necessary as it provides the most useful information on the severity of valvular lesions, LV contractility, EF, and verification of causes of HF.

  It is necessary to exclude radiologic mimics of cardiogenic pulmonary edema:
  (a) Circulatory overload.
  (b) Lung infection—viral and other pneumonias.
  (c) Allergic pulmonary edema: heroin and nitrofurantoin.
  (d) Lymphangitic carcinomatosis.
  (e) Uremia.
  (f) Inhalation of toxic substances.
  (g) Increased cerebrospinal fluid (CSF) pressure.
  (h) Drowning.
  (i) High altitude.
  (j) Alveolar proteinosis.

3. BNP: Rapid testing of brain natriuretic peptide (BNP) in the emergency room helps differentiate cardiac from pulmonary causes of acute dyspnea and has proved useful (Maisel et al. 2002). The popularity of BNP or amino-terminal pro-BNP as an aid to the diagnosis of HF continues to increase.

Table 12-2
Echocardiography, the most useful test to evaluate patients with proven heart failure

Asses left ventricular (LV) function and provide a sufficiently
   accurate ejection fraction (EF)[a] for guidance of therapy
Screen for regional or global hypokinesis
Gives accurate cardiac dimensions; replaces radiology for
   cardiac chamber dilation
Assess regional LV wall motion abnormalities that indicate
   ischemia and significant coronary heart disease
Asses hypertrophy, concentric or other
Left atrial enlargement common with valvular heart disease and
   early sign of LV hypertrophy
Assess valvular heart disease
Congenital heart disease
Diastolic dysfunction: assess after confirmation of normal
   systolic function and absence of valvular disease
Pericardial disease, effusion, tamponade
Myocardial disease

[a]Gated nuclear imaging is more accurate for EF in the *absence of atrial fibrillation* but does not assess values, hypertrophy, or items 3–11

4. Echocardiography is the single most useful diagnostic test to
   evaluate the causes of HF and the heart function in patients confirmed to have HF clinically radiologically or by BNP (see
   Table 12-2). The echocardiographic measurement of EF carries
   a substantial error but is sufficient for patient management and
   comparison.

In patients in whom it is crucial to obtain an accurate EF,
a gated radionuclide study should be requested after the
results of echocardiography, except in patients with atrial
fibrillation. Echocardiography is the key investigation
because correctable causes of HF such as valvular disease,
pericardial, and other problems can be rapidly documented.
Adequate information on LV function is provided, e.g., a
poorly contractile ventricle, and fractional shortening should

suffice. An EF < 45 % is in keeping with decreased LV systolic function. Values of 20–30–35–40–% have some meaning to those who are used to these numbers. Also, the numbers assist with reference to published articles that do not use fractional shortening. A radionuclide cardiac scan is more accurate for the determination of EF but does not evaluate hypertrophy or valvular, pericardial, and other diseases. The cost of a second test is not justifiable.

PATHOPHYSIOLOGY

- It is most important to have a clear knowledge of the pathophysiology of HF, in particular how LV work is dictated by systemic vascular resistance (SVR; see Fig. 12-1).
- Decrease neurohormonal activation; inhibition of the renin–angiotensin–aldosterone system.
- Inhibit LV remodeling.
- Improve myocardial hemodynamics.
- Increase cardiac output to deliver oxygenated blood to vital organs and to meet the metabolic needs of the tissues, especially during normal activities and exercise.
- The cardiac output (CO) is reduced and filling pressure is increased. The low CO results in a number of compensatory responses, as outlined in Fig. 12-1.

The following definitions are relevant:

- Cardiac output = stroke volume × heart rate (HR). Stroke volume is a reflection of preload (filling pressure), myocardial contractility, and afterload (arterial impedance).
- LV work and myocardial oxygen consumption depend on
  (a) HR × blood pressure (BP) (rate-pressure product).
  (b) BP = cardiac output × SVR.

The resistance or arterial impedance (afterload) against which the left ventricle must eject is an important determinant of LV workload. A reduced SVR requires less energy and less force of myocardial contraction to produce an increase in stroke volume.

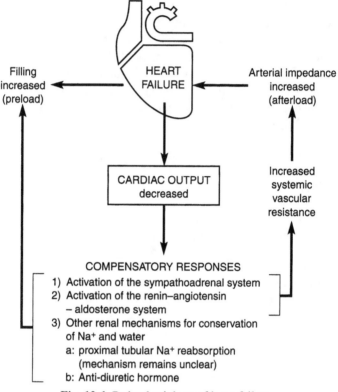

Fig. 12-1 Pathophysiology of heart failure.

SVR is automatically increased early in the development of HF and remains unchanged or increases with increasing HF. This reaction is a necessity and is a normal compensatory adjustment to maintain blood pressure and vascular homeostasis.

The compensatory adjustments are initiated by:

- Sympathetic stimulation that causes an increase in
  (a) Heart rate
  (b) The force of myocardial contraction
  (c) SVR

- Activation of the renin–angiotensin–aldosterone system (RAAS), which causes
  (a) Intense arterial constriction and therefore an increase in SVR and blood pressure
  (b) An increase in aldosterone, which produces distal sodium and water retention

The important proximal tubular reabsorption of sodium is believed to be caused by a combination of the preceding points and other as yet undetermined mechanisms (see Fig. 12-1).

- The renal response to a low CO in the normal subject is to maintain the blood pressure by causing vasoconstriction and sodium and water reabsorption (saline autotransfusion). We cannot expect the kidney to change its program when HF occurs. The kidney is behaving appropriately in the wrong circumstances. Clearly, we can prevent the kidney from carrying out its program only if we switch off the initiating cause of the renal reflex, that is, by increasing the cardiac output. Therefore, any drug that will increase CO will reduce the renal response and lower SVR and further improve CO. An alternative strategy is to reset the neurohormonal imbalance by the use of ACE inhibitors and aldosterone antagonists.

Note: Inotropic agents, digoxin or dobutamine, improve cardiac output and, therefore, cause a fall in SVR. Similar acting agents, but with minimal side effects, are needed.

Management Guide

Four golden rules dictate the efficient management of HF:

1. Ensure that the diagnosis of HF is correct, eliminating conditions that may mimic HF.
2. Determine and treat the basic cause of the heart disease. The rare surgical or medical cure is worth the effort.
3. Search for the precipitating factors; remove or treat and prevent their recurrence to avoid further episodes of HF.

Withdraw drugs known to worsen HF: NSAIDs and notably calcium antagonists commonly administered to patients with hypertension and CHD.

4. The specific treatment of HF requires sound and up-to-date knowledge of the pathophysiology of HF and the actions, indications, and side effects of the pharmacologic agents used in its management.

Relieve symptoms and signs of HF by reducing raised filling pressures to near normal. Therapeutic goals:

- Shift the cardiac function curve to the left and upward, decreasing the filling pressure yet increasing stroke volume.
- Arrest or cause amelioration of the disease process.

This can be achieved by the judicious use of

- Loop diuretics.
- Angiotensin-converting enzyme (ACE) inhibitors or angiotensin II receptor blockers (ARBs).
- Beta-blockers.
- Digoxin: this old drug still has a role and is underused; toxicity is very rare if used by a watchful physician: keep levels 0.6–1.0 nmol/l (0.5–0.9 ng/ml). See later discussion.
- Aldosterone antagonists: eplerenone, if not available use spironolactone or amiloride.

VASODILATORS

ACE Inhibitors/Angiotensin II Receptor Blockers

These agents are discussed in Chap. 3. ACE inhibitors play a major role in the management of HF. When there is intolerance to ACE inhibitor therapy, selected ARBs are administered.

Activation of the RAAS is an early manifestation of HF. The prime role of angiotensin II is to support systemic blood pressure by:

- Causing systemic vasoconstriction, and increase in SVR.
- Stimulation of the central and peripheral effects of the sympathetic nervous system (NOVEL DRUG 2014).

- Causing retention of sodium and water in the proximal nephron and directly by stimulation of aldosterone production.
- Stimulating thirst and enhancing synthesis of vasopressin, thereby increasing total body water.

In addition, angiotensin II preserves cerebral blood flow. Renal blood flow is preserved by selective vasoconstriction of the postglomerular (efferent) arterioles. Thus, the influence of angiotensin II allows patients with severe HF to maintain blood pressure for cerebral, renal, and coronary perfusion, and relatively normal values for serum creatinine and blood urea nitrogen concentration also prevail. ACE inhibitors may cause a dramatic decrease in glomerular filtration rate and increase azotemia in patients with HF and hypotension. This deleterious effect can be minimized by reducing the patient's dependence on the renin–angiotensin system by reducing the dose of diuretic used. Initially it is best to choose an ACE inhibitor with a short action so as to allow brief restoration of the normal homeostatic actions of the renin–angiotensin system (Packer 1985). Long-acting agents may produce prolonged hypotensive effects that may compromise cerebral and renal function and thus may have disadvantages in such cases compared with short-acting agents. Initial low-dose enalapril, 2.5 mg, caused a low 3.2 % incidence of hypotension in a Scandinavian study, proving the drug's safe profile (CONSENSUS 1987).

If ACE inhibitors or ARBs are not tolerated or are contraindicated, the combination of hydralazine/isosorbide dinitrate (ISDN) should be tried; this combination is preferred over ACE inhibitors in black patients as indicated in the Veterans Administration Heart Failure Trial (A-HeFT et al. 2004).

Data from the Veterans Administration Vasodilator Heart Failure Trial (V-HeFT) suggested that patients with chronic HF could be considered for treatment with hydralazine (25 mg three or four times daily) and ISDN (Cohn et al. 1987), but use of captopril or enalapril is preferred.

In V-HeFT, the 2-year reduction in mortality rate was 25 %. Hydralazine and ISDN were poorly tolerated and were withdrawn in 19 % of patients. Only 55 % of patients were taking full doses of both drugs 6 months after randomization (Cohn et al. 1986). Improvement in survival was observed mainly in patients with New York Heart Association (NYHA) class II HF. In this subset, 48 (24 %) of 200 patients treated with enalapril and 66 (31 %) of 210 patients treated with hydralazine/ISDN died (V-HeFTII et al. 1991).

The following studies have tested the effect of ACE inhibitors:

CONSENSUS 1987: The Cooperative North Scandinavian Enalapril Survival Study showed that 6 months of enalapril therapy produced a reduction in mortality rate in patients with NYHA class IV, severe HF. Total mortality 68 in the placebo arm and 50 in the treated subjects ($P = 0.003$). This is significant but a modest effect.

The drug, when given as a 2.5-mg initial dose, was well tolerated. Patients were receiving optimal treatment with digitalis (~94 % of subjects) and diuretics. Treatment with enalapril or an identical placebo was started in the hospital with a dose of 5 mg twice a day. After 1 week, the dosage was increased to 10 mg twice a day if the patient did not have symptoms of hypotension or other side effects. According to the clinical response, a further increase in dosage could occur up to a maximal dose of 20 mg twice a day.

SOLVD 1991 studied the effect of the ACE inhibitor, enalapril, on mortality and hospitalization in patients with chronic heart failure and ejection fractions ≤ 0.35. Patients receiving conventional treatment for heart failure were randomly assigned to receive either placebo ($n = 1,284$) or enalapril ($n = 1,285$) at doses of 2.5–20 mg per day in a double-blind trial. Approximately 90 % of the patients were in New York Heart Association functional classes II and III. The follow-up averaged 41.4 months. Only about 8 % received beta-blockers and 68 % digoxin.

Results. There were 510 deaths in the placebo group (39.7 %), as compared with 452 in the enalapril group (35.2 %). **A modest reduction in risk, 16 %, was observed** ($P = 0.0036$).

SAVE 1992 In the Survival and Ventricular Enlargement trial, 36,630 *post-MI patients* were screened. Within 3–16 days after MI 2,231 patients with ejection fractions of 40 % or less but without overt heart failure or symptoms of myocardial ischemia were randomly assigned to receive double-blind treatment with either placebo (1,116 patients) or captopril (1,115 patients) and were followed for an average of 42 months.

275 of the 1,116 patients (25 %) in the placebo group and 228 of 1,115 (20 %) in the captopril group died; **the reduction in the risk of death from all causes was small 19 %** ($P = 0.019$). Follow-up at 3.5 years **showed a 22 % decrease in the risk of requiring hospitalization for HF**. But only ~36 % of subjects received a beta-blocker (thus current optimal therapy was lacking).

AIRE (1993): In the Acute Infarction Ramipril Efficacy study, ramipril was shown to improve prognosis in post-MI patients with clinical evidence of HF.

Drug name:	**Captopril**
Trade name:	Capoten
Supplied:	12.5, 25, 50, 100 mg
Dosage:	*See* text

Dosage: Withdraw diuretics and other antihypertensives for 24–48 h; give a test dose of 3–6.5 mg and then the same dose twice daily, increasing to 12.5 mg two or three times daily, preferably 1 h before meals (on an empty stomach)

The maximum suggested daily dose is 75–150 mg

In renal failure, the dose interval is increased according to the creatinine clearance (see Chap. 3 for a detailed account of adverse effects, cautions, interactions, and pharmacokinetics).

Drug name:	**Enalapril**: Vasotec, Innovace (UK)
Supplied:	2.5, 5, 10, 20 mg
Dosage:	2.5-mg test dose; 8–12 h later start 2.5 mg twice daily, increasing over days to weeks to 10–20 mg once or twice daily

Contraindications, side effects, and other considerations are discussed in Chap. 3 (see Table 3-1). Notably, the drug's onset of action is delayed 2–4 h as opposed to captopril (½–1 h). Withdrawal of diuretics does not always prevent marked hypotension or syncope (Cleland et al. 1985), so caution is required with captopril and enalapril. A RCT indicates that 20 mg of enalapril is as beneficial as 40 mg daily for HF treatment (Nanas et al. 2000).

Drug name:	**Lisinopril**
Trade names:	Prinivil, Zestril, Carace (UK)
Supplied:	5, 10, 20, 40 mg
Dosage:	2.5-mg test dose, then titrate dosage; 5–10 mg once daily, average 10–20 mg daily. If no hypotension or adverse effects, the dose may be increased to 30–35 mg daily

The high dose was used in the Assessment of Treatment with Lisinopril and Survival (ATLAS 1999) study. Unfortunately, the ATLAS study compared 2.5–5 mg with 32.5–35 mg lisinopril daily. It would make more clinical sense to have compared the dose commonly used in clinical practice (i.e., 10–20 mg) as the low dose. The results of the study showed a marginal difference; the high dose decreased modestly the risk of hospitalization but not total mortality.

Drug name:	**Ramipril**
Trade names:	Altace, Tritace (UK)
Supplied:	1.25, 2.5, 5, 10 mg
Dosage:	1.25–2.5 mg daily, increasing over weeks to 5–10 mg once daily or two divided doses

For other ACE inhibitors and ARBs, see Chap. 3.

In the AIRE (1993) trial, ramipril administered to patients within 3–10 days of acute MI with transient signs and symptoms of HF caused a significant 27 % reduction in the risk of death at 15 months, a benefit that was maintained for 5 years.

Angiotensin-Receptor Blockers

ARBs are advisable if ACE inhibitors are not tolerated, but they have not been shown to significantly decrease total mortality. These agents are overused; trial results are as follows:

CHARM (2003). In this study, 2,028 patients were studied to examine the effects of the ARB candesartan in patients with reduced left ventricular ejection fraction (<40 %) who were intolerant of ACE inhibitors. Treated patients received candesartan 4–8 mg titrated to 32 mg once daily plus the treatment given to placebo patients. Standard heart failure therapy included diuretics, beta-blockers, digoxin, and spironolactone (85 %, 54 %, 45 %, and 24 %, respectively).

Results: Total mortality was not significantly reduced by the ARB candesartan. There were 265 deaths from any cause in the candesartan group and 296 in the placebo group.

$P = 0.11$. Hospitalization for heart failure occurred in 207 (20.4 %) in the candesartan group and 286 (28.2 %) in the placebo group, a modest 27 % reduction in admissions to hospital, $P = 0.0001$. Digoxin and beta blockers were underused.

- **In CHARM—Alternative** (2003). 7,599 patients [with left-ventricular ejection fraction (LVEF)] 40 % or less, and mainly class 11 and 111 HF, who were not receiving ACE inhibitors because of previous intolerance were randomly assigned candesartan ($n = 3,803$, titrated to 32 mg once daily) or matching placebo. Median follow-up was 37.7 months. **Total mortality was not reduced: 886 (23 %) patients in the candesartan and 945 (25 %) in the placebo group died $p = 0.055$. In this negative trial ~50 % of subjects had a previous MI**.

In Val-HeFT (2001). A total of 5,010 patients with HF class II, III, or IV were randomly assigned to receive 160 mg of valsartan or placebo twice daily. There was no reduction in all-cause mortality. The incidence of the combined end point, however, was a modest 13.2 % lower with valsartan than with placebo ($P = 0.009$), predominantly because of a lower number of patients hospitalized for heart failure: 455 (18.2 %) in the placebo group and 346 (13.8 %) in the valsartan group ($P < 0.001$). **Overall mortality was not reduced by valsartan administration**. Unfortunately less than 36 % of subjects received a beta-blocker and ~68 % received digoxin.

TRANSCEND (2008)

- **There was no reduction in total mortality**.
- Investigators studied the effects of telmisartan on cardiovascular events in high-risk patients intolerant to ACE inhibitors. Telmisartan therapy for 56 months, although shown in ONTARGET (2008) to be equivalent to ramipril surprisingly, had no significant effect on the primary outcome, hospitalizations for HF.

The drug was not effective for stroke prevention in the PROFESS RCT

- **Yet these agents are widely prescribed**.

HYDRALAZINE

Drug name:	Hydralazine; Apresoline
Supplied:	25, 50 mg
Dosage:	25 mg (average 50 mg) three times daily, max. 200 mg daily

V-HeFT II (1991) indicated that hydralazine with ISDN is inferior to ACE inhibitor therapy in achieving improved survival in patients with NYHA class II HF. More than 33 % of patients cannot tolerate hydralizine because of headaches, dizziness, and other side effects. Adverse effects were similar in V-HeFT I and II. Hydralizine/ISDN may be used if an ACE inhibitor or ARB is contraindicated.

In A-HeFT (2004) **the combination significantly reduced mortality and hospitalizations in patients of African origin** (see Chap. 22).

CALCIUM ANTAGONISTS

Amlodipine

The Prospective Randomized Amlodipine Survival Evaluation PRAISE-2 (1996) study showed that amlodipine caused neither benefit nor harm in patients with CHF. In PRAISE-2, amlodipine increased the occurrence of pulmonary edema in patients with low EF. **Calcium antagonists should be avoided in patients with HF, and in all patients with EF < 40 %, because HF may be precipitated.**

DIURETICS

Indications and Guidelines

Heart failure precipitated by acute MI: In this situation, the cautious use of titrated doses of furosemide remains most useful.

Furosemide 20–40 mg intravenously (IV) followed by 40 mg, 30 min to 1 h later, is given. If symptoms persist, diuresis is not established, and if the BP is stable, 80 mg is given.

Ensure that the serum K^+ level remains normal; do not wait to see it fall to <3.5 mEq (mmol)/L before adding potassium chloride (KC1) or preferably an aldosterone antagonist (eplerenone or spironolactone).

In patients with moderate and severe HF who are predicted to have recurrent bouts of HF and who are receiving digitalis, give furosemide 80–160 mg once daily.

Metolazone: 2.5–5 mg once daily with close monitoring of renal function and watch for low serum potassium.

- The combination of furosemide and metolazone (Kiyingi et al. 1990) increases diuresis and should be given a trial in patients refractory to furosemide or other loop diuretics. In patients with refractory HF with severe renal failure, furosemide 160–320 mg along with metolazone may be required to promote adequate diuresis.
- The addition of metolazone can decrease hyperkalemia precipitated by aldosterone antagonists.

Note that the diuretic and antihypertensive actions of furosemide and thiazides are reduced by drugs that are prostaglandin inhibitors, in particular indomethacin and other NSAIDs.

Torsemide (Demadex): 10–20 mg IV. Maximum single dose 100–200 mg.

Bumetamide: 1.0 mg, maximum 4–8 mg.

ALDOSTERONE ANTAGONISTS

Figure 12-1 indicates the role of increased aldosterone production in the pathophysiology of HF (see also Chap. 7). It is necessary to block aldosterone completely because it causes:

- Na and water retention. This effect continues when the effects of short-acting, poorly absorbed loop diuretics, such as furosemide, have dissipated.
- K^+ and Mg loss.

- Myocardial and vascular fibrosis.
- Norepinephrine release and increased myocardial uptake of norepinephrine that can contribute to sudden death; myocardial fibrosis that contributes to progressive HF.
- Although aldosterone antagonists have proved successful in reducing adverse outcomes in patients with HF, their use in patients with impaired renal function is a risk factor for hyperkalemia.
- Most important, elderly patients with a serum creatinine in the normal range often have renal impairment, and the various formulas for assessing glomerular filtration rate (GFR) have drawbacks, particularly in patients older than age 75.

Drug name:	**Spironolactone**; Aldactone
Dosage:	Initial 12.5 mg if serum assess K^+ 5.0 or less and reassess in 3 days and at 1 week; if K^+ <5.0 mEq/L, give 25 mg once daily

Reassess at 1 month and then every 3 months: maintain K^+ 4 to maximum 5.2 mEq/L (mmol/L)

Use cautiously with close monitoring of serum potassium in patients with serum creatinine 1.2–1.5 mg/dL (106–133 μmol/L) or estimated GFR 50–59 mL/min (Stevens et al. 2006)

Avoid in patients with more severe renal dysfunction: estimated GFR < 50 or creatinine clearance <50 mL/min

The 50 mg dose should only be administered to patients with normal renal function eGFR > 70 mL/min

In the RALES (1999) RCT the drug caused a 30 % reduction in the risk of death among patients with HF and EF < 35 % treated with loop diuretics, an ACE inhibitor, and digoxin. Hospitalization for recurrent HF was significantly reduced. The dosage of ACE inhibitor used was smaller than that used in modern clinical practice: mean dose captopril 63 mg, enalapril 15 mg, and lisinopril 14.3 mg. Larger doses can cause a high occurrence of hyperkalemia

- Spironolactone causes gynecomastia and other androgenic effects. Eplerenone, which does not have these effects, has proved effective in an RCT.

- The dose of spironolactone used in the RALES trial was 25 mg.
- Caution is required in patients with abnormal renal function and in type II diabetes with hyporeninemic hypoaldosteronism because severe hyperkalemia may ensue.
- If the serum K^+ reaches 5.0–5.1 mEq/L, the dose of ACE inhibitor should be decreased and loop diuretic increased before reducing the 25-mg dose of spironolactone.
- Serum K^+ should be evaluated at 3 days and 1–2 weeks after starting treatment and then about 3 monthly. If the K^+ reaches 5.1 mEq/L, spironolactone should be discontinued. Caution: Spironolactone or eplerenone should be used with close monitoring of serum potassium in patients with serum creatinine 1.2–1.5 mg/dL (106–133 μmol/L) or estimated GFR 50–59 mL/min.

Adverse effects; rarely: hyperkalemia (discontinue), hepatotoxicity; gynecomastia, benign breast tumor, breast pain, menstrual disturbances, changes in libido; agranulocytosis, thrombocytopenia; leg cramps; alopecia, hirsutism, rash, and Stevens–Johnson syndrome

- Avoid in patients with moderate renal dysfunction: estimated GFR or creatinine clearance <50 mL/min.
- Elderly patients with a creatinine 1.2–1.4 mg/dL (102–123 μmol/L) within the normal range may have a markedly reduced creatinine clearance (estimated GFR) of 50–59 mL/min.
- In patients aged >75 years, a normal serum creatinine does not indicate normal renal function. It is necessary to assess the GFR using a 24 h urine collection.
- Caution is needed because the formula to determine estimated GFR gives inaccurate results in patients older than age 70; in blacks a correction is required: multiply by 1.2.
- Avoid concomitant use of NSAIDS or cyclooxygenase-2 inhibitors.

Drug name:	**Eplerenone**: Inspra; Supplied tablets 25 mg
Dosage:	If baseline K^+ <5.1 mEq/L, 12.5 mg once daily

Assess K^+ in 3 days and at 1 week; if <5.0 mEq/L, increase to 25 mg once daily

Reassess K^+ at 1 month and then every 3 months: maintain K^+ 4 to maximum 5.1 mEq/L (mmol/L) max. 50 mg once daily, and watch serum potassium closely

- Use cautiously 25 mg maximum with close monitoring of serum potassium in patients with serum creatinine 1.2–1.5 mg/dL (106–133 µmol/L) or estimated GFR 50–59 mL/min.
- Avoid in patients with more severe renal dysfunction: eGFR or creatinine clearance <50 mL/min.
- Avoid concomitant use of NSAIDS or cyclooxygenase-2 inhibitors.

Adverse effects: diarrhea, nausea; hypotension; dizziness; hyperkalemia; rash; less commonly, dyslipidemia, pharyngitis, headache, insomnia, gynecomastia, asthenia, malaise, back pain, leg cramps, impaired renal function, azotemia, sweating, and pruritus.

BETA-BLOCKERS

Beta-blockers are the mainstay of therapy for heart failure. They decrease total mortality, an effect only modestly provided by ACE inhibitors, and not at all by ARBS. See discussion under ARBs.

- Two beta-blocking drugs have been approved worldwide for the management of HF: carvedilol and bisoprolol. Metoprolol succinate extended release (Toprol XL) is also approved in the US.
- Beta-blockers play a major role in the management of patients with HF and are strongly recommended for the management of class I–III HF and also for compensated class IV patients.
- Beta-blocker therapy is initiated as soon as possible after the diagnosis of HF provided the patient is free from fluid overload.

Some specialists have advocated the commencement of a beta-blocker prior to ACE inhibition in the hypotensive patient because this may cause an improvement in LV function, thus allowing initiation (or an increase in dosage) of the ACE inhibitor (Hass and Abraham 2005).

Beta-blockers are most effective in patients with ischemic heart disease and dilated cardiomyopathy.

Transmyocardial measurements have documented that the failing human heart is exposed to increased adrenergic activity. Chronic adrenergic activation has adverse effects on the natural course of heart muscle disease (Bristow et al. 1985; Packer et al. 1996).

These agents partially block RAAS and augment atrial and brain natriuretic peptide. It is often forgotten that beta-blockers significantly reduce renin secretion from the juxtaglomerular cells of the kidney, which causes a decrease in angiotensin levels and reduced aldosterone production; this action adds to their life-saving potential in patients with HF, but a mild increase in K^+ may occur and potentiate that caused by spironolactone or eplerenone.

Use of 1 of the 3 beta-blockers proven to reduce mortality (e.g., bisoprolol, carvedilol, and sustained-release metoprolol succinate) is recommended for all patients with current or prior symptoms of HF with reduced EF, unless contraindicated, to reduce morbidity and mortality (Level of Evidence: A, ACCF/AHA 2013).

Drug name:	**Carvedilol**
Trade names:	Coreg, Eucardic (UK)
Supplied:	12.5, 25 mg
Dosage:	3.125-mg test dose and then twice daily with food for 2 weeks; increase to 6.25 mg twice daily wk 3–4; then 9.375 mg twice daily during weeks 5–8; then if tolerated 12.5 mg twice daily. Increase slowly to the highest level tolerated; max. 25 mg twice daily. See text for further advice

Carvedilol should be taken with food to slow the rate of absorption and reduce the incidence of orthostatic effects. If dizziness, light-headedness, or hypotension occurs, the dose of diuretic or ACE inhibitor should be reduced to allow up-titration of carvedilol or other beta-blocker. If symptoms persist, the dose of carvedilol should be reduced.

In an RCT the drug resulted in a significant reduction in mortality rate in patients with HF treated with diuretics and an ACE inhibitor; almost all patients were taking digoxin (Packer et al. 1996). Importantly ARBs, despite their widespread use, have not been shown to decrease total mortality in any of three large RCTs (CHARM, 2003; Val-HeFT 2001; TRANSCEND 2008).

The Carvedilol Postinfarct Survival Controlled Evaluation (CAPRICORN 2001) study in patients after MI with a mean EF of 33 % found a 23 % relative reduction in mortality, identical to the result of a meta-analysis of 22 long-term RCTs in post-MI patients. Notably, a similar benefit—a 2.3 % absolute reduction in risk—was observed in SAVE, AIRE, and TRACE with ACE inhibitors, i.e., 43 patients treated to save one life.

The Carvedilol Prospective Randomized Cumulative Survival Study (COPERNICUS 2001) trial studied 2,289 patients with severe HF, EF 16–24 %, but free from overt fluid retention or recent treatment with IV diuretics or positive inotropic drugs. The results showed a highly significant 35 % reduction in all-cause mortality with carvedilol (see Chap. 22).

Beta-blocking drugs such as carvedilol have proved useful in improving survival and decreasing the number of hospitalizations for worsening HF. Carvedilol is indicated for the management of NYHA class II–III HF. Compensated class IV HF patients free of fluid overload have shown benefit and should be treated, judiciously, with carvedilol with up-titration of doses over 4–6 weeks. Most patients with class 1 V heart failure should be treated with an appropriate dose of diuretic, ACE inhibitor (not ARB), digoxin (with close monitoring of renal function and digoxin level), and when compensated carvedilol is strongly advisable.

Drug name:	**Bisoprolol**; Zebeta
Dosage:	1.25 mg test dose; then once daily; increase in 2–3 weeks to 3.75 mg; at 5–6 weeks if tolerated 5-mg maintenance dose at >12 weeks, if needed max. dose 10 mg provided that the BP is >110 mmHg systolic and heart rate >50 beats/min

In the Cardiac Insufficiency Bisoprolol Study II (CIBIS II) (1999), bisoprolol resulted in a significant decrease in mortality in patients with NYHA class III HF and EF < 35 %. CIBIS II involved 2,647 patients aged 18–80 year with class III or IV HF. Study patients received ACE inhibitor and diuretic (digitalis was allowed) for at least 2 months prior to bisoprolol or placebo. Bisoprolol, initial dose 1.25 mg daily, was titrated at weekly intervals in 1.25-mg increments for 4 weeks and then up to a maximum of 10 mg daily. Bisoprolol therapy reduced all-cause mortality by 32 % ($P = 0.00005$) and sudden death by 45 % ($P = 0.001$). A 30 % reduction in hospitalization occurred in the bisoprolol-treated group. Treatment withdrawals in the bisoprolol- and placebo-treated patients were similar (approx 15 %).

Drug name:	**Metoprolol succinate** Extended-release Metoprolol CR/XL
Supplied:	50, 100 mg
Dosage:	12.5 mg test dose and then once daily for 2 weeks; then 25 mg; titrate over 4–8 weeks to 100 mg usual maintenance dose; maximum 200 mg see MERIT-HF

- MERIT-HF (2000): The Metoprolol Extended-Release Randomized Intervention Trial in Heart Failure trial involved patients with class II and III HF, mean EF 28 %. Patients were randomized to metoprolol CR/XL, 25 mg once per day (NYHA class II), or 12.5 mg once per day (NYHA class III or IV), titrated for 6–8 weeks up to a target dosage of 200 mg once per day ($n=1,990$), or matching placebo ($n=2,001$). Treatment resulted in risk reduction of 33 % for total mortality or worsening HF. This is a combined end point, however. **The total mortality was not given in the article and it appears therefore that total deaths were not significantly reduced.**
- **Metoprolol tartrate used worldwide also includes a long-acting formulation that does not cover a full 24 h and both formulations are not recommended for HF in the UK or by the author.**
- **Only carvedilol and bisoprolol are approved for HF in the UK. Nebivolol is approved in the UK for HF in patients 70 and older.**

Drug name:	**Nebivolol**
Trade name:	Bystolic/US; Nebilet/UK
Dosage:	5 mg daily; for the elderly, initially 2.5 mg daily for a few days to weeks then 5 mg daily.
Dosage:	For mild-to-moderate heart failure, mainly in patients 70 years and older: initially 1.25 mg once daily, then if tolerated increased at intervals of 1–2 weeks to 2.5 mg once daily, then to 5 mg once daily, and then to max. 10 mg once daily

Cautions: reduce dose in renal impairment, in the elderly, and in hepatic dysfunction. Avoid if serum creatinine greater than 250 µmol/L. Nebivolol is a novel beta-blocker with several important pharmacologic properties that distinguish it from traditional beta-blockers (Gray and Ndefo 2008).

This highly selective beta1-adrenergic receptor blocker is the only beta-blocker known to induce vascular production of nitric oxide, the main endothelial vasodilator.

Nebivolol induces nitric oxide production via by stimulating the beta3-adrenergic receptor-mediated production of nitric oxide in the heart; this stimulation results in a greater protection against heart failure (Maffei and Lembo 2009).

- In addition, nebivolol increases NO by decreasing its oxidative inactivation (Cominacini et al. 2003). The drug stimulates the endothelial L-arginine/nitric oxide pathway and thus causes vasodilation (Cockcroft et al. 1995). Nebivolol should find a role in the management of heart failure, particularly in patients with normal or slightly reduced EF.

SENIORS study (Flather et al. 2005; van Veldhuisen et al. 2009) 2,111 patients; 1,359 (64 %) had impaired (35 %) EF (mean 28.7 %) and 752 (36 %) had preserved (>35 %) EF (mean 49.2 %).

During follow-up of 21 months the primary end point occurred in 465 patients (34.2 %) with impaired EF and in 235 patients (31.2 %) with preserved EF. The effect of nebivolol on the primary end point [hazard ratio (HR) of nebivolol versus placebo] was 0.86 (95 % confidence interval: 0.72–1.04) in patients with impaired EF and preserved EF ($P=0.720$ for subgroup interaction). Effects on all secondary end points were similar between groups.

Conclusions: The effect of beta-blockade with nebivolol in elderly patients with HF in this study was similar in those with preserved and impaired EF (van Veldhuisen et al. 2009).

Nebivolol reduces P-wave dispersion on the electrocardiogram, which would attenuate the risk of atrial fibrillation (Tuncer et al. 2008). Time to maximum concentration is 0.5–2 h, and half-life is 11 h in extensive metabolizers; these values are about three times longer in poor metabolizers.

Nebivolol appears to have a minor, if any, effect on libido and sexual performance, which likely ensues from a compensatory effect of the increased NO release (Boydak et al. 2005). In contrast with metoprolol, nebivolol improves secondary sexual activity and erectile dysfunction scores (Brixius et al. 2007). Particularly, comparative trials on the efficacy of nebivolol versus other beta-blockers and/or other antihypertensive drugs are awaited (Münzel and Gori 2009). This is a finding of paramount importance because all current HF agents (carvedilol, bisoprolol, ACE inhibitors) are not effective in patients with HFPEF.

The drug should be tried as the beta-blocker of choice in all patients with HFPEF.

INOTROPIC AGENTS

Drug name:	Digoxin; Lanoxin
Supplied:	0.625, 0.125, 0.25 mg
Dosage:	See text

Digoxin Studies

Hemodynamics: A study by Arnold and colleagues (1980) demonstrated that patients with proven HF show improvement in hemodynamics during acute and long-term administration as well as during exercise. Withdrawal of digoxin in that study produced a significant increase in pulmonary capillary wedge pressure, heart rate, and SVR and a fall in stroke work index and EF. After acute retreatment, all parameters improved, including exercise hemodynamics. Gheorghiade and colleagues (1987: 42) have confirmed these hemodynamic effects of digoxin.

Withdrawal of digoxin: The Randomized Assessment of Digoxin on Inhibitors of ACE (RADIANCE) study included 178 patients with chronic HF and sinus rhythm who were clinically stable with diuretics, an ACE inhibitor, and digoxin (Packer and Cohn 1999). Most patients (70 %) were in NYHA class II. In patients withdrawn from digoxin for 3 months, there was a sixfold worsening of HF. Patients taking a placebo had a higher incidence of deterioration and worsening HF (23 versus 4 patients) and more deterioration in quality of life. The dose of digoxin in the RADIANCE study was 0.38 mg daily, and serum digoxin levels ranged from 0.9 to 2.0 ng/mL.

In a double-blind placebo-controlled study of patients with documented HF and no reversible etiology, 16 of the 46 patients deteriorated between 4 days and 3 weeks after stopping digoxin (Dobbs et al. 1977).

ANALYSIS OF THE DIGOXIN STUDY

The results of the DIG study (1997) provided some answers to 200 years of controversy regarding the use of digitalis.

Digoxin was assigned to 3,397 patients, and 3,403 received diuretics and an ACE inhibitor. The mean EF was 28 ± 9 %. The average follow-up was 37 months. Fewer patients in the digoxin group were hospitalized for worsening HF: 26.8 % versus 34.7 % in the placebo group ($P < 0.001$; see Table 12-3).

- **Most important, the risk associated with the combined outcome of death related to HF or hospitalization related to HF was significantly lower in the digoxin group (1,041 versus 1,291 patients, $P < 0.01$), but this result is considered nonsignificant because it is an additive result. But additive results are used for most other agents claimed effective including ACE inhibitors and ARBs.**
- DIGOXIN RESULTS ARE similar to that observed for ACE inhibitors in SAVE (see Table 12-3).
- ARBs in CHARM 2003 and Val-HeFT (2001) showed no meaningful decrease in mortality; a significant effect materializes because of addition of significant rehospitalization and negative mortality effect.

Table 12-3
Effect of digoxin on mortality and morbidity in patients with heart failure

	Digoxin (n = 3,397)	Placebo (n = 3,403)	(%) reduction	P	Risk ratio[a]
Worsening CHF	910	1,180	22.9	<0.001	
Death plus CHF	1,041	1,291	19.3	<0.001	
Death owing to worsening CHF	394	449		0.06	
Death or hospitalization owing to CHF EF<0.25	428/1,127	556/1,130	23.0		0.68 (0.60–0.70)
Class III or IV Class IV only 2 % of study group	438/1,118	552/1,105	20.6		0.70 (0.61–0.79)
Cardiothoracic ratio	441/1,176	567/1,170	22.2		0.69 (0.61–0.79)

Modified from the Digitalis Investigation Group. The effect of digoxin on mortality and morbidity in patients with heart failure. N Engl J Med 1997:336:525

[a]Values in parentheses are 95 % confidence intervals. CHF, congestive heart failure; EF, ejection fraction. The 19–23 % reduction in outcomes is similar to that observed for ARBs in CHARM 2003 and Val-HeFT 2001

The DIG study showed that in patients with EF < 0.30.

- Death or hospitalization related to worsening HF occurred in 428 of 1,127 in the digoxin group and in 556 of 1,130 in the placebo group, a 23.0 % reduction.
- In patients with NYHA class III HF, death or hospitalization occurred in 438 of 1,118 in the digoxin group and in 552 of 1,105 in the placebo group, a 20.6 % reduction {risk ratio 0.70 [95 % confidence (CI) interval 0.61–0.79]}.
- Hospitalization for recurrent HF continues worldwide in the absence of digoxin administration. Logic is perhaps lost by our professors and those who write editorials.
- A 19 % reduction was observed for the risk of death, CHF, or hospitalization ($P = 0.001$) a result that is far better than observed for ARB therapy that is widespread.
- A 22 % decrease in death or hospitalization was observed in patients with cardiothoracic ratio > 0.55.

The study indicated that digoxin significantly decreases death or hospitalization caused by worsening HF in patients with class II–III and IV HF with EF < 0.30 or with cardiothoracic ratio > 0.55 this result is far better than that obtained with ARB therapy. A comprehensive post hoc analysis of the DIG trial offered new insights (Ahmed et al. 2006)

- The drug is highly recommended in patients with class 11, III, and IV HF, with EF < 40 %, also in those with increased LV volume and cardiothoracic ratio > 0.55. This is advisable particularly if the systolic blood pressure is < 115 mmHg caused by ACE inhibitors and beta-blockers. Digoxin does not cause a decrease in BP, a welcome asset for clinicians who use logic in choosing medications.
- Digoxin levels must remain in the range 0.5–0.9 ng/mL. (0.6–1 nmol/L). Patients maintained within this range showed maximum benefit. These levels must not be exceeded, particularly in females.

Levels > 1.1 ng/ml increases risk and may increase mortality.

INDICATIONS

- Atrial fibrillation with ventricular response 90–150/min is the most clear-cut indication, particularly if HF or left ventricular dysfunction is present; or if HF in recent past or if the EF is <40 %. In this setting a beta-blocker (carvedilol or bisoprolol) and digoxin are advisable.
  - HF related to poor LV contractility, systolic HF. If a third heart sound gallop (S3) is heard, and EF<40 % digoxin is advisable and is proven effective.
- HF persisting or a recurrence due to a failure of diuretics and vasodilator therapy.
- HF accompanied by hypotension: systolic BP~110 or less often limits the use of vasodilators (ACE inhibitors, ARBs) and an increase in diuretic dose that can cause falls resulting in injuries, particularly in the elderly.
  - Digoxin has a role in this category of patients. Digoxin is indicated for all patients with impaired systolic function and NYHA class III and IV HF because these patients are at high risk for recurrent heart failure and hospitalization.

Digoxin is not usually recommended, or is of limited value, for the management of HF resulting from or accompanied by:

- Acute MI, except from day 4 if HF is not easily controlled by furosemide, nitrates, ACE inhibitor, dobutamine, or nitroprusside.
- Advanced first-degree, second-degree, and complete atrioventricular (AV) block. (It is preferable with second- and third-degree AV block to pace the patient and then use digitalis.)
  - Mitral stenosis, normal sinus rhythm.
- Hypertrophic cardiomyopathy (HCM), except if HF is moderate or severe. (The drug is potentially dangerous in HCM.)
- Cor pulmonale, except for the management of atrial fibrillation with a fast ventricular response or in patients with added severe LV failure exhibiting a low cardiac output and both central and peripheral cyanosis.

Mechanism of Action

1. Digoxin increases the force and velocity of myocardial contraction in both the failing and the nonfailing heart. It inhibits
   the function of the sodium pump, resulting in an increase in
   intracellular sodium accompanied by an increase in cellular
   calcium. Digoxin causes the Frank–Starling function curve
   to move upward and to the left, i.e., an improved ventricular
   function curve. Improvement in cardiac output produces a
   favorable alteration of the compensatory responses of HF
   including the neurohormonal response (see Fig. 12-1).
2. Electrophysiologic effects:
   (a) Decreases conduction velocity in the AV node, i.e., the
       drug sets up a "traffic jam" in the AV node, producing an
       important reduction in ventricular response in atrial
       fibrillation.
   (b) Increases the slope of phase 4 diastolic depolariza-
       tion and therefore increases automaticity of ectopic
       pacemakers.
3. Vasoconstrictor: The drug has a mild vasoconstrictor effect
   that increases total systemic resistance. In the failing heart,
   however, the drug increases cardiac output, which counter-
   acts the reflex stimulation of the sympathetic and angiotensin systems, resulting in vasodilation and a fall in total
   systemic resistance, i.e., afterload reduction.
4. Neurohormonal
   Digoxin favorably alters the neurohormonal imbalance that
   contributes to HF. It is, therefore, rational to use the triple
   combination of diuretics, ACE inhibitors, and digoxin to
   manage LV failure and improve symptoms, survival, and
   quality of life in virtually all patients with class III–IV HF.
5. Reduction in myocardial fibrosis
   A salutary interaction of digoxin and spironolactone: These two
   now have an important role in the management of class III and
   IV HF. Na entry into Na channels in myofibroblasts is enhanced
   by aldosterone and is the trigger for myocardial fibrosis. When
   digoxin is added, there is a reduction in fibrosis because digoxin
   blocks sodium–potassium adenosine triphosphatase (Na^+, K^+-
   ATPase) and thus decreases Na entry into fibroblasts and

decreases fibrosis. In the RALES spironolactone study, 72 % of patients received digoxin.

Dosage Considerations

Before writing an order for digoxin, review the indications and reassess renal function and conditions that increase sensitivity (Table 12-4).

1. Loading Dose (Initial Dose)
   For adults and children over 10 years and in the absence of conditions that may increase sensitivity:
   - 0.5 mg immediately and 0.25 mg every 12 h for two doses (1 mg/24 h).
                         OR
   - 0.25 mg twice daily at **bedtime** for 2 days and then maintenance: if in sinus rhythm.
       - **Patients older than 70**: maintenance usually 0.0625– 0.125 mg **at bedtime** once daily depending on renal function

Table 12-4

Conditions in which there is an increased sensitivity to digoxin and conservative dosing is recommended

Elderly patients (age > 75 year)
Renal dysfunction; creatinine > 1.2 mg/dl (106 μmol/L)
Estimated GFR < 50 mL/h
Thin patients, low skeletal mass
Hypokalemia
Hyperkalemia
Hypoxemia
Acidosis
Acute myocardial infarction
Hypomagnesemia
Hypercalcemia
Myocarditis
Hypothyroidism
Amyloidosis

Note: A low skeletal mass means less binding to skeletal muscle receptors, and therefore a smaller loading dose is required in the thin or elderly patient and in women. For a more rapid effect (e.g., atrial fibrillation, heart rate 130–50/beats/min) give 0.5 mg immediately and then 0.25 mg every 6 h for two or three doses.

Intravenous: Mainly for atrial fibrillation, in the presence of HF, heart rate 140–170/beats/min in the absence of digoxin therapy within the last 2 weeks. Give either:

- 0.5 mg IV slowly over 5 min (or infusion) and then 0.25 mg every 2 h for two doses, total 1 mg under electrocardiography (ECG) cover, reassessing the patient before each dose is given.

OR

- Advised in the UK when rapid control is needed. 0.75–1.0 mg as an infusion over 2 h or more, and then maintenance by mouth

2. Maintenance Dose

Digoxin is mainly excreted unchanged by the kidney, with an average half-life of 36 h. In normal renal function, as a general rule give the following:

- Age < 70 year: usually 0.25 mg daily, normal renal function (occasionally 0.125 mg) **preferably at bedtime** to allow appropriate sampling for digoxin levels.
- Age > 70 year: 0.0625–0.125 mg daily, and a reduced dose if renal impairment is present: 0.0625 mg alternate day in some if eGFR 50–60 ml/min],
  - Monitor dosing and levels **to maintain a level 0.5 to maximum 0.9 ng/mL. (0.6–1.0 nmol/L).**
  - **It is rare to observe digoxin toxicity if renal function is normal and above dosing schedule is used.**
  - **Avoid digoxin if e GFR < 40 ml/min.**

Caution:

- Serum digoxin levels >1.0 ng/ml appear to increase mortality in women.

- In renal failure, the dose interval is increased depending on the creatinine clearance. The serum creatinine level is not an accurate measure of the creatinine clearance. It is advisable to estimate the GFR, but this is a rough measure of renal function. Despite such calculations, digoxin toxicity may develop if renal dysfunction is present. The use of digitalis in the presence of moderate or severe renal failure represents a controversial area because the risk of toxicity is common.

The bioavailability of digitalis is reduced in malabsorption syndrome and by the following drugs:

- Cholestyramine, colestipol
- Neomycin
- Antacids
- Metoclopramide
- Diphenylhydantoin
- Phenobarbital
- Phenylbutazone

Caution: Atorvastatin, quinidine, calcium antagonists, and amiodarone increase serum digoxin levels. Decreased renal elimination of digoxin results from a quinidine-induced decrease in tubular secretion of digoxin (Schenck-Gustafsson et al. 1982). Verapamil causes a significant increase in digoxin levels that may result in severe bradycardia or asystole (Zatuchni 1984). Interaction with diltiazem is minimal and with nifedipine insignificant. Amiodarone reduces clearance of digoxin and causes a 25–75 % increase in digoxin levels. A reduction of the dose of digoxin by 50 % is recommended when quinidine, quinine, verapamil, or amiodarone is given concurrently (Marcus 1985).

Clinicians may consider adding digoxin in patients with persistent symptoms of HF reduced EF. Digoxin may also be added to the initial regimen in patients with severe symptoms who have not yet responded symptomatically. When administered with attention to dose and factors that alter its metabolism, digoxin is well tolerated by most patients with HF (ACCF/AHA 2013).

Clinical studies indicate that there is no clear-cut serum level that establishes the presence of toxicity. The serum digoxin level is useful when interpreted relative to the serum potassium level and the clinical situation. The serum K^+ concentration increases with digitalis toxicity.

If digoxin toxicity is suspected, it is advisable to discontinue digoxin if:

- Serum digoxin level is >1.1 ng/mL with a serum K^+ level of 2.5–3.5 mEq (mmol)/L.
- Serum potassium level is <3 mEq (mmol)/L. In this case, digoxin should be withheld regardless of the serum digoxin concentration.

Potassium depletion must be corrected before recommencing digoxin. This seems a reasonable course of action because there are other treatments for the management of HF.

Digitalis Toxicity

- The incidence of digoxin toxicity decreased during the 1990s, and toxicity occurs in about one episode for every 20 years of treatment. In large digoxin trials, adverse effects have been no different than with placebo.
- The incidence of toxicity is rare with the lowered dose currently advised if renal function digoxin blood levels and serum potassium are monitored every 3 months.
- The ECG may be nonspecific, but symptoms may provide enough clues, especially when combined with knowledge of the results of the serum creatinine or creatinine clearance and the maintenance dose of digoxin. This information should enable the physician to reach a decision about whether or not the patient has digoxin toxicity. There is no need to await notification of digoxin levels. If you suspect toxicity, withhold the drug for at least 48 h—there are other effective treatments for HF or atrial fibrillation, and withholding a few doses of digoxin will not be detrimental.

Symptoms of Toxicity

- Gastrointestinal: anorexia, nausea, vomiting, diarrhea, and weight loss.
- Central nervous system: visual hallucinations, mental confusion, psychosis, restlessness, insomnia, drowsiness, and extreme weakness; blue-green-yellow vision, blurring of vision, and scotomas.

Cardiac Dysrhythmias

1. Ventricular premature beats: bigeminal or multifocal.
2. AV block:
   (a) Second degree (Wenckebach).
   (b) Atrial tachycardia with AV block, ventricular rate commonly 90–120/min, so often missed clinically, and the ECG may be misread because the P-waves can be buried in the T-waves. Be on the alert when there is steady moderate tachycardia without obvious cause.
   (c) Rarely, complete heart block.
   (d) A very slow ventricular response <50/min; an intermittently regular rhythm at a slow rate in a patient with atrial fibrillation.
3. Tachycardias:
   (a) Nonparoxysmal junctional tachycardia with AV dissociation or accelerated AV junctional rhythm.
   (b) Ventricular tachycardia and ventricular fibrillation.
4. Bradyarrhythmias:
   (a) Sinus bradycardia alone is a poor predictor of toxicity.
   (b) Sinus arrest and sinoatrial block.

Management of Toxicity

General measures:

- Stop the drug.
- Discontinue diuretics or, if they are necessary, use a potassium-sparing diuretic or ample K supplements.
- Measure serum digoxin levels and serum K.
- Recheck the dose used and correlate with weight, age, and creatinine clearance.

- Record baseline ECG. If arrhythmia is present, monitor the cardiac rhythm.
- Search for and correct factors that can precipitate digitalis toxicity, e.g., physician error, giving too big a dose in the presence of renal insufficiency or hypokalemia.

Hyperkalemia may be owing to digitalis toxicity, and it is believed to result from inhibition by digitalis of the Na^+, K^+-ATPase enzyme causing a release of intracellular potassium into the extracellular space. Other predisposing factors are as listed in Table 12-2. Advise the patient in the future to bring all medications, to be rechecked at each hospital or office visit.

Tachyarrhythmias: Ventricular tachycardia, multifocal premature ventricular contractions (PVCs), and atrial tachycardia with block are managed as follows:

1. Potassium intravenously: 40–60 mEq (mmol) in 1 L of normal or half-normal saline is given over 4 h, except:
   (a) In patients with a raised serum K^+ concentration (>5 mEq (mmol)/L).
   (b) In renal insufficiency.
   (c) In patients with AV block because increasing K^+ concentration may increase the degree of the AV block.
       If more than 10 mEq (mmol)/h of KC1 is infused, cardiac monitoring is necessary. KC1 in 5 % dextrose/water is used if HF is present.
2. Lidocaine (lignocaine) is reasonably effective for the management of ventricular tachycardia and multifocal PVCs. The short duration of action and relatively low toxicity are major advantages. A bolus of 1–1.5 mg/kg is given simultaneously with a continuous infusion of 2–3 mg/min.
3. Phenytoin may be effective in the management of digitalis-induced ventricular arrhythmias but should be reserved for nonresponders to lidocaine or K^+ because more careful supervision is required during its administration and severe toxic side effects do occur.
       Dosage: IV 250 mg at a rate of 25–50 mg/min given in 0.9 % saline through a caval catheter or utilizing a central vein. Phenytoin is useful as it depresses ventricular

automaticity without slowing intraventricular conduction. The decrease in AV conduction produced by digitalis may be reversed. The drug has a relatively mild negative inotropic effect in comparison with procainamide or disopyramide.

Caution
- Hypotension, heart block, asystole, and ventricular fibrillation have occurred, especially with increase in the infusion rate of phenytoin.
- 250-mg vials contain 40 % propylene glycol as a diluent with a pH of 11. Do not mix with dextrose. Pain, inflammation, or venous thrombosis may occur.

4. Magnesium deficiency may coexist with hypokalemia. Magnesium sulfate parenterally may be indicated.

5. Beta-blockers are reserved for nonresponders to measures 1–4. The drug may be useful for PVCs or supraventricular tachycardia (SVT) in the absence of AV block. The use of beta-blockers has appropriately dwindled with the advent of digoxin-specific Fab antibody.

Bradyarrhythmias: Sinoatrial dysfunction causing syncope or hemodynamic deterioration can be managed with atropine IV 0.4, 0.5, or 0.6 mg every 5 min to a maximum of 2.4 mg. Failure to respond to atropine is an indication for temporary pacing.

Cardioversion: Ventricular fibrillation requires the usual energy levels (200 J, if necessary up to 320 J). IV amiodarone is of value in the management of recurrent ventricular fibrillation. If other arrhythmias are life threatening, phenytoin or lidocaine followed if necessary by cardioversion using a low energy of 5–20 J initially is tried.

Drug name:	Digoxin Immune Fab (Digoxin-specific antibody)
Trade name:	Digibind
Supplied:	Vial 40 mg (38 mg)
Dosage:	2–6 vials; infusion of six vials (228–240 mg) is adequate to reverse most cases of toxicity; see text for further advice

There is little doubt that this method of treatment is effective for the management of life-threatening arrhythmias not responding to conventional therapy. The treatment is especially useful in the presence of hyperkalemia. Skin testing to avoid allergic reactions to the digoxin-specific Fab from sheep is recommended.

Beta-Stimulants

DOBUTAMINE

Dosage: 250 mg/20 mL vial—diluted in 5 % dextrose/water and infused at a rate of 2.5–10 µg/kg/min. Dobutamine is a direct myocardial beta1- and a mild beta2-stimulant. The positive inotropic effect is equal to that of isoproterenol.

The reduction in SVR with dobutamine may rarely cause hypotension, and the drug is contraindicated in patients who are hypotensive.

Increase in cardiac output occurs with only minimal increase in heart rate at infusion rates <5 µg/kg/min.

Dobutamine increases cardiac output while reducing left ventricular filling pressure (LVFP) with little or no increase in heart rate or blood pressure. Except at low doses, dopamine produces an increase in LVFP, heart rate, SVR, and blood pressure and therefore increases myocardial oxygen demand. Dobutamine is thus superior to dopamine in patients with a very high LVFP. Advantages of dobutamine include a short half-life <3 min, which allows rapid dissipation of adverse effects.

Importantly low doses are currently advised: 1 µg/kg/min with increase to 2 µg; a dose of 5 µg/kg/min is often excessive. This lower recommended dose avoids adverse effects.

- Dopamine increases SVR, and cardiac output may not increase despite its inotropic effect.

In patients with peripheral vascular disease, gangrene of the digits may be precipitated.

NEW DEVELOPMENTS

Spironolactone

- In patients with heart failure and a preserved ejection fraction, treatment with spironolactone did not significantly reduce the incidence of the primary composite outcome of death from cardiovascular causes, aborted cardiac arrest, or hospitalization for recurrence of heart failure (Pitt et al. TOPCAT 2014)

Istaroxime

Gheorghiade et al. (2008) suggest that istaroxime is a novel IV inotropic and lusitropic agent; studies are under way.

The addition of SERCA2a pump activation appears to improve diastolic function and ameliorates adverse effects of increased intracellular calcium. Small trials have assessed IV istaroxime. A study of 120 patients admitted for acute HF showed decreased pulmonary wedge pressure and improved diastolic function (Gheorghiade et al. 2008). Importantly, there was no precipitation of arrhythmias or hypotension. Istaroxime is intriguing as a potential inotrope which avoids the adverse effects associated with conventional inotropic agent (Francis et al. 2014), but IV medications are not the solution for significantly preventing death or rehospitalizations.

Omecamtiv mecarbil

Non-glycoside agents
Cardioactive agents with actions similar to digoxin and stimulation of the sarcoplasmic reticulum calcium (SERCA2a) pump (inotropic and lusitropic agents) are being studiedKrum and Teerlink (2011)).

The small omecamtiv mecarbil molecule increases the efficiency of heart muscle contraction via selectivity for a subset of cardiac myosins. Omecamtiv mecarbil does not appear to drive oxygen consumption as does most inotropes, which is a unique attribute (Francis et al. 2014), and is a new potential therapy for heart failure (Teerlink et al. 2011).

SERCA2a

Two clinical trials are currently targeting sarcoplasmic reticulum Ca2þ-ATPase (SERCA2a), one in patients implanted with left ventricular assist devices and another examining the effect on cardiac remodeling (Francis et al. 2014).

Serelaxin

Serelaxin is a recombinant form of the pregnancy hormone relaxin-2. The hormone regulates maternal adaptations to improve arterial compliance, cardiac output, and renal blood flow.

- The RELAX-AHF trial tested the hypothesis that serelaxin-treated patients would have greater dyspnea relief compared with patients treated with standard care and placebo.
- This double-blind, placebo-controlled trial randomly assigned 1,161 patients admitted to hospital for acute HF to serelaxin ($n=581$) or placebo ($n=580$). Subjects were assigned to standard care plus 48-h intravenous infusions of placebo or serelaxin (30 µg/kg per day) within 16 h from presentation (Teerlink et al. 2013).
- All patients had dyspoea, congestion on chest radiograph, and increased brain natriuretic peptide (BNP)
- Serelaxin improved the primary dyspnea end point (448 mm×h,; $P=0.007$) compared with placebo, but had no significant effect on the other primary end point. No significant effects were observed for the secondary end points of cardiovascular death or readmission to hospital for HF. Serelaxin treatment was well tolerated; a reduced 180-day mortality was observed (Teerlink et al. 2013). Early administration of serelaxin was associated with a reduction of 180-day mortality, and this occurred with fewer signs of organ damage and more rapid relief of congestion during the first days after admission (Metra et al. 2013).

Rosuvastatin

In CORONA trial when repeat events were included, rosuvastatin was shown to reduce the risk of HF hospitalizations approximately 15–20 %, equating to approximately 76 fewer admissions per 1,000 patients treated over a median 33 months of follow-up (Rogers et al. 2014).

LCZ696

A novel drug LCZ696, a dual inhibitor of angiotensin II receptor and neprilysin proved to be more effective than enalapril, (Jessup 2014). A total of 711 patients (17.0 %) receiving LCZ696 and 835 patients (19.8 %) receiving enalapril died P<0.001); of these patients, 558 (13.3 %) and 693 (16.5 %), respectively, died from cardiovascular causes (McMurray et al. 2014, see Chap. 22).

MANAGEMENT OF PULMONARY EDEMA

Pulmonary edema is not a diagnosis. Its cause is usually cardiogenic or noncardiogenic.

Cardiogenic

- Usually owing to LV failure, often caused by complications of ischemic heart disease, tachyarrhythmias, hypertension, valvular heart disease, or congestive dilated cardiomyopathy.
- Mitral stenosis and, rarely, left atrial myxoma.

OR Noncardiogenic

- Adult respiratory distress syndrome in which there is altered alveolar-capillary membrane permeability caused by pneumonia, toxins, allergens, smoke inhalation, gastric aspiration, radiation pneumonitis, and hemorrhagic pancreatitis.
- Other causes include drugs, narcotic overdose, severe hypoalbuminemia, uremia, and neurogenic and lymphangitic carcinomatosis.

Treatment of Cardiogenic Pulmonary Edema

1. Oxygen, to maintain an adequate PO2.
2. Morphine or diamorphine, provided severe respiratory insufficiency is absent, because either drug may cause respiratory depression or even arrest.

   Dosage: A dilute solution of morphine sulfate 1 mg/mL is administered IV at a rate of 1 mg/min in a dose of 3–5 mg. Repeat as needed at 15- to 30-min intervals to a total dose of 10–15 mg. The average patient may require 30 mg in 24 h. Diamorphine 2–5 mg, repeated once if necessary, is often used in the UK. The beneficial effects of the opiates result from:
   (a) venous pooling and therefore preload reduction.
   (b) the allaying of anxiety and reduction in tachypnea.
   (c) an increase in ventricular fibrillation threshold.

   Vomiting and aspiration should be avoided. An antiemetic such as cyclizine or metoclopramide 5 mg is useful when given 15 min before the dose of morphine is repeated. Naloxone (Narcan) 0.4 mg IV repeated at 4-min intervals is given if respiratory depression occurs (maximum 1.2 mg).
3. Furosemide 40–80 mg IV slowly repeated in 30 min if symptoms persist and the blood pressure is stable.

   Warning: In patients with normal or low blood volume, an initial dose of 40 mg or more may cause severe hypotension, especially when morphine and nitrates are used concomitantly. Improvement in dyspnea usually occurs within 10 min of furosemide administration as a result of its venodilator action. Failure to respond to the second dose is an indication for preload- or afterload-reducing agents.
4. Nitroglycerin (glyceryl trinitrate) can be of immediate benefit. Nitroglycerin is given sublingually along with a transdermal preparation. In severe pulmonary edema IV nitrate or nitroprusside is indicated.

   If hypotension is present, dopamine 2.5–10 µg/kg/min and nitrate are indicated.

REFERENCES

ACCF/AHA Guideline for the Management of Heart Failure: Executive Summary. A Report of the merican College of Cardiology Foundation/ American Heart Association Task Force on Practice Guidelines 2013.

A-HeFT, Taylor AL, Ziesche S, Yancy C, et al. Combination of isosorbide dinitrate and hydralazine in blacks with heart failure. N Engl J Med. 2004;351:2049–57.

Ahmed A, Rich MW, Love TE, et al. Digoxin and reduction in mortality and hospitalization in heart failure: a comprehensive post hoc analysis of the DIG trial. Eur Heart J. 2006;27:178–86.

AIRE: Acute Infarction Ramipril Efficacy (AIRE) Study Investigators. Effect of ramipril on mortality and morbidity of survivors of acute myocardial infarction with clinical evidence of heart failure. Lancet. 1993;342:821.

Arnold SB, Byrd RC, Meister W, et al. Long-term digitalis therapy improves left ventricular function in heart failure. N Engl J Med. 1980;303:1443.

ATLAS Study Group, Packer M, Poole-Wilson PA, Armstrong P, et al. Comparative effects of low and high doses of angiotensin-converting inhibitor, lisinopril, on morbidity and mortality in chronic heart failure. Circulation. 1999;100:2312.

Boydak B, Nalbantgil S, Fici F, et al. A randomised comparison of the effects of nebivolol and atenolol with and without chlorthalidone on the sexual function of hypertensive men. Clin Drug Investig. 2005;25:409–16.

Bristow MR, Kantrowitz NE, Ginsburg R, et al. Beta-adrenergic function in heart muscle disease and heart failure. J Mol Cell Cardiol. 1985;17:41.

Brixius K, Middeke M, Lichtenthal A, et al. Nitric oxide, erectile dysfunction and beta-blocker treatment (MR NOED study): benefit of nebivolol versus metoprolol in hypertensive men. Clin Exp Pharmacol Physiol. 2007;34:327–31.

CAPRICORN Investigators. Effect of carvedilol on outcome after myocardial infarction in patients with left-ventricular dysfunction. Lancet. 2001;357:1385.

CHARM Investigators and Committees, Granger CB, McMurray JJV, Yusuf S, et al. Effects of candesartan in patients with chronic heart failure and reduced left ventricular systolic function intolerant to angiotensin converting enzyme inhibitors; the CHARM-alternative trial. Lancet. 2003;362:772–6.

CIBIS-II. The Cardiac Insufficiency Bisoprolol Study II (CIBIS-II). A randomized trial. Lancet. 1999;353: 9–13.

Cleland JGF, Dargie HJ, McAlpine H, et al. Severe hypotension after first dose of enalapril in heart failure. BMJ. 1985;291:1309.

Cockcroft JR, Chowienczyk PJ, Brett SE, et al. Nebivolol vasodilates human forearm vasculature: evidence for a L-arginine/No-dependent mechanism. J Pharmacol Exp Ther. 1995;274:1067–71.

Cohn JN, Archibald DG, Francis GS, et al. Veterans Administration Cooperative Study on Vasodilator Therapy of Heart Failure: Influence of prerandomization variables on the reduction of mortality by treatment with hydralazine and isosorbide dinitrate. Circulation. 1987;75:IV49.

Cohn JN, Archibald DG, Ziesche S, et al. Effect of vasodilator therapy on mortality in chronic congestive heart failure. Results of a Veterans Administration Cooperative Study. N Engl J Med. 1986;314:1547.

Cominacini L, Pasini AF, Garbin U, et al. Nebivolol and its 4-keto derivative increase nitric oxide in endothelial cells by reducing its oxidative inactivation. J Am Coll Cardiol. 2003;42:1838–44.

CONSENSUS: Consensus Trial Study Group. Effects of enalapril on mortality in severe congestive heart failure: results of the Cooperative North Scandinavian Enalapril Survival Study (Consensus). N Engl J Med. 1987;316:1429.

Dobbs SM, Kenyon WI, Dobbs RJ. Maintenance digoxin after an episode of heart failure: placebo-controlled trial in outpatients. BMJ. 1977;1:749.

Flather MD, Shibata MC, Coats AJ, et al. Randomized trial to determine the effect of nebivolol on mortality and cardiovascular hospital admission in the elderly patients with heart failure. Eur Heart J. 2005;26:215–25.

Francis GS, Bartos JA, Adatya S, et al. Inotropes. J Am Coll Cardiol. 2014;63:2069–78.

Gheorghiade M, Blair JE, Filippatos GS, et al. Hemodynamic, echocardiographic, and neurohormonal effects of istaroxime, a novel intravenous inotropic and lusitropic agent: a randomized controlled trial in patients hospitalized with heart failure. J Am Coll Cardiol. 2008;51:2276–85.

Gheorghiade M, St Clair J, St Clair C, et al. Hemodynamic effects of intravenous digoxin in patients with severe heart failure initially treated with diuretics and vasodilators. J Am Coll Cardiol. 1987;9:849.

Hass GJ, Abraham WT. The challenge of heart failure. J Am Coll Cardiol. 2005;46:2052–3.

Jessup M. Neprilysin inhibition – a novel therapy for heart failure. N Engl J Med. 371:1062–64. http://www.nejm.org/toc/nejm/371/11/. Accessed 11 Sep 2014.

Khan MG. Clinical trials. In: Cardiac drug therapy. Philadelphia, PA: WB Saunders/Elsevier; 2003. p. 502

Khan MG. Hypertension. In: Encyclopedia of heart diseases. 2nd ed. New York: Springer; 2011. p. 556.

Khan MI. Treatment of refractory congestive heart failure and normokalemic hypochloremic alkalosis with acetazolamide and spironolactone. Can Medl Assoc J. 1980;123:883–7.

Kiyingi A, Field MJ, Pawsey CC, et al. Metolazone in treatment of severe refractory congestive cardiac failure. Lancet. 1990;336:29.

Krum H, Teerlink JR. Medical therapy for chronic heart failure. Lancet. 2011;378(9792):713–21.

Little WC. Enhanced load dependence of relaxation in heart failure: clinical implications. Circulation. 1992;85:2326.

Maffei A, Lembo G. Nitric oxide mechanisms of nebivolol. Ther Adv Cardiovasc Dis. 2009;3(4):317–27.

Maisel AS, Krishnaswamy P, Nowak RM, et al. Rapid measurement of B-type natriuretic peptide in the emergency diagnosis of heart failure. N Engl J Med. 2002;347:l6l.

Marcus FI. Pharmacokinetic interactions between digoxin and other drugs. J Am Coll Cardiol. 1985;5:82A.

MERIT/HF: The Metoprolol CR/XL Randomized Intervention Trial in Congestive Heart Failure. Effects of controlled-release metoprolol on total mortality, hospitalizations, and well-being in patients with heart failure. JAMA. 2000;283:1295.

Metra M, Cotter G, Davison BA, et al. Effect of serelaxin on cardiac, renal, and hepatic biomarkers in the relaxin in acute heart failure (RELAX-AHF) development program: correlation with outcomes. J Am Coll Cardiol. 2013;61(2):196–206.

Münzel T, Gori T. Nebivolol: The somewhat-different b-adrenergic receptor blocker. J Am Coll Cardiol. 2009;54:1491–9.

Nanas JN, Alexopoulos G, Anastasiou-Nana MI, et al. Outcome of patients with congestive heart failure treated with standard versus high doses of enalapril: a multicenter study. J Am Coll Cardiol. 2000;36:2090.

NOVEL DRUG, McMurray JJV, Packer M, Desai AS, et al. Angiotensin-neprilysin inhibition versus enalapril in heart failure. N Engl J Med. 2014;371:993–1004.

The ONTARGET Investigators. Telmisartan, ramipril, or both in patients at high risk for vascular events Randomized. N Engl J Med. 2008;358:1547–59. http://www.nejm.org/doi/full/10.1056/NEJMoa0801317. Accessed 10 Apr 2008.

Packer M, Bristow MR, Cohn JN, et al. The effect of carvedilol on morbidity and mortality in patients with chronic heart failure. N Engl J Med. 1996;334:1349.

Packer M, Coats JS, Fowler MB, for the Carvedilol Prospective Randomized Cumulative Survival Study Group, et al. Effect of carvedilol on survival in severe chronic heart failure. N Engl J Med. 2001;344:1651.

Packer M, Cohn JN. Consensus recommendations for the management of chronic heart failure. Am J Cardiol. 1999;83:1A.

Packer M, Gheorghiade M, Young JB, for the RADIANCE study, et al. Withdrawal of digoxin from patients with chronic heart failure treated with angiotensin-converting-enzyme inhibitors. N Engl J Med. 1993; 329:1.

Packer M. Is the renin-angiotensin system really unnecessary in patients with severe chronic heart failure?: The price we pay for interfering with evolution. J Am Coll Cardiol. 1985;6:171.

Pitt B, Pfeffer MA, Assmann SF, for the TOPCAT Investigators. Spironolactone for heart failure with preserved ejection fraction. N Engl J Med. 2014;370:1383–92.

PRAISE, Packer M, O'Connor CM, Ghali JK, et al. Effect of amlodipine on morbidity and mortality in severe chronic heart failure. For the Prospective Randomized Amlodipine Survival Evaluation Study Group. N Engl J Med. 1996;335:1107.

RALES, Pitt B, Zannad F, Remme WJ, et al. The effect of spironolactone on morbidity and mortality in patients with severe heart failure: for the Randomized Evaluation Study Investigators. N Engl J Med. 1999;341:709.

Rogers JK, Jhund PS, Perez A. Effect of rosuvastatin on repeat heart failure hospitalizations: the CORONA trial (controlled rosuvastatin multinational trial in heart failure). JCHF. 2014;2(3):289–97.

SAVE, Pfeffer MA, Braunwald E, Moye LA, et al. Effect of captopril on mortality and morbidity in patients with left ventricular dysfunction after myocardial infarction. Results of the Survival and Ventricular Enlargement trial. For the SAVE Investigators. N Engl J Med. 1992;327:669.

Schenck-Gustafsson K, Jublin-Dannfelt A, Dahlquist R. Renal function and digoxin clearance during quinidine therapy. Clin Physiol. 1982;2:401.

SENIORS Investigators, van Veldhuisen DJ, Cohen-Solal A, Bohm MA, et al. Beta-blockade with nebivolol in elderly heart failure patients with impaired and preserved left ventricular ejection fraction: data from SENIORS (Study of Effects of Nebivolol Intervention on Outcomes and Rehospitalization in Seniors with Heart Failure). J Am Coll Cardiol. 2009;53:2150–8.

SOLVD Investigators. Effect of enalapril on survival in patients with reduced ventricular ejection fractions and congestive heart failure. N Engl J Med. 1991;325:293.

Stevens LA, Coresh J, Green T. Assessing kidney function—measured and estimated glomerular filtration rate. N Engl J Med. 2006;354:2473–83.

Teerlink JR, Cotter G, Davison BA. Serelaxin, recombinant human relaxin-2, for treatment of acute heart failure (RELAX-AHF): a randomised, placebo-controlled trial. Lancet. 2013;381(9860):29–39.

Teerlink JR, Clarke CP, Sailkali KG, et al. Dose-dependent augmentation of cardiac systolic function with the selective cardiac myosin activator, omecamtiv mecarbil: a first-in-man study. Lancet. 2011;378:667–75.

The Digitalis Investigation Group. The effect of digoxin on mortality and morbidity in patients with heart failure. N Engl J Med. 1997;336:525.

TRANSCEND Investigators, Yusuf S, Teo K, Anderson C, et al. Effects of the angiotensin-receptor blocker telmisartan on cardiovascular events in high-risk patients intolerant to angiotensin converting enzyme inhibitors: a randomised controlled trial. Lancet. 2008;372:1174–83.

Tuncer M, Fettser DV, Gunes Y, et al. Comparison of effects of nebivolol and atenolol on P-wave dispersion in patients with hypertension [in Russian]. Kardiologiia. 2008;48:42–5.

Val-HeFT Cohn JN, Tognoni G. A randomized trial of the angiotensin-receptor blocker valsartan in chronic heart failure. N Engl J Med. 2001;345:1667–75.

V-HeFTII, Cohn JN, Johnson G, Ziesche S, et al. A comparison of enalapril with hydralazine-isosorbide dinitrate in the treatment of chronic congestive heart failure. N Engl J Med. 1991;325:303.

Waagstein F, Hjalmarson A, Swedberg K, et al. Beta-blockers in dilated cardiomyopathies: they work. Eur Heart J. 1993;4(Suppl A):173–8.

Yancy CW, Jessup M, Bozkurt B, et al. A report of the American College of Cardiology Foundation/American Heart Association Task Force on Practice Guidelines for the management of heart failure. Executive summary. J Am Coll Cardiol. 2013;62(16):e147–239.

Zatuchni J. Verapamil-digoxin interaction. Am Heart J. 1984;108:412.

13 Heart Failure Controversies

ARE ARBS AS EFFECTIVE AS ACE INHIBITOR THERAPY FOR HEART FAILURE?

The carefully run RCTs CHARM (2003), Val-HeFT (2001), and TRANSCEND (2008) did not show a decrease in total mortality in heart failure (HF) subjects (see Chaps. 4 and 12). This surprising finding was observed in patients intolerant to ACE inhibitor administration. It is abundantly clear that ARBs are not as effective as ACE inhibitor therapy for HF, hypertension, or stroke. The salutary effects of ARBs are probably less than that observed with digoxin, yet these agents are used widely and excessively. In **Val-HeFT** valsartan when combined with a beta-blocker caused significantly more cardiac events. A total of 5,010 patients with HF class II, III, or IV were randomly assigned to receive 160 mg of valsartan or placebo twice daily.

- The incidence of the combined end point was a modest 13.2 % lower with valsartan than with placebo), predominantly because of a lower number of patients hospitalized for heart failure: 455 (18.2 %) in the placebo group and 346 (13.8 %) in the valsartan group.
- **"Overall mortality was not reduced by valsartan administration"** (Cohn and Tognoni 2001); see results for digoxin.

Unfortunately, less than 36 % of subjects received a beta-blocker and ~68 % received digoxin.

"The post hoc observation of an adverse effect on mortality and morbidity in the subgroup receiving valsartan,

© Springer Science+Business Media New York 2015
M. Gabriel Khan, *Cardiac Drug Therapy*, Contemporary Cardiology,
DOI 10.1007/978-1-61779-962-4_13

an ACE inhibitor, and a beta-blocker raises concern about the potential safety of this specific combination" (Cohn and Tognoni 2001).

Often in patients with HF, a beta-blocker is needed as proven therapy. Thus an ACE inhibitor must be used, not an ARB; telmisartan also failed in HF trials.

Caution: valsartan should not be combined with a beta-blocker.

In **VALIANT 2003**: a clinical trial of valsartan, captopril, or both in MI complicated by HF, left ventricular dysfunction, or both, during a median follow-up of 24.7 months, **total mortality was not reduced by valsartan**: 979 patients in the valsartan group died, as did 941 patients in the valsartan-and-captopril group and 958 patients in the captopril group. There was no placebo group.

Caution: valsartan therapy does not decrease mortality and is not advisable in HF patients because in this large number of patients, a beta-blocker is a needed therapy.

ARBs are administered only if there is intolerance to ACE inhibitor therapy. Telmisartan and olmesartan are not advisable. Telmisartan failed to significantly reduce mortality or hospitalizations in the large RCT TRANSCEND (See Chaps. 3 and 12).

MANAGEMENT OF HEART FAILURE PRESERVED EJECTION FRACTION

- Heart failure preserved ejection fraction (HFPEF) is not uncommon in elderly women. Atrial fibrillation is common in the elderly, and ventricular rates even when not very rapid (120–140) may precipitate HFPEF. Is it preferable to adopt the term HFPEF rather than diastolic HF? Not all patients with HFPEF show definite diagnostic diastolic abnormalities. Controversies abound, however, among the experts.

Mauer et al. (2004 stated that HF with normal ejection fraction is preferred over the term diastolic heart failure (DHF) mainly because:

- Doppler-derived diastolic parameters do not provide specific information on intrinsic passive diastolic properties; thus, diastolic dysfunction cannot be diagnosed reliably by Doppler echocardiography.
- Delayed relaxation and/or stiffened passive properties may not be the unifying pathophysiologic mechanisms in all patients who present with HF and normal EF.

Nonetheless, abnormal diastolic function is a common cause of HFPEF if atrial fibrillation as a cause is excluded.

Oh et al. (2006) criticized Mauer and colleagues and emphasized that diastolic HF is easily diagnosed by echocardiography in a patient with a preserved left ventricular (LV) EF with evidence of abnormal relaxation, decreased compliance, increased filling pressure, and normal LV dimensions. However, Oh et al. describe the situation that exists in most sophisticated diagnostic laboratories with highly trained echocardiographers and clinicians and that does not represent the real world of medicine.

The diagnosis of probable diastolic HF can be made by using the criteria of Vasan and Levy (2000).

Differential diagnosis and mimics include:

1. Incorrect diagnosis or incorrect measurement of EF. The echocardiographic assessment of EF is fraught with errors but remains a useful guide to diagnosis and management of systolic HF.
2. Valvular disease.
3. Pericardial constriction and left atrial myxoma are rare and do not genuinely represent HFPEF; in this setting there is simply restriction to ventricular filling.
4. Severe hypertension can cause both systolic HF and HFPEF.
5. Myocardial ischemia more commonly causes systolic HF but can cause a combination of both types of HF and rarely pure HFPEF.

Age and the diseases listed appear to cause changes in cross-linking of intercellular connective tissue. The heart fills less and empties less, and the percentage ejected may be relatively normal, but the stroke output and cardiac index are decreased; thus, the renin-angiotensin-aldosterone system (RAAS) is stimulated. Systolic dysfunction impairs the ability of the left ventricle to relax and fill at low pressure. Thus, systolic dysfunction is a principal cause of diastolic dysfunction.

TREATMENT

Importantly, the treatment of HFPEF is treatment of the cause. With systolic HF, medications help considerably to improve outcomes versus HFPEF, in which medications are unproved except for symptomatic improvement enhanced by judicious diuretic therapy.

- The judicious use of diuretics is recommended to relieve symptoms.
- Beta-blockers decrease heart rate, and the longer diastolic interval might improve ventricular filling. **Nebivolol proved effective for both systolic HF and HF with normal EF (see Seniors study** 2009 **in Chap. 12).**
  ACE inhibitors are not effective:
- Aldosterone antagonists: Spironolactone is effective for heart failure with reduced EF (Pitt et al. 1999) but in patients with heart failure and a preserved ejection fraction. Treatment with spironolactone did not significantly reduce the incidence of the primary composite outcome of death from cardiovascular causes, aborted cardiac arrest, or hospitalization for recurrence of heart failure (Pitt et al. TOPCAT 2014).
- Because a decrease in preload exists, the overzealous use of preload-reducing agents, including loop diuretics, ACE inhibitors, and nitrates, may cause hemodynamic and clinical deterioration. Usually dosages are 50–75 % lower than those used for systolic HF, and diuretics except eplerenone 25 mg may not be required except during the symptomatic

congestive phase that may last a few weeks. Loop diuret-ics are contraindicated in pericardial diseases and restric-tive cardiomyopathy and relatively contraindicated in hypertrophic cardiomyopathy (HCM) and in hypertensive HCM of the elderly with impaired ventricular relaxation (Topol et al. 1985).

DIGOXIN IS NOT USEFUL FOR HFPEF: TRUE OR FALSE?

Ahmed et al. (2006) did a comprehensive post hoc analysis of the randomized-controlled Digitalis Investigation Group trial ($n = 7,788$) (Eichhorn and Gheorghiade 2002) and focused on 5,548 patients: 1,687 with digoxin levels drawn randomly at 1 month, and 3,861 placebo patients, alive at 1 month. Findings: **Digoxin at 0.5–0.9 ng/mL reduced mortality and hospitalizations in all HF patients,** *including those with HFPEF. Yet the drug is rarely administered.*

Is CHARM-Preserved a Clear Study of HFPEF?

It must be emphasized that the EF should be >45 % deter-mined within 3 days of the episode of HF to be diagnostic of HFPEF. Thus, Candesartan in Heart Failure Assessment in Reduction of Mortality (CHARM)-Preserved (2003), which studied patients with EF >40 %, was not a true study of patients with HFPEF. An EF of 40–45 % cannot be assumed to be normal LV systolic function.

- CHARM-Preserved randomized 3,025 patients with EF >40 %. There was an 18 % reduction in the number of patients with investigator-reported hospitalizations for HF with candesartan (230 versus 279, $p = 0.017$), but there was no decrease in total mortality. The primary end points of cardiovascular disease (CVD) death and hospitalization were not met (11 %, $p = 0.051$; total hospitalization, 912 patients versus 922, $p = 0.99$), a result not superior to that observed fro digoxin.

DOES AN ACE INHIBITOR COMBINED WITH AN ARB IMPROVE OUTCOMES?

The Valsartan Heart Failure Trial (Val-HeFT 2001) compared valsartan (160 mg/day)+ACE inhibitor with placebo in approx 5,000 patients with class II–III HF. There was a 28 % reduction in hospitalization for HF but no reduction in mortality.

- **Importantly, in 794 patients given an ACE inhibitor, a beta-blocker, and a valsartan, there was a significant increase in mortality [129 versus 97 deaths; hazard ratio (HR), 1.42; 95 % $p=0.009$], compared with 806 patients treated with an ACE inhibitor, a beta-blocker, and a placebo.**

Beta-blocker therapy is an integral component of HF therapy. An angiotensin receptor blocker (ARB) added to ACE inhibitor/beta-blocker therapy is not advisable. Extensive RAAS blockade appears to be harmful; CHARM-Added used the same entry criteria as Val-HeFT: mainly patients with class III HF and virtually no class IV patients.

- In patients treated with beta-blockers in addition to an ACE inhibitor, 175 (25 %) of 702 died in the candesartan group, and 195 (27 %) of 711 died in the placebo group ($p=0.22$) (CHARM-Added).
- Hyperkalemia was observed in 3 % of treated patients and 1 % in the placebo arm; caution is required.
- The combination of an ACE inhibitor and an ARB is not advisable. Also, patients should not receive aldosterone antagonists when this combination is used because the incidence of hyperkalemia is significantly increased. It is more beneficial to add an aldosterone antagonist to an ACE inhibitor than to add an ARB.

HEART FAILURE IN BLACKS:
DO DIFFERENCES EXIST?

- Heart failure has a 50 % higher incidence in the African-American population than is observed in the general population.
- ACE inhibitors have not shown as great a benefit in black patients with HF as found in the white population. Also, angioedema is more common in black versus white patients treated with ACE inhibitors.
- In the Veterans Administration Heart Failure Trial (VHeFT), hydralazine combined with isosorbide dinitrate *was not shown* to be significantly effective in reducing cardiac mortality in mainly white patients (see Chap. 12).

An RCT of 1,050 black patients with class III/IV HF was conducted using *isosorbide dinitrate and hydralazine along with a standard HF regimen. Treatment resulted in a 43 % decrease in total mortality*, which led to premature termination of the trial. Time to first hospitalization was improved (Taylor et al. 2004).

ARE STATINS RECOMMENDED
FOR PATIENTS WITH HEART FAILURE?

Two large RCTs have shown no beneficial effects. The CORONA (Controlled Rosuvastatin Multinational Trial in Heart Failure) trial was a multicenter, randomized-controlled, placebo-controlled trial of 5,011 older patients randomized to either rosuvastatin at 10 mg daily or placebo and received a median of 2.7 years follow-up. The study did not reach the primary combined end point, Kjekshus et al. (2007). In CORONA trial when repeat events were included, rosuvastatin was shown to reduce the risk of HF by approximately 15–20 %, equating to approximately 76 fewer admissions per 1,000 patients treated over a median of 33 months of follow-up (Rogers et al. 2014).

In the GISSI-HF (Gruppo Italiano per lo Studio della Sopravvivenza nell'Infarto Miocardico-Insufficienza Cardiaca) trial, rosuvastatin did not demonstrate a reduction in mortality or cardiovascular hospitalizations (GISSI-HF 2008).

REFERENCES

Ahmed A, Rich MW, Love TE, et al. Digoxin and reduction in mortality and hospitalization in heart failure: a comprehensive post hoc analysis of the DIG trial. Eur Heart J. 2006;27:178–86.

CHARM alternative trial, Granger CB, McMurray JJV, Yusuf S, et al. for the CHARM Investigators and Committees. Effects of candesartan in patients with chronic heart failure and reduced left ventricular systolic function intolerant to angiotensin converting enzyme inhibitors. Lancet. 2003;362:772–776.

CHARM, McMurray JJV, Östergren J, Swedberg K, Granger CB. Effects of candesartan in patients with chronic heart failure and reduced left-ventricular systolic function taking angiotensin-converting-enzyme inhibitors: Lancet. 2003;362:767–71.

CHARM Preserved Trial, Yusuf S, Pfeffer MA, Swedberg K, et al. Effects of candesartan in patients with chronic heart failure and preserved left-ventricular ejection fraction. Lancet. 2003;362:777–81.

Cohn JN, Tognoni G. A randomized trial of the angiotensin-receptor blocker valsartan in chronic heart failure. N Engl J Med. 2001;345: 1667–75.

CORONA, Kjekshus J, Apetrei E, Barrios V et al for the CORONA Group. Rosuvastatin in older patients with systolic heart failure. N Engl J Med. 2007;357:2248–61.

Eichhorn EJ, Gheorghiade M. Digoxin—new perspective on an old drug. N Engl J Med. 2002;47:1394.

GISSI-HF Investigators. Effect of rosuvastatin in patients with chronic heart failure (the GISSI-HF trial): a randomised, doubleblind, placebo-controlled trial. Lancet. 2008;372:1231–9.

Mauer MS, Spevack D, Burkhoff D, Kronzon I. Diastolic dysfunction: can it be diagnosed by Doppler echocardiography? J Am Coll Cardiol. 2004;44:1543–9.

Oh JK, Hatle L, Tajik AJ, et al. Diastolic heart failure can be diagnosed by comprehensive two-dimensional and Doppler echocardiography. J Am Coll Cardiol. 2006;47:500–6.

Pitt B, Pfeffer MA, Assmann SF. for the TOPCAT Investigators. Spironolactone for heart failure with preserved ejection fraction. N Engl J Med. 2014;370:1383–92.

RALES, Pitt B, Zannad F, Remme WJ, et al. for the Randomized Evaluation Study Investigators. The effect of spironolactone on morbidity and mortality in patients with severe heart failure. N Engl J Med. 1999;341:709.

Rogers JK, Jhund PS, Perez A. Effect of rosuvastatin on repeat heart failure hospitalizations: the CORONA trial (controlled rosuvastatin multinational trial in heart failure). JCHF 2014;2(3):289–97.

SENIORS study, van Veldhuisen DJ, Cohen-Solal A, Bohm MA et al. SENIORS Investigators. Beta-blockade with nebivolol in elderly heart failure patients with impaired and preserved left ventricular ejection fraction: data from (study of effects of nebivolol intervention on outcomes and rehospitalization in seniors with heart failure). J Am Coll Cardiol. 2009;53:2150–58.

Taylor AL, Ziesche S, Yancy C, et al. Combination of isosorbide dinitrate and hydralazine in blacks with heart failure. N Engl J Med. 2004; 351:2049–57.

Topol EJ, Traill TA, Fortuin NJ. Hypertensive hypertrophic cardiomyopathy of the elderly. N Engl J Med. 1985;312:277.

TRANSCEND, Yusuf S, Teo K, Anderson C et al. For the TRANSCEND Investigators. Effects of the angiotensin-receptor blocker telmisartan on cardiovascular events in high-risk patients intolerant to angiotensin-converting enzyme inhibitors: a randomised controlled trial. Lancet 2008;372:1174–83.

Val-HeFT Cohn JN, Tognoni G. A randomized trial of the angiotensin-receptor blocker valsartan in chronic heart failure. N Engl J Med. 2001;345:1667–75.

Vasan RS, Levy D. Defining diastolic heart failure. A call for standardized diagnostic criteria. Circulation. 2000;101:2118.

VALIANT, Pfeffer MA, McMurray JJV, Velazquez EJ, et al. Valsartan, captopril, or both in myocardial infarction complicated by heart failure, left ventricular dysfunction, or both. N Engl J Med. 2003;349:1893–906.

14 Arrhythmias

The rational basis of antiarrhythmic therapy ideally requires a knowledge of:

1. **The mechanism of the arrhythmia**:
   - Disturbances in impulse generation (enhanced automaticity or ectopic tachyarrhythmia).
   - Disturbances of impulse conduction (reentrant arrhythmias). Most of the evidence suggests that reentry is the mechanism for sustained ventricular tachycardia (VT).
   - The site or sites where such disturbances are present.
2. **The mode of action of the drug** with which control of the arrhythmia is to be attempted
3. **The clinical situation**:
   - Acute, persistent, or paroxysmal
   - Associated with a low blood pressure <90 mmHg, congestive heart failure (HF), or distressing symptoms
   - Associated with cardiac pathology, accessory pathway or secondary to hypoxemia, acute blood loss, electrolyte or acid-base imbalance, extracardiac conditions as diverse as thyrotoxicosis, chronic obstructive pulmonary disease, or acute conditions such as pyrexial illness, pneumothorax, or even rupture of the esophagus

Prevention of episodes of arrhythmia and treatment of the acute attack are considered separately.

Except in emergency, the first step in therapy is to remove or correct a precipitating cause when this is feasible, thus reducing the need for antiarrhythmic medication. Precipitating factors include heart failure (HF), ischemia, digoxin toxicity or administration of beta-stimulants or

© Springer Science+Business Media New York 2015
M. Gabriel Khan, *Cardiac Drug Therapy*, Contemporary Cardiology,
DOI 10.1007/978-1-61779-962-4_14

theophylline, sick sinus syndrome, atrioventricular (AV) block, thyrotoxicosis, hypokalemia, hypomagnesemia, hypoxemia, acute blood loss, acid-base disturbances, and infection.

Not all arrhythmias require drug treatment, and the need for therapy is considered carefully for each individual bearing in mind the limited effectiveness of drugs and the occurrence of adverse effects, which is particularly important during long-term management and the occasional unexpected proarrhythmic effect of some drugs.

In addition, especially in the management of ventricular arrhythmias that are difficult to control, it is important to achieve target plasma concentrations known to be associated with suppression of the arrhythmia. This requires careful titration of dosage dictated by salutary effects and sometimes by concentration monitoring.

Note: Plasma concentration for some drugs does not reflect the full activity of the drug or metabolites.

CLASSIFICATION

Antiarrhythmic drugs may be considered from three distinct points of view:

1. According to their **site of action**.
2. According to their **electrophysiologic action** on isolated cardiac fibers [classes I–IV, as proposed by Vaughan Williams (1970)].

   Class IA (quinidine, disopyramide, procainamide) are membrane stabilizing; they inhibit fast sodium channel causing restriction of sodium current and slowing phase 0 of the action potential; the duration of the action potential is thus slightly prolonged.

   IB drugs (lidocaine, mexiletine) are rapidly attached to sodium channels during the action potential. Thus, few channels are available for activation at the commencement of diastole, and the effective refractory period (ERP) is prolonged. During diastole, however, the drugs are rapidly detached. At the end of diastole, most channels are drug free. Thus, there is no slowing of conduction velocity in the ventricle or His–Purkinje system. There is minimal slowing of phase 0.

Class IC drugs, flecainide and propafenone, detach very slowly from their binding to the channels during diastole. This action eliminates some sodium channels, producing slower conduction; ERP is not prolonged. The duration of the action is unaffected or a slight effect results in minimal slowing of phase 0.

Class II (beta-blockers) inhibit sympathetic stimulation; the main in vitro antiarrhythmic effect of beta-blockers is the depression of phase 4 diastolic depolarization. They are therefore effective in abolishing arrhythmias produced by increased catecholamines. See figure under section Antiarrhythmic Drugs.

Class III (amiodarone, sotalol) cause delayed repolarization, and the duration of the action is prolonged as major action. Amiodarone has class I, II, and III actions. Sotalol has a beta-blocker action and a unique class III effect.

Class IV (verapamil, diltiazem) inhibit slow calcium channel, causing restriction of calcium current.

The experience during the past 20 years indicates that drug actions are much more complex than those given in this classification, but the classification is retained because it has been used worldwide for several years, and it simplifies our understanding of drug action.

DIAGNOSIS OF ARRHYTHMIAS

The following advice on diagnosis is confined to relevant clinical clues and is of necessity brief. The diagnosis is usually established by careful examination of multiple leads of the electrocardiogram and information derived from carotid massage as appropriate in doubtful cases.

Figure 14-1 gives the differential diagnosis of narrow and wide QRS tachycardias.

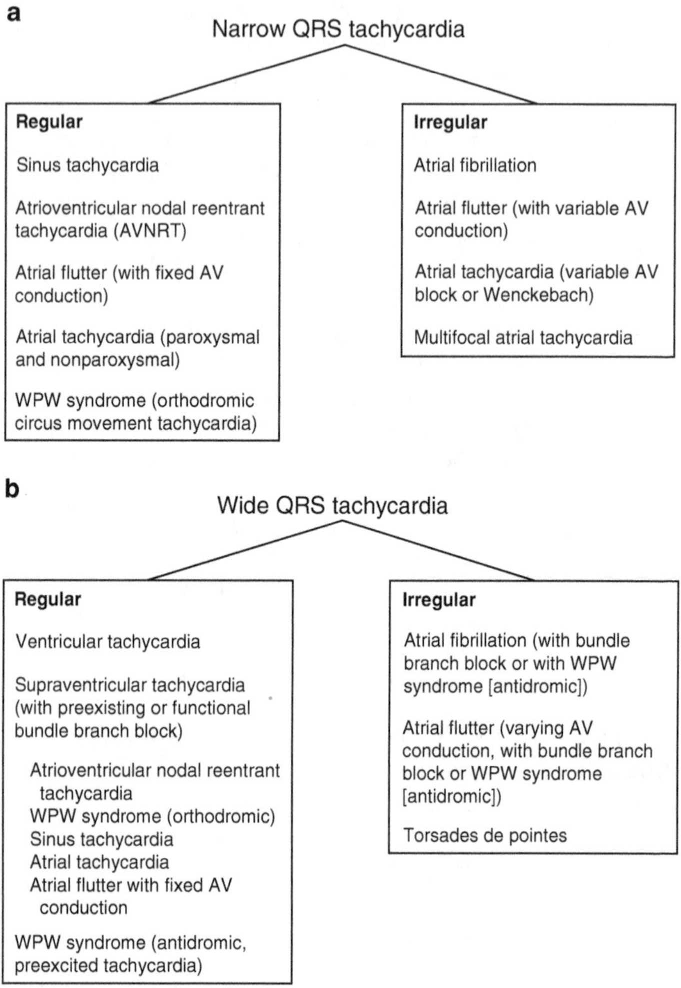

a

Narrow QRS tachycardia

Regular	Irregular
Sinus tachycardia	Atrial fibrillation
Atrioventricular nodal reentrant tachycardia (AVNRT)	Atrial flutter (with variable AV conduction)
Atrial flutter (with fixed AV conduction)	Atrial tachycardia (variable AV block or Wenckebach)
Atrial tachycardia (paroxysmal and nonparoxysmal)	Multifocal atrial tachycardia
WPW syndrome (orthodromic circus movement tachycardia)	

b

Wide QRS tachycardia

Regular	Irregular
Ventricular tachycardia	Atrial fibrillation (with bundle branch block or with WPW syndrome [antidromic])
Supraventricular tachycardia (with preexisting or functional bundle branch block)	Atrial flutter (varying AV conduction, with bundle branch block or WPW syndrome [antidromic])

Atrioventricular nodal reentrant tachycardia
  WPW syndrome (orthodromic)
  Sinus tachycardia
  Atrial tachycardia
  Atrial flutter with fixed AV conduction
	Torsades de pointes

WPW syndrome (antidromic, preexcited tachycardia)	

Fig. 14-1. Differential diagnosis of narrow QRS tachycardia (**a**) and wide QRS tachycardia (**b**). Reproduced with permission from Khan MG, *Rapid ECG Interpretation*, 3rd edition. New York: Humana Press/Springer Science + Business Media; 2008. With kind permission from Springer Science + Business Media.

Arrhythmias with Narrow QRS Complex

1. Regular
   (a) *Ventricular rate 140–240/min*: Consider **AV nodal reentrant tachycardia** (**AVNRT**) (>70 % of regular SVTs). Retrograde P waves are usually buried within the QRS or at the end of the QRS complex, with a short R–P interval causing pseudo-S waves in II, III, and aVF and pseudo r^1 that mimics Rsr^1 in V_1. See Fig. 14.2.
   (b) *Ventricular rate 100–140/min*: Consider **atrial tachycardia**. P-wave morphology is identical to that during normal sinus rhythm. The arrhythmia accounts for about 5 % of cases of supraventricular tachycardia (SVT).
   (c) **Paroxysmal atrial tachycardia** (PAT) with block: The P wave is often buried in the preceding T wave.
   (d) **Wolff–Parkinson–White (WPW) syndrome** with AV reentry (about 15 % of SVTs). See Figs. 14-3 and 14-4.
   (e) **Atrial flutter.**
   (f) Ectopic atrial tachycardia.
2. **Irregular**
   (a) **Atrial fibrillation** (AF). See Figs. 14-5, 14-6, and 14-7.
   (b) **Atrial flutter** (when AV conduction is variable). See Figs. 14-8 and 14-9.
   (c) **Multifocal atrial tachycardia** (chaotic atrial tachycardia). Varying P-wave morphology, P–P intervals vary, and atrial rate 200–130/min.

Key diagnostic clues for the diagnosis of supraventricular tachycardias are given in Fig. 14-10.

Arrhythmias with Wide QRS Complex

1. **Regular rhythm**
   A wide QRS complex regular tachycardia is usually caused by VT or SVT with functional aberrant conduction (SVT with preexisting bundle branch block and preexcited tachycardia/SVT with anterograde conduction over an accessory pathway).

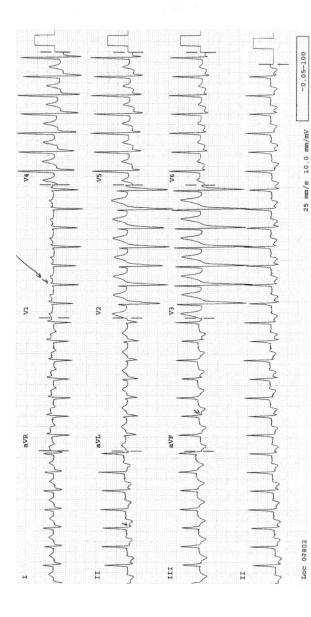

Loc 09802

25 mm/s 10.0 mm/mV

~0.05-100

Fig. 14-2. AV nodal reentrant tachycardia. Note the pseudo-s-wave in lead III (*arrow*), and pseudo-r¹ in V₁ (*arrow*). Reproduced with permission from Khan MG, *Encyclopedia of Heart Diseases*, 2nd edition. New York: Springer Science + Business Media; 2011. With kind permission from Springer Science + Business Media.

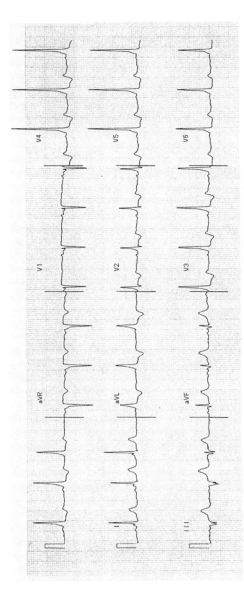

Fig. 14-3. Sinus rhythm; WPW pattern; short PR and delta wave. Reproduced with permission from Khan MG, *Encyclopedia of Heart Diseases*, 2nd edition. New York: Springer Science + Business Media; 2011. With kind permission from Springer Science + Business Media.

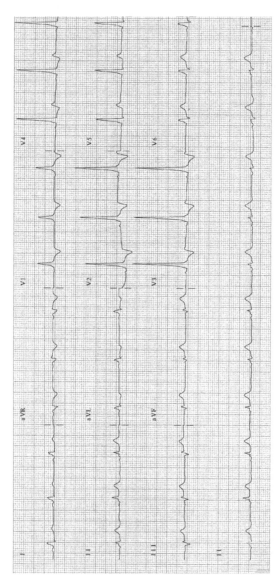

Fig. 14-4. Tall R-waves V_1–V_3; type A WPW syndrome. Reproduced with permission from Khan MG, *Encyclopedia of Heart Diseases*, 2nd edition. New York: Springer Science + Business Media; 2011. With kind permission from Springer Science + Business Media.

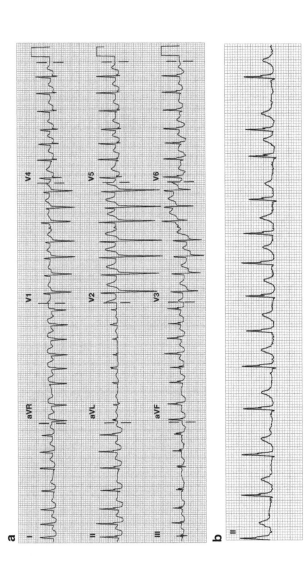

Fig. 14-5. (a) Atrial fibrillation with a rapid ventricular rate of 175 bpm. (b) Atrial fibrillation, same patient as in (a); controlled ventricular rate of 108 bpm. Lenient study rate control goal 70–109/min (Van Gelder et al. 2010). The European Society of Cardiology (ESC) recommends a resting heart rate target of <110 bpm for heart rate control, the ACCF/AHA/HRS recommends this only if the ejection fraction is >40 %, and the Canadian Cardiovascular Society (CCS) recommends <100 bpm. Reproduced with permission from Khan MG, *Rapid ECG Interpretation*, 3rd edition. New York: Humana Press/Springer Science + Business Media; 2008. With kind permission from Springer Science + Business Media.

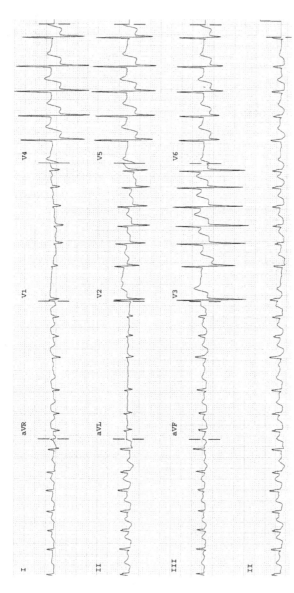

Fig. 14-6. Atrial fibrillation with rapid ventricular response 152 BPM; marked ST-segment depression in $V_2–V_6$, in keeping with subendocardial ischemia, probable non-ST-segment elevation MI. Reproduced with permission from Khan MG, *Encyclopedia of Heart Diseases*, 2nd edition. New York: Springer Science + Business Media; 2011. With kind permission from Springer Science + Business Media.

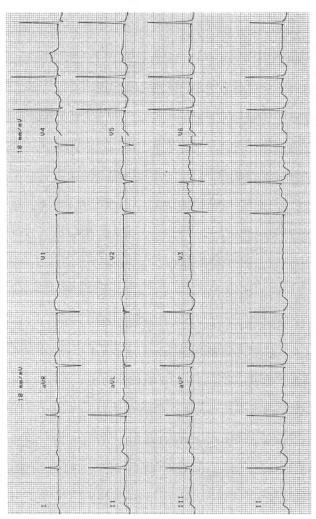

Fig. 14-7. Atrial fibrillation, slow ventricular response 60/min: ST–T changes, probable digitalis effect (digoxin level maintained very low at <0.9 ng/ml). This rate should be adjusted to goal rate 70–100/min. The patient is treated with bisoprolol 2.5 mg and digoxin 0.125 mg daily following an episode of heart failure >2 years ago. Reproduced with permission from Khan MG, *Encyclopedia of Heart Diseases*, 2nd edition. New York: Springer Science + Business Media; 2011. With kind permission from Springer Science + Business Media.

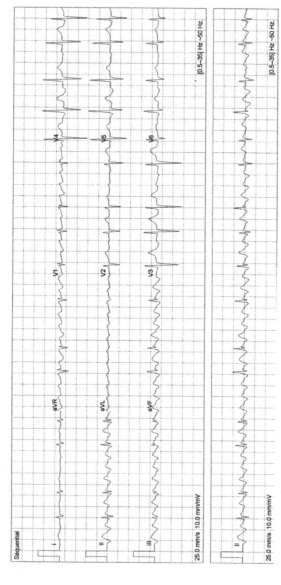

Fig. 14-8. Atrial flutter; typical flutter waves in leads II, III, and aVF, note the absence of flutter waves in lead I and V$_6$. Reproduced with permission from Khan MG, *Encyclopedia of Heart Diseases*, 2nd edition. New York: Springer Science + Business Media; 2011. With kind permission from Springer Science + Business Media.

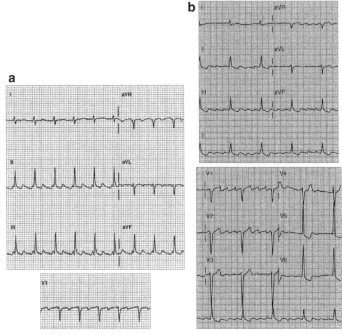

Fig. 14-9. (a) Atrial flutter: atrial rate, 270 BPM; ventricular rate, 135 BPM. Note: The downward deflection of F waves in leads II, III, and aVF has a gradual slope followed by an abrupt upward deflection. This causes the sawtooth pattern. Alternate F waves coincide with the QRS complex, and the diagnosis may be missed. Note: The deformity of the T-waves by the flutter wave revealed in leads II, III, and aVF is absent in lead I, a clue to the presence of atrial flutter. (b) Flutter waves in leads II, III, and aVF; spiky F waves in V_1, and notably absence of the sawtooth deformities in lead I, V_5, and V_6. Reproduced with permission from Khan MG, *Rapid ECG Interpretation*, 3rd edition. New York: Humana Press/Springer Science + Business Media; 2008. With kind permission from Springer Science + Business Media.

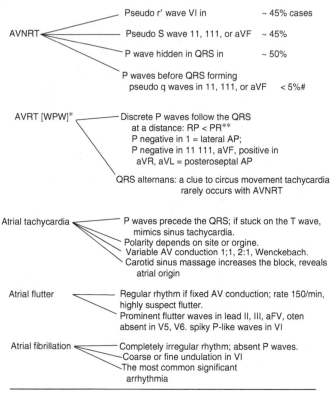

*common circus movement tachycardia uses the fast accessory pathway [AP]; rare
form uses the slow AP and the RP is >PR.
**May occur with atrial tachycardia.
#rare form: negative Ps follow the QRS with RP > PR.

Fig. 14-10. Supraventricular arrhythmias: key diagnostic clues.
(*Single asterisk*) common circus movement tachycardia uses the fast
accessory pathway (AP); rare form uses the slow AP and the RP
is>PR. (*Double asterisk*) may occur with atrial tachycardia. # rare
form: negative Ps follow the QRS with RP>PR. Reproduced with
permission from Khan MG, *Encyclopedia of Heart Diseases*, 2nd
edition. New York: Springer Science + Business Media; 2011. With
kind permission from Springer Science + Business Media.

Regular wide QRS tachycardia is considered VT if the following clues apply (Steurer et al. 1994):

- Predominantly negative QRS complexes in the precordial leads V_4–V_6: diagnostic for VT (Fig. 14-11).
- Presence of a QR complex in one or more of the precordial leads V_2–V_6: certainly VT.
- Absence of an RS complex in all precordial leads: Negative QRS complexes in all precordial leads V_1–V_6 and negative concordance V_1–V_6=VT (Fig. 14-11).
- AV relationship different from 1:1: more QRS complexes than P waves; consider VT. Consider SVT with aberrant conduction only in the absence of any of (a) or (b) and with the following present:
- QRS morphology similar to intraventricular conduction defect (IVCD) apparent on electrocardiography (ECG) while not in tachycardia.
- In basic sinus rhythm.
- Visible on atrial ectopic beats=SVT with aberrant conduction. Fixed relationship with P waves, or the presence of a q in V_6, suggests but does not prove a supraventricular origin.
- Other clues in favor of VT include lead V_6: QS or rS; r/S ratio less than 1. Lead V_1, V_2: If the tachycardia has an LBBB shape and an R wave that is smaller than the r when in sinus rhythm or notched or slurred downslope of the S wave, the left "rabbit-ear" is taller than the right. Figure 14-12 shows salvos of VPBs and ventricular tachycardia.

Figure 14-13 gives ventricular tachycardia: key diagnostic clues.

Alternative diagnoses to VT or SVT with aberrance:
(a) Atrial flutter and WPW conduction
(b) WPW tachycardia (rare type with anterograde conduction, through accessory pathway, preexcited tachycardia)
2. Irregular rhythm
Atrial fibrillation (AF) and WPW syndrome with a rapid conduction, rate 200–300/min. Figure 14-14 shows AF with preexcited wide QRS tachycardia in a patient with WPW syndrome.

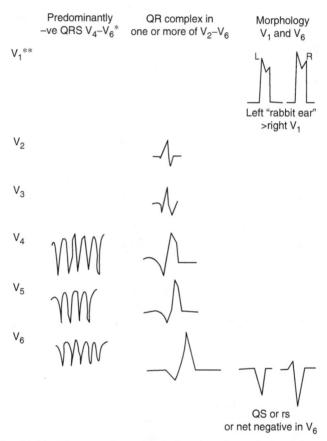

Fig. 14-11. Electrocardiographic hallmarks of ventricular tachycardia. (*Single asterisk*) or concordant negativity in leads V_1–V_6; positive concordance in leads V_1–V_6 can be caused by ventricular tachycardia or Wolff–Parkinson–White antidromic (preexcited) tachycardia. (*Double asterisk*) it is necessary to study the entire 12 lead tracing with particular emphasis on leads V_1–V_6; lead 2 may be useful for assessment of P waves and AV dissociation. Reproduced with permission from Khan MG, *Rapid ECG Interpretation*, 3rd edition. New York: Humana Press/Springer Science + Business Media; 2008. With kind permission from Springer Science + Business Media.

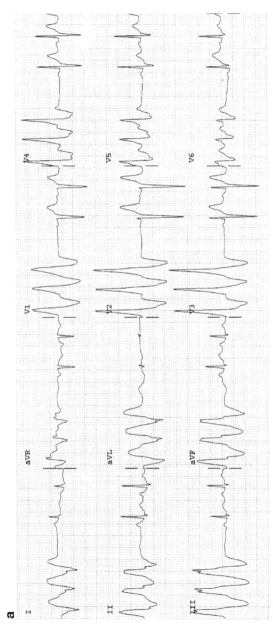

Fig. 14-12. (a) Salvos of three VPBs. The above trace is (b) The same patient as in Fig. 14a; ECG taken 1 min later shows ventricular tachycardia. (c) Salvos five VPBs, nonsustained VT; complexes in the V leads show negative concordance; typical features diagnostic for VT. Reproduced with permission from Khan MG, *Encyclopedia of Heart Diseases*, 2nd edition. New York: Springer Science + Business Media; 2011. With kind permission from Springer Science + Business Media.

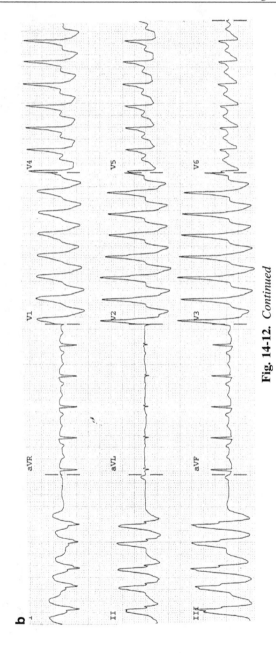

Fig. 14-12. *Continued*

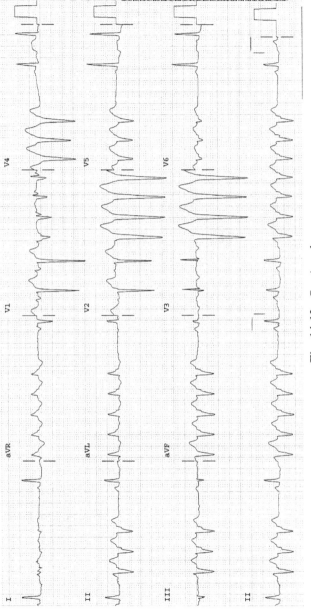

Fig. 14-12. *Continued*

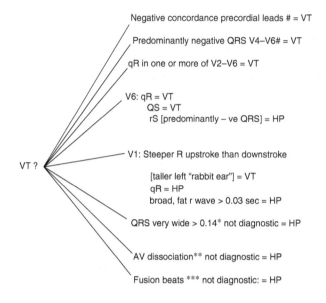

Negative concordance precordial leads # = VT

Predominantly negative QRS V4–V6# = VT

qR in one or more of V2–V6 = VT

V6: qR = VT
    QS = VT
    rS [predominantly – ve QRS] = HP

V1: Steeper R upstroke than downstroke

    [taller left "rabbit ear"] = VT
    qR = HP
    broad, fat r wave > 0.03 sec = HP

QRS very wide > 0.14* not diagnostic = HP

AV dissociation** not diagnostic = HP

Fusion beats *** not diagnostic: = HP

VT ?

HP = High probability VT.
#: Excludes a preexcited WPW antidromic tachycardia.
*QRS: if know in recent past to be normal duration.
**Only observed in <45% VT, and can occur with junctional tachycardia with LBBB.
***Observed in only ~15% of VT and fusion of aberrantly conducted junctional impulses with simultaneous sinus impulses do occur.

Fig. 14-13. Ventricular tachycardia: key diagnostic clues. HP=high probability VT. (*Number sign*) excludes a preexcited WPW antidromic tachycardia. (*Single asterisk*) QRS: if known in recent past to be normal duration. (*Double asterisk*) only observed in <45 VT and can occur with junctional tachycardia with LBBB. (*Triple asterisk*) observed in only ~15 % of VT and fusion of aberrantly conducted junctional impulses with simultaneous sinus impulses do occur. Reproduced with permission from Khan MG, *Rapid ECG Interpretation*, 3rd edition. New York: Humana Press/Springer Science+Business Media; 2008. With kind permission from Springer Science+Business Media.

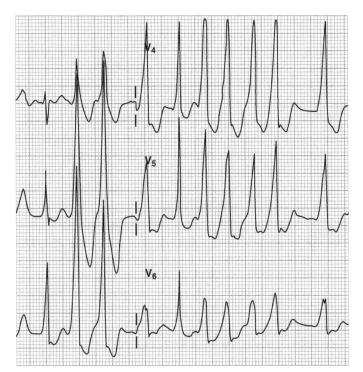

Fig. 14-14. Atrial fibrillation with preexcited wide QRS tachycardia in a patient with WPW syndrome: antidromic tachycardia. Reproduced with permission from Khan MG, *Rapid ECG Interpretation*, 3rd edition. New York: Humana Press/Springer Science + Business Media; 2008. With kind permission from Springer Science + Business Media.

Note: The rapidity of the ventricular response (regular or irregular, narrow or wide) should alert the physician to the diagnosis of WPW. AV block or dissociation excludes the presence of a bypass tract:

• AF and IVCD; a previous ECG is needed for comparison.

MANAGEMENT OF SUPRAVENTRICULAR ARRHYTHMIAS

AV Nodal Reentrant Tachycardia

SVT usually arises from reentry mechanisms involving the AV node (AVNRT) and occasionally an accessory pathway, AV reciprocating tachycardia (AVRT), the sinus node, or the atrium. Consequently, drug therapy is directed toward slowing or blocking conduction at some point within the reentry circuit. Whenever the AV node or sinus node is involved directly in the reentry circuit, as is usually the case, SVT is frequently terminated by maneuvers or drugs that increase vagal activity or drugs that slow the velocity of propagation of impulses in the region of the sinoatrial (SA) or AV nodes.

AVNRT in patients aged <35 years usually occurs in an otherwise normal heart, with a good prognosis. It may occur in patients with organic heart disease, e.g., ischemic or rheumatic heart disease, and can be life threatening. The episode is characterized by an abrupt onset and termination. The heart rate varies from 140 to 240/beats/min and the rhythm is regular (Fig. 14-2).

Termination of the Acute Attack of **AVNRT**

Vagal Maneuvers. Many patients learn to terminate the arrhythmia by gagging or by the Valsalva maneuver (expiration against a closed glottis) or Müller maneuver (sudden inspiration against the closed glottis) or facial immersion in cold water. The Valsalva maneuver is effective in approx 50 % of patients with AVNRT.

Warning. Eyeball pressure has also been used to cause reflex vagal stimulation but is not recommended as retinal detachment may occur.

Carotid sinus massage either causes a reversion to sinus rhythm or has no effect at all. This all-or-none effect is in contrast to the slowing that results when atrial flutter or fibrillation is present. Carotid sinus massage is not recommended in the elderly or in patients with known carotid artery disease. In patients over age 35 years, if a history of carotid disease is suggested by transient ischemic attacks or carotid bruits on auscultation, do not massage the carotid.

The patient must be supine with the head slightly hyperextended and turned a little toward the opposite side. Locate the right carotid sinus at the angle of the jaw. Using the first and second fingers, apply firm pressure in a circular or massage fashion for 2–6 s. Carotid massage is discontinued immediately upon termination of the arrhythmia because prolonged asystole may otherwise supervene in rare patients. If unsuccessful, massage the left carotid sinus.

Warning. Never massage for more than 10 s and do not massage the right and left carotid simultaneously.

In some patients, restoration of sinus rhythm is clearly a matter of great urgency because of hemodynamic deterioration or angina, and direct current (DC) cardioversion is performed either before any drug is given or when the need becomes apparent following unsuccessful drug therapy.

Drug Management in the Acute Situation

1. Adenosine (Adenocard) 0.05–0.25 mg/kg given IV is an effective and relatively safe agent for the termination of acute reentrant SVT. Adenosine terminates AVNRT and AVRT in up to 90 % of cases (DiMarco et al. 1990; Rankin and McGovern 1991). The 6-mg and 12-mg doses cause a 60–80 % and 90–95 % termination, respectively. The drug has both therapeutic and diagnostic value. The drug has replaced verapamil when very rapid conversion of the arrhythmia is required, as in cases with HF or hemodynamic compromise, thus avoiding DC countershock in many individuals. It can be given to patients with known SVT and aberration; little harm ensues if the diagnosis is in fact VT, whereas verapamil use is detrimental. Nonetheless, the drug is contraindicated in patients with a wide QRS complex tachycardia unless the diagnosis of SVT with aberrancy is

certain (Delacrétaz 2006). The drug has no appreciable hypotensive or negative inotropic effect and slows AV nodal conduction.

Dosage: Usually IV bolus 6 mg (0.05–0.25 mg/kg) over 2 s, rapidly flushed into a peripheral vein, followed by a bolus of 20 ml of fluid should cause reversion to sinus rhythm in 1 min; the action of the drug is only about ½ min and, if needed, a 12-mg second bolus injection is given approximately 2 min after the first injection. A further 12-mg dose may be repeated in 3–5 min, as the arrhythmia occurs in 10–33 % of cases. The very short half-life, less than 2 s, allows rapid dose titration to be achieved. Because adenosine may excite atrial and ventricular tissue, it causes atrial fibrillation in up to 12 % of patients and nonsustained VT in rare cases (Strickberger et al. 1997). It should be administered only when a cardiac monitor is being used and a defibrillator is on hand.

Interactions: Dipyridamole potentiates the effects of adenosine. Thus, the dose of adenosine must be reduced in patients taking dipyridamole; significant hypotension may be caused by the combination. Theophylline is an antagonist.

Adverse effects: Transient headache, facial flushing, and dyspnea, but bronchospasm may last more than a half hour in asthmatics. The drug has minor proarrhythmic effects and may cause atrial and ventricular premature beats; rarely SVT or atrial flutter may degenerate to AF (Jaeggi et al. 1999). Atrial flutter is not an indication for adenosine; 1:1 conduction and extreme tachycardia may ensue.

Contraindications: Asthma, severe chronic obstructive lung disease (COPD), and wide QRS complex if the diagnosis of SVT with aberrancy is uncertain and in heart transplant recipients.

2. **Verapamil** IV is effective in more than 90 % of episodes of AVNRT (narrow complex).

Contraindications: Verapamil is contraindicated in patients with wide QRS tachycardia, WPW syndrome, severe hypotension, HF, acute MI, known sick sinus syndrome, digitalis toxicity, and concurrent use of beta-blockers or disopyramide.

Dosage: IV 0.075–0.15 mg/kg, i.e., 5–10 mg, is given slowly over 1–2 min. The depressant effect on the AV node may persist for up to 6 h, and a second dose may produce complications. If the arrhythmia persists following Valsalva maneuver or right carotid massage or recurs without hemodynamic deterioration in patients with a normal heart, a second dose not exceeding 5 mg may be considered after 30 min. If restoration of sinus rhythm is clearly urgent, adenosine is tried and then, if needed, DC conversion. IV infusion 1 mg/min to a total of 10 mg or 5–10 mg over 1 h; 100 mg in 24 h. Prolongation of AV conduction induced by verapamil can be reversed by atropine. Calcium gluconate or chloride is useful in the management of hypotension, circulatory collapse, or asystole owing to sinus arrest or AV block. Atropine may be of value in this situation.

3. **Propranolol** 1 mg IV given slowly and repeated every 5 min to a maximum of 5 mg; the usual dose required is 2–4 mg. Metoprolol is given in a dose of 5 mg at a rate of 1–2 mg/min repeated after 5 min if necessary to a total dose of 10–15 mg.

4. **Diltiazem** IV is as effective as verapamil and causes fewer adverse effects; both agents cost approximately $15 per treatment compared with $100 for two 6-mg doses of adenosine. Diltiazem has a role in patients who have well-defined SVT.

   Dosage: Initial bolus 0.25 mg/kg over 2 min and, if needed, rebolus 0.35 mg/kg.

5. **Phenylephrine** (Neo-Synephrine) is an alpha-sympathetic agonist. The drug is now rarely used because of better alternatives, especially adenosine. The drug has a role only in young patients with a normal heart, when adenosine has failed, when the blood pressure is <90 mmHg, and when cardioversion is considered undesirable. The resulting increase in blood pressure stimulates the baroreceptor reflexes and increases vagal activity, often resulting in termination of the arrhythmia.

   Contraindications: Patients with MI, severe cardiac pathology, and narrow-angle glaucoma.

   Dosage: Phenylephrine is administered as repeated IV bolus injections; 0.1 mg is diluted with 5 mL 5 % dextrose and water

(D/W) and given over 2 min. Blood pressure is measured at 30-s intervals. Arterial blood pressure must not be allowed to exceed 140 mmHg. Sufficient time (1–2 min) should elapse after each bolus to allow the blood pressure to return to its base-line value before subsequent doses are administered. Dose range: 0.1–0.5 mg. Higher doses have been used but are not recommended. Administration by IV drip infusion may result in variation in drug rates that may cause an unacceptable increase in blood pressure.

Chronic Drug Management of AVNRT

Recurrent prolonged or frequent episodes may require chronic drug therapy. The following may be tried:

1. **Digoxin**. This drug is especially useful in patients with left ventricular dysfunction (LV) and in those with resting systolic blood pressure <110 mmHg in whom beta-blockers, vera-pamil, or diltiazem may cause symptomatic hypotension or bradycardia. Also, the drug is inexpensive and available as a one-a-day tablet. It is not used in patients with WPW syndrome.
2. **A beta-blocker**. Choose a once-daily preparation: bisoprolol 5–10 mg daily, metoprolol succinate sustained release (Toprol-XL) 50 mg. Atenolol is not recommended (see Chap. 1) If AVNRT recurs on this regimen, verapamil 80–120 mg orally usually aborts the attack within 1 h and avoids bothersome emergency room visits.
3. **Digoxin plus a beta-blocker** may be necessary in patients resistant to (1) and (2).
4. **Verapamil** SR 120–180 mg daily or diltiazem 180–240 mg may be tried but is effective in <50 % of patients and is an expensive therapy.
5. **Pill in the pocket**. No prophylactic treatment is given. At the onset of an episode, the patient takes verapamil 80–120 mg or a beta-blocker, e.g., metoprolol tartrate (rapid acting) 50 mg or bisoprolol 5 mg orally.
   • **The combination of diltiazem and propranolol** termi-nated 80 % of SVT episodes within 2 h of administration (Alboni et al. 2001).

These regimens are safe and efficacious in patients with normal hearts. Recurrent AVNRT resistant to pharmacologic therapy should prompt consideration of catheter ablation.

Multifocal Atrial Tachycardia (Chaotic Atrial Tachycardia)

This arrhythmia is caused by frequent atrial ectopic depolarizations. The arrhythmia is characterized by variable P-wave morphology and P–P and PR interval. The atrial rate is usually 100–130/min, and the ventricular rhythm is irregular. The diagnosis is made by demonstrating three or more different P-wave morphologies in one lead. The arrhythmia is usually precipitated by acute infections, exacerbation of COPD, electrolyte and acid-base imbalance, theophylline, beta1-stimulants, and, rarely, digitalis toxicity. Digitalis is usually not effective, and treatment of the underlying cause is most important. If the ventricular response is excessively rapid, slowing may be achieved with verapamil given orally. Magnesium sulfate is an effective alternative if verapamil is contraindicated. **Adenosine is ineffective**.

Paroxysmal Atrial Tachycardia with Block

Episodes are usually associated with severe cardiac or pulmonary disease. PAT is a common manifestation of digitalis toxicity. The atrial rate is commonly 180–220/min. AV conduction is usually 2:1. The rhythm is usually regular. The ventricular rate of 90–120/min may not cause concern, and the P waves are often buried in the preceding T wave, so the diagnosis is easily missed.

If the ventricular rate is 90–120/min and the serum potassium (K^+) level is normal, digoxin and diuretics should be discontinued, and often no specific treatment is required. If the serum K^+ concentration is <3.5 mEq (mmol)/L and a high degree of AV block is absent, IV potassium chloride 40 mEq (mmol) in 500 mL 5 % D/W is given over 4 h through a central line. If the serum K^+ level is <2.5 mEq (mmol)/L, KC1 is best given in normal saline to improve the serum potassium level quickly. Other therapies are outlined under treatment of digitalis toxicity.

Atrial Premature Contractions

Atrial premature contractions (APCs) often occur without apparent cause. Recognized causes include stimulants, drugs, anxiety, hypoxemia, HF, ischemic heart disease, and other cardiac pathology. APCs in themselves require no drug therapy. Treatment of the underlying cause is usually sufficient. In patients with no serious underlying cardiac disease, reassurance is of utmost importance. Stimulants such as caffeine, theophylline, nicotine, nicotinic acid, and other cardiac stimulants as well as alcohol should be avoided.

When heart or pulmonary disease is present, APCs may predict runs of SVT, AF, or atrial flutter, and the resulting increase in heart rate may be distressing to the patient. Digoxin may be useful and, rarely, disopyramide may be necessary. If mitral valve prolapse is associated, sedation or a beta-blocker may be useful.

Atrial Flutter

Underlying heart disease is usually present; however, hypoxemia owing to a pneumothorax, atelectasis, and other noncardiac causes may precipitate the arrhythmia. Atrial flutter tends to be unstable, either degenerating into AF or reverting to sinus rhythm.

The atrial rate is usually 240–340/min. The ventricular rate is often 150/min with an atrial rate of 300, i.e., 2:1 conduction. Therefore a ventricular rate of 150/min with a regular rhythm should alert the clinician to a diagnosis of atrial flutter. The sawtooth pattern in lead II should confirm the diagnosis. See Figs. 14-8 and 14-9.

Carotid sinus massage may increase the degree of AV block, slow the ventricular response, and reveal the sawtooth P waves as opposed to P waves separated by isoelectric segments in PAT with block. Rarely a 1:1 conduction with a rapid ventricular response is seen, especially in patients with preexcitation syndromes or in patients receiving a class I antiarrhythmic agent.

Treatment: Atrial flutter is easily converted to sinus rhythm by synchronized DC shock at low energies of 25–50 J. Electrical cardioversion is often indicated and should be performed if the patient is hemodynamically compromised or if the ventricular response is >200/min or the patient is known or suspected to have WPW syndrome. If the patient is hemodynamically stable with a ventricular response <200/min, propranolol may be used to slow the ventricular response. The benefit of propranolol or metoprolol is that patients who can undergo electrical cardioversion may do so easily, whereas following digoxin DC shocks have been reported to be hazardous. If underlying heart disease is present, digoxin has a role in the acute and chronic management. Digoxin converts atrial flutter to AF, and the ventricular response is nearly always slowed to an acceptable level provided sufficient digoxin is used. Removal of underlying causes may be followed by spontaneous reversion to sinus rhythm. Verapamil or diltiazem is effective in slowing the ventricular response and may occasionally cause conversion to sinus rhythm. Digoxin, verapamil, and beta-blockers are contraindicated in patients with WPW syndrome presenting with atrial flutter. Quinidine, procainamide, or disopyramide must not be used alone for the conversion of atrial flutter to sinus rhythm because these drugs, especially quinidine, increase conduction in the AV node and may result in a 1:1 conduction with a ventricular response exceeding 220/min. If quinidine is administered, it must be preceded by adequate digitalization to produce a sufficient degree of AV block.

Propafenone and flecainide have been shown to convert atrial flutter to sinus rhythm in 20 % and 33 % of patients, respectively.

Atrial Fibrillation

The AHA/ACC provided sound guidelines in 2014. AF is the most common sustained arrhythmia observed in clinical practice. Among patients with a recent crypto-genic stroke or TIA who were 55 years of age or older, noninvasive ambulatory ECG monitoring for a target of 30 days significantly improved the detection of atrial fibrilla-tion by a factor of more than five and nearly doubled the rate of anticoagulant treatment. Atrial fibrillation lasting 30 s or longer was detected in 45 of 280 patients (16.1 %) in the intervention group, as compared with 9 of 277 (3.2 %) in the control group monitored for 24 h (Gladstone et al. 2014).

A prospective study and dose–response meta-analysis indicate that alcohol consumption, even at moderate intakes, is a risk factor for atrial fibrillation (Larsson et al. 2014).

In most patients, drug action to control the ventricular response provides adequate therapy. A ventricular response <60/min in an untreated patient should raise the suspicion of disease of the AV node or concomitant sick sinus syndrome, particularly in the elderly. AF with a slow ventricular rate that becomes regular, indicative of the presence of a junc-tional pacemaker, should raise the suspicion of digitalis toxicity.

ATRIAL FIBRILLATION OF RECENT ONSET

In acute AF, with a fast ventricular rate, especially if there is hemodynamic compromise or with rates exceeding 220/min, WPW syndrome may be the cause, and drugs that block the AV node are contraindicated. Drug therapy to slow the ventricular response in patients with AF, in whom conduction using the accessory pathway can be excluded, includes the following:

1. **Diltiazem** IV is the drug of choice for urgent rate control in patients with AF; a constant IV infusion brings the ventricular response under control reliably. Sinus rhythm is achieved in only about 15 %, and hypotension occurs in up to 33 % of patients. Diltiazem IV followed by procainamide IV bolus may cause reversion to sinus rhythm.
2. **Esmolol** slows the rate adequately over 20 min, and sinus rhythm may ensue. The drug causes hypotension in up to 40 % of patients. Esmolol and digoxin are effective, and hypotension is much less common than when esmolol alone is used. Digoxin appears to protect from hypotension.

PAROXYSMAL ATRIAL FIBRILLATION

Paroxysmal atrial fibrillation is a major clinical problem that is difficult to manage. The patient should be anticoagulated to prevent embolization. IV disopyramide (not approved in the USA) or procainamide given with digoxin may restore sinus rhythm in <33 %. If the rate <150 is well tolerated, it is advisable to observe the rhythm for 8–12 h because spontaneous rhythm is common, particularly if the patient has taken an extra dose of sotalol (40–80 mg) prior to coming to the emergency room. DC cardioversion should be immediately available if drug therapy fails, when the ventricular rate is rapid, or when hypotension and HF ensue. For the prevention of recurrent episodes, low-dose sotalol 40–60 mg is beneficial in 40–50 % of patients. Although low-dose amiodarone is more effective than sotalol (approx 75 %) and pulmonary side effects run approx 3 %, other side effects may emerge.

Fortunately life-threatening paroxysmal atrial fibrillation is rare. Even severe cases can be rapidly brought under control in the ER, and recurrences in the majority occur after 1–5 years. These patients are anticoagulated with warfarin or preferably rivaroxaban (the latter may prevent MI).

Sotalol 80–160 mg or bisoprolol 5–10 mg combined with digoxin to maintain a digoxin level 0.5–0.9 ng/ml (0.6–1.0 nmol/L) should result in a ventricular rate <140/min if a paroxysm occurs patients with stroke with undetermined cause (cryptogenic) may have underlying undetected paroxysmal atrial fibrillation. Monitoring for a target of 30 days significantly improved the detection of atrial fibrillation by a factor of more than five and nearly doubled the rate of anticoagulant treatment, Atrial fibrillation lasting 30 s or longer was detected in 45 of 280 patients (16.1 %) in the intervention group, as compared with 9 of 277 (3.2 %) in the control group monitored for 24 h (Gladstone et al. 2014).

CATHETER ABLATION

In patients with paroxysmal atrial fibrillation, it is only necessary to rapidly obtain a ventricular rate of <140/min during a paroxysm; a rate 120–150/min is well tolerated by most patients. In patients with left ventricular dysfunction or an ejection fraction of <45 %, a rate >140 may precipitate HF. In such selected patients ablation should be considered. Fortunately this scenario is rare. The rush to ablation should be halted because anticoagulation is still necessary when sinus rhythm is restored and many complications are been reported.

Caution: 83 % of centers reported the use of oral anticoagulants following ablation; death (0.05 %) and stroke (0.28 %) were observed in 6 % of 11,762 procedures (Cappato et al. 2005). This report covered a period during which skill and technologic devices were being developed. Significant PV stenosis and stroke occurred in 1.3 % and 0.2 % of patients, respectively. About half of the PV stenoses required interventional treatment, a strategy that does not necessarily abolish symptoms. Constrictive pericarditis has been reported (Ahsan et al. 2008). Tamponade may occur. Intracranial emboli which typically presents as a transient ischemic attack (TIA) or stroke occurs (Steinberg and Mittal 2011).

A worldwide survey on catheter ablation of AF reported a 0.71 % incidence of TIA and 0.23 % incidence of stroke.

Periprocedural complications occurred in 1 of 20 patients undergoing AF ablation, and all-cause and arrhythmia-related rehospitalizations were common (Shah et al. 2012). Among 4,156 patients who underwent an initial AF ablation, 5 % had periprocedural complications, most commonly vascular, and 9 % were readmitted within 30 days. Less hospital experience with AF ablation were associated with higher adjusted risk of complications and/or 30-day readmissions. The rate of all-cause hospitalization was 38.5 % by 1 year. The rate of readmission for recurrent AF, atrial flutter, and/or repeat ablation was 21.7 % by 1 year and 29.6 % by 2 years (Shah et al. 2012). The recurrence rate for atrial fibrillation after the first year is 6–9 % per year (Hussein et al. 2011; Weerasooriya et al. 2011; Ouyang et al. 2010).

Haines emphasized that the real-world success rate of this procedure is unknown but is likely considerably lower than published reports from single-center studies. Also complication rates are significant, as are late hospitalization rates. Data from many investigations in AF ablation and other interventional procedures have demonstrated that operator and hospital procedure volume are inversely correlated with poor outcomes (Haines 2012).

CHRONIC ATRIAL FIBRILLATION

In most patients with chronic AF of more than 1 year's duration, slowing of the ventricular response will suffice.

- **A beta-blocker is a good choice** even in patients with class I–III HF or asymptomatic LV dysfunction.
- **Verapamil or a beta-blocker** slows the ventricular rate during exercise, whereas digoxin may fail to do so in a few patients. Beta-blockers are preferred.
- **Combination of digoxin and a beta-blocker** [bisoprolol 5–10 mg or metoprolol long acting (Toprol-XL) 50 mg] is often beneficial.

- **Sotalol** is not advisable for chronic AF because it carries a risk of TDP and is no more effective than other beta-blockers in controlling the ventricular rate. The three drugs are contraindicated in patients with WPW syndrome and AF or atrial flutter.
- **Digoxin** is inexpensive and is suitable in many elderly people who do not engage in much physical activity. If the patient is asymptomatic, the rate at rest is <110, and on a 4-min walk the rate is <120; digoxin should suffice. Verapamil should be avoided in the elderly because it causes bothersome constipation and may cause HF in some. The ventricular rate may be slow in the elderly because of concomitant AV node disease. Sick sinus syndromes should be anticipated, and pacing may be considered. The majority of patients older than age 70 can be controlled with a small dose of digoxin or a small dose beta-blocker; rarely both drugs are needed particularly if left ventricular dysfunction or HF is a problem; see Fig. 14-7.

Atrial Fibrillation Post Surgery

Colchicine appears to offer a new way to prevent atrial fibrillation after heart surgery. The relative risk of developing post-op Afib was reduced to 42.1 % if patients were treated with colchicine rather than placebo ($P = 0.002$).

The incidence of atrial fibrillation at 12 months was 8.9 % in patients given colchicine compared with 21.1 % among patients randomized to placebo (Imazio et al. 2011).

Synchronized DC Cardioversion

The advisability of attempting DC conversion of AF is always considered carefully. In selected acute cases, reversion to sinus rhythm may be warranted. One should first consider whether it would be worthwhile to restore sinus rhythm with DC conversion. The question is necessary because reversion to sinus rhythm may cause embolization, or AF may recur because the underlying heart disease is unchanged. The incidence of embolization following cardioversion is about 2 %.

Except in special circumstances, cardioversion is usually contraindicated in patients with:

- AF of duration >1 year. Valvular heart disease in patients due to undergo surgery within the next few weeks. Digitalis-induced arrhythmias. Sick sinus syndrome.
- Advanced AV block. Left atrium > 5 cm, as sinus rhythm is usually not maintained.

If AF is of <48 h duration, anticoagulants are believed not to be necessary. If AF is of >3 days duration, administer warfarin for 3 weeks before and for 8–12 weeks after elective cardioversion. Digoxin is maintained for the period before conversion and is interrupted 24–48 h before conversion. Sotalol or quinidine is commenced immediately after conversion when there is believed to be a high probability of recurrence of AF. Sotalol is more effective than quinidine in the prevention of recurrent AF and for the maintenance of sinus rhythm (see below). Amiodarone may be commenced before conversion if this drug is selected.

Cardioversion is considered only when conditions contra-indicating its use are absent or the patient's life is threatened by the rapidity of the ventricular response or loss of atrial transport function, such as:

- Heart rate >150/min believed to be causing HF, chest pain, or cardiogenic shock
- Patients with hypertrophic cardiomyopathy or severe aortic stenosis (in whom atrial transport function is of great importance)
- AF in patients with WPW syndrome

Rate Control Versus Rhythm Control

No clear advantage exists between rhythm control and rate control. In five RCTs, no significant differences were recorded in primary end points. Adverse outcomes with a rhythm-control approach were seen in the two largest studies (Opolski et al. 2004; Wyse et al. 2002). Antiarrhythmic used to maintain sinus rhythm produces unacceptable side effects.

Dronedarone is a modified version of amiodarone. The FDA has issued a safety alert on the antiarrhythmic dronedarone because of cases of severe liver injury associated with the drug. Two cases required liver transplants. The use of dronedarone should be curtailed. Analysis of the halted PALLAS trial turned up a 2.29-fold excess in stroke, MI, systemic embolism, and death from cardiovascular causes combined among patients on the rhythm-control drug ($P = 0.002$).

Hospitalization for heart failure was increased 81 % compared with placebo ($P = 0.02$), all-cause mortality (25 versus 13 events, hazard ratio 1.94, $P = 0.049$), and cardiovascular mortality (21 versus 10, HR 2.11, $P = 0.046$).

Arrhythmia-related death (13 versus 4, HR 3.26, $P = 0.03$). Stroke (23 versus 10, HR 2.32, $P = 0.02$). Unplanned hospitalization for cardiovascular causes (113 versus 59, HR 1.97, $P < 0.001$). Conclusion: Dronedarone increased rates of heart failure, stroke, and death from cardiovascular causes in patients with permanent atrial fibrillation. The data show that this drug should not be used in such patients (Connolly et al. 2011a, b). In clinical trials and the real world of practice, the strongest risk factor for stroke was a lack of anticoagulation, because of the tendency to stop anticoagulants in patients who reverted to sinus rhythm, resulting in increased stroke rate. This is also true following catheter ablation for atrial fibrillation.

Lenient rate control is simple in the vast majority of patients with atrial fibrillation. A resting heart rate of 80–100/min is appropriate.

Van Gelder and colleagues randomly assigned 614 patients with permanent atrial fibrillation to undergo a lenient rate-control strategy (resting heart rate <110/min (80–109/min)) or a strict rate-control strategy (resting heart rate <80/min; >75 % of participants attained a rate of 65–80/min) and heart rate during moderate exercise (<110 BPM). The primary outcome was a composite of death from cardiovascular causes, hospitalization for heart failure, and stroke and systemic embolism.

Results: The estimated cumulative incidence of the primary outcome at 3 years was 12.9 % in the lenient-control group and 14.9 % in the strict-control group, with an absolute difference with respect to the lenient-control group of −2.0 % points $P < 0.001$ for the prespecified non-inferiority margin. The frequencies of the components of the primary outcome were similar in the two groups. More patients in the lenient-control group met the heart rate target or targets [304 (97.7 %) versus 203 (67.0 %) in the strict-control group; $P < 0.001$] with fewer total visits [75 (median, 0) versus 684 (median, 2); $P < 0.001$]. The frequencies of symptoms and adverse events were similar in the two groups (Van Gelder et al. 2010). In practice a resting rate 70–100 is acceptable and simple to achieve. See Fig. 14-7.

ANTICOAGULANTS FOR AF

Approximately 70 % of AF occurs at age 65–85. The risk of stroke in patients with AF who have one or more risk factors for stroke is approx 5 %, and anticoagulants are recommended to keep the international normalized ratio (INR) at 2–3. Bleeding occurrence is associated in virtually all cases with an INR > 3.

Risk factors include:

• Significant valvular heart disease, particularly mitral stenosis and moderate mitral regurgitation, LV dysfunction, HF, hypertension, prior stroke or transient ischemic attack, and age >75 years

In patients <65 years with lone AF (no cardiac abnormality risk factors), the risk of stroke is low (<1 %), and coated acetylsalicylic acid (ASA) 325 mg is recommended. In patients age 65–75 with lone AF, the risk is approx 2 %, and ASA versus warfarin should be determined on an individual basis because trials have not yielded clear answers. All patients with risk factors should receive anticoagulants, but patients older than 75 have an increased risk of intracranial hemorrhage, and the INR should be closely monitored to keep it between 1.8 and 2.8.

NEWER ANTICOAGULANTS

Rivaroxaban (Xarelto): In patients with atrial fibrillation, rivaroxaban was noninferior to warfarin for the prevention of stroke or systemic embolism. There was no significant between-group difference in the risk of major bleeding, although intracranial and fatal bleeding occurred less frequently in the rivaroxaban group. The FDA has approved the oral direct factor Xa inhibitor rivaroxaban for prevention of stroke in patients with nonvalvular atrial fibrillation. The Rivaroxaban Once Daily Oral Direct Factor Xa Inhibition Compared with Vitamin K Antagonism for Prevention of Stroke and Embolism Trial (ROCKET AF, Patel et al. 2011). was a large, double-blind, randomized trial comparing rivaroxaban 20 mg once daily or a reduced dose of 15 mg once daily for patients with creatinine clearance of 30–49 mL/min with warfarin (goal INR 2.0–3.0) in 14 264 patients with nonvalvular AF. Rates for the primary outcome of all stroke (ischemic or hemorrhagic) or systemic embolism were 1.71 % per year in the rivaroxaban group and 2.2 % per year in the warfarin group (Patel et al. 2011).

Approximately 51 % of an oral dose of rivaroxaban is metabolized primarily by CYP 3A4/5. Thus, blood level of the drug is increased (Patel et al. 2011). The drug was used successfully in patients following an acute MI (Mega et al. 2012).

Caution: Rivaroxaban is **36 %** renally eliminated as unchanged drug (Patel et al. 2011) and should not be administered to patients with creatinine clearance <20 mL/min. Caution is needed in patients older than age 75 because serum creatinine levels and eGFR are inaccurate. The 15-mg dose is suggested if a reliable creatinine clearance is in range 30–50 ml/min. A 24 h creatinine clearance is very necessary. The author does not recommend the drug if the GFR is < 40 ml/min.

Apixaban (Eliquis): The direct factor Xa inhibitor apixaban was better than warfarin at preventing stroke in patients with atrial fibrillation. In ARISTOTLE (Granger et al. 2011), a total of 18,201 subjects with nonvalvular atrial fibrillation and at least one additional risk factor for stroke were enrolled in the trial and were randomly assigned to receive the direct factor Xa inhibitor apixaban (at a dose of 5 mg twice daily) or warfarin [target international normalized ratio (INR), 2.0–3.0]. Apixaban was not only noninferior to warfarin but actually superior, reducing the risk of stroke or systemic embolism by 21 % and the risk of major bleeding by 31 %. This remarkable agent, as compared with warfarin, reduced the risk of death from any cause by 11 %.

Elimination is only **25 % renal** and allows some safety in the elderly. Cytochrome P450 3A4 is involved with the metabolism so that strong inhibitors substantially increase drug levels (Eikelboom JW, Weitz 2010).

Dabigatran: this agent was shown to be noninferior to warfarin for the prevention of stroke in patients with atrial fibrillation in the absence of valvular heart disease (Connolly et al. 2009). Dabigatran should be started when the INR is <2.0. Dose 150 mg twice daily if creatinine clearance is normal >60 ml/min.

The drug, however, carries some risk, increased intracranial bleeding, and a probable increased risk for MI, which although small and stated by some to be insignificant renders this mainly renal-eliminated agent a poor choice.

Caution: Chronic atrial fibrillation is mainly a disease of the elderly. This drug elimination is ~ 80 % renal; thus caution is needed in patients over age 75 and those with creatinine clearance <50 mL/min. In many patients older than age 75 and in diabetics of long-standing, the creatinine clearance is <50 ml/min. See Chap. 22.

GENETICALLY MEDIATED ARRHYTHMIC DISORDERS

Wolff–Parkinson–White Syndrome

During sinus rhythm, the short PR interval and delta wave are characteristic (see Figs. 14-3 and 14-4). Patients with WPW syndrome may present with atrial flutter or AF as well as with AVRT. A circus movement through the AV node with retrograde conduction along the accessory bundle, reaching the AV node again via the atria, produces the typical AVRT pattern. This variety usually responds to verapamil. However, verapamil should not be given to prevent paroxysmal tachycardia until proven safe by electrophysiologic (EP) testing because the drug has been reported to accelerate the ventricular response following the development of AF or atrial flutter.

In some patients with AF or flutter with WPW conduction, the impulses are conducted at high frequency through the accessory pathway. A rapid ventricular response of 240–300/min can occur with a risk of precipitating ventricular fibrillation. The rapidity of the ventricular response should alert the clinician to the diagnosis of WPW syndrome. In this subset of patients with WPW syndrome, drugs that block impulses through the AV node (digoxin, verapamil, diltiazem, and beta-blockers) do not slow the response and are contraindicated. Furthermore, digoxin and verapamil may dangerously accelerate the ventricular rate. Verapamil or digoxin may precipitate VF.

DC conversion is indicated, and drugs that block conduction in the bypass tract—flecainide, disopyramide, procainamide, aprindine, propafenone, and especially amiodarone—slow the response. IV amiodarone can rarely increase the ventricular rate or cause hypotension and caution is required. Lidocaine could occasionally increase the ventricular response in patients with WPW syndrome presenting with AF or flutter. EP testing is advisable in symptomatic patients and in those with AF, flutter, or rates exceeding 220/min. Patients shown to be at risk of sudden death should have the bypass tract obliterated cryothermally or by other ablation techniques that produce a cure. Fortunately, serious life-threatening arrhythmias are rare. Asymptomatic patients in whom the delta wave disappears rarely have problems.

Long QT Syndrome

In the congenital prolonged QT syndrome, beta-blockers are of proven value, and a dose of propranolol 40–60 mg three times daily is often effective. Chockalingam et al. (2012), based on a multicenter study, recommend treatment of symptomatic long QT (LQT1) and LQT2 patients with either propranolol or nadolol. The investigators state, "clearly not all beta-blockers are equal in their antiarrhythmic efficacy in LQTS. Propranolol was superior to both nadolol and metoprolol in terms of shortening the cardiac repolarization time, particularly in high-risk patients with markedly prolonger QTc". The above finding is not surprising. Propranolol is more lipophilic than nadolol and metoprolol and thus attains higher brain concentration than nadolol, metoprolol, and atenolol. The author does not recommend atenolol for any cardiac problem (*see* Chap. 1).

Genetic testing can identify patients at risk, aids in identifying patients who are not carriers, and therefore assigns them to a low-risk group. But the best-case scenario is not always the clinical scenario (Webster and Berul 2013).

Phenytoin has a role if beta-blockers are contraindicated. For resistant cases, permanent pacing plus beta-blockers or left stellate ganglionectomy is of value.

Treatment of the acquired prolonged QT syndrome is correction of the underlying cause and avoidance of the class I antiarrhythmics, especially quinidine, disopyramide, procainamide, and sotalol. A short-coupled variant of TDP has been described. This variant responds to verapamil IV and not to beta-blockers or amiodarone; because of the high incidence of sudden death in this variant of torsades, an ICD is strongly recommended (Leenhardt et al. 1994).

BRUGADA SYNDROME

Brugada and Brugada described a cardiac condition typified by an electrocardiographic pattern and a high incidence of sudden death particularly in young individuals (Brugada and Brugada 1992; Brugada et al. 2002). The Brugada syndrome is a congenital disorder of sodium cardiac channel function (Antzelevitch et al. 2003, 2005; Antzelevitch 2007). Southeast Asia is endemic for Brugada syndrome. About 60 % of the affected individuals are of Asian origin.

Although rare in the rest of the world, sudden unexpected death syndrome in East Asia and Southeast Asia is a major cause of death in young men without known underlying cardiac diseases (Nademanee et al. 1997). About 80 % of the clinically affected patients are male. Malignant arrhythmias occur and sudden death typically occurs at night. Most patients had a family history of syncope, sudden death, or abnormal ECG changes. Atrial fibrillation is the most common atrial arrhythmia (Francis and Antzelevitch 2008).

The curious ECG pattern may be intermittent and shows a distinctive type of atypical right bundle branch block: The ST segment is elevated in chest leads V_1, V_2, and V_3 where the right bundle branch pattern is usually seen. Figures 14-15 and 14-16 show the ECG findings in patients with Brugada syndrome. The elevated ST segment has a curious convex curve or a coved and saddleback shape.

MANAGEMENT

Individuals with Brugada syndrome and their family members who are genetic carriers of a sodium channelopathy should be aware that some substances or medications (such as cocaine, methadone, procainamide, propofol,

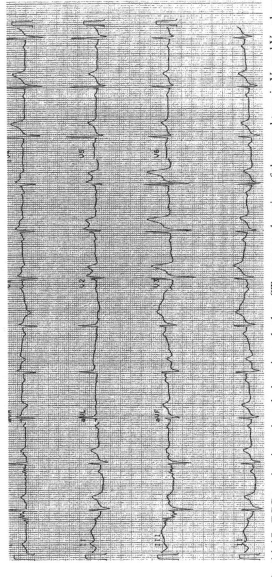

Fig. 14-15. ECG tracing in patient during sinus rhythm: ST-segment elevation of the coved type in V_1 and V_2, characteristic of Brugada syndrome. Reproduced with permission from Khan MG, *Encyclopedia of Heart Diseases*, 2nd edition. New York: Springer Science + Business Media; 2011. With kind permission from Springer Science + Business Media.

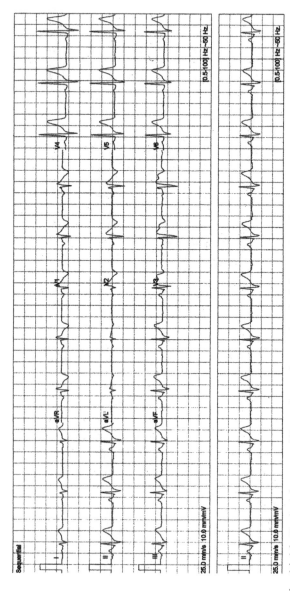

Fig. 14-16. Typical features of Brugada syndrome. Atypical, incomplete right bundle branch block with a curious (odd shape) ST-segment elevation/deformity in V_1–V_3, described as the coved (in V_1, V_2) and saddleback patterns (V_3). Note there is no widened S wave in V_5 or in V_6, as seen in true incomplete or complete RBBB. Thus, if you recognize an atypical RBBB, think of Brugada syndrome and reassess for the characteristic features of this rare but important diagnosis. ECG from a 40-year-old man with episodes of syncope/collapse. No recurrence of syncope over 3 years following ICD. Reproduced with permission from Khan MG, *Rapid ECG Interpretation*, 3rd edition. New York: Humana Press/Springer Science + Business Media; 2008. With kind permission from Springer Science + Business Media.

antidepressants, and antihistamines), fevers, and some disease states may increase their risk of arrhythmias.

Mizusawa et al. (2006) from a study suggest that a dosage of quinidine (300–600 mg a day) may be effective in preventing ventricular fibrillation. Viskin et al. (2007) in an editorial emphasized that for patients with short QT syndrome, Brugada syndrome, and idiopathic VF, the sudden unavailability of quinidine supplies, because of a halt in production, is potentially life threatening. These investigators appear convinced that quinidine is the most effective—and in many cases the only effective—antiarrhythmic therapy for patients suffering from unique malignant ventricular arrhythmias including the short QT syndrome, Brugada syndrome, and idiopathic VF (Kaufman 2007; Belhassen et al. 2004).

Zipes et al. (2006a, b) for the American College of Cardiology/American Heart Association guidelines recommend the placement of an implantable cardioverter-defibrillator (ICD) in Brugada syndrome patients with a previous history of cardiac arrest and who are receiving optimal medical therapy.

VENTRICULAR ARRHYTHMIAS

Ventricular arrhythmias are best considered under benign, potentially fatal, and fatal arrhythmias.

Premature Ventricular Contractions: Benign Arrhythmias

The Cardiac Arrhythmia Suppression Trial (CAST 1989) indicated that treatment of post-MI PVCs and potentially fatal arrhythmias with flecainide or encainide caused an increase in mortality. Beta-blockers are the only safe antiarrhythmic agents that have been shown to improve survival in patients with postinfarction ventricular arrhythmias regardless of their ability to suppress PVCs. Amiodarone has been shown to have a modest beneficial effect.

VENTRICULAR TACHYCARDIA

VT is a regular wide QRS complex tachycardia. In general, consider regular wide QRS complex tachycardia as ventricular unless there is strong evidence to the contrary; if there is doubt about the diagnosis (VT versus SVT with aberrant conduction), treat as VT; the accurate diagnosis of VT is sometimes difficult. The salient diagnostic points for VT were discussed earlier in this chapter (see Figs. 14-1, 14-11, and 14-13).

Nonsustained ventricular tachycardia (NSVT) may occur in patients with significant heart disease but may be observed in healthy individuals. The prognostic significance of NSVT is debatable in individuals with no detectable heart disease. When detected during exercise, and especially at recovery, NSVT indicates increased cardiovascular mortality within the next decades (Katritsis et al. 2012). In trained athletes, NSVT is usually benign when suppressed by exercise. In patients with non-ST-segment elevation MI, NSVT occurring beyond 48 h after admission indicates an increased risk of cardiac and sudden death, especially when associated with myocardial ischemia (Katritsis et al. 2012).

In the treatment of VT, cardioversion is frequently employed, especially in patients with acute MI or when the rate is over 200/min or there is hemodynamic disturbance or coronary insufficiency. Drugs are used cautiously to terminate the attack because of the combined effect of the arrhythmia and the drug on blood pressure. Cardioversion is immediately available during drug treatment. It is quite legitimate to use DC conversion as first-line elective therapy.

Fatal Ventricular Arrhythmias

- VF outside hospital
- Recurrent sustained VT
- Torsades de pointes

EP testing. EP testing may result in selection of a drug or combination that is more efficacious than empirical therapy (Buxton et al. 1986; Josephson 1986) and that does not include amiodarone or sotalol.

- Clinical studies support the empirical use of amiodarone and sotalol to prevent recurrent VT and sudden death, especially in patients with CHD and previous infarction. Amiodarone does not appear to be as effective in patients with HF or hypertrophic cardiomyopathy, and sotalol has not been sufficiently studied (see discussion under amiodarone).
- Flecainide and propafenone are sodium channel blocking agents that may be considered for idiopathic ventricular tachycardias but are contraindicated in patients with heart disease (Zipes et al. 2006a, b). Unfortunately, they have negative inotropic effects, and thus heart failure may be precipitated. Flecainide increased mortality when given to survivors of myocardial infarction (Zipes et al. 2006a, b).
- Amiodarone toxicities restrict long-term use in more than 20 % of patients (Connolly et al. 2006). In patients with LVEF of 35 % or less, amiodarone had no effect on mortality in class II heart failure but was associated with increased mortality in class III heart failure (Bardy et al. 2005).

Torsades de pointes is a life-threatening arrhythmia and is associated with prolongation of the QT interval. The rate is usually 200–250/min. The amplitude and shape of the QRS complexes progressively vary, and they are dramatically spindle-shaped. The peaks of the R-wave direction change from one side to the other of the isoelectric line. This twisting appearance resulted in the name torsades de pointes. The normally conducted complexes show a prolonged QT interval or a prominent U wave. The QT interval is usually >500 ms. The episode of TDP commonly lasts 5–30 s and may end with a return to normal rhythm, extreme bradycardia, or ventricular standstill or may degenerate to VF. The patient usually complains of syncope. Palpitations may be present.

The many precipitating causes of TDP (Smith and Gallagher 1980, 19, 20) include:

- Antiarrhythmics: disopyramide, procainamide, sotalol, and amiodarone (Lazzara 1989). In the absence of hypokalemia, amiodarone does not appear to cause torsades. The drug has been used successfully to treat torsades and can be used as treatment of arrhythmias in patients who have had recurrent TDP (Mattioni et al. 1989; Rankin et al. 1990a, b).
- Coronary vasodilators: prenylamine and lidoflazine.
- Astemizole, terfenadine, and pentamidine.
- Psychotropic: tricyclic antidepressants and phenothiazines.
- Electrolyte disturbances: hypokalemia and hypomagnesemia.
- Bradycardia owing to complete heart block, sinoatrial block, or sinus bradycardia.
- Congenital QT prolongation syndromes (with or without deafness).

Rare causes include subarachnoid hemorrhage, ischemic heart disease, mitral valve prolapse, and liquid protein diet.

Treatment. Because TDP is a brady-dependent arrhythmia, accelerating the heart rate is the simplest and quickest method to shorten the QT interval and usually results in control of the attacks. Temporary atrial or ventricular pacing (AV sequential pacing is preferable to ventricular pacing) should be instituted as soon as possible. Pacing rates within the range of 70–90/min are usually effective. Occasionally, higher rates up to 120/min are required. While preparing for pacing or when pacing is not available, a trial of isoproterenol IV infusion 2–8 μg/min may be given, and control is sometimes achieved within a few minutes.

Isoproterenol is contraindicated in acute MI, angina, or severe hypertension. Magnesium sulfate bolus injection, 2 g

(10 mL of a 20 % solution) over 1 min, causes reversion to sinus rhythm in some patients, particularly in patients with an acquired form of TDP (Tzivoni et al. 1988).

ANTIARRHYTHMIC AGENTS

Class IA

Drug name:	**Quinidine**
Supplied:	Quinidine sulfate: 200, 300 mg
	Quinidine bisulfate: 250 mg
Dosage:	See text

The use of quinidine has decreased greatly since 1975, especially since the advent of other antiarrhythmic agents. Viskin et al. (2007) in an editorial emphasized that for patients with short QT syndrome, Brugada syndrome, and idiopathic VF, the sudden unavailability of quinidine supplies, because of a halt in production, is potentially life threatening. **These investigators appear convinced that quinidine is the most effective—and in many cases the only effective antiarrhythmic therapy—for patients suffering from unique malignant ventricular arrhythmias including the short QT syndrome, Brugada syndrome, and idiopathic VF** (Kaufman 2007; Belhassen et al. 2004). Mizusawa et al. (2006) from a study suggest that a dosage of quinidine (300–600 mg a day) may be effective in preventing ventricular fibrillation in these patients.

Dosage: Quinidine sulfate, 200 mg test dose to detect hypersensitivity reactions. If there are no adverse effects, give 200–400 mg every 3 h for three or four doses, then 6-hourly. Introduce controlled-release preparations only after suppression of the arrhythmia. Quinidine bisulfate

(Biquin, Kinidin Durules): 250 mg; usual maintenance 500 mg twice daily. Sustained-release tablets: Quinaglute Dura-Tabs 324 mg; 1–2 tablets, two or three times daily.

Action: Quinidine inhibits the fast sodium channel, slows phase 0 of the action potential, and depresses spontaneous phase 4 diastolic depolarization (see Fig. 14-17). Quinidine also inhibits the outward K$^+$ current and thus prolongs the

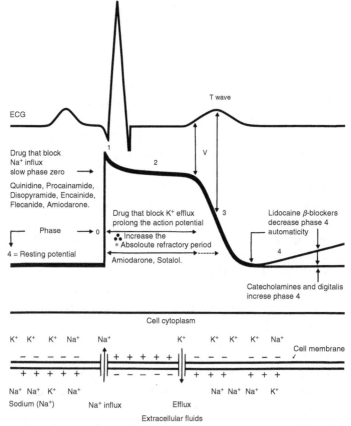

Fig. 14-17. Antiarrhythmic drug action. Reproduced with permission from Khan, MG, Cardiovascular system pharmacology. In Dulbecco R (ed) *Encyclopedia of Human Biology*, 2nd ed. Academic Press, San Diego; 1997.

duration of the action potential. Type I agents in general are potent local anesthetics on nerves and produce a depressant effect on myocardial membrane. The added antivagal action can cause acceleration of AV nodal conduction.

Pharmacokinetics

- Absorption from the gut is about 70 %.
- Peak plasma concentrations are achieved in 1–3 h.
- The half-life is 7–9 h, but slow-release preparations are available. In liver or renal disease, the half-life is increased; in HF the half-life is relatively unchanged.
- Protein binding is 80–90 %.
- Metabolized mainly in the liver by hydroxylation; a small amount is excreted by the kidneys.
- Plasma levels for antiarrhythmic effects are 2–5 µg/mL (3–5.5 µmol/L).

ADVICE, ADVERSE EFFECTS, AND INTERACTIONS

Sinus arrest, SA block, AV dissociation, excessive QRS, and QT prolongation with the precipitation of TDP or other reentry arrhythmias can occur. The risk of torsades may be decreased by giving quinidine only to patients with a normal serum K^+ level and a QT interval <400 ms (8,30). Other adverse effects include nausea, vomiting and diarrhea, and thrombocytopenia. The idiosyncratic reaction and rate precipitation of ventricular fibrillation, especially in those undergoing medical cardioversion for AF, are well known.

The drug decreases ventricular fibrillation threshold, and it does not seem reasonable to give priority to a drug that may increase the risk of VF. Quinidine may precipitate VT and cardiac arrest.

The drug is contraindicated in WPW syndrome associated with atrial flutter or AF. Quinidine increases the serum digoxin level, and the digoxin dose should be decreased by 50 %. The effect of coumarin anticoagulants is enhanced.

Drug name:	**Disopyramide**
Trade names:	Norpace, Rythmodan, Dirythmin SA (UK)
Supplied:	Ampules: 100 mg in 5 mL
	100, 150 mg and controlled release (CR-SR)
	See text for further details
Dosage:	Oral: 300 mg initially, and then 100–150 mg every 6 h; max. 200 mg every 6 h
	Sustained action: 150–300 mg twice daily IV, 2 mg/kg over 15 min and then 1–2 mg/kg by infusion over 45 min (max. 300 mg in first hour; 800 mg daily); maintenance 0.4 mg/kg/h
Sustained release:	Norpace CR 150 mg; Rythmodan Retard 250 mg; Dirythmin 100–150 mg; Dirythmin SA 150 mg

Indications: ventricular arrhythmias and supraventricular arrhythmias.

Adverse effects: Urinary retention, constipation, and worsening of glaucoma are bothersome adverse effects. The drug has a very significant negative inotropic effect, which is much greater than that of any other available antiarrhythmics. CHF may be precipitated, and this is a major drawback to the use of the drug in patients with poor ventricular function. HF, sinus node depression, dry mouth, and blurred vision are not uncommon sequelae. TDP or VF may also occur. Do not use in combination with diltiazem or verapamil.

Contraindications: second- and third-degree heart block and sinus node dysfunction (unless pacemaker fitted), cardiogenic shock, and severe uncompensated heart failure. Do not use in the presence of severe renal failure or HF or in patients with poor LV contractility. Glaucoma, myasthenia gravis, hypotension, and significant hypertrophy of the prostate causing urinary retention are contraindications.

Absorption from the gut is adequate; bioavailability is about 80 %.

Peak plasma concentration is achieved in 1–2 h. The therapeutic range is 2–5 mg/L (2–5 µg/mL, 6–12 µmol/L). Half-life is 6–8 h; 50 % of the drug is excreted unchanged by the kidney; about half is metabolized, and the metabolites may have some activity. One metabolite is powerfully anticholinergic.

The drug is indicated for the management of VT in the acute setting. It is used after trials of other agents such as lidocaine and procainamide have resulted in failure. The drug along with other class I agents does not decrease the incidence of VF in the acute phase of MI and does not reduce the incidence of cardiac death in the post-MI patient. Disopyramide acts selectively on the accessory bundle and may result in a clinically useful decrease in ventricular response or may terminate the episode of atrial flutter or fibrillation in WPW syndrome. The drug may be combined with digoxin in the management of supraventricular arrhythmias. The drug has a limited role in the management of recurrent ventricular arrhythmias and in general is not administered in combination with other antiarrhythmic agents, apart from digoxin. Disopyramide appears to have a role in the management of hypertrophic cardiomyopathy because of its negative inotropic effect. Caution side effects: VT, VF, or torsades de pointes.

Dosage: By slow IV injection, 2 mg/kg over at least 5 min to a max. of 150 mg, with ECG monitoring, followed immediately either by 200 mg by mouth, then 200 mg every 8 h for 24 h, or 400 micrograms/kg/h by intravenous infusion; max. 300 mg in first hour and 800 mg daily.

Drug name:	**Procainamide**
Trade names:	Pronestyl, Procanbid
Supplied:	Oral capsules: 250, 375, 500 mg
	Sustained release (Procanbid): 500, 1,000 mg tablets
	IV ampules: 100 mg/mL, 10 mL vial
Dosage:	*See* text

This old Class I antiarrhythmic slightly prolongs the duration of the action potential (see Fig. 14-17). The drug is indicated for the acute management of VT when lidocaine fails.

Dosage: IV 100-mg bolus at a rate of 20 mg/min and then 10–20 mg/min, maximum 24 mg/min to a maximum of 1 g over the first hour. Maintenance 1–4 mg/min. IV doses exceeding 24 mg/min commonly cause hypotension. Oral administration is not recommended; severe neutropenia may occur (Ellrodt et al. 1984).

Class IB

Lidocaine, Lignocaine

Indicated for ventricular arrhythmias, especially after myocardial infarction.

Dosage: IV, initial bolus 1.0–1.5 mg/kg (75–100 mg). After 5–10 min, administer a second bolus of 0.75–1.0 mg/kg. Halve dose in the presence of severe hepatic disease or reduced hepatic blood flow as in cardiogenic shock, severe HF, during concurrent cimetidine administration, and in patients over age 65 years. Blood levels are increased by concomitant administration of hepatic metabolized beta-blockers and halothane. The initial bolus is given simultaneously with the commencement of the IV infusion of lidocaine so that a lag between the bolus and the infusion does not occur. Commence the infusion at 2 mg/min.

If arrhythmias recur, administer a third bolus of 50 mg and increase the infusion rate to 3 mg/min. Carefully reevaluate the clinical situation and rationale before increasing the rate to the maximum of 4 mg/min. Maximum dose in 1 h = 300 mg, IM 400 mg.

Preparation of IV infusion: 1 g lidocaine for IV use is added to 500 mL or 1 L of 5 % D/W. The major action is depression of spontaneous phase 4 diastolic depolarization. There is little effect on action potential duration or conduction in normal circumstances, but conduction in diseased myocardium or following premature stimulation may be depressed.

The drug is more effective in the presence of a relatively high serum K^+ level, so hypokalemia should be corrected to obtain the maximum effect of lidocaine or other class I antiarrhythmics. A single bolus is effective for only 5–10 min. Clearance is related to the hepatic blood flow and to hepatic function. Clearance is prolonged in the elderly in cardiac failure and hepatic disease. Therapeutic blood levels are 1.4–6 mg/L (1.4–6 µg/mL or 6–26 µmol/L). Central nervous system side effects, including seizures, may occur at concentrations >5 mg/L.

In the UK by intravenous injection, in patients without gross circulatory impairment, 100 mg as a bolus over a few minutes (50 mg in lighter patients or those whose circulation is severely impaired), followed immediately by infusion of 4 mg/min for 30 min, 2 mg/min for 2 h, then 1 mg/min; reduce concentration further if infusion continued beyond 24 h.

If an intravenous infusion is not immediately available, the initial intravenous injection of 50–100 mg can be repeated if necessary once or twice at intervals of not less than 10 min. The main indication for lidocaine is in the acute management of VT. In the early post-MI patient, proven prophylactic therapy requires the use of high doses of lidocaine. Prophylactic lidocaine remains controversial and is not cost-effective; most centers in the USA and Europe do not routinely use the drug.

Ventricular arrhythmias caused by digitalis intoxication, phenothiazines, or tricyclic antidepressants are managed effectively by lidocaine. Lidocaine crosses the placenta after IV or epidural administration. The drug appears to be safe during pregnancy if used in the smallest effective dose for the suppression of VT (Rotmensch 1983).

Class IC

Drug name:	**Flecainide**
Trade name:	Tambocor
Supplied:	400, 600 mg (UK 100, 200 mg)
Dosage:	100 mg twice daily, increasing if needed to 200 mg twice daily, reducing the dose after 3–5 days if possible. Elderly: 50 mg twice daily, max. 100 mg twice daily; reduce dose in renal or hepatic dysfunction

- Flecainide is well absorbed and is metabolized.
- The half-life is about 20 h; half-life is prolonged with renal failure. Therapeutic levels are 400–800 mg/mL. The drug is effective in suppressing ventricular premature beats and nonsustained VT and blocks the accessory pathways in WPW syndrome. The drug is poorly effective against sustained VT, especially in patients with ventricular dysfunction. In this subset, the drug increases the frequency of sustained VT that is poorly tolerated and difficult or impossible to terminate even with prolonged resuscitation (Roden and Woosley 1986).

Flecainide is effective in the prevention of recurrent AVNRT and AVRT. An overall efficacy for long-term control of PSVT (81 % for AVNRT and 74 % for AVRT) has been observed (Anderson et al. 1988). Another study indicated that flecainide was effective in 74 % of cases of AVNRT and in 66 % of AVRT (Benditt et al. 1991). The incidence of such serious drug-induced arrhythmia is about 20 %. Among 588 patients, 33 developed new or worsened VT or VF, and there was difficulty resuscitating some patients. Other side effects include precipitation of or worsening HF, dizziness, and visual problems.

The increase in mortality rate owing to flecainide observed in the CAST study has caused the drug to be removed from use for benign or potentially fatal ventricular arrhythmias. Flecainide is occasionally used for the prevention of atrial flutter or fibrillation or acute conversion, but caution is necessary because 1:1 conduction may occur as with quinidine if treatment with digoxin is not enforced.

In the UK indications/dosage: AV nodal reciprocating tachycardia, arrhythmias associated with accessory conducting pathways (e.g., Wolff–Parkinson–White syndrome). Slow intravenous injection, 2 mg/kg over at least 5 min to a max of 150 mg, with ECG monitoring, followed immediately either by 200 mg by mouth, then 200 mg every 8 h for 24 h or 400 micrograms/kg/h by intravenous infusion; max. 300 mg in first hour and 800 mg daily.

Contraindications. Patients with CHF or LV dysfunction, benign or potentially fatal ventricular arrhythmias.

Drug name:	**Propafenone**
Trade names:	Rythmol, Arythmol (UK)
Supplied:	150, 225, 300 mg
Dosage:	Oral: For patients >70 kg, 150 mg three times daily after meals; lower dose in elderly or patients <70 kg; increase if needed in 3–7 days to 300 mg two or three times daily IV (not in the USA): 2 mg/kg followed by an infusion of 2 mg/min. Administer under hospital supervision with ECG monitoring and blood pressure assessment

This class IC drug blocks the fast sodium channel, membrane-stabilizing activity, prolongation of the PR interval owing to blocking at the AV node, and prolongation of the PR and QRS intervals owing to prolonged ventricular conduction but with no effect on QT. Oral use is restricted and not advisable.

Indications in UK: Ventricular arrhythmias and paroxysmal supraventricular tachyarrhythmias which include paroxysmal atrial flutter or fibrillation and paroxysmal reentrant tachycardias involving the AV node or accessory pathway, where standard therapy is ineffective or contraindicated. It has complex mechanisms of action, including weak beta-blocking activity (therefore caution is needed in obstructive airways disease—contraindicated if severe).

Flecainide and propafenone have negative inotropic effects, and thus heart failure may be precipitated.

Cautions: not advisable following myocardial infarction, heart failure, elderly, pacemaker patients, potential for conversion of paroxysmal atrial fibrillation to atrial flutter with 2:1 or 1:1 conduction block.

Class II

BETA-BLOCKERS

Many arrhythmias are provoked by exertion or sympathetic stimulation and respond favorably to beta-blockers. Their favorable safety profile places them as first-line therapy for most symptomatic ventricular arrhythmias (John et al. 2012).

From the EP standpoint, beta-blockers produce depression of phase 4 diastolic depolarization (Fig. 14-15). Sympathetically mediated acceleration of impulses through the AV node is blocked, and beta-blockers are therefore effective in abolishing arrhythmias induced or exacerbated by increased catecholamine levels. There is a variable but often fairly potent effect on ventricular arrhythmias that may be abolished if they result from increased sympathetic activity such as may occur in myocardial ischemia and other situations. Beta-blockers cause a significant increase in VF threshold. Intravenous propranolol (Norris et al. 1984), metoprolol, and timolol have been shown to reduce the incidence of VF during acute infarction. Beta-blockers and amiodarone are the only antiarrhythmics proved to reduce cardiac mortality. They suppress VT without complete suppression of VPCs.

Drug name:	**Sotalol**
Trade names:	Betapace, Sotacor, Beta-Cardone (UK)
Supplied:	40, 80, 160 mg
Dosage:	40–80 mg once or twice daily; max 240 mg, rarely 320 mg daily

Sotalol is a unique beta-blocker with additional class III activity. The drug is a more effective antiarrhythmic agent than other beta-blockers.

Sotalol is effective in suppressing ventricular couplets and frequent ventricular ectopy; in a randomized study, a 99 % reduction in ventricular couplets was achieved with sotalol and 49 % with propranolol (Kubac et al. 1988).

Sotalol should not be used with potassium-wasting diuretics or other agents that cause hypokalemia or prolong the QT interval because TDP may be precipitated. Torsades caused by sotalol do occur, albeit rarely, in the absence of hypokalemia.

Sotalol reduces ventricular and atrial arrhythmias that can lead to ICD shocks (Connolly et al. 2006).

Class III

Drug name:	**Amiodarone**
Trade names:	Cordarone, Cordarone X (UK)
Supplied:	Tablets, 200 mg; ampules, 150 mg
Dosage:	See text

Amiodarone is a benzofuran derivative that has two atoms of iodine and structural similarities to thyroxine (T4) and triiodothyronine (T3).

Indications: Amiodarone is indicated for paroxysmal supraventricular, nodal, and ventricular tachycardias, atrial fibrillation and flutter, and ventricular fibrillation. In the UK but not in the USA, the drug is indicated for the management of patients with WPW syndrome who have life-threatening arrhythmias and is given IV in these situations.

Amiodarone reduces ventricular and atrial arrhythmias that can lead to ICD shocks (Connolly et al. 2006). Amiodarone toxicities restrict long-term use in more than 20 % of patients (Connolly et al. 2006). In patients with LVEF of 35 % or less, amiodarone had no effect on mortality in class II heart failure but was associated with increased mortality in class III heart failure (Bardy et al. 2005). Amiodarone is a reasonable consideration for patients who have had sustained ventricular tachycardia or fibrillation but who have a contraindication to or refuse an ICD (Zipes et al. 2006a, b).

Dosage **IV** (indicated only for recurring VF, unstable VT): 5 mg/kg (in glucose 5 %), over 20–120 min with ECG monitoring, subsequent infusion given maximum 1.2 g/24 h.

Repeat if needed for 2 days, for life-threatening arrhythmias. Severe hypotension may occur with the IV preparation. Incompatible with sodium chloride infusion; avoid equipment containing the plasticizer di-2-ethylhexyl phthalate.

Oral: A low-dose regimen is used, 200 mg three times daily for 1 week reduced to 200 mg twice daily for a further week or two and then maintenance of 200 mg daily or the minimum dose required to control the arrhythmia after 4 weeks. A 5 days/week regimen may suffice in some. The total daily dose of drug should be lower in patients with HF. After 4 weeks, aim for a serum level of 2 µg/mL amiodarone and 2 µg/mL of the active metabolite desethylamiodarone (Somberg 1987). Initial loading with IV amiodarone 5 mg/kg followed by oral dosing can shorten the time to optimal arrhythmic control (Kerin et al. 1985).

Administer only under hospital or specialist supervision. The drug causes little or no myocardial depression; this is a major asset in the management of malignant arrhythmias that often occur in the setting of poor myocardial contractility. Amiodarone IV acts relatively rapidly. Intravenous injection of amiodarone can be used in cardiopulmonary resuscitation for ventricular fibrillation or pulseless tachycardia unresponsive to other interventions.

Electrophysiologic and antiarrhythmic effects: Oral administration of amiodarone lengthens the action potential duration and thus the ERP in all cardiac tissues including accessory pathways. The drug has been labeled a class III antiarrhythmic agent because of the aforementioned major action. Its effects, however, overlap those of other classes of antiarrhythmics, e.g., class IA. Amiodarone produces potent sodium channel blockade during phases 2 and 3 of the cardiac action potential. Thus, the drug depresses myocardial and His–Purkinje conduction.

The salutary antiarrhythmic effects are accompanied by a consistent lengthening of the QT interval (Nademanee et al. 1983). The latter effect, if conspicuous, may arouse suspicion of imminent side effects such as precipitation of VF or TDP. EP studies do not consistently predict the drug's clinical effect on ventricular arrhythmias. Horowitz and colleagues (1985, 69) and others (Naccarelli et al. 1985; McGovern et al. 1984) noted a predictable effect.

Hemodynamic consequences are usually negligible. Vasodilation produces a mild decrease in systemic vascular resistance. There is a very mild negative inotropic effect, and in clinical practice the drug does not usually precipitate HF (Mason 1987), except in rare circumstances associated with cardiac slowing.

- Absorption from the gut is about 50 %; bioavailability ranges from 22 to 86 %. The drug undergoes extensive hepatic metabolism. Peak plasma levels are reached 6–8 h after an oral dose. The therapeutic effect is not well defined by plasma levels. However, after 4 weeks of therapy, levels between 1.0 and 2.5 µg/mL appear to be associated with therapeutic effect and lowered toxicity.
- The volume of distribution is high (approx 5,000 L). The drug is almost completely bound to protein and binds extensively with virtually all body tissues. The concentration in the myocardium is 10–15 times that in plasma, and the concentration in the liver, lung, and adipose tissue is much higher. Because of the large volume of distribution, the drug is preferably given as a loading dose when used orally, if prompt control of arrhythmia is required.
- Half-life is 30–110 days. Therapeutic effect generally occurs within 10–15 days of oral therapy but may take 3–6 weeks with the use of low loading doses. At high loading doses, a response may be seen within 48 h. Activity persists for more than 50 days after stopping the drug.

Adverse Effects

1. Corneal microdeposits of yellow–brown granules occur in 50–100 % during long-term therapy. They do not affect vision, are reversible on discontinuing the drug, and constitute clinical evidence of the drug's impregnation. Periodic eye examinations are recommended during long-term use. There is some evidence that the deposits can be diminished by withdrawal of therapy for 1–2 weeks or by ophthalmic drops containing sodium–iodine heparinate; optic neuritis and blindness have been reported.

2. Rashes, especially photosensitivity; permanent grayish blue discoloration of the skin occurs in over 10 % of patients after approx 18 months of high-dose therapy but is rare with current low-dose regimens. On discontinuing amiodarone, the discoloration regresses. Patients should be advised to use a sunscreen and to shield their skin from light.

3. Mild bradycardia, but rare precipitation of severe bradyarrhythmia in patients with sick sinus syndrome, may occur. Asystole and sinus arrest have occurred in patients with therapeutic serum concentrations of amiodarone.

4. Precipitation of TDP is rare and occurs mainly in patients with hypokalemia and with drugs that prolong the QT interval. Amiodarone has been used successfully to treat TDP (Rankin et al. 1990a, b) but cannot be recommended as first-line (Rankin et al. 1990a, b) or second-line treatment.

5. Pulmonary toxicity; infiltrates and pulmonary fibrosis occur in 5–20 % of patients receiving chronic doses, 400–800 mg/day (Morady et al. 1983; Marchlinski et al. 1982). The incidence is <1 % with low dosage. Periodic pulmonary function tests, in particular diffusion capacity (DCO), reveal early cases. Discontinuation of amiodarone and steroid therapy causes regression of pulmonary complications in some patients.

6. Hypothyroidism or hyperthyroidism occurs in about 3–7 % of patients. The T4 concentration is mildly raised, the T3 level is very mildly decreased, and there is a marked rise in reverse T3 levels in patients without clinical thyroid disturbance.

7. Proximal muscle weakness and neurologic problems, especially ataxia, are not uncommon.

Drug interaction: with anticoagulants has been well documented. Amiodarone potentiates, and the combination may lead to serious bleeding. The maintenance dose of warfarin should be halved when amiodarone and warfarin are used together. A significant interaction between amiodarone and digoxin occurs. Serum digoxin concentration usually doubles, but ventricular dysrhythmias are suppressed by amiodarone. Halve the dose of digoxin when the two drugs are given together. The combination of amiodarone and verapamil or diltiazem should be avoided because severe depression of SA and AV nodes may occur. Interactions have been noted with flecainide, phenytoin, and theophylline and colchicine. See Chap. 21. Drugs that prolong the QT interval should not be combined with amiodarone: sotalol, class IA antiarrhythmics, tricyclic antidepressants, and phenothiazines. Potassium-losing diuretics must not be given concomitantly, as torsades may be precipitated.

A 5-year follow-up of 242 amiodarone-treated patients (Smith et al. 1986, 90) revealed the following: 59 % adverse effects and withdrawal in 26 % and 25 % discontinued the drug. Few patients tolerated the drug on a long-term basis. In addition, blindness appears to be a rare but alarming adverse effect. Before commencing amiodarone, the physician must be aware of the amiodarone withdrawal problem (Mason 1987). If the drug is discontinued because of a serious side effect, the effect may persist for months.

REFERENCES

Ahsan SY, Moon JC, Hayward MP, et al. Constrictive pericarditis after catheter ablation for atrial fibrillation. Circulation. 2008;118:e834–5. 10.1161.

Alboni P, Tomasi C, Menozzi C, et al. Efficacy and safety of out-of-hospital self-administered single-dose oral drug treatment in the management of infrequent, well-tolerated paroxysmal supraventricular tachycardia. J Am Coll Cardiol. 2001;37:548–53.

Anderson JL, Jolivette DM, Fredell PA. Summary of efficacy and safety of flecainide for supraventricular arrhythmias. Am J Cardiol. 1988;62:62D.

Antzelevitch C, Brugada P, Brugada J, et al. Brugada syndrome: 1992–2002: a historical perspective. J Am Coll Cardiol. 2003;41:1665–71.

Antzelevitch C, Brugada P, Borggrefe M, et al. Brugada syndrome: report of the second consensus conference: endorsed by the heart rhythm society and the European heart rhythm association. Circulation. 2005;111:659–70.

Antzelevitch C. Genetic basis of Brugada syndrome. Heart Rhythm. 2007;4:756–7.

Bardy GH, Lee KL, Mark DB, et al. Amiodarone or an implantable cardioverter-defibrillator for congestive heart failure. N Engl J Med. 2005;352:225–37.

Belhassen B, Glick A, Viskin S. Efficacy of quinidine in high-risk patients with Brugada syndrome. Circulation. 2004;110:1731–7.

Benditt DG, Dunnigan A, Buetikofer J, et al. Flecainide acetate for long-term prevention of PSVT. Circulation. 1991;83:345.

Brugada P, Brugada J. Right bundle branch block, persistent ST segment elevation and sudden cardiac death: a distinct clinical and electrocardiographic syndrome. J Am Coll Cardiol. 1992;20:1391–6.

Brugada J, Brugada R, Antzelevitch C, et al. Long-term follow-up of individuals with the electrocardiographic pattern of right bundle branch block and ST-segment elevation in precordial leads V1 to V3. Circulation. 2002;105:73–8.

Buxton AE, Marchlinski FE, Flores BT, et al. Non-sustained ventricular tachycardia in patients with coronary artery disease: role of electrophysiological study. Circulation. 1986;75:1178.

Cappato R, Calkins H, Chen S, et al. Worldwide survey on the methods, efficacy, and safety of catheter ablation for human atrial fibrillation. Circulation. 2005;111:1100–5.

Chockalingam P, Crotti L, Girardengo G, et al. Not all beta-blockers are equal in the management of long QT syndrome types 1 and 2: higher recurrence of events under metoprolol. J Am Coll Cardiol. 2012;60:2092–9. doi:10.1016/j.jacc.2012.07.046.

Connolly SJ, Dorian P, Roberts RS, et al. Comparison of beta-blockers, amiodarone plus beta-blockers, or sotalol for prevention of shocks from implantable cardioverter defibrillators—the OPTIC Study: a randomized trial. JAMA. 2006;295:165–71.

Connolly SJ, Eikelboom J, Joyner C, et al. Apixaban in patients with atrial fibrillation. Engl J Med. 2011a;364:806–17.

Connolly SJ, Ezekowitz MD, Yusuf S, et al. The RE-LY Steering Committee and Investigators. Dabigatran versus warfarin in patients with atrial fibrillation. N Engl J Med. 2009;361:1139–51. (RE-LY).

Connolly S, Camm AJ, Halperin JL, For the PALLAS Investigators, et al. Dronedarone in high-risk permanent atrial fibrillation. N Engl J Med. 2011b;365:2268–76.

Delacrétaz E. Supraventricular tachycardia. N Engl J Med. 2006;354:1039–51.

DiMarco JP, Miles W, Akhtar M. Adenosine for paroxysmal supraventricular tachycardia: dose ranging and comparison with verapamil.

Assessment in placebo-controlled, multicenter trials. Ann Intern Med. 1990;113:104.

Ellrodt AG, Murata GH, Riedinger MS, et al. Severe neutropenia associated with sustained release procainamide. Ann Intern Med. 1984; 100:197.

Eikelboom JW, Weitz JI. New anticoagulants. Circulation. 2010;121:1523–32.

Francis J, Antzelevitch C. Atrial fibrillation and Brugada syndrome. J Am Coll Cardiol. 2008;51:1149–53.

Gladstone DJ, DJ S, Dorian P, et al. Atrial fibrillation in patients with cryptogenic stroke. N Engl J Med. 2014;370:2467–77.

Granger CB, Alexander JH, McMurray JJV, et al. Apixaban versus warfarin in patients with atrial fibrillation (ARISTOTLE). N Engl J Med. 2011;365:981–92.

Haines DE. Atrial fibrillation ablation in the real world. J Am Coll Cardiol. 2012;59(2):150–2.

Horowitz LN, Greenspan AM, Spielman SR, et al. Usefulness of electrophysiologic testing in evaluation of amiodarone therapy for sustained ventricular tachyarrhythmias associated with coronary heart disease. Am J Cardiol. 1985;55:367.

Hussein AA, Saliba WI, Martin DO, et al. Natural history and long-term outcomes of ablated atrial fibrillation. Circ Arrhythm Electrophysiol. 2011;4:271–8.

Imazio M, Brucato A, Ferrazzi P, et al. Colchicine reduces postoperative atrial fibrillation: results of the Colchicine for the Prevention of the Postpericardiotomy Syndrome (COPPS) atrial fibrillation substudy. Circulation. 2011a;124:2290–5.

Imazio M, Brucato A, Ferrazzi P, et al. Colchicine reduces postoperative atrial fibrillation: results of the Colchicine for the Prevention of the Postpericardiotomy Syndrome (COPPS) atrial fibrillation substudy. Circulation. 2011b;22(124):2290–5.

Jaeggi E, Chiu C, Hamilton R, et al. Adenosine induced atrial pro arrhythmia in children. Can J Cardiol. 1999;15:169.

John RM, Tedrow UB, Koplan BA, et al. Ventricular arrhythmias and sudden cardiac death. The Lancet. 2012;380(9852):1520–9.

Josephson ME. Treatment of ventricular arrhythmias after myocardial infarction. Circulation. 1986;74:653.

Katritsis DG, Zareba W, John Camm AJ. Nonsustained ventricular tachycardia. J Am Coll Cardiol. 2012;60(20):1993–2004.

Kaufman ES. Quinidine in short QT syndrome: an old drug for a new disease. J Cardiovasc Electrophysiol. 2007;18:665–6.

Kerin NZ, Blevins RD, Frumin H, et al. Intravenous and oral loading versus oral loading alone with amiodarone for chronic refractory ventricular arrhythmias. Am J Cardiol. 1985;55:89.

Kubac G, Klinke WP, Grace M. Randomized double blind trial comparing sotalol and propranolol in chronic ventricular arrhythmia. Can J Cardiol. 1988;4:355.

Larsson SC, Drca N, Wolk A. Alcohol consumption and risk of atrial fibrillation: a prospective study and dose-response meta-analysis. J Am Coll Cardiol. 2014;64:281–9.

Lazzara R. Amiodarone and torsades de pointes. Ann Intern Med. 1989;111:549.

Leenhardt A, Glasser E, Burguera M, et al. Short-coupled variant of torsade de pointes: a new electrocardiographic entity in the spectrum of idiopathic ventricular tachyarrhythmias. Circulation. 1994;89:206.

Marchlinski FE, Gansher TS, Waxman HL, et al. Amiodarone pulmonary toxicity. Ann Intern Med. 1982;98:839.

Mason JW. Drug therapy: amiodarone. N Engl J Med. 1987;316:455.

Mattioni TA, Zheutlin TA, Sarmiento JJ, et al. Amiodarone in patients with previous drug-mediated torsade de pointes. Ann Intern Med. 1989;111:574.

McGovern B, Hasan G, Malacoff RF, et al. Long-term clinical outcome of ventricular tachycardia or fibrillation treated with amiodarone. Am J Cardiol. 1984;53:1558.

Mega JL, Braunwald E, Wiviott SD, et al. Rivaroxaban in patients with a recent acute coronary syndrome. N Engl J Med. 2012;366:9–19.

Mizusawa Y, Sakurada H, Nishizaki M, et al. Effects of low-dose quinidine on ventricular tachyarrhythmias in patients with Brugada syndrome: low-dose quinidine therapy as an adjunctive treatment. J Cardiovasc Pharmacol. 2006;47:359–64.

Morady F, Sauve MJ, Malone P, et al. Long-term efficacy and toxicity of high-dose amiodarone therapy for ventricular tachycardia or ventricular fibrillation. Am J Cardiol. 1983;52:975.

Naccarelli GV, Fineberg NS, Zipes DP, et al. Amiodarone: risk factors for recurrence of symptomatic ventricular tachycardia identified at electrophysiologic study. J Am Coll Cardiol. 1985;6:814.

Nademanee K, Singh BN, Hendrickson J, et al. Amiodarone in refractory life-threatening ventricular arrhythmias. Ann Intern Med. 1983; 98:577.

Nademanee K, Veerakul G, Nimmannit S, et al. Arrhythmogenic marker for the sudden unexplained death syndrome in Thai men. Circulation. 1997;96:2595–600.

Norris RM, Barnaby PF, Brown MA, et al. Prevention of ventricular fibrillation during acute myocardial infarction by intravenous propranolol. Lancet. 1984;2:883.

Opolski G, Torbicki A, Kosior DA, et al. Rate control vs rhythm control in patients with nonvalvular persistent atrial fibrillation: the results of the Polish How to Treat Chronic Atrial Fibrillation (HOT CAFE) study. Chest. 2004;126:476–86.

Ouyang F, Tilz R, Chun J, et al. Long-term results of catheter ablation in paroxysmal atrial fibrillation: lessons from a 5-year follow-up. Circulation. 2010;122:2368–77.

ROCKET AF, Patel MR, Mahaffey KW, Garg J, et al. Rivaroxaban versus warfarin in nonvalvular atrial fibrillation. N Engl J Med. 2011;365:883–91.

Rankin AC, McGovern BA. Adenosine or verapamil for the acute treatment of supraventricular tachycardia? Ann Intern Med. 1991;114:513.

Rankin AC, Pringle SD, Cobbe SM, et al. Amiodarone and torsades de pointes. Am Heart J. 1990a;120:1482.

Rankin AC, Pringle SD, Cobe SM. Acute treatment of torsades de pointes with amiodarone: proarrhythmic and antiarrhythmic association of QT prolongation. Am Heart J. 1990b;19:185.

Roden DM, Woosley RL. Drug therapy: flecainide. N Engl J Med. 1986;315:36.

Rotmensch HH, Elkayam U, Frishman W. Antiarrhythmic drug therapy during pregnancy. Ann Intern Med. 1983;98:487.

Ruskin JN. The cardiac arrhythmia suppression trial (CAST). N Engl J Med. 1989;321:85.

Shah RU, Freeman JV, Shilane D, et al. Procedural complications, rehospitalizations, and repeat procedures after catheter ablation for atrial fibrillation. J Am Coll Cardiol. 2012;59:143–9.

Smith WM, Gallagher JJ. "Les torsades de pointes": an unusual ventricular arrhythmia. Ann Intern Med. 1980;93:578.

Smith WM, Lubbe WF, Whitlock RM, et al. Long-term tolerance of amiodarone treatment for cardiac arrhythmias. Am J Cardiol. 1986;57:1288.

Somberg JC. Antiarrhythmic drags: making sense of the deluge. Am Heart J. 1987;113:408.

Steinberg SJ, Mittal S. Intracranial emboli associated with catheter ablation of atrial fibrillation: has the silence finally been broken? J Am Coll Cardiol. 2011;58:689–91.

Steurer G, Gursoi S, Frey B, et al. Differential diagnosis on the electrocardiogram between ventricular tachycardia and preexcited tachycardia. Clin Cardiol. 1994;17:306.

Strickberger SA, Man KC, Daoud EG, et al. Adenosine-induced atrial arrhythmia: a prospective analysis. Ann Intern Med. 1997;127:417–22. Erratum, Ann Intern Med. 1998;128:511.

Task Force of the Working Group on Arrhythmias of the European Society of Cardiology. The Sicilian gambit. A new approach to the classification of antiarrhythmic drugs based on their actions on arrhythmogenic mechanisms. Circulation. 1991;4:1831.

Tzivoni D, Banai S, Schuger C, et al. Magnesium sulfate therapy for sustained monomorphic ventricular tachycardia. Circulation. 1988;77:392.

Van Gelder IC, Groenveld HF, Crijns HJGM, For the RACE II Investigators, et al. Lenient versus strict rate control in patients with atrial fibrillation. N Engl J Med. 2010;362:1363–73.

Vaughan Williams EM. Classification of antiarrhythmic drugs. In: Sandhoe E, Flensted-Jensen E, Olesen KH, editors. Symposium on cardiac arrhythmias. Sodertalje: AB Astra; 1970. p. 449.

Viskin S, Antzelevitch C, Marquez MF, et al. Quinidine: a valuable medication joins the list of "endangered species". Europace. 2007;9(12):1105–6.

Webster G, Berul CI. An update on channelopathies. From mechanisms to management. Circulation. 2013;127:126–40.

Weerasooriya R, Khairy P, Litalien J, et al. Catheter ablation for atrial fibrillation: are results maintained at 5 years of follow-up? J Am Coll Cardiol. 2011;57:160–6.

Wyse DG, Waldo AL, DiMarco JP, Atrial Fibrillation Follow-up Investigation of Rhythm Management (AFFIRM) Investigators, et al. A comparison of rate control and rhythm control in patients with atrial fibrillation. N Engl J Med. 2002;347:1825–33.

15 Cardiac Arrest

Sudden cardiac death accounts for >50 % of all coronary artery disease deaths and 15–20 % of all deaths (Gillum 1990; Myerburg et al. 2004). Thus cardiac arrest prevention represents a major opportunity to further reduce mortality (Deo and Albert 2012).

Survival to hospital discharge was estimated to be only 7.9 % among out-of-hospital (OOH) cardiac arrests that were treated by emergency medical services personnel (Nichol et al. 2008). Importantly, the majority of cardiac arrests occur at home, mostly unwitnessed. Thus, automated external defibrillators (AEDs) that improve resuscitation rates for witnessed arrests have limited effectiveness on reducing overall mortality. Should most homes with occupants older than age 50 deemed to be at risk carry a defibrillator?

Dr J.F. Pantridge initiated coronary care ambulances in Belfast in 1966 (Pantridge and Geddes 1967) and was instrumental in developing portable defibrillators. He advocated that a cardiac defibrillator should be considered in the same light as a *fire extinguisher* and thus should be available in most homes, place of work, and sports arenas (J.F. Pantridge, 1974 personal conversation).

"TIME IS OF THE ESSENCE"

In the majority of cases of cardiac arrest, ventricular fibrillation (VF) is the only correctable rhythm. Thus, there is no need to waste precious time checking for a pulse or for

© Springer Science+Business Media New York 2015
M. Gabriel Khan, *Cardiac Drug Therapy*, Contemporary Cardiology,
DOI 10.1007/978-1-61779-962-4_15

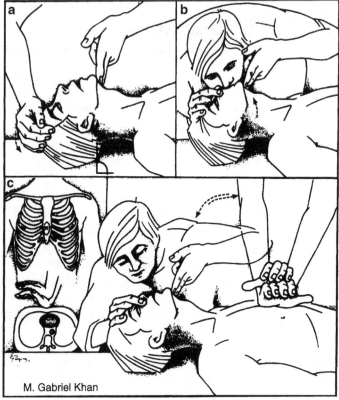

Fig. 15-1 Sequence is CAB, not the old ABC. Compress hard and fast, 100/min, until an AED is available for immediate defibrillation; then continue compressions until circulation restored. Following defibrillation, rescuers should not interrupt chest compressions to check circulation (e.g., evaluate rhythm or pulse) until after approximately 2 min of CPR. No need for rescue breath until after the fourth minute (in the United Kingdom 6 min.). Note the position and shape of the applied hands

the rhythm prior to defibrillation. Just get on with 100 compressions/min and continue for 4 min (Bray et al. 2011) while someone grabs a defibrillator and rapidly defibrillate. Only halt the 100/min compressions when the defibrillator is charged and ready to apply. See Fig. 15-1.

A "dispatcher should provide instructions assertively on compression-only CPR. Thus the 'kiss of life' should be replaced by 'Keep It Simple, Stupid', which is broadly consistent with the practice of many emergency medical dispatchers in the UK" (Nolan and Soar 2010).

Following defibrillation, immediately continue compressions.

No need for rescue breath until after the fourth minute (in the United Kingdom 6 min).

Approx 50 % of patients with VF survive cardiopulmonary resuscitation (CPR) if a defibrillator is available, versus <10 % for other rhythms, represented by asystole and pulseless electrical activity. The incidence of VF in most surveys of cardiac arrest is approx 50 %. Thus chest compression and immediate defibrillation remains the mainstay of therapy for cardiac arrest.

TWO CARDIAC RHYTHMS

There are only two cardiac arrest rhythms:

1. Ventricular fibrillation/pulseless ventricular tachycardia (VF/VT). VF is defined as a pulseless chaotic disorganized rhythm with an undulating irregular pattern that varies in size and shape and a ventricular waveform >150/min.
2. Non-VF/VT: asystole and pulseless electrical activity.

Individuals who can be saved from cardiac arrest are usually in VF.

The widespread distribution of AEDs has helped to accomplish early defibrillation programs and has definitely saved lives particularly in crowded stadiums.

All first-responding emergency personnel, both hospital and nonhospital (e.g., physicians, nurses, emergency medical technicians, paramedics, firefighters, volunteer emergency personnel), must be trained and permitted to operate a defibrillator, which should be readily available in all emergency ambulances or emergency vehicles that engage in the transit of cardiac patients and should be available in many areas including shopping centers and sports arenas. Availability of the AED is thus of paramount importance.

Modern biphasic defibrillators have a high first-shock efficacy in more than 90 % (White et al. 2005; Morrison et al. 2005); thus, VF is usually eliminated with one shock of 360 J.

In a study of 168 consecutive cases of sudden coronary death (within 6 h of onset of symptoms), Davies (1992) showed that 74 % had a recent coronary thrombotic lesion. These patients had warning chest pain prior to arrest. In 52 patients without chest pain or infarction, 48 % had coronary thrombi. In patients with previous infarction, the absence of warning chest pain before arrest selects for a primary arrhythmia caused by preexisting hypertrophy or scarring or both. In a study of successfully resuscitated cardiac arrest victims, 40 of 84 (48 %) had coronary artery occlusion on angiography; successful angioplasty was achieved in 28 of 37 of these patients (Spaulading et al. 1997).

Atheroma complicated by erosion, fissuring, or minute rupture initiates thrombus formation and cardiac arrest; thus the author recommends daily aspirin 75–81 mg non-enteric coated to be taken after the evening meal to all who are at risk, typically:

- Men over age 45 with family history of MI prior to age 75 (old concept < age 55)
- Cigarette smokers
- Patients with mild to moderate hypertension
- Sedentary men > age 45
- Male > age 40 and female > age 50 with LDL cholesterol > 3.5 mmol/l ~ 140 mg/dl
- Male > age 45 and female > age 50 with stressful occupation
- Male > age 45 and female > age 50 who spend > 1 h/day in cities driving in high-volume traffic and cannot avoid

pollution from automobile exhaust fumes (see Chap. 11 for details)

- Diabetics > age 40

Hopefully the antithrombotic effects of aspirin may prevent enlargement of thrombus, by ameliorating platelet aggregation. This scenario will never be tested in an RCT but is logical therapy. Individuals with known peptic disease or GI bleeding should not consider this strategy.

Cardiac deaths in young athletes are usually caused by hypertrophic cardiomyopathy (Maron 1997) (35 %) and anomalous origin of the left main coronary artery from the right sinus of Valsalva (20 %). Other conditions causing sudden cardiac death include arrhythmogenic right ventricular dysplasia, prolonged QT syndromes, and Brugada syndrome (See Chap. 14).

When multiple rescuers are present, one rescuer can perform compression CPR while the other readies the defibrillator, thereby providing both immediate compressions and early defibrillation.

- A change from a three-shock sequence to one shock followed immediately by compressions.
- The consensus recommendation for initial and subsequent monophasic waveform doses is 360 J.
- Modern biphasic defibrillators have a high first-shock efficacy (defined as termination of VF for at least 5 s after the shock), averaging more than 90 %, so that VF is likely to be eliminated with one shock.

BASIC LIFE SUPPORT

Adult basic life support (BLS) (AHA Guidelines 2010a, b, 2012) requires:

- Rapid recognition of cardiac arrest (assessing responsiveness and the absence of normal breathing); victims of cardiac arrest may initially have gasping respirations or even appear to be having a seizure. The lay rescuer should not attempt to check for a pulse and should assume that cardiac arrest is present if an adult suddenly collapses, is unresponsive, and is not breathing or not breathing normally (i.e., only gasping).

- Activation of the emergency response system.
- Rapid commencement of high-quality chest compression.

See Fig. 15-1. Place the heel of one hand over the lower half of the sternum but at least 1½ in. (two fingerbreadths) away from the base of the xiphoid process. The heel of the second hand is positioned on the dorsum of the first, both heels being parallel. The fingers are kept off the rib cage; if the hands are applied too high, ineffective chest compression may result, and fractured ribs are more common with this hand position:

- Position of the hands on each other is crucial to obtain downward pressure.
- No bend at the elbows.
- Hand on the chest avoiding the rib cage (see Fig. 15. 1).
- THE bystander or trained person should push hard and fast on the patient's chest with the goal of compressing at a rate of at least 100 times/min at a depth of at least 2 in. (AHA Scientific Statement 2012).
- Rapid defibrillation.
- The recommended depth of compression for adult victims has increased from a depth of 1–2 in. to a depth of at least 2 in.

The arms are kept straight at the elbow (locked elbows), and pressure is applied as vertically as possible. The resuscitator's shoulders should be directly above the victim's sternum. The rescuer should compress at the center of the chest at the nipple line.

Chest compressions are straight down and thus easily carried out by forceful movements of the shoulders and back, so the maneuver is less tiring. The sternum is depressed 2 in. toward the spine using the heel of both hands. CPR should never be interrupted for more than 10 s. This interval should be sufficient to allow defibrillation. Cessation should not exceed 30 s for endotracheal intubation.

The 2010 AHA Guidelines for CPR is a change in the BLS sequence of steps from "A-B-C" (airway, breathing, chest compressions) to "C-A-B" (chest compressions, airway, breathing) for adults (see studies : Svensson et al. 2010, Rea et al. 2010a).

Studies indicate that an AED must be available within 5 min of the arrest to engage the shockable rhythm or the result is a poor outcome. In the majority of cases of cardiac arrest, when an AED is available somewhere in the facility, it usually takes >5 min to obtain the AED at the side of the victim, and thus bystanders who witness the arrest must be encouraged to learn and initiate chest compressions within seconds of the witnessed patient collapse and to give 100 compressions/min until the defibrillator is in readiness to apply a shock (4–6 min).

Compressions (200) are recommenced immediately following defibrillation without concern for the airway and mouth-to-mouth breathing.

Bystanders do rarely start CPR because they are uncomfortable with giving rescue breaths, panic, or fear that they will cause harm or do CPR incorrectly. What we do know is that bystander CPR is important (Nolan and Soar 2010). Dispatcher-assisted bystander CPR increases survival by about 50 % compared with no CPR (Rea et al. 2010b).

Hüpfl and colleagues (2010) conducted a primary meta-analysis that included three randomized trials of dispatcher-assisted chest-compression-only CPR versus dispatcher-assisted standard CPR. The three dispatcher-CPR studies were of high quality and used similar methods. Each trial showed a slightly increased survival to hospital discharge with compression alone compared with standard CPR, but the associations were not significant.

One weakness of all three dispatcher-assisted CPR studies is that standard CPR was done with a compression/ventilation ratio of 15:2 instead of 30:2 (Nolan and Soar 2010).

A secondary meta-analysis (Hüpfl et al. 2010) included seven observational cohort studies of bystander CPR that compared compression-only CPR with standard CPR and excluded the three randomized studies of dispatcher-assisted CPR. This meta-analysis showed no difference in survival to hospital discharge at 1 week or 30 days. Nolan and Soar (2010) provided advice:

- Hüpfl et al.'s (2010) interpretation of observational studies is flawed because of likely undetected confounders. The results of both meta-analyses should affect practice as follows:
- If the information from a caller suggests sudden adult cardiac arrest, the dispatcher should provide instructions assertively on compression-only CPR.
- Animal and human studies have reported that blood flow is greatest with chest compression rates near 120/min. Idris et al. (2012) from a study using compression rate 112 ± 19/min observed that chest compression rate was not significantly associated with survival to hospital discharge.
- In the United Kingdom: For adult cardiac arrest, the bystander gives 600 compressions (over about 6 min) = 100/min followed by two rescue breaths and then a compression ventilation ratio of 100:2.

  Rescue breathing is unnecessary in the first few minutes after sudden cardiac arrest—the lungs will contain sufficient oxygen at the time of cardiac arrest, and gasping, which is present initially in a third of cardiac arrests, might provide some ventilation (Bobrow et al. 2008).

Defibrillation

The following points need to be borne in mind for successful defibrillation:

1. Defibrillation should be accomplished as quickly as possible.
2. Paddle placement should be as follows:

- One paddle electrode is positioned to the right of the upper sternum below the clavicle (right second intercostal space).
- The other paddle is placed to the left of the left nipple with the center of the electrode in the midaxillary line. In the United Kingdom, the latter paddle is placed over the points designated as V4–V5 for the electrocardiogram—a little outside the position of the normal apex beat. The paddle should be placed at least 5 in. away from a pacemaker generator.

3. Conducting gel pads are preferred to jelly but should be removed between shocks.
4. Heavy arm pressure must be applied on each paddle.
5. Defibrillation should take place when the victim's phase of ventilation is in full expiration.
6. Energy setting: First shock 360 J. Subsequent shocks: 360 J.
7. Both paddle buttons should be discharged simultaneously.

PROCEDURE FOR DEFIBRILLATION

Defibrillation should be accomplished at the earliest opportunity when VF is present.

- Turn on defibrillator power (be certain defibrillator is not in synchronous mode).
- Select energy and charge the capacitor.

Properly place paddles on right chest second interspace ~ lead V1 area and left paddle over V5–V6 ECG area (United Kingdom: V4–V5 area).

- Because VF is the only rhythm that is amenable to treatment in a cardiac arrest adult victim, there is no need to waste time checking the rhythm on monitor. Just hurry up/halt compression for the 10 s needed.
- Clear area and check that no personnel are directly or indirectly in contact with the patient. The operator must ensure that he or she is not touching the patient when the shock is delivered.

- Apply firm arm pressure (approximately 10 kg or 25 lb) on each paddle with a squeezing action. (Do not lean on paddles—they may slip.)
- Deliver countershock by depressing both paddle discharge buttons simultaneously. (If no skeletal muscle contraction is observed, check equipment.)
- Recommence CPR.

If an organized rhythm has been restored, check for an effective pulse. If no pulse is present, resume BLS.

VF may masquerade as asystole. The monitoring electrodes should be rotated from their original position to ensure that VF is not present. Asystole or electromechanical dissociation is usually owing to irreversible myocardial damage and inadequate myocardial perfusion; pacing is ineffective in this poor prognostic setting.

DRUG THERAPY

Vasopressors, antiarrhythmics, and sequence of actions during treatment of cardiac arrest:

- Despite the widespread use of epinephrine and several studies of vasopressin, no placebo controlled study has shown that any medication or vasopressor given routinely at any stage during human cardiac arrest increases rate of survival to hospital discharge.
- A meta-analysis of five randomized out-of-hospital trials showed no significant differences between vasopressin and epinephrine for return of spontaneous circulation, death within 24 h, or death before hospital discharge (Aung and Htay 2005).

Given this lack of documented effect of drug therapy in improving long-term outcome from cardiac arrest, the sequence for CPR de-emphasizes drug administration and reemphasizes chest compression and rapid defibrillation.

Amiodarone 300 mg IV push (cardiac arrest dose). If VF/pulseless VT recurs, consider administration of a second dose of 150 mg IV. Maximum cumulative dose: 2.2 g over 24 h.

Lidocaine (class indeterminate) 1.0–1.5 mg/kg IV push. Consider repeat in 3–5 min to a maximum cumulative dose of 3 mg/kg. A single dose of 1.5 mg/kg in cardiac arrest is acceptable.

Magnesium sulfate 1–2 g IV in polymorphic VT (torsades de pointes) and suspected hypomagnesemic state.

Epinephrine; adrenaline

Dosage:	IV: 1 mg, 0.01 mg/kg (10 mL of a 1:10,000 solution) repeated at 3–5-min intervals as needed; ILCOR recommendation is every 3 min. Give a 20-mL flush of IV fluid to ensure delivery of the drug centrally
Tracheobronchial:	1 mg, 10 mL of a 1:10,000 solution. The epinephrine solution can be instilled directly into the tracheobronchial tree through an endotracheal tube. Chest compression should be interrupted for no more than 30 s, while epinephrine is introduced through the endotracheal tube. Positive-pressure ventilation is then applied and chest compression resumed

Hagihara et al. (2012) in a study observed that "among patients with out-of-hospital (OOH) cardiac arrest in Japan, use of prehospital epinephrine was significantly associated with increased chance of return of spontaneous circulation before hospital arrival but decreased chance of survival and good functional outcomes 1 month after the event." **Epinephrine use for in-hospital arrests must continue until further studies prove the drug useless.**

Asystole and Pulseless Idioventricular Rhythms

Electromechanical dissociation. Epinephrine should continue to be used as the primary vasopressor for the management of cardiac arrest. Epinephrine is an alpha- and beta-adrenergic agonist. It stimulates spontaneous cardiac contractions. Peripheral vascular effects cause a marked increase in systemic vascular resistance resulting in an increased aortic diastolic perfusion pressure and thus improving coronary blood flow. It is relevant that epinephrine constricts peripheral vessels but preserves flow to vital organs, and, importantly, coronary artery dilation occurs.

Isoproterenol Is Contraindicated in the Treatment of Cardiac Arrest

Vasopressin

Dosage:	40 U IV single dose, one time only
Indication:	Only for VF/pulseless VT; if no response in 5 min, resume epinephrine IV 1 mg

Beta-Blockers

Beta-blockers have a role in patients with recurrent VF and several countershocks are required; an intravenous beta-blocker may occasionally be useful, especially with electrocution (Sloman et al. 1965; Rothfeld et al. 1968). In general, beta-blockers as well as all other agents that have a negative inotropic effect should be avoided in cardiac arrest.

REFERENCES

AHA Scientific Statement, Lerner EB, Rea TD, Bobrow BJ, et al. Emergency medical service dispatch cardiopulmonary resuscitation prearrival instructions to improve survival from out-of-hospital cardiac arrest: a scientific statement from the American heart association. Circulation. 2012;125(4):648–55.

AHA guidelines, Hazinski MF, Nolan JP, Billi JE et al. Part 1: Executive summary: 2010 international consensus on cardiopulmonary resuscitation and emergency cardiovascular care science with treatment recommendations. Circulation 2010; 122:S250–75.

AHA guidelines, Part 1: Executive summary: 2010 American Heart Association Guidelines for Cardiopulmonary Resuscitation and Emergency Cardiovascular Care. Circulation 2010;122:S640–56.

Aung K, Htay T. Vasopressin for cardiac arrest: a systematic review and meta-analysis. Arch Intern Med. 2005;165:17–24.

Bobrow BJ, Zuercher M, Ewy GA, et al. Gasping during cardiac arrest in humans is frequent and associated with improved survival. Circulation. 2008;118:2550–4.

Bray JE, Deasy C, Jamie Walsh J, et al. Changing EMS dispatcher CPR instructions to 400 compressions before mouth-to-mouth improved bystander CPR rates. Resuscitation. 2011;82(11):1393–8.

Davies MJ. Anatomic features in victims of sudden coronary death; coronary artery pathology. Circulation. 1992;85 Suppl 1:1.

Deo R, Albert CM. Sudden cardiac death. Epidemiology and genetics of sudden cardiac death. Circulation. 2012;125:620–37.

Gillum RF. Geographic variation in sudden coronary death. Am Heart J. 1990;119:380–9.

Hagihara A, Hasegawa M, Abe T, et al. Prehospital epinephrine use and survival among patients with out-of-hospital cardiac arrest. JAMA. 2012;307(11):1161–8.

Hüpfl M, Selig HF, Nagele P. Chest-compression-only versus standard cardiopulmonary resuscitation: a meta-analysis. Lancet. 2010; 376(9752):1552–7.

Idris AH, Guffey D, Aufderheide TP, et al. Relationship between chest compression rates and outcomes from cardiac arrest. Circulation. 2012;125:3004–12.

Maron BJ. The young competitive athlete with heart disease. Cardiol Rev. 1997;5:220.

Morrison LJ, Dorian P, Long J, et al. Out-of-hospital cardiac arrest rectilinear biphasic to monophasic damped sine defibrillation waveforms with advanced life support intervention trial (ORBIT). Resuscitation. 2005;66:149–57.

Myerburg RJ, Interian A, Simmons J, Castellanos A. Sudden cardiac death. In: Zipes DP, editor. Cardiac electrophysiology: from cell to bedside. Philadelphia, PA: WB Saunders; 2004. p. 720–31.

Nichol G, Thomas E, Callaway CW, Hedges J, Powell JL, Aufderheide TP, Rea T, Lowe R, Brown T, Dreyer J, Davis D, Idris A, Stiell I. Regional variation in out-of-hospital cardiac arrest incidence and outcome. JAMA. 2008;300:1423–31.

Nolan JP, Soar J. Dispatcher-assisted bystander CPR: a KISS for a kiss. Lancet. 2010;376(9752):1522–4.

Pantridge JF, Geddes JS. A mobile intensive-care unit in the management of myocardial infarction. Lancet. 1967;2:270–3.

Rea TD, Eisenberg MS, Culley LL, Becker L. Dispatcher-assisted cardio-pulmonary resuscitation and survival in cardiac arrest. Circulation. 2010a;104:2513–6.

Rea TD, Fahrenbruch C, Culley L, et al. CPR with chest compressions alone or with rescue breathing. N Engl J Med. 2010b;363:423–33.

Rothfeld EL, Lipowitz M, Zucker IR, et al. Management of persistently recurring ventricular fibrillation with propranolol hydrochloride. JAMA. 1968;204:546.

Sloman G, Robinson JS, McLean K. Propranolol (Inderal) in persistent ventricular fibrillation. BMJ. 1965;1:895.

Spaulading CM, Joly LM, Rosenberg A, et al. Immediate coronary angi-ography in survivors of out-of-hospital cardiac arrest. N Engl J Med. 1997;336:1629.

Svensson L, Bohm K, Castrèn M, et al. Compression-only CPR or stan-dard CPR in out-of-hospital cardiac arrest. N Engl J Med. 2010;363:434–42.

White RD, Blackwell TH, Russell JK, Snyder DE, Jorgenson DB. Transthoracic impedance does not affect defibrillation, resuscitation or survival in patients with out-of-hospital cardiac arrest treated with a non-escalating biphasic waveform defibrillator. Resuscitation. 2005;64:63.

16 Infective Endocarditis

Infective endocarditis (IE) most often results from bacterial infection, but infections caused by fungi, Coxiella, or Chlamydia are not rare. Infection usually involves heart valves not always previously known to be abnormal, in particular a bicuspid aortic valve, mitral valve prolapse, or (rarely) a septal defect or ventricular aneurysm. Coarctation of the aorta, patent ductus arteriosus, aneurysms, or arteriovenous shunts may be the site of infective endarteritis. Prosthetic valves may be involved, and infection at the site of implantation of foreign material including devices poses a particularly difficult problem.

- The old fashioned terms acute and subacute bacterial endocarditis (SBE) are still clinically useful, although they no longer hold prominence because pathogens such as *Staphylococcus aureus* and streptococci can cause either fulminant or indolent disease in different patients.
- The term SBE or subacute IE used in a patient who is not critically ill refers to a subacute syndrome, with minimal signs of toxicity, which is usually caused by viridans streptococci, enterococci, coagulase-negative staphylococci, or gram-negative coccobacilli. These organisms cause a slow, low-grade infection that evolves clinically over weeks to months, thus allowing the clinician to delay therapy for a few days while awaiting the results of blood cultures and other diagnostic tests.
- Acute IE is accompanied by marked toxicity with progression over days to a few weeks resulting in valvular destruction, hemodynamic deterioration, heart failure (HF), and metastatic infection and is caused mainly by *S. aureus*, which carries about a 40 % rate of HF.

© Springer Science+Business Media New York 2015
M. Gabriel Khan, *Cardiac Drug Therapy*, Contemporary Cardiology,
DOI 10.1007/978-1-61779-962-4_16

Rheumatic valvular heart disease is now uncommon in developing countries, and IE is encountered mainly in patients with prosthetic heart valves, bicuspid aortic valves, particularly in men over age 60, and degenerative valvular disease (aortic sclerosis). Mitral valve prolapse (MVP) accounts for approximately 18 % of native valve IE, with an increased risk in men older than 45. The risk of IE in patients with MVP is significant mainly if a regurgitant murmur is heard or if there is documented thickening of valve leaflets >5 mm. Intravenous (IV) drug abusers represent a special group with right-sided IE.

CLASSIFICATION AND DIAGNOSIS

A logical classification of IE is as follows:

- Native valve IE; acute or subacute presentation.
- Prosthetic valve IE.
- Right-sided endocarditis, observed particularly in IV drug users.
- Culture-negative IE.

The European Society of Cardiology (ESC 2009) provided a statement: "The epidemiology of IE has changed, now more often affecting elderly patients and occurring as a result of health care-associated procedures. IE can be categorized as left-sided native valve IE, left-sided prosthetic valve IE, right-sided IE, or device-related IE."

Diagnostic Guidelines

Diagnostic criteria are as follows:

- Conformation of persistent bacteremia resulting from organisms.
- Evidence of cardiac valvular involvement: documentation of vegetation, new murmur of valvular regurgitation, or paravalvular abscess.
- Supporting findings include: fever, risk factors for IE, vascular or immune complex phenomena, or intermittent bacteremia or fungemia.

The diagnosis of IE requires a high index of suspicion. The condition should be considered and carefully excluded in all patients with a heart murmur and pyrexia of undetermined origin. The Duke criteria utilize echocardiographic findings as a major criterion for diagnosis and have merit for diagnosis of native valve endocarditis; the utility of the Duke criteria has not yet been adequately assessed, however, for suspected prosthetic valve endocarditis. Diagnosis is made in the majority by blood cultures and echocardiography.

Echocardiography: Transesophageal echocardiography (TEE) is superior to transthoracic assessment in the search for infected vegetations located on heart valves and is crucial for the diagnosis of endocarditis. See Fig. 16-1.

Transthoracic two-dimensional Doppler echocardiography gives poor detection of prosthetic heart valves, especially in the mitral position and of calcific sclerotic native valves. Vegetations that are less than 5 mm, 6–10 mm, or greater than 10 mm are observed in 25 %, 65 %, and 70 %, respectively, by transthoracic technique. This is 100 % for all lesions using TEE.

Two-dimensional transthoracic endocardiography (TTE) can miss 25 % of vegetations <10 mm and 75 % of those <5 mm. (TEE) is more sensitive than TTE for detecting vegetations and cardiac abscess.

High-risk echocardiographic features include

- Large and/or mobile vegetations.
- Valvular insufficiency.
- Suggestion of perivalvular extension.
- Secondary ventricular dysfunction.

Need for surgery

- Heart failure is an immediate indication. Features that suggest potential need for surgical intervention (Baddour et al./AHA 2005) are as follows:
- Abscess formation.
- Staph infection.
- Persistent vegetation after systemic embolization.

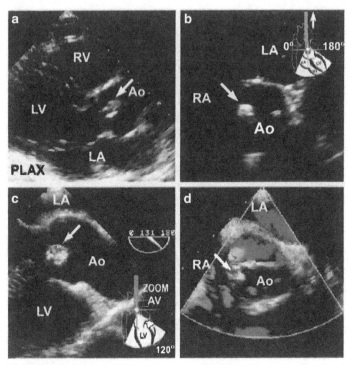

Fig. 16-1. A 40-year-old heroin user presenting with a leg pain, visual disturbances, fever, and a murmur. Transthoracic still frames showing a vegetation on the tip of an aortic cusp (*arrow*, **a**). This was believed responsible for the patient's extracardiac complications. No tricuspid vegetations were observed. Transesophageal images revealed a circumscribed vegetation (*arrows*, **c**, **d**). Mild aortic regurgitation was seen on Color Doppler examination (**d**). Reproduced with permission from Anavekar NS, Averbach M, Bulwer BE: Infective Endocarditis. In: Solomon SD, Bulwer BE, editors. *Essential Echocardiography: A Practical Handbook*. Totowa, NJ: Humana Press, 2007; p. 292. With kind permission of Springer Science + Business Media.

- Anterior mitral leaflet vegetation, particularly with size >10 mm.
- One or more embolic events during first 2 weeks of antimicrobial therapy.
- Increase in vegetation size >1.5 cm despite appropriate antimicrobial therapy.

- Acute aortic or mitral insufficiency with signs of ventricular failure.
- Valve perforation or rupture, valvular dehiscence, or fistula.
- Large abscess or extension of abscess despite appropriate antimicrobial therapy.
- New heart block.
- Combination of large vegetation size and positive antiphospholipid antibody.

Precipitating and predisposing factors

- If prior to dental work, the usual organism producing IE is *S. viridans* or, rarely, *S. faecalis*. If an acute presentation emerges after dental work, one must suspect *Staphylococcus* or the extremely rare *Fusobacterium*, which is not uncommon in gingival crevices and the oropharynx.
- With genitourinary instrumentation or in other surgical procedures, gram-negative bacteria are the rule.
- Prosthetic heart valve.
- Narcotic addicts: mainly right heart endocarditis, owing to *S. aureus*, *Pseudomonas aeruginosa*, *P. cepacia*, and *Serratia marcescens*.

Blood cultures: Adequate cultures and as wide as possible a range of sensitivities must be obtained. Approximately 90 % of the causative organisms can be isolated if there has been no previous antibiotic therapy. The past two decades have seen an increasing incidence of staphylococci and enterococci, often resistant to penicillin. The incidence of gram-negative organisms has also increased. If the organism is to be isolated at all, four to six blood cultures carry a 98 % chance of success.

Three separate sets of blood cultures should be taken, each from a separate venipuncture site, over 24 h. Ten milliliters of blood drawn should be put in each of two blood culture bottles, one containing aerobic and the other anaerobic medium (Towns and Reller 2002).

If the presentation is acute and the patient's status is critical with a high suspicion of *S. aureus* infection, another view is to take four blood cultures over a period of 1–2 h, after which antibiotic treatment should begin and should on no account be withheld pending a bacteriologic diagnosis. The presence of echocardiographically visible vegetations greatly increases the urgency of commencing treatment, as does the presence of infection on prosthetic valves.

Aids in identifying the organism:

- Cultures must be incubated both aerobically and anaerobically; the latter is necessary especially for *Bacteroides* and anaerobic streptococci.
- Serological tests (complement fixation tests (CFTs)) are of value in patients with *Brucella*, *Candida*, *Cryptococcus*, *Coxiella*, or *Chlamydia*.
- Examination of a Gram stain of the "buffy" coat of the peripheral blood.
- In cases other than group A *Streptococcus*, it is advisable to monitor the serum bactericidal titer (SBT) 1:8 or higher, the minimum inhibitory concentration (MIC), and the minimum bactericidal concentration (MBC).

A discussion of the case with the microbiologist is often helpful. Some organisms such as *Haemophilus influenzae* and variants of streptococci require enriched media. *Neisseria gonorrhoeae* and *N. meningitidis* require 5–10 % of CO_2, and *Pseudomonas* grows poorly in unvented bottles. Fungi require a medium containing broth and soft agar and are seldom identified by culture. The culture of an arterial embolus may reveal a fungal etiology.

THERAPY

Initial choice of appropriate antibiotic prior to laboratory determination of the infecting organism is guided by the following parameters:

1. Native valve: a subacute presentation, SBE, is caused by *S. viridans* in approximately 80 %, *S. faecalis* in 10 %, and other organisms in 10 %.

2. Native valve, elderly endocarditis: *S. faecalis* is commonly seen, but *S. viridans* is implicated in about 50 % of cases.
3. Prosthetic valve endocarditis.
   - Early infection after operation is usually caused by *Staphylococcus epidermidis* or *S. aureus.*
   - Late after operation the organisms are similar to those seen in SBE or acute endocarditis with the additional probability of fungal infection, but *S. epidermidis* is not uncommon. Following abdominal surgery, gram-negative and anaerobic infections are not uncommon.
4. Acute bacterial endocarditis (ABE) is usually caused by *S. aureus.*
5. Endocarditis in narcotic addicts: right-sided endocarditis.
6. Culture-negative endocarditis is often caused by:
   - The usual bacterial organisms, which are masked by previous antibiotic therapy.
   - Slow-growing penicillin-sensitive streptococci with fastidious nutritional tastes.
   - *Coxiella* and *Chlamydia.*

S. aureus *Endocarditis*

This most harmful organism accounts for nearly all cases of native valve acute bacterial endocarditis and approximately 50 % of prosthetic valve IE.

For penicillinase-producing staphylococci, nafcillin, oxacillin, or flucloxacillin with the optional addition of gentamicin is given for 6 weeks, the latter for only 1 week (see Table 16-1). An aminoglycoside is not added in the United Kingdom. Other regimens advised for penicillinase-producing staphylococci include:

- Vancomycin
- Cephalosporins: cephalothin, cephradine, cefuroxime
- Rifampin plus aminoglycoside; rifampin plus cloxacillin; rifampin plus vancomycin
- Clindamycin and cephalosporin

Table 16-1
Treatment of Staphylococcus aureus Endocarditis

Type	Antibiotic	Dosage
Native valve	Nafcillin +	2 g IV every 4 h for 6 weeks
	Optional	1–1.4 mg/kg IV every 8 h for 1 week
	Gentamicin	
Methicillin-resistant staphylococci	Vancomycin	15 mg/kg IV every 12 h for 6 weeks
Prosthetic valve	Nafcillin +	2 g every 4 h for >6 weeks
	Rifampin	300 mg orally every 8 h for 6 weeks
	Gentamicin	1–1.4 mg/kg IV every 8 h for 2 weeks
Methicillin-resistant staphylococci	Vancomycin +	15 mg/kg IV every 12 h for 6 weeks
	Rifampin	300 mg orally every 8 h for >6 weeks
	Gentamicin	1–1.4 mg/kg IV every 8 h for 2 weeks

Vancomycin and cephalothin are effective alternatives when penicillin is contraindicated. Cephalothin is more active than other cephalosporins against *S. aureus*. Clindamycin is relatively effective but is not advisable because it is bacteriostatic or less bactericidal than penicillin or cephalosporins; also, pseudomembranous colitis may supervene. If metastatic infection is present, rifampin is usually added at a dose of 600–1,200 mg daily and continued until abscesses are drained and excised. For methicillin-resistant staphylococci, vancomycin 1 g every 12 h is the treatment of choice. Care should be taken in patients over age 65 years and/or those with renal impairment or eighth nerve dysfunction. Vancomycin serum levels should be maintained at <50 µg/mL. There appears to be no advantage in adding an aminoglycoside or rifampin. If vancomycin is contraindicated, no suitable alternatives have been tested: trimethoprim–sulfamethoxazole (Bactrim, Septra) has been used with some success. Rifampin must not be used alone because resistant strains quickly emerge. Fusidic acid 500 mg four times daily with rifampin has been used and provides a reasonable alternative.

Generally, 4–6 weeks of antibiotic therapy is considered adequate for methicillin-resistant staphylococci, but some patients require extended treatment.

Prosthetic Valve Endocarditis

Methicillin-resistant strains are common, and vancomycin is the agent of choice. Combination with an aminoglycoside and rifampin improves the cure rate but increases the incidence of drug toxicity and resistant strains. The infection is usually invasive, destructive, and often difficult to eradicate, with a mortality rate exceeding 50 %. TEE is crucial for the diagnosis. Prognosis is poor, especially if HF supervenes; thus, surgery is frequently necessary.

Native Valve Endocarditis Caused by Staphylococci

Oxacillin-susceptible strains: Nafcillin or oxacillin 12 g/24 h IV in 4–6 equally divided doses for 6 weeks.

Oxacillin-resistant strains: Vancomycin 30 mg/kg per 24 h IV in two equally divided doses for 6 weeks. Adjust vancomycin dosage to achieve 1-h serum concentration of 30–45 µg/mL and trough concentration of 10–15 µg/mL (Baddour et al./AHA 2005).

Native valve endocarditis caused by *S. viridans* and *Streptococcus bovis* sensitive to penicillin.

Native Valve Endocarditis

Non-staph endocarditis: it is advisable to commence antibiotic treatment in hospital for 1 week and then proceed to outpatient therapy.

In patients <65 years old with normal renal function: 18–30 million U/24 h IV either continuously or in six equally divided doses plus gentamicin 1 mg/kg every 8 h for 4–6 weeks or ampicillin 12 g/24 h IV in six equally divided doses for 4–6 weeks (Baddour et al./AHA 2005). The use of ceftriazone constitutes the biggest advance in antibiotic therapy during the past two decades.

Ceftriaxone 2 g IV or IM once daily can be given to selected patients as outpatient therapy for 4 weeks.

- Native valve: 4-week therapy recommended for patients with symptoms of illness ≤3 months; 6-week therapy recommended for patients with symptoms >3 months
- In patients older than 65 years and/or in those with renal impairment or impairment of eighth cranial nerve function: Crystalline penicillin G sodium; 12–18 million U/24 h IV either continuously or in four or six equally divided doses for 4 weeks **or**
- Ceftriaxone sodium: 2 g/24 h IV/IM in 1 dose, for 4 weeks (Baddour et al./AHA 2005).

Prosthetic Valve Endocarditis Caused by Susceptible S. viridans *or* S. bovis *Infections*

Penicillin and gentamicin should be given for 4–6 weeks at doses given above with close monitoring for gentamicin toxicity.

S. viridans or *S. bovis* relatively resistant to penicillin should be treated with ampicillin and gentamicin for 4 weeks and then amoxicillin orally 500 mg every 6 h for 2 weeks. In patients allergic to penicillin, give vancomycin 12.5 mg/kg every 12 h.

Vancomycin may cause ototoxicity, thrombophlebitis, or nephrotoxicity. Thus, an approximate cephalosporin may be used cautiously except in patients who have had angioedema, anaphylaxis, or definite urticarial reactions to penicillin. *S. bovis* accounts for about 20 % of cases of penicillin-sensitive streptococcal endocarditis. *S. bovis* bacteremia usually arises in patients with gastrointestinal lesions, in particular inflammatory bowel disease, bleeding diverticula, polyposis, villous adenoma, and (rarely) carcinoma of the colon. Thus, gastrointestinal investigations should be undertaken to exclude these lesions.

NATIVE VALVE *ENTEROCOCCAL ENDOCARDITIS*

Therapy of native valve *Enterococcal endocarditis* remains difficult.

IV ampicillin 1.5–2 g every 4 h or penicillin 3–6 million U every 4 h plus gentamicin 1–1.4 mg/kg every 8 h for 4–6 weeks **or**

Ceftriaxone sodium 2 g/24 h IV/IM in one dose for 4 weeks plus gentamicin 3 mg/kg per 24 h IV in three equally divided doses for 2 weeks.

Enterococcal endocarditis is usually caused by *S. faecalis* and rarely by *S. faecium* or *S. durans*. These organisms are relatively resistant to most antibiotics. Penicillin and vancomycin are only bacteriostatic, and in this situation many strains are resistant to penicillin as well as streptomycin.

Vancomycin dose: 30 mg/kg per 24 h IV in two equally divided doses not to exceed 2 g/ 24 h. Vancomycin therapy is recommended only in the presence of normal renal function and for patients unable to tolerate penicillin or ceftriaxone therapy.

No single antibiotic consistently produces bactericidal activity against enterococci in vivo or in vitro. However, bactericidal synergy between the penicillins and streptomycin or gentamicin has been well documented. Thus, antibiotic combinations are necessary to eradicate the infection. A combination of penicillin or ampicillin and/or gentamicin is standard therapy. There is some evidence that amoxicillin is more rapidly bactericidal than ampicillin and may be more active against *S. faecalis*. Gentamicin is more effective than streptomycin and is more conveniently given IV. Thus, it is the aminoglycoside of choice.

Enterococcal endocarditis in the penicillin-allergic patient: A combination of vancomycin and gentamicin for 6 weeks is recommended, notwithstanding the potential toxicity of the combination. Unfortunately, "third-generation" cephalosporins are relatively inactive against enterococci.

Other Bacteria Causing IE

Other bacteria and suggested antibiotics include:

- Nutritionally variant viridans streptococci (NVVS), for example, *Streptococcus mitis*, *S. anginosus*, and other strains may be missed if blood cultures are not quickly subcultured on special media that support the growth of NVVS. These organisms were believed to be the cause of some cases of "culture-negative" endocarditis. Treatment is similar to that for Enterococcal endocarditis with ampicillin or penicillin and gentamicin for 4–6 weeks.
- *H. influenzae* and *H. parainfluenzae* are best treated with ampicillin and gentamicin IV for 6 weeks or more.
- *P. aeruginosa*: Tobramycin with carbenicillin is one combination of value.
- *P. cepacia* is often sensitive to trimethoprim–sulfamethoxazole.
- *Chlamydia psittaci* endocarditis is very rare. Treatment includes the use of tetracycline or doxycycline 200 mg orally daily; valve replacement is suggested as necessary in most cases.
- The Q fever organism is difficult to eradicate with tetracycline. A combination of cotrimoxazole and rifampin is advisable, but surgery may be finally required.

Right-Sided Endocarditis

IE in IV drug users is right sided in approximately 63 % and is caused by *Staphylococcus* in approximately 77 %, streptococci in approximately 5 %, and enterococci in only approximately 2 %; it is polymicrobial in approximately 8 % with absence of fungi. By contrast, left-sided IE occurs in approximately 37 % with approximately 23 % caused by *Staphylococcus*, approximately 15 % by streptococci, >24 % by enterococci, gram-negatives by approximately 13 %, and fungi by approximately 12 %. Right-sided endocarditis has increased in incidence because of IV drug abuse. *S. aureus* is the commonest infecting organism, followed by *P. aeruginosa* in some cities and, less commonly, streptococci, *Serratia marcescens*, gram-negatives, and *Candida*. The tricuspid valve is commonly affected and occasionally the pulmonary valve. The murmur of tricuspid regurgitation is commonly missed; the murmur can be augmented by deep inspiration and hepatojugular reflux. Also, pleuropneumonic symptoms may mask and delay diagnosis.

Therapy: Empirical therapy is commenced as outlined earlier and adjusted when culture and sensitivities are available. TEE differentiation of vegetations into less or greater than 1.0 cm diameter is helpful in directing surgical intervention. Vegetations <1.0 cm are usually cured by antibiotic therapy for 4–6 weeks, as well as about two-thirds of cases seen with vegetations >1.0 cm. If in the latter category fever persists beyond 3 weeks without a cause such as abscess, phlebitis, drug fever, or inadequate antibiotic levels, valve replacement should be contemplated.

Gentamicin and Tobramycin

Dosage:	1.5–2 mg/kg loading dose and then 3–5 mg/kg daily in divided doses every 8 h
Predose level (trough):	<2 µg/mL (2 mg/L)
Postdose level (peak):	<10 µg/mL (10 mg/L)

The normal dose interval every 8 h can vary (e.g., every 24 h), depending on creatinine clearance, age, sex, and lean body weight. Despite the use of nomograms, errors are not unusual and it is advisable to have repeated aminoglycoside serum concentrations (ASCs) to achieve adequate peak levels and therefore therapeutic success without causing nephrotoxicity or ototoxicity. Gentamicin trough concentrations >2 mg/L appear to be more important than high peak concentrations in the causation of ototoxocity.

The usual recommended dose of gentamicin of 3 mg/kg/day may not achieve optimal peak and trough ASCs in more than 50 % of patients with normal renal function. In young adults the dose may need to be given every 6 h. Do not rely on the serum creatinine level as an estimate of glomerular filtration rate (GFR). If the estimated GFR is 40–70 mL/min, give the dose every 12 h; 20–39 mL/min every 24 h; and 5–19 mL/min every 48 h. Beyond age 70 the estimated GFR formula is inaccurate. Caution is needed to avoid toxicity effects of these antibiotics. In such difficult cases, it is advisable to obtain the assistance of an ID specialist and to warn the patient of the dangers of the therapy.

Troughs and Peaks. The trough ASC is best taken immediately before the dose and the peak 30 min after the end of an IV infusion. If the ASC trough is too high (>2 μg/mL), extend the dosing interval. If the peak is too high (>10 μg/mL), decrease the dose. Peak levels must not exceed 14 μg/mL (14 μg/L).

Fungal Endocarditis

Major predisposing factors for the development of fungal endocarditis are previous valve surgery and IV drug abuse. Most commonly infection is caused by *Candida* (66 %) or occasionally *Aspergillus* or *Histoplasma*, and rarely *Coccidioides* and *Cryptococcus*. Except for *Candida*, fungi are difficult to grow from blood cultures. Thus, diagnosis may be difficult. Sometimes the diagnosis is made from examination of an arterial embolus. Serological tests (CFT) for *Candida*, *Histoplasma*, and *Cryptococcus* are useful in monitoring therapy and may be the clue to deep fungal infection.

The diagnosis of fungal endocarditis is often impossible to establish. The clinical circumstances (e.g., previous prolonged course of antibiotics) sometimes lead to suspicion, as does failure to detect other organisms or failure to respond to other antimicrobial agents. Amphotericin exerts antifungal activity by binding to ergosterol in fungal cell walls.

Side effects can be minimized by IV administration of hydrocortisone 100 mg and diphenhydramine 50 mg before each dose. Monitor renal function, blood count, and platelets. Hypokalemia and hypomagnesemia may occur.

Drug name:	**Amphotericin B**
Trade names:	Amphocil, Fungizone
Dosage:	IV: 1-mg test dose over 4 h; if tolerated, give 10-mg dose in 500 mL 5 % dextrose over 12 h and then 0.25 mg/kg/day. Increase by 0.25 mg/kg/day to reach 0.5–1 mg/kg/day. Usually 25–50 mg is given in 500 mL 5 % dextrose over 6 h once daily. Maximum dose range: 35–50 mg/day. **Do not** exceed 90 mg/day. *See* text for further advice

If the organism is sensitive to flucytosine (5-fluorocytosine), this drug can be added in a dose of 37.5 mg/kg every 6 h (dose and interval to be altered, depending on creatinine clearance). When used in combination with flucytosine, the dose of amphotericin B should be reduced to 0.3 mg/kg/day (Cohen 1982).

The toxicity of the drugs and the resistance of the organisms often necessitate valve replacement, especially in patients with a prosthetic valve. Valve replacement is strongly recommended. The prognosis is generally poor.

Histoplasma is the only infection that is often successfully managed medically.

Anticoagulant Therapy in Endocarditis

- Avoid heparin except when absolutely necessary.
- If warfarin is used, keep the prothrombin time to 1.25–1.5 times the normal control value or the International Normalized Ratio (INR) to 2–3. This may be necessary in patients with prosthetic heart valves who were previously taking anticoagulants.

Indications for surgery: the decision to operate and the timing of operation are of critical importance, especially in patients with prosthetic heart valves and most patients with gram-negative endocarditis.

Heart Failure Complicating Endocarditis

HF is associated with a grave prognosis with medical or surgical therapy. In the presence of HF, the decision to delay surgery to prolong the duration of preoperative antibiotic therapy carries with it the risk of permanent ventricular failure and is not recommended. Evaluation with TEE helps to delineate the causes and severity of HF.

Suggested indications for early surgical intervention are:

- The development of or deterioration in left or right heart failure. Native valve endocarditis complicated by HF has a high mortality rate that can be improved significantly by early surgical intervention.
- Sudden onset or worsening of aortic or mitral incompetence with precipitation of HF.
- Patients with prosthetic valve endocarditis: advise surgical intervention after infection has been brought under control because of the poor chance of achieving a long-term cure with antibiotics alone. Immediate surgery without delay for:
- Precipitation of HF.
- Dehiscence.
- Abscess formation.
- Fungal infection, especially of a prosthetic valve, is virtually never cured medically and requires early intervention.

- Gram-negative infection (mostly cannot be cured with antibiotics).
- Resistant organism or recurrent infection.
- Accessible mycotic aneurysms.
- Most patients with left-sided gram-negative endocarditis are rarely completely cured with antibiotics and may present a difficult decision.
- Rare organisms, e.g., *Brucella* or Q fever (*Coxiella*), known to be difficult to eradicate and showing no response after 3 weeks of treatment.
- Relapse after 6 weeks of adequate medical therapy.
- Aneurysm of the sinus of Valsalva.
- Septal abscess (suggested by increasing degree of atrioventricular block).
- Valve ring abscesses.
- Patients with repeated arterial embolization. (Embolization, Osler nodes, change in murmur, or congestive heart failure may develop, however, during adequate medical therapy or when treatment/cure has been established.) Right-sided endocarditis is associated with a 70–100 % incidence of pulmonary emboli; such recurrent emboli are not an indication for surgery.

PROPHYLAXIS OF BACTERIAL ENDOCARDITIS

Bacterial endocarditis is hard to prevent. Endocarditis occurred in 6 % of 304 patients with prosthetic valves undergoing 390 procedures without prophylaxis. No cases of endocarditis occurred in 229 patients undergoing 287 procedures with prior prophylaxis (Horstkotte et al. 1991). About 20 % of cases of IE are believed to be of dental origin, and in approximately 60 % of cases the portal of entry cannot be identified (MacMahon et al. 1986).

In over 40 % of cases, infection occurs on valves not known to be abnormal, especially on bicuspid aortic valves and in patients with MVP. Except for prosthetic valves, prophylaxis is aimed at streptococci, which account for only about 65 % of all cases of endocarditis.

Prophylaxis is not indicated for dental work in cardiac patients with pacemakers, implantable cardioverter defribillators (ICDs), and stents.

The American Heart Association (AHA) guidelines include the following:

The guidelines (AHA 2007) advise prophylaxis only for high-risk cases. This high-risk group includes:

1. Patients with a prosthetic heart valve or prosthetic material used for valve repair.
2. Patients with a past history of infective endocarditis.
3. Patients with cardiac valvulopathy after cardiac transplantation.
4. Specific patients with congenital heart disease.

The guidelines have been modified somewhat, however, during 2008 to pacify many clinicians.

- The list is clinically flawed.
- In select circumstances, the committee also understands that some clinicians and some patients may still feel more comfortable continuing with prophylaxis for infective endocarditis, particularly for those with bicuspid aortic valve or coarctation of the aorta, severe mitral valve prolapsed, or hypertrophic obstructive cardiomyopathy (ACC/AHA 2008).

Thus, some clinicians including the author will continue to prescribe antibiotic coverage for patients with aortic stenosis and rheumatic valvular disease, including significant mitral valve prolapse causing definite regurgitation. The guidelines are not applicable to developing and undeveloped countries.

Several notable experts in the field have criticized the new guidelines. These are only guidelines, and all practitioners in all circumstances need not necessarily follow them Bach (2009). The notion of individually weighing risks and benefit is not irrational, especially in a setting where there are no data that refute a time-honored standard of care.

When given a choice, most of my patients remain comfortable continuing to use antibiotic prophylaxis. If and when prospective, randomized trials are performed, rethinking individual decisions will again make sense. The author agrees with this advice.

Maron and Lever (2009) emphasized that the "New" recommendations, which represent a striking change from the original guidelines followed for more than 50 years, are based largely on two risk versus benefit assumptions: significant mortality or morbidity (e.g., anaphylaxis) associated with prophylactic antibiotic therapy and a lack of evidence (particularly, randomized trials) supporting the efficacy of antibiotic prophylaxis in the prevention of infective endocarditis. Withholding antibiotics from patients with HCM will unavoidably have the effect of unnecessarily creating several new cases of IE each year.

- We are at a loss to understand how these AHA recommendations, which we believe should be revised, are in the best interests of the HCM patient population, and for many other valvular disorders (Maron and Lever 2009).

In the UK: Prophylaxis against infective endocarditis: antimicrobial prophylaxis against infective endocarditis in adults and children undergoing interventional procedures see NICE 2008.

Older Regimen Acceptable to Many

- Prior to the 2007–2008 ACC/AHA practice guidelines, patients with valvular heart disease (low to high risk) were given antibiotics 1 h prior to all dental or surgical procedures. Fortunately, this old regimen may continue in several countries worldwide and are presented below because the ACC/AHA practice guidelines address patient populations (and healthcare providers) residing in North America and lacks clear thinking (Khan 2011).
- There is little doubt that IE can and does occur in patients with valvular heart disease following dental procedures.

Antibiotic Prophylaxis

- General prophylaxis: amoxicillin (adults)—2 g; children—50 mg/kg administered orally 1 h before the procedure.
- For patients unable to take oral medications, give ampicillin 2 g intramuscularly or intravenously; children—50 mg/kg IM or IV within 30 min before the procedure.
- For patients allergic to penicillin: clindamycin is recommended 600 mg orally for adults; children—20 mg/kg IV within 30 min before procedure; or azithromycin 500 mg for adults; children—15 mg/kg orally 1 h before procedure.

Prophylactic Regimens for Genitourinary, Gastrointestinal Procedures Are Follows:

- High-risk patients should be given ampicillin, 2 g intramuscularly or intravenously, plus gentamicin 1.5 mg/kg not to exceed 120 mg within 30 min of starting the procedure; 6 h later ampicillin 1 g IM or IV, or amoxicillin 1 g orally.
- For high-risk patients and for patients allergic to penicillin or amoxicillin, give vancomycin 1 g IV over 1–2 h; complete the infusion within 30 min of starting the procedure.

Antibiotic is given orally for dental work done under local anesthetic. It is given intravenously for patients with prosthetic valves, patients with highest risk of developing endocarditis, or patients who are having a general anesthetic.

- All dental procedures that are likely to result in gingival bleeding such as extractions, root canal, scaling and cleaning, surgery in the oral cavity, biopsies, and many surgical operations and tests such as cystoscopy require antibiotic coverage to prevent endocarditis.

The guideline advises oral antibiotic therapy, amoxicillin 2 g to be administered 1 h prior to the procedure when a local anesthetic is used.

Patients allergic to penicillin usually receive clindamycin 600 mg 1 h prior to the procedure. For surgery on the intestine or the genitourinary systems, other antibiotics are required intravenously.

- For high-risk patients, prophylaxis is reasonable for all dental procedures that involve manipulation of either gingival tissue or the periapical region of teeth or perforation of oral mucosa.

Prophylaxis is no longer recommended for prevention of infective endocarditis for GI or GU procedures, including diagnostic esophago-gastroduodenoscopy or colonoscopy. But it can be acceptable for colonoscopy and removal of polyps or other lesions in patients with prosthetic valves and those with rheumatic valvular disease.

However, in high-risk patients with infections of the GI or GU tract, it is reasonable to administer antibiotic therapy to prevent wound infection or sepsis. For high risk patients undergoing elective cystoscopy or other urinary tract manipulation who have enterococcal urinary tract infection or colonization, antibiotic therapy to eradicate enterococci from the urine before the procedure is reasonable.

There is no evidence to recommend using antibiotics before procedures on the gastrointestinal or urinary tracts (Punnoose et al. 2012).

- The British Society for Antimicrobial Chemotherapy did differ with the ACC/AHA 2008 in continuing to recommend prophylaxis for high-risk patients before gastrointestinal (GI) or genitourinary (GU) procedures associated with bacteremia (ESC 2009).

The Guideline Development Group (GDG) comprised NICE's short clinical guidelines technical team and experts from many branches of medicine and dentistry, "The GDG were unanimous in their conclusions about which patients

with preexisting cardiac lesions are at risk of developing
IE. They also agreed that the body of clinical and cost-
effectiveness evidence reviewed in this guideline supported
a recommendation that at-risk patients undergoing interventional procedures should no longer be given antibiotic prophylaxis against IE. In particular, the GDG were convinced
by the evidence suggesting that current antibiotic prophylaxis
regimens might result in a net loss of life" (NICE 2008).

On the basis of data complete through 2010, there has been
no perceivable increase in the incidence of veridans Group
Streptococci **in Olmsted County, Minnesota, since the publication of the 2007 American Heart Association endocarditis prevention guidelines** (DeSimone et al. 2012).

REFERENCES

ACC/AHA 2008: Nishimura RA, Carabello BA, Faxon DP, et al. ACC/
    AHA 2008 guideline update on valvular heart disease: focused update
    on infective endocarditis: a report of the American College of
    Cardiology/American Heart Association Task Force on Practice
    Guidelines. J Am Coll Cardiol. 2008;52:676–85.
Bach DS. Perspectives on the American College of Cardiology/American
    Heart Association guidelines for the prevention of infective endocar-
    ditis. J Am Coll Cardiol. 2009;53:1852–4.
Cohen J. Antifungal chemotherapy. Lancet. 1982;2:1323.
DeSimone DC, Tleyjeh IM, de Sa Correa DD, et al. Incidence of infective
    endocarditis caused by viridans group streptococci before and after
    publication of the 2007 American heart association's endocarditis
    prevention guidelines. Circulation. 2012;126:60–4.
ESC: Endorsed by the European Society of Clinical Micro, Authors/Task
    Force Members, Habib G, Hoen B, Tornos P, et al. Guidelines on the
    prevention, diagnosis, and treatment of infective endocarditis (new
    version 2009): the task force on the prevention, diagnosis, and treat-
    ment of infective endocarditis of the European society of cardiology
    (ESC). Eur Heart J. 2009;30(19):2369–413.
Horstkotte D, Sick P, Bircks W, et al. Effectiveness of antibiotic prophy-
    laxis to prevent prosthetic valve endocarditis: evidence in humans.
    J Am Coll Cardiol. 1991;71:2125.
Khan MG. Endocarditis. In: Encyclopedia of heart diseases. New York:
    Springer; 2011. p. 471.

MacMahon SW, Hickey AJ, Wilcken DEL, et al. Risk of infective endocarditis in mitral valve prolapse with and without precordial systolic murmurs. Am J Cardiol. 1986;58:105.

Maron BJ, Lever H. In defense of antimicrobial prophylaxis for prevention of infective endocarditis in patients with hypertrophic cardiomyopathy. J Am Coll Cardiol. 2009;54(24):2339–40.

NICE Short Clinical Guidelines Technical Team. Prophylaxis against infective endocarditis: antimicrobial prophylaxis against infective endocarditis in adults and children undergoing interventional procedures. London: National Institute for Health and Clinical Excellence; 2008.

Punnoose AR, Lynm C, Golub RM. TOPICS: antibiotics, bacterial endocarditis. JAMA. 2012;308(9):935.

Towns ML, Reller LB. Diagnostic methods as current best practices and guidelines for isolation of bacteria and fungi in infective endocarditis. Infect Dis Clin North Am. 2002;16:363.

Wilson W, Taubert KA, Gewitz M, et al. Prevention of infective endocarditis. Guidelines from the American heart association. A guideline from the American heart association rheumatic fever, endocarditis, and Kawasaki disease committee, council on cardiovascular disease in the young, and the council on clinical cardiology, council on cardiovascular surgery and anesthesia, and the quality of care and outcomes research interdisciplinary working group. Circulation. 2007;116:1736–54.

2014 AHA/ACC guideline for the management of patients with valvular heart disease: a report of the American College of Cardiology/American Heart Association Task Force on Practice Guidelines Circulation 2014;129:e521–643.

17 Dyslipidemias

DIAGNOSIS

Persons with a marked increase in serum levels of cholesterol to >350 mg/dL (9 mmol/L) represent a very small group of individuals in the population at very high risk for developing atherosclerotic coronary disease. Less than 20 % of these individuals (0.1 % of the population) have a genetic abnormality, characterized by cellular low-density lipoprotein cholesterol (LDL-C) receptor deficiency (Brown and Goldstein 1979). Thus, emphasis is now correctly placed on the vast population of individuals with a total serum cholesterol concentration in the range of 200–265 mg/dL (5.5–6.9 mmol/L), in whom the majority of heart attacks occur.

FASTING OR NON-FASTING LDL-C?

Patients enrolled in the National Health and Nutrition Examination Survey III (NHANES III), a nationally representative cross-sectional survey performed between 1988 and 1994, were stratified based on fasting status (≥8 h or <8 h) and followed for a mean of 14.0 years.

Conclusion—Non-fasting LDL-C has similar prognostic value as that of fasting LDL-C. National and international agencies should consider reevaluating the recommendation that patients fast before obtaining a lipid panel (Doran et al. 2014). The author advise fasting −12 hr for LDL-C in diabetics and for all with elevated triglycerides.

© Springer Science+Business Media New York 2015
M. Gabriel Khan, *Cardiac Drug Therapy*, Contemporary Cardiology,
DOI 10.1007/978-1-61779-962-4_17

The LDL-C is the main marker and discussion and clinical practice is centered around goal levels depending on risk. The recent guidelines have demoted the LDL-C somewhat; there advice is flawed.

Boekholdt et al. (2014) report a patient-level meta-analysis of data from large statin trials as follows: "in terms of risk reduction, there was a clear relationship between LDL-C level attained and cardiovascular risk, with the major cardiovascular event rate at 1 year increasing incrementally from 4.4 % in those with LDL-C levels <50 mg/dL, to 10.9 % for LDL-C between 50 and <70 mg/dL, 16 % between 70 and <100 mg/dL (1.8 mmol/L), and up to 34.4 % in those with LDL-C 190 mg/dL (4.9 mmol/L). This relationship supports the premise that 'lower is better' when it comes to LDL-C goals" (Ben-Yehuda and DeMaria 2014).

- The focus should not be on total cholesterol, HDL-C levels, ratios, or calculation of risk.
- Most national guidelines agree that the recommended lipoprotein targets of therapy remains the LDL-cholesterol.
- It is important to identify the number of CHD risk factors: Framingham 10-year absolute CHD risk, as advised (Goff et al. 2014, the 2013 ACC/AHA guideline). But calculation of risk without LDL numbers is not logical.
- Managing risk related to LDL-C is vital in therapy for patients at risk for atherosclerotic cardiovascular disease events given its important etiologic role in atherogenesis (Morris et al. 2014).
- Dyslipidemia, particularly increased LDL-C, is the major culprit underlying the development of atheroma in arteries. But why some individuals with severe atheromatous disease do not succumb to acute MI while others with mild to moderate atherosclerotic disease are hit by an acute MI is largely unknown.
- The evidence for heritability of AMI is striking, with a positive family history being one of the most important risk factors for this complex trait (Wang et al. 2004). Genetic studies indicate that the heritability of AMI is much more

impressive than that of atherosclerotic CAD (Willett 2002; Topol et al. 2001), which in the majority remains stable and without plaque erosion or rupture.

- Although more than 50 million American adults have some atheromatous coronary artery disease (CAD), only a small fraction will ever develop erosion, fissuring, or plaque rupture that culminates in AMI (Topol 2005) or sudden death (see Chap. 15 cardiac arrest).
- Lifestyle changes must be made to reduce risk (Eckel et al. 2014).
- An ideal LDL-C level that carries a reduced risk for CAD events is <100 mg/dL (2.6 mmol/L) for all asymptomatic adults ages 30–80.
- Stable CAD, established atherosclerosis, and presence of several risk factors including family history of MI necessitates an LDL-C<2 mmol/L (77 mg/dL). In many, this ideal is difficult to achieve without drug therapy. For patients with acute coronary syndrome (ACS) or proven ischemia, a level of 1.2–1.6 mmol/L (45–62 mg/dL) is advisable.
- HDL-C<1.0 mmol/L (38 mg/dL) appears to increase CAD risk but is unproven. The LDL-C remains the main marker of risk. Low HDL-C is a novel lipid phenotype that appears to be more prevalent among Asian populations, in whom it is associated with increased coronary risk (Huxley et al. 2011).

Conversion Formula for mg to mmol

- LDL-C is calculated by the laboratory, utilizing the total cholesterol (TC) and >12-h fasting triglyceride (TG) as follows: LDL-C mg/dL=TC−HDL-C−(TG÷5). For LDL-C using mmol/L, divide by 2.2 instead of 5. If the TG level is >400 mg/dL (4 mmol/L), the calculation is not valid.
- To convert total-C, LDL-C, or HDL-C from mg/dL to mmol/L, divide by 38.5 or multiply by 0.02586.

Secondary Causes of Dyslipidemias

A secondary cause commonly accounts for dyslipidemia, and the following conditions must be sought and treated or regulated:

- Dietary
- Diabetes mellitus
- Hypothyroidism
- Nephrotic syndrome
- Chronic liver disease
- Obesity
- Dysgammaglobulinemia (monoclonal gammopathy)
- Obstructive jaundice
- Biliary cirrhosis
- Pancreatitis
- Excess alcohol consumption
- Estrogens/progesterone
- Glycogen storage disorders
- Lipodystrophy
- Medications

1. Dietary: Excessive carbohydrate intake; weight gain; increased saturated fat or alcohol intake.
2. Diseases: Diabetes mellitus, hypothyroidism, pancreatitis, nephrotic syndrome, liver disease (obstructive jaundice, biliary cirrhosis), and monoclonal gammopathy.
3. Medications: Oral contraceptives and diuretics may unfavorably alter cholesterol and HDL-C cholesterol. The serum lipid alterations produced by beta-blockers have been exaggerated and perhaps exploited. Acebutolol with weak intrinsic sympathomimetic activity (ISA) caused no significant changes in total or HDL-C cholesterol at 24 months.

In the Norwegian timolol multicenter study, timolol decreased total cardiac and sudden deaths regardless of serum lipid levels (Gundersen et al. 1985). Some studies indicate that non-ISA beta-blockers cause no significant alteration of HDL-C (Valimaki et al. 1986), whereas others indicate a small decrease of 5 %. There is no evidence to support the notion that a 5 % decrease in HDL-C increases risks. The variable and mild decrease in the HDL-C (1–7 %) caused by a beta-blocking drug should not persuade against their use because these agents have important salutary effects and a proven role in prolongation of life. Thus, when needed, it is advisable to combine a beta-blocker with statin in patients at high risk for CHD events. Beta-blockers may increase triglyceride levels in some individuals. The evidence linking triglycerides with an increased risk of CHD remains elusive. Markedly raised levels of triglycerides >200 mg/dl appear to be a significant risk factor in women but is unproven. Low HDL-C is a novel lipid phenotype that appears to be more prevalent among Asian populations; it is associated with increased coronary risk.

DIETARY THERAPY

Dietary therapy is necessary in all patients with hyperlipidemia. In individuals without evidence of CHD or cardiovascular disease, drugs are utilized only after a concerted effort by the physician and patient to lower serum cholesterol adequately. Fortunately, raised levels of triglycerides are virtually always controlled by carbohydrate and alcohol restriction, weight reduction, and exercise. There is no need to add niacin or a fibrate to control triglyceride levels because the risk of myopathy is not justifiable.

1. Phase I diet: Fat intake reduced to 30 % of food energy with approximately 15 % from saturated fats and 10 % from polyunsaturated. Cholesterol intake should be <300 mg, carbohydrate 55 %, and protein 15 % of calories daily. This modification is recommended for the general population.
2. Phase III: Intake of fat 20 %, approx 7 % total daily calories from saturated fats, cholesterol 100–150 mg, carbohydrate 65 %, and protein 15 % of calories. The ratio of polyunsaturated fat to saturated fat (P/S) should be near 1.0. The recommendations in the United Kingdom are not as restrictive. For the general population or those at risk, the recommendation is an intake of fat of 35 %, with saturated fat 11 % of food energy. Polyunsaturated acids should reach 7 % with P/S ratio about 0.45 % (10). The UK panel claims that the effects on the population of a P/S ratio of 1.0 or beyond are unknown (Trustwell 1984).

In constructing diets, the following points should be considered. Most studies show that saturated and monounsaturated fats modestly raise the HDL-C concentration; high consumption of polyunsaturated fats lowers the level of HDL-C slightly (Pietinen and Huttunen 1987). A reduction in saturated fat intake from 35–40 % to 20–25 % of energy intake lowers HDL-C concentration irrespective of the type of fat (Pietinen and Huttunen 1987). Depending on the dose, marine (*n*-3 polyunsaturated) oils may modestly increase HDL-C levels and decrease serum cholesterol and TG levels and platelet aggregation (Sanders and Roshanai 1983). The favorable effects are not consistent, and occasionally a fall in HDL-C concentration occurs (Nestel et al. 1984; Illingworth et al. 1984).

• Diets containing 200 g of mackerel raised HDL-C levels in two studies (Singer et al. 1985; Van Lossonczy et al. 1985). However, 1 or 2 g of fish consumed twice weekly for 3 months produced no changes in HDL-C in a large group of subjects (Fehily et al. 1983).

Care is needed to avoid overindulgence because marine oils also contain a significant amount of cholesterol. One hundred grams of cod liver oil contain approximately 19 g of omega-3 fatty acids but 570 mg of cholesterol (Hepburn et al. 1986: 18). One hundred grams of salmon or herring or commercial fish body oils contain approximately 485, 766, and 600 mg cholesterol, respectively. Noncholesterol foods with abundant omega-3 fatty acids include purslane (*Portulaca oleracea*) (Exler and Wehlrauch 1986), common beans, soybeans, walnuts, walnut oil, wheat-germ oil, butternuts, and seaweed.

• A Mediterranean-type diet is strongly recommended: no day without fruit; abundant fresh vegetables, olive oil, avocado, more fiber, fish, nuts, and less meat; butter and cream replaced by polyunsaturated/monounsaturated margarine, non-trans fatty acids. A trial comparing a Mediterranean-based alpha-linolenic acid-rich diet with a postinfarct low-fat diet in the secondary prevention of CHD reported a risk ratio of 0.24 for cardiovascular death and 0.30 for total mortality in the linolenic acid group at 27 months of follow-up (de Lorgeril et al. 1994: 20). The Lyon Heart Study confirmed post-myocardial infarction protection (de Lorgeril et al. 1999).

- Nuts such as almonds, walnuts, hazelnuts, and pecans are high in beneficial poly- and monounsaturated fat as well as arginine, the precursor of nitric oxide (NO), which causes vasodilation. Arginine/NO appears to improve endothelial dysfunction and may improve performance in some patients with claudication and also angina (Maxwell et al. 2002).

- Trans fatty acids increase LDL-C and must be curtailed. Major sources of food containing trans isomers include margarine, cookies (biscuits), cake and white bread, shortening, some margarine, fried foods, and cookies prepared with these fats (Willett et al. 1994: 24). The effect of intake of trans fatty acids was evaluated in the Nurses' Health Study of 85,095 women without diagnosed CHD, stroke, or dyslipidemia in 1980. At 8-year follow-up, intake of trans isomers was directly related to the risk of CHD (Willett et al. 1994).

DRUG THERAPY

- The assignment to three categories of risk by the Adult Treatment Panel (ATP 2004) III includes an important 10-year risk score of >20 % or <20 %, which remains clinically helpful (Grundy et al. Expert Panel 2004). The recent guidelines (2013) are complicated and flawed.

- Because approximately 66 % of diabetics die of cardiovascular disease, they are considered CHD risk equivalent and to have a 10-year risk for a CHD event >20 %, so do patients with abdominal aortic aneurysm (AAA), peripheral vascular disease (PVD), and significant carotid disease. Guidelines for drug therapy are given in Table 17-1.

- The recent guidelines deal mainly with risk assessment and place too much attention on this and unfortunately less emphasis on LDL-C (Goff et al. 2014, the 2013 ACC/AHA guideline).

Table 17-1

Guidelines for the management of elevated LDL-C cholesterol: when to use drug therapy

CAD[a]	Several risk factors[b]	Average risk (one or two risk factors)	Low risk
LDL-C	LDL-C	LDL-C	LDL-C
>100 mg/dL	>130 mg/dL	>160 mg/dL	>180 mg/dL[c]
(2.5 mmol/L)	(3.5 mmol/L)	(4 mmol/L)	(4.5 mmol/L)
Drug therapy	Drug therapy	Drug therapy	Consider drug therapy
Goal	Goal	Goal	Goal
<80 mg/dL	<100 mg/dL	<120 mg/dL	<130 mg/dL
(<2 mmol/L)	(<2.5 mmol/L)	(<3.0 mmol/L)	(<3.5 mmol/L)
Very high risk[d]			
Goal			
<1.8 mmol/L[e]			
<70 mg/dL			

See Chap. 22
LDL-C low-density lipoprotein cholesterol
[a]Coronary artery disease or diabetes
[b]Including established atherosclerosis
[c]After 6 months dietary therapy
[d]Acute coronary syndrome
[e]Rosuvastatin achieved goal in SATURN (Nicholls et al. 2011)

• Many agree that the guidelines should be modified. The guide advises that statins should be commenced in patients whose risk of a heart attack, stroke, or death from CHD (coronary heart disease) in the next 10 years is at least 7.5 %. The risk-factor calculation uses sex, age, race, total cholesterol level, HDL cholesterol level, systolic blood pressure, treatment for high blood pressure, diabetes, and smoking. Strangely, no target on-treatment LDL cholesterol levels are given specified.

STATINS

The management of dyslipidemia has been revolutionized with the expanded use of statins (3-hydroxy-3-methylglutaryl coenzyme A (HMG CoA) reductase inhibitors). The statins are competitive inhibitors of HMG-CoA reductase, the key enzyme catabolizing the early rate-limiting step in the biosynthesis of cholesterol within the hepatocyte. The lowering of intracellular cholesterol levels, resulting in a small increase in the number of receptors on the hepatocyte through the process of upregulation, results in increased clearance of circulating LDL-C cholesterol and a decrease in total serum cholesterol levels.

Pleiotropic effects of statins include antithrombotic, anti-inflammatory, decreased hsCRP, and antioxidant-reduced endothelial dysfunction. Violi et al. present experimental data in support of the ability of statins to interfere directly with the clotting system and platelet activation, as well as the clinical settings that suggest that statins exert beneficial effects related to their antithrombotic properties (Violi et al. 2013).

Available statins include atorvastatin, fluvastatin, lovastatin, simvastatin, pravastatin, and rosuvastatin. The more powerful LDL-C-lowering agents, rosuvastatin and atorvastatin, are effective in reducing:

- LDL-C cholesterol to goal levels in the majority of patients
- Mortality in patients with CHD
- The incidence of MI in patients with CHD
- The degree of obstructive atheroma in coronary arteries (ASTEROID 2006; SATURN 2011)
- Regression in atheroma volume; see ASTEROID AND SATURN trials (Chap. 22)
- The risk of stroke

Statins Possess Subtle Differences

- The only hydrophilic agent excreted by the kidney is pravastatin. Thus, fewer adverse effects occur from drug interactions compared with lipophilic statins, which are hepatically metabolized see Chap. 21 Interactions.
- Lipophilic agents (atorvastatin, lovastatin, and simvastatin) are hepatically metabolized. Interactions may occur with cimetidine, cyclosporine, and other agents that use the cytochrome P-450 pathway (3A4).
- Rosuvastatin and fluvastatin engage hepatic 2C9; thus, caution is required particularly with cyclosporine, warfarin, and phenytoin. Rosuvastatin is partly renally eliminated and caution is needed in patients with eGFR < 40 ml/min. Atorvastatin is the only statin recommended for the management of mixed dyslipidemia; the drug decreases triglyceride levels ~10 %.
- Atorvastatin has been shown to raise fibrinogen levels by 22 % (Wierbicki et al. 1998).

Contraindications include hepatic dysfunction and concomitant use of nicotinic acid or fibrates, cyclosporin, other cytotoxic drugs, and erythromycin and similar antibiotics.

- **Avoid in women of childbearing age**. They are contraindicated in pregnancy and during lactation.

Advice and Adverse Effects

- Hypothyroidism should be managed adequately before starting treatment with a statin.
- Increase in hepatic transaminases greater than three times the upper limit of normal occurs in 1–2 % of patients receiving average maintenance and maximum dosages of these agents, respectively.

Monitoring of transaminase levels should be done every 4 months, and the drug should be discontinued if levels of these enzymes are raised. If drug treatment is considered essential, patients with an increase less than three times normal can be observed at least twice monthly. Increases of up to fivefold with or without myalgia occur in up to 3 % of patients, and levels >10 times normal with myalgia are observed in <1 %. Myalgia without an increase in creatine kinase (CK) concentration is not uncommon.

- Severe myositis with rhabdomyolysis with the risk of renal failure has occurred with the combination of HMG-CoA reductase inhibitors with gemfibrozil, fibrates and also with cyclosporine and colchicine. See Table 17-2.
- It is advisable to give the individual administered a statin a requisition for an emergency blood test for CK and creatinine and a urinalysis if muscle pains occur without associated upper respiratory tract infection (URTI) symptoms. The statin is discontinued immediately pending results of these tests.

Statins can rarely cause hepatitis and jaundice, hepatic failure, and pancreatitis. Statins can cause interstitial lung disease albeit rarely. Patients should report immediately if cough, dyspnea, or weight loss is not easily explained.

Gastrointestinal disturbances, headache, peripheral neuropathy, amnesia, arthralgia, visual disturbance, alopecia, and rarely lupus erythematosus-like reactions have been reported.

- Myopathy has been noted with erythromycin and similar antibiotics combination, and other antibiotic interactions in seriously ill patients may ensue. Angioedema has been reported.
- Caution: it is necessary to discontinue these lipid-lowering agents during serious intercurrent illness and sepsis when other drugs that interact are being used.
- The anticoagulant effect of warfarin may be slightly enhanced by simvastatin administration, and digoxin levels may show a small increase: approx 10 % for simvastatin and approx 20 % for atorvastatin.
- Headaches are bothersome in up to 10 % of patients. A switch from one HMG-CoA reductase inhibitor to another may resolve headaches, chest or abdominal pain, or rash. Thrombocytopenia has been reported.

Table 17-2
Statins: pharmacokinetics and drug interactions

	Atorvastatin	Fluvastatin	Pravastatin	Rosuvastatin	Simvastatin
Pharmacokinetics					
Lipophilic (L) or hydrophilic (H)	L	Both	H	Both	L
Renal excretion	No	~10 % renal, ~90 % fecal	~60	~20 % renal, ~80 % fecal	No
Renal excretion patient in a renal failure or elderly patient[a]	No	Yes, if GFR <30 mL/min	Yes; caution if GFR <50 mL/min	Yes, if GFR <30 mL/min: use cautiously if GFR is 31–45 mL/min	No
Cytochrome P-450	3A4	2C9	Not known (multiple pathways)	2C9	3A4
Drug interactions					
Warfarin[b]—INR increased	No	Yes	No	Yes	No
Digoxin level increased	Yes (20 %)	<10 %	No	No	<10 %
Macrolide[c] antibiotics	Yes	No	No	No	Yes

Antifungal agents	Yes	No	No	Yes
Antiviral agents	Yes	No	No	Yes
Cyclosporine	Yes	Yes	Yes[d]	Yes
Fluoxetine and similar agents	Yes	No	No	Yes
Fibrates[e] or niacin[e]	Yes	Yes	Yes	Yes
Grapefruit juice	Yes	No	No	Yes
Phenytoin	No	Yes	Yes	No
Verapamil, diltiazem	Weak	No	No	Weak
Amiodarone		No	No	Yes[f]

Antacids may lower levels of rosuvastatin

Ranolazine: plasma concentration of simvastatin increased by ranolazine

Ticagrelor: plasma concentration of simvastatin increased

Colchicine combination with statin to be avoided/can cause myopathy

Modified from Khan, M Gabriel. *On Call Cardiology*. Philadelphia, Elsevier, 2006, p. 441

H hydrophilic, *INR* international normalized ratio, *L* lipophilic

[a] Contraindicated if severe renal failure, GFR <30 mL/min. Relatively contraindicated—the elderly (age >70) often have diminished renal function yet a normal serum creatinine, yet GFR 50–55 mL/min

[b] See Table 19.4 warfarin interactions

[c] Erythromycin, clarithromycin, troleandomycin, azithromycin

[d] Avoid concomitant use

[e] **Caution:** myopathy and rare rhabdomyolysis (combination of statin and fibrate or nicotinic acid, niacin is not recommended by the author)

[f] Warning: serious myopathy

- Lens opacities have been noted only in dogs given very high doses of these agents but have not been observed in patients. Current clinical data indicate that these agents do not cause cataracts (Tobert et al. 1990), but long-term effects beyond 15 years are unknown.
- Statins are less effective in patients with familial hypercholesterolemia because these individuals have very low or absent LDL-C receptor activity. In these patients, combination therapy is necessary.

CLINICAL TRIALS

- 4S: Scandinavian Simvastatin Survival

This hallmark study enrolled 4,444 patients with angina or previous heart attacks (79 %) and a **high total cholesterol 5.5–8 mmol/L.** The subjects were randomized to a double-blind treatment with simvastatin or placebo.

All patients followed a lipid-lowering diet. **Median follow-up was 5.4 years.**

Results: 256 patients (12 %) in the placebo group died, compared with 182 (8 %) in the simvastatin group. The relative risk of death in the simvastatin group was 0.70 $p=0.0003$). There were 189 coronary deaths in the placebo group and 111 in the simvastatin group, while noncardiovascular causes accounted for 49 and 46 deaths, respectively. 622 patients (28 %) in the placebo group and 431 (19 %) in the simvastatin group had one or more major coronary events. Other benefits of treatment included a 37 % reduction ($p<0.00001$) in the risk of undergoing myocardial revascularization procedures. Simvastatin administration caused a 25 % decrease in cholesterol and 35 % reduction in LDL cholesterol, a reduction that was meaningful. **Long-term treatment with simvastatin improves survival in CHD patients with hyperlipidemia** (Shepherd et al. 4S 1995).

- West of Scotland Study (Shepherd et al. 1995).
  In the so-called healthy Scottish men with **a high mean cholesterol level of 272** mg/dL, (7 mmol/L), **total mortality**

was not significantly decreased. Only nonfatal MIs were decreased significantly. *On probabilities these MI s could have been prevented by the use of daily aspirin*. Thus, it is not justifiable to apply the results of the West of Scotland trial to healthy men with cholesterol concentration in the range of ~200–240 mg/dL (5–6.2 mmol/L).

- CARE 1996: The Cholesterol and Recurrent Events *study involved post MI patients with cholesterol concentration in the low range (209±17 mg/dL*; 5.4–5.8 mmol/L) that is commonly seen in patients with acute coronary syndrome.

There was no decrease in total mortality rate. The number of fatal MIs was 38 versus 24 ($p = 0.07$). This is stated as a relative risk reduction of 37 %. Clinicians should not accept percentage relative risk reduction as significant if the p value is not expressed or is 0.04 or greater. Note that breast cancer occurred in 12 pravastatin-treated patients versus 1 in the control group ($p = 0.002$). It is important in women to evaluate the use of statins, particularly in patients who have a positive family history of breast cancer.

- LIPID study 1998: In the long-term intervention with pravastatin in ischemic disease, the effects of pravastatin (40 mg daily) were compared with those of a placebo over a **mean follow-up period of** 6.1 years in 9014 patients who were 31–75 years of age. The patients had a history of MI or hospitalization for unstable angina and initial plasma total cholesterol levels of 155–271 mg/dL (4.0–7.0 mmol/L). Baseline cholesterol was much higher than in the CARE study.

Results: Overall mortality was (633) 14.1 % in the placebo group and (498) 11.0 % in the pravastatin group (relative reduction in risk, 22 %; $p < 0.001$).

Deaths from CHD, the primary end point: 373 versus 287; pravastatin reduced the risk for CHD mortality by 24 % ($p < 0.001$) and significantly reduced nonfatal MIs and coronary revascularization (SATURN 2011 see Chap. 11).

Individual Statins

Simvastatin:

Drug name:	**Simvastatin**
Trade name:	Zocor
Supplied:	5, 10, 20, 40, 80 mg
Dosage:	5 or 10 mg with evening meal. Monitor hepatic transaminases and CK in 3–4 months with repeat serum cholesterol; if needed, increase to 20 mg once daily; max. 60 mg daily

Use other treatments if patients' LDL targets are not met with the 40-mg simvastatin dose. See the many interactions listed below. **The 80-mg dose has been abandoned; myopathy has been reported to be higher with this dose that resulted in an FDA warning.**

CAUTION: Do not use statins, particularly simvastatin, with medications that inhibit the enzyme (CYP3A4): they can increase the blood level of simvastatin:

- Amiodarone
- Itraconazole
- Ketoconazole
- Erythromycin-like antibiotics, azithromycin
- Clarithromycin
- Telithromycin
- HIV protease inhibitors
- Nefazodone

Do not use more than 10 mg of simvastatin, or avoid use with these medications:

- Gemfibrozil
- Cyclosporine
- Danazol
- Diltiazem or verapamil
- Colchicine
- Amiodarone

Among the statins, simvastatin has the most interactions (*see* Table 17-2).

Nonetheless high-dose simvastatin reduced the annualized rate of whole-brain atrophy in patients with secondary progressive multiple sclerosis compared with placebo and was well tolerated. These results support the advancement of this treatment to phase 3 testing (Chataway et al. 2014).

Pravastatin

Drug name:	**Pravastatin**
Trade names:	Pravachol, Lipostat
Supplied:	10-, 20-, 40-mg tablets
Dosage:	10–20 mg with evening meal, increasing in 3–4 months as required; max. 40 mg daily, with the same precautions as for lovastatin. Do not use if renal failure is present; maximum dose 10 mg in the elderly or if the GFR is 50–70 mL/min

Results of the Pravastatin Limitations of Atherosclerosis in the Coronary Arteries (PLAC) I trial (Pitt et al. 1995: 33) indicate that pravastatin therapy reduced progression of CHD by 40 % compared with placebo and caused a 54 % reduction in fatal and nonfatal infarctions. The study included 408 patients with a <50 % angiographically determined coronary stenosis. Patients were randomly assigned to pravastatin or placebo and followed up for 3 years with repeated angiography performed in 323 patients and determination of clinical events. Baseline characteristics: cholesterol level of about 230 mg/dL (5.9 mmol/L), LDL-C cholesterol of 162–165 mg/dL (4.2–4.3 mmol/L), HDL-C cholesterol of 41 mg/dL (1.1 mL/L). After 3 years of treatment, LDL-C cholesterol was reduced 28 %, and an 8 %

increase in HDL-C cholesterol was observed. There were 15 new lesions in the pravastatin group, compared with 33 in the placebo patients. It appears that pravastatin inhibits platelet mural thrombosis at the site of arterial injury. A histologic study of patients' arteries showed that pravastatin decreased platelet formation in the arterial wall in hypercholesterolemic patients.

Drug name:	**Atorvastatin**
Trade name:	Lipitor
Supplied:	Tablets: 10, 20, 40, 60, 80 mg
Dosage:	10–40 mg daily after the evening meal; max. 80 mg: mainly for acute coronary syndrome

Atorvastatin 10, 40, and 80 mg has been shown to cause a 38, 46, and 54 % decrease in LDL-C cholesterol, respectively.

In the atorvastatin versus revascularization treatment (AVERT) study, treatment with 80-mg atorvastatin caused a 36 % reduction in nonfatal MI, revascularization, and worsening angina compared with patients receiving angioplasty followed by usual care. In the Myocardial Ischemia Reduction with Aggressive Cholesterol Lowering (MIRACL) study, atorvastatin reduced early recurrent ischemic events in non-ST-elevation MI (NSTEMI) ACS patients treated within 14 days of an event (Schwartz et al. 2001, 4). In PROVE-IT TIMI 22, ACS patients showed a significant reduction in CAD outcomes when treated with atorvastatin 80 mg daily (Cannon et al. 2004 see Chap. 22 results).

ADVERSE EFFECTS AND INTERACTIONS

Flatulence and headaches occurred in 2 % of patients in trials. As with other statins metabolized by the cytochrome P-450 system (3A4), interactions occur with grapefruit juice and agents such as cimetidine and erythromycin series of antibiotics, and digoxin levels may increase 20 % but warfarin is not affected. **Colchicine caution with all statins**

Drug name:	**Rosuvastatin**
Trade name:	Crestor
Supplied:	10, 20, 40 mg
Dosage:	10–40 mg once daily. Do not use if severe renal failure is present

__In elderly or of Asian origin, start with 5 mg once daily__, if necessary to 10 mg max. 20 mg daily.

Caution: if renal failure is present. Commence at 5 mg; monitor closely at 10-mg dose; maximum 20 mg/day in patients age >75 or if GFR is 50–60 mL/min. Avoid if GFR is < 40 ml/min. UK advice: avoid if eGFR is less than 30 mL/min. Do not add fibrate to this drug particularly if renal dysfunction is present (see overuse of fibrates).

Rosuvastatin is the most powerful statin currently available. The drug has been shown to cause a 40–65 % reduction in LDL-C and ~ a 12 % increase in HDL-C beyond that of atorvastatin. The drug avoids the cytochrome P-450, 3A4 pathway, resulting in no interactions with drugs that use this pathway.

Caution: Cytochrome P-450, 2C9 is involved; thus caution is required, particularly with cyclosporine, warfarin, and phenytoin. Lovastatin, simvastatin, and atorvastatin use the 3A4 pathway. Rosuvastatin and fluvastatin engage 2C9.

• Warning: The active metabolite is approx 90 % fecal and 10 % renal eliminated. In individuals with renal failure, GFR < 30 mL/min, there is a threefold increase in plasma concentrations and the drug is contraindicated. Caution is also needed in those with GFR 31–50 mL/min and in individuals older than age 75 who may have a normal serum creatinine but a GFR 50–55 mL/min.

Rosuvastatin at 20–40 mg daily should allow more patients to attain LDL-C goals (see SATURN TRIAL 2011 in Chap. 22).

In the CORONA trial, when repeat events were included, rosuvastatin was shown to reduce the risk of HF hospitalization by ~15 to 20 %, equating to approximately 76 fewer admissions per 1,000 patients treated over a median 33 months of follow-up (Rogers et al. 2014).

CHOLESTEROL ABSORPTION INHIBITORS

Drug name:	**Ezetimibe**
Trade names:	Zetia, Ezetrol (C)
Supplied:	Tablets, 10 mg
Dosage:	10 mg once daily, with or without food

Ezetimibe is a class of cholesterol absorption inhibitors. The drug localizes and appears to act at the brush border of the small intestine and inhibits cholesterol absorption. Ezetimibe 10 mg combined with simvastatin 40 mg resulted in a mean LDL-C lowering of 20 %. Combination with a statin further decreases LDL-C. Useful for homozygous familial hypercholesterolemia in which statins are poorly effective. The statins and ezetimibe have rendered cholestyramine and colestipol bile acid-binding resins obsolete.

Adverse effects: headache, gastrointestinal disturbances; myalgia; rarely arthralgia, hepatitis; very rarely pancreatitis, cholelithiasis, cholecystitis, raised creatine kinase, myopathy, and rhabdomyolysis; hypersensitivity reactions (including rash, angioedema, and anaphylaxis), also see discussion of cancer risk.

CANCER RISK

Simvastatin and Ezetimibe in Aortic Stenosis (SEAS) study randomized 1,873 patients to receive either a combination of simvastatin (40 mg daily) and ezetimibe (10 mg daily) or a matching placebo. After a median of 52.2 months of follow-up, LDL levels in the combined therapy group were reduced by 53.8 %, compared with 3.8 % in the placebo group, but no between-group difference was observed in the primary end point, a composite of events resulting from aortic valve disease, atherosclerotic disease, or both.

- At a 4-year follow-up, the incidence of cancer was significantly higher in the combined therapy group than in the placebo group [105 (11.1 %) versus 70 (7.5 %); $p=0.01$].

A 67 % increase was seen in the rate of cancer deaths [39 (4.1 %) versus 23 (2.5 %); $p=0.05$]. No specific cancer at any particular site accounted for this excess (Rossebø et al. for the SEAS Investigators 2008).

Shor et al. in a small study found that the low serum LDL cholesterol level was associated with increased risks of hematological cancer, fever, and sepsis. Each 1 mg/dl increase in LDL was associated with a relative reduction of 2.4 % in the odds of hematologic cancer (OR 0.976, $p=0.026$). Low LDL levels also increased the odds (Shor et al. 2007).

NICOTINIC ACID

Drug name:	Nicotinic acid; niacin
Supplied:	50, 100, 250 mg (500 mg US)
Dosage:	100 mg three times daily with meals for 1 week and then 200 mg three times daily for 1–4 weeks; average 500 mg three times daily; see text for further advice

Nicotinic acid inhibits lipolysis of adipose tissue. Also, the drug inhibits secretion of lipoproteins from the liver, causing a reduction in LDL-C and TGs.

The Atherothrombosis Intervention in Metabolic Syndrome with Low HDL/High Triglycerides: Impact on Global Health Outcomes trial (AIM-HIGH) randomized 4,414 patients to simvastatin (Zocor, 40–80 mg) in combination with high-dose niacin (1,500–2,000 mg) or a placebo spiked with 50 mg niacin per tablet to cause flushing to maintain blinding.

Extended-release niacin (Niaspan) was associated with a clinical event rate of 16.4 % compared with 16.2 % in the control group, for a slim 2 % relative risk reduction that was not significant at $p=0.79$ in the AIM-HIGH trial.

The trial was halted for futility and a small excess of ischemic strokes in the niacin group (AIM-HIGH Investigators 2011). See Chap. 22.

This drug should be considered obsolete; use is not justifiable yet continues to be prescribed.

Adverse Effects and Interactions

Adverse effects include flushing, pruritus, nausea, abdominal pain, diarrhea, significant hepatic dysfunction and cholestatic jaundice, exacerbation of diabetes mellitus, hyperuricemia and exacerbation of gouty arthritis, palpitations, arrhythmias, dizziness, and rashes.

Cautions. Hypotension may occur in combination with other medications. Should not be combined with HMG-CoA reductase inhibitors (statins).

- **Avoid in patients with AMI, heart failure (HF)**, gallbladder disease, past history of jaundice, liver disease, peptic ulcer, and diabetes mellitus. **If a drug is not safe to be used in patients with acute MI, that should be evidence for non-usage of the drug.**
- **Hepatic necrosis has been reported and because of the adverse effects with little gain for patients, the drug is not recommended by the author and it should not be combined with statins. It is time to retire niacin (Giugliano** 2011).

FIBRATES

These agents are overused. The use of fenofibrate in the United States more than doubled between 2002 and 2009 despite the absence of clear supporting evidence (Goldfine et al. 2011). They have a small role in managing patients solely with triglyceride elevations. They are indicated for LDL-C lowering only if statins are not tolerated. The drug has a role to manage elevated triglyceride levels > ~300 mg/dl that has failed to respond to dietary restriction, weight loss, and cessation of alcohol.

- Avoid combination with statins.
- On the basis of the FDA review and committee deliberations, we conclude that the benefit of adding a fibrate to statin therapy in reducing the risk of cardiovascular events in patients with type 2 diabetes remains unproven (Goldfine et al. 2011). In diabetics it should suffice to lower LDL-C to goal levels with a statin and reduce triglycerides if >200 mg/dl by diet, weight reduction, and avoidance of alcohol and fibrates.

Adverse effects include gastrointestinal disturbances, cholestasis, *rarely* gallstones, weight gain, headache, renal impairment, raised serum creatinine (unrelated to renal impairment), erectile dysfunction, myalgia—risk increased in patients with renal dysfunction and in the elderly, leucopenia, alopecia, toxic epidermal necrolysis, and Stevens–Johnson syndrome.

Drug name:	**Bezafibrate**
Trade names:	Bezalip, Bezalip Mono
Supplied:	200 mg (Mono 400 mg)
Dosage:	200 mg three times daily with or after food

Mono formulation one tablet daily in the evening

Drug name:	**Fenofibrate**
Trade names:	Lipidil Supra, Lipantil, Supralip (UK)
Supplied:	100, 145 mg
Dosage:	100–145 mg once daily with the main meal; max. 100 mg in renal dysfunction, with monitoring

Avoid if creatinine >1.5 mg/dL 132 μmol/L or estimated GFR <60 mL/min

This drug has been shown to decrease LDL-C cholesterol levels by up to 15 % and to increase HDL-C concentration by about 20 %. In the FIELD trial (2005, 43) (see Chap. 22), fenofibrate did not significantly reduce the risk of the primary outcome of coronary events. It did reduce total cardiovascular events, mainly owing to fewer nonfatal MIs.

- Fenofibric acid has not been shown to reduce the risk of heart attack or stroke.
- **Data from a substudy of the ACCORD 2010 (Action to Control Cardiovascular Risk in Diabetes) trial found no extra benefit in clinical outcomes from a combination of fenofibric acid and simvastatin (Zocor) compared with simvastatin alone.**

The ACCORD data covered about 5,500 patients randomized to the combination or to simvastatin alone. After a median of 4.7 years of follow-up, the addition of fenofibric acid reduced major cardiovascular events by a statistically insignificant 8 % ($p=0.32$).The drug has a small role if any in the treatment of patients with elevated LDL-C. Goal LDL-C is most often not achieved. **Fibrates are overprescribed and not recommended by the author except for management of very high triglyceride levels >4 mmol/L (~400 mg/dL) that fail to respond to strict dietary and alcohol restrictions.**

HDL LOWERING

Some genetic mechanisms that raise plasma HDL cholesterol do not lower risk of MI. These data challenge the concept that raising of plasma HDL cholesterol will uniformly translate into reductions in risk of MI (Voight et al. 2012).

Evacetrapib

Nicholls et al. (2011) examined the biochemical effects, safety, and tolerability of evacetrapib, as monotherapy and in combination with statins, in patients with dyslipidemia. This RCT was conducted among 398 patients with elevated low-density lipoprotein cholesterol (LDL-C) or low high-density lipoprotein cholesterol (HDL-C) levels. Following dietary lead-in, 398 patients with elevated LDL-C or low HDL-C levels were randomly assigned to receive placebo ($n = 38$); evacetrapib monotherapy, 30 mg/day ($n = 40$), 100 mg/day ($n = 39$), or 500 mg/day ($n = 42$); or statin therapy ($n = 239$) (simvastatin, 40 mg/day; atorvastatin, 20 mg/day; or rosuvastatin, 10 mg/day) with or without evacetrapib, 100 mg/d, for 12 weeks.

The mean baseline HDL-C level was 55.1 mg/dL and the mean baseline LDL-C level was 144.3 mg/dL. As monotherapy, evacetrapib produced dose-dependent increases in HDL-C of 30.0–66.0 mg/dL (53.6–128.8 %) and decreases in LDL-C of −20.5 to −51.4 mg/dL.

In combination with statin therapy, evacetrapib, 100 mg/day, produced increases in HDL-C of 42.1–50.5 mg/dL (78.5–88.5 %; $p < 0.001$ for all compared with statin monotherapy) and decreases in LDL-C of −67.1 to −75.8 mg/dL (−11.2 to −13.9 %; $p < 0.001$ for all compared with statin monotherapy). Compared with placebo or statin monotherapy, evacetrapib as monotherapy or in combination with statins increased HDL-C levels and decreased LDL-C levels; no adverse effects were observed.

REFERENCES

ACC/AHA: Goff Jr DC, Lloyd-Jones DM, Bennett G, et al. 2013 ACC/ AHA guideline on the assessment of cardiovascular risk: a report of the American college of cardiology/American heart association task force on practice guidelines. J Am Coll Cardiol. 2014;63:2935–59.

ACC/AHA: Stone NJ, Jennifer G. Robinson JG, Lichtenstein AH et al. A Guideline on the Treatment of Blood Cholesterol to Reduce Atherosclerotic Cardiovascular Risk in Adults: A Report of the American College of Cardiology/American Heart Association Task Force on Practice Guideline2013s. Am Coll Cardiol. 2014;63(25_PA): 2889–2934.

ACCORD Study Group. Effects of combination lipid therapy in type 2 diabetes mellitus. N Engl J Med. 2010;362:1563–74.

AIM-HIGH Investigators. Niacin in patients with low HDL cholesterol levels receiving intensive statin therapy. N Engl J Med. 2011; 365:2255–67.

ASTEROID, Nissen SE, Nicholls SJ, Sipahi I, et al. Effect of very high-intensity statin therapy on regression of coronary atherosclerosis: the ASTEROID trial. JAMA. 2006;295:1556–65.

ATP: Expert Panel, Grundy SM, Cleeman JI, Merz CN, et al. Implications of recent clinical trials for the national cholesterol education program adult treatment panel III guidelines. Circulation. 2004;110:227–39 (Erratum, Circulation 2004;110:763).

Ben-Yehuda O, DeMaria AN. LDL-C targets after the ACC/AHA 2013 guidelines; evidence that lower is better. J Am Coll Cardiol. 2014; 64(5):495–7.

Boekholdt SM, Hovingh GK, Mora S, et al. Very ow levels of atherogenic lipoproteins and the risk for cardiovascular events: a meta-analysis of statin trials. J Am Coll Cardiol. 2014;64:485–94.

Brown MS, Goldstein JL. A receptor-mediated pathway for cholesterol homeostasis. Science. 1979;323:361.

Cannon CP, Braunwald E, McCabe CH, et al. Intensive versus moderate lipid lowering with statins after acute coronary syndromes. N Engl J Med. 2004;350:1495–504.

CARE: For the Cholesterol and Recurrent Events Trial Investigators. The effect of pravastatin on coronary events after myocardial infarction in patients with average cholesterol levels. N Engl J Med. 1996;335:1001.

Chataway J, Schuerer N, Alsanousi A. Effect of high-dose simvastatin on brain atrophy and disability in secondary progressive multiple sclerosis (MS-STAT): a randomised, placebo-controlled, phase 2 trial. Lancet. 2014;383(9936):2213–21.

de Lorgeril M, Renaud S, Mamelle N, et al. Mediterranean alpha-linolenic acid rich diet in secondary prevention of coronary heart disease. Lancet. 1994;343:1454.

de Lorgeril M, Salen P, Maril JL, et al. Mediterranean diet: traditional risk factors, and the rate of cardiovascular complications after myocardial infarction: final report of the Lyon Diet Heart Study. Circulation. 1999;99:779.

Doran B, Guo Y, Xu J. Prognostic value of fasting vs. non-fasting low density lipoprotein cholesterol levels on long-term mortality: insight from the national health and nutrition survey III (NHANES-III). Circulation. 2014;130:546–53.

Eckel RH, Jakicic JM, Ard JD, et al. 2013 AHA/ACC guideline on lifestyle management to reduce cardiovascular risk: a report of the American college of cardiology/American heart association task force on practice guidelines. J Am Coll Cardiol. 2014;63:2960–84.

Effects of long-term fenofibrate therapy on cardiovascular events in 9795 people with type 2 diabetes mellitus (the FIELD study): randomised controlled trial. The FIELD study investigators. Lancet. 2005; 366:1849–1861.

Exler J, Wehlrauch JL. Provisional table on the content of omega-3 fatty acids and other fat components in selected seafoods (Publication HNIS/PT-103). Washington, DC: US Department of Agriculture; 1986.

Fehily AM, Burr ML, Phillips KM, Deadman NM. The effect of fatty fish on plasma lipid and lipoprotein concentrations. Am J Clin Nutr. 1983;38:349.

Giugliano RP. Niacin at 56 years of age—time for an early retirement? N Engl J Med. 2011;365:2318–20.

Goldfine AB, Kaul S, Hiatt WR. Fibrates in the treatment of dyslipidemias—time for a reassessment. N Engl J Med. 2011;365:481–4.

Gundersen T, Kjekshus J, Stokke O, et al. Timolol maleate and HDL cholesterol after myocardial infarction. Eur Heart J. 1985;6:840.

Hepburn FN, Exler J, Weihrauch JL. Provisional tables on the content of omega-3 fatty acids and other fat components of selected foods. J Am Diet Assoc. 1986;86:788.

Huxley RR, Barzi F, Lam TH, et al. An individual participant data meta-analysis of 23 studies in the Asia-Pacific region. Circulation. 2011;124:2056–64.

Illingworth DR, Harris WS, Connor WE. Inhibition of low density lipoprotein synthesis by dietary omega-3 fatty acids in humans. Arteriosclerosis. 1984;4:270.

Lipid Research Clinics Coronary Primary Prevention Trial Results. I. Reduction in incidence of coronary heart disease. II. The relationship of reduction in incidence of coronary heart disease to cholesterol lowering. JAMA. 1984;251:351.

LIPID Study Group. Prevention of cardiovascular events and death with pravastatin in patients with coronary heart disease and a broad range of initial cholesterol levels. N Engl J Med. 1998;339:1349–57.

Maxwell AJ, Zapien MP, Pearce GL, et al. Randomized trial of a medical food for the dietary management of chronic, stable angina. J Am Coll Cardiol. 2002;39:37.

Morris PB, Ballantyne CM, Birtcher KK, State-of-the-Art Review. Review of clinical practice guidelines for the management of LDL-related risk. J Am Coll Cardiol. 2014;64:196–206.

Nestel PH, Connor WE, Reardon MF, et al. Suppression by diets rich in fish oil on very low density lipoprotein production in man. J Clin Invest. 1984;74:82.

Nicholls SJ, Brewer HB, Kastelein JJP, et al. Effects of the CETP inhibitor evacetrapib administered as monotherapy or in combination with statins on HDL and LDL cholesterol: a randomized controlled trial. JAMA. 2011;306(19):2099–109.

Pietinen P, Huttunen JK. Dietary determinants of plasma high-density lipoprotein cholesterol. Am Heart J. 1987;113:620.

Pitt B, Mancini GBJ, Ellis SG, et al. Pravastatin limitation of atherosclerosis in the coronary arteries. J Am Coll Cardiol. 1995;26:1133.

PROVE IT-TIMI 22. Murphy SA, Cannon CP, Wiviott SD, et al. Reduction in recurrent cardiovascular events with intensive lipid-lowering statin therapy compared with moderate lipid-lowering statin therapy after acute coronary syndromes: from the PROVE IT–TIMI 22 (Pravastatin or Atorvastatin Evaluation and Infection Therapy – Thrombolysis in Myocardial Infarction 22) trial. J Am Coll Cardiol. 2009b;54:2358–62.

Rogers JK, Jhund PS, Perez A. Effect of rosuvastatin on repeat heart failure hospitalizations: the CORONA trial (controlled rosuvastatin multinational trial in heart failure). JCHF. 2014;2(3):289–97.

Sanders TAB, Roshanai F. The influence of different types of n-3-polyunsaturated fatty acids on blood lipids and platelet function in healthy volunteers. Clin Sci. 1983;64:91.

Saturn Nicholls SJ., Ballantyne CM, Barter PJ, et al. Effect of Two Intensive Statin Regimens on Progression of Coronary Disease N Engl J Med December 1, 2011; 365:2078–2087. http://www.nejm.org/doi/full/10.1056/NEJMoa1110874.

Scandinavian Simvastatin Survival Study Group (4S). Randomized trial of cholesterol lowering in 4444 patients with coronary heart disease. Lancet 1994;344:1383.

Schwartz GG, Olsson AG, Ezekowitz MD, et al. for the Myocardial Ischemia Reduction with Aggressive Cholesterol Lowering (MIRACL) Study Investigators. Effects of atorvastatin on early recurrent ischemic events in acute coronary syndromes. The MIRACL STUDY: a randomized controlled trial. JAMA 2001;285:1711–1718.

SEAS: Rossebo AB, Pedersen TR, Boman K et al. the SEAS Investigators. Intensive lipid lowering with simvastatin and ezetimibe in aortic stenosis. NEJM 2008;359:1343–1356.

Shepherd J, Cobbe SM, Ford I, et al. Prevention of coronary heart disease with pravastatin in men with hypercholesterolemia. N Engl J Med. 1995;333:1301.

Shor R, Wainstein J, Oz D. Low serum LDL cholesterol levels and the risk of fever, sepsis, and malignancy. Ann Clin Lab Sci. 2007;37(4):343–8.

Singer P, Wirth M, Voigt S, et al. Blood pressure and lipid-lowering effect of mackerel and herring diet in patients with mild essential hypertension. Atherosclerosis. 1985;56:223.

Tobert JA, Sheer CL, Chremos AN, et al. Clinical experience with lovastatin. Am J Cardiol. 1990;65:23F.

Topol EJ, McCarthy J, Gabriel S, et al. GeneQuest Investigators. Single nucleotide polymorphisms in multiple novel thrombospondin genes may be associated with familial premature myocardial infarction. Circulation 2001;104:2641–2644.

Topol EJ. The genomic basis of myocardial infarction. J Am Coll Cardiol. 2005;46:1456–65.

Trustwell AS. End of a static decade for coronary disease? BMJ. 1984;289:509.

Valimaki M, Maass L, Harno K, et al. Lipoprotein lipids and apoproteins during beta-blocker administration: comparison of penbutolol and atenolol. Eur J Clin Pharmacol. 1986;30:17.

Van Lossonczy TO, Ruiter A, Bronsgeest-Schoute HC, et al. The effect of a fish diet on serum lipids in healthy human subjects. Am J Clin Nutr. 1985;31:1340.

Violi F, Calvieri C, Ferro D, et al. Statins as antithrombotic drugs. Circulation. 2013;127:251–7.

Voight BF, Peloso GM, Orho-Melander M. Plasma HDL cholesterol and risk of myocardial infarction: a mendelian randomisation study. Lancet. 2012;380(9841):572–80.

Wang Q, Rao S, Shen G-Q, et al. Premature myocardial infarction novel susceptibility locus on chromosome 1p34-36 identified by genome-wide linkage analysis. Am J Hum Genet. 2004;74:262–71.

Wierbicki AS, Lumb PJ, Semra YK, et al. Effect of atorvastatin on plasma fibrinogen. Lancet. 1998;351:569.

Willett WC, Stamper MJ, Manson JE, et al. Intake of trans fatty acids and risk of coronary heart disease among women. Lancet. 1994;341:581.

Willett WC. Balancing life-style and genomics research for disease prevention. Science. 2002;296:695–8.

18 Endocrine Heart Diseases

ACROMEGALY

Enlargement of the heart, premature coronary artery disease (CAD), heart failure, hypertension, intraventricular conduction defects, and cardiac arrhythmias may require management by a cardiologist. Mild hypertension occurs in more than 50 % of patients. Rarely acromegalic cardiomyopathy occurs. There is myocyte hypertrophy and an increase in the collagen content per gram of heart compared with normal myocardium. The defect in the myocardium causes arrhythmias, which weaken the myocardial force that leads to heart failure.

Management

Treatment of patients with somatostatin analogues that inhibit the secretion of growth hormone, octreotide and lanreotide, have shown beneficial effects in small studies. In some patients, when heart failure has been completely controlled the left ventricle mass index and mean wall thickness have shown improvement with this therapy. In patients with long-standing acromegaly, there is nonreversible interstitial fibrosis with little recovery. Hypertension can be controlled with diuretics and other antihypertensive agents.

Acromegalic cardiomyopathy may show some amelioration with the administration of octreotide. Treatment of the lesion with heavy particle, proton beam irradiation, or surgery is usually curative.

© Springer Science+Business Media New York 2015
M. Gabriel Khan, *Cardiac Drug Therapy*, Contemporary Cardiology,
DOI 10.1007/978-1-61779-962-4_18

CARCINOID SYNDROME

Carcinoid heart disease may occur in patients with carcinoid syndrome. The main symptoms of flushing, diarrhea, and bronchospasm are caused mainly by 5-hydroxytryptamine or serotonin, which is liberated from carcinoid tumors that originate from chromaffin cells (neuroendocrine cells) of the terminal ileum. Neurosecretory granules release amines that include serotonin, histamine, bradykinins, tachykinins, and prostaglandins. Involvement of the heart occurs in about 50 % of carcinoid syndrome cases and is usually a late manifestation seen mainly in patients with malignant tumors that have metastasized to the liver. In carcinoid heart disease, 5-hydroxytryptamine is metabolized by monoamine oxidase to 5-hydroxyindoleacetic acid (5-HIAA). Elevated levels of 5-HIAA in the urine confirm the diagnosis. Echocardiography reveals thickening of the tricuspid and pulmonary valves with tricuspid and pulmonary valve regurgitation and, in some cases, pulmonary valve stenosis. The lesions in the heart cause right heart failure. Because the tricuspid valve leaks, blood regurgitates into the veins of the neck and back toward the liver, which becomes pulsatile with each heartbeat. Examination of the jugular venous pulse reveals prominent pulsatile V waves of tricuspid regurgitation. A right ventricular lift or heave is often detected. Findings include a pansystolic murmur of tricuspid regurgitation, an early diastolic murmur of pulmonary regurgitation, and a systolic murmur of pulmonary stenosis best heard at the left sternal edge. Murmurs may be soft because of low output from the right ventricle. Ascites becomes prominent prior to mild edema of the ankles. When tricuspid regurgitation is prominent the enlarged liver is visibly pulsatile.

Management: There is no specific treatment for carcinoid heart disease. Octreotide reduces flushing diarrhea and urinary levels of 5-HIAA. Cardiac surgery offers definitive therapy for symptoms. Marked symptomatic improvement, of >1 New York Heart Association class, occurs after valve replacement (Castillo et al. 2008; Connolly et al. 1995, 2001).

CUSHING'S SYNDROME

This disorder is caused by either an ACTH-dependent adenoma or an ACTH-independent adenoma. Manifestations include truncal obesity that involves the abdomen, chest, and the upper back causing a buffalo hump. Cardiovascular complications such as hypertension may be severe. Diabetes may occur, and along with hypertension, this increases the risk for myocardial infarction. Accelerated atherosclerosis is a common finding in patients not treated early in the course of this disease.

Management: Cushing's disease requires transsphenoidal pituitary surgery and adrenal tumors require adrenalectomy. Ectopic ACTH syndrome occurs and requires treatment of the underlying tumor. Correction of hypokalemia with potassium replacement and spironolactone or eplerenone and drugs that block steroid synthesis may be required.

DIABETES AND THE HEART

Patients with type 2 diabetes mellitus without a history of myocardial infarction (MI) have the same risk of a coronary event as patients without diabetes who do have a history of MI (Haffner et al. 1998). Much of their care therefore involves the prescriptions used for the management of patients with angina or post-acute coronary syndrome. Cardiologist and clinicians who care for cardiac patients, thus, have a role to play. The ACCORD trial on blood pressure (2008), and the ACCORD trials on intensive blood glucose control (2008) have failed to show that intensive glucose control in type 2 diabetes reduces the risk for CVD events.

Which Cardiovascular Drugs Are Best ACE Inhibitors/ARBS?

Angiotensin-converting enzyme (ACE) inhibitors and angiotensin II receptor blockers (ARBs) are touted to cause a slightly reduced incidence of diabetes, but this has not been proven without doubt in RCTs. These inaccurate assumptions are based on secondary analyses of clinical trials. More importantly, many trialists fail to understand that the finding of glucose intolerance does not indicate a proven diagnosis of diabetes mellitus.

Nathan (2010) in an editorial emphasized that the only clinical trial that directly examined whether ACE inhibition would prevent diabetes failed to show that diabetes was prevented (The DREAM Trial Investigators 2006) or that there were any beneficial effects on insulin resistance or beta-cell function (Hanley et al. 2010). See Chaps. 3 and 4.

Beta-Blockers Underused in Diabetics

Because the majority of patients with long-standing type 2 diabetes over age 50 develop atheromatous obstructive CHD culminating in sudden cardiac death or fatal or nonfatal MI, it is necessary to maintain type 2 diabetics on a beta-blocker for hypertension control. Nebivolol, bisoprolol, or in non-brittle diabetics carvedilol are advisable. Also a statin, an ACE inhibitor, and chewable aspirin should be administered. The commonly used atenolol is not recommended because it is poorly effective; this widely prescribed beta-blocker should become obsolete (Khan 2011); see Chap. 1. Many type 2 diabetics older than age 50 unknown to have CHD are at high risk for CHD events. These agents do not cause diabetes, an unproved notion held by many learned physicians worldwide (see Chap. 2). Sudden death appears to be more common in diabetics than in non diabetic patients with known CHD. Only timolol and propranolol have been shown in soundly conducted RCTs to prevent sudden cardiac death (see Chap. 1). Guideline experts appear to be unaware of these facts.

Aspirin

- Chewable soft aspirin 75–81 mg once daily after meal is strongly recommended for diabetics older than age 50 and is more reliably efficacious than enteric coated aspirin which should be used only if stomach irritation occurs with chewable aspirin. The enteric coated drug is often not 100 % absorbed, and aspirin resistance is incorrectly blamed. Absorption proved very variable and caused up to 49 % apparent resistance to a single dose of enteric coated aspirin but not to immediate release aspirin (0 %); pharmacologic resistance to aspirin is rare; the study failed to identify a single case of true aspirin resistance. Pseudoresistance, reflecting delayed and reduced drug absorption, complicates enteric coated but not immediate release aspirin administration (Grosser et al. 2013).

  The author abandoned the use of enteric coated aspirin in 2007 and instead prescribes soft chewable aspirin 81 mg for CVD prevention.

  - In addition if chest pain occurs the patient needs to take 3–4 chewable aspirin (not coated) while awaiting ambulance transport to an emergency.

Dyslipidemia in Diabetics

Diabetic patients with elevated LDL-C (>200 mg/dl, 4.0 mmol/l), mild elevation of triglycerides (<250 mg/dl), and lowered are best managed with atorvastatin. If triglycerides are not elevated rosuvastatin is advisable to attain goal LDL-C levels but should not be used if the eGFR is <40 ml/min. Reduce the dose in patients with mild renal dysfunction, the elderly, Asians, and patients with hypothyroidism. In diabetics with known CVD the LDL goal is <70 mg/dl (1.8 mmol/l). In the absence of CVD, an LDL goal of <2.6 mmol/l (100 mg/dl) is advisable.

- Simvastatin is not recommended because of many interactions that can occur with this proven useful drug (see Chaps. 17 and 21).
- Fenofibrates should not be combined with statins.

- In ACCORD Lipid (2010) the combination of fenofibrate and simvastatin did not reduce the rate of fatal cardiovascular events, nonfatal MI, or nonfatal stroke, as compared with simvastatin alone.

Blood Pressure Control

The ACCORD Study Group Diabetic Blood Pressure Trial (2010) showed that among patients with type 2 diabetes at high risk for cardiovascular events, a target systolic BP of <120 mmHg was not superior to a target of <140 mmHg. This intensive target did not reduce composite cardiovascular events. In the intensive systolic BP group there were more serious adverse events, hypokalemia, and elevated serum creatinine.

The UKPDS 9-year follow-up showed that tight BP control was most useful. Importantly BP >160 mmHg was reduced only to <144 mm.

- The notion commonly held in North America that the systolic BP should be decreased to <125 mmHg is false.
- **If kidney function is normal, and atherosclerotic disease is not present, a goal of systolic BP < 140 or diastolic < 90 is appropriate and avoids the use of 3–4 antihypertensive agents**. Polypharmacy must be avoided.
- If renal failure or atherosclerotic disease is present a BP < 135/85 mmHg appears appropriate until further trials are conducted. The UK and other guidelines suggest <130/80.
- An ambulatory 24-h BP assessment is useful if home and clinic BP control is difficult to achieve.

Appropriate drugs include ACE inhibitors, calcium antagonists, beta-blockers, and diuretics.

- Experts who formulate National guidelines express the view that diuretics and beta-blockers should be avoided because these commonly used drugs cause diabetes. Interestingly. The British guideline, and British national formulary 2011 state: "Beta-blockers, especially when combined with a thiazide diuretic, should be avoided for the routine treatment of uncomplicated hypertension in patients with diabetes or in those at high risk of developing diabetes."

The notion that these agents cause genuine diabetes mellitus is false (see Chap. 2).

Murphy et al. (1982) reported on the results of a much-prolonged 14-year follow-up in hypertensive patients treated with a diuretic, showing a major increase in the incidence of glucose intolerance. But this effect was promptly reversed on discontinuation of the diuretic in more than 60 % of the individuals who had developed elevated glucose levels beyond the top limit of normal. Most important, this glucose elevation proved reversible (Murphy et al. 1982).

• It must be emphasized that based solely on the finding of glucose intolerance, these knowledgeable clinicians did not classify their subjects who exhibited fasting glucose levels above normal as diabetics. These subjects developed benign reversible glucose intolerance which disappeared on discontinuing the long-term diuretic therapy. The doses used were far greater than that used during the past 30 years. The remaining 40 % of the individuals who exhibited elevated plasma glucose levels developed true diabetes because they were pre-diabetics. A similar reversible metabolic disturbance may occur in a few patients on long-term treatment with a beta-blocker. This trial information appears to have been missed by Trialists, and this article is not quoted by editorialists or investigators who have reviewed the topic. See Chap. 2.

ORAL DIABETIC AGENTS

Metformin

This old agent remains a mainstay of treatment, and is also particularly useful in patients administered insulin. The drug's effect on peripheral insulin-sensitive tissues requires the presence of insulin for its full action. Renal failure needs dose titration: the dose should be reduced if eGFR is <50 ml/min; avoid if eGFR < 35 ml/min.

- **"Among patients with diabetes who were receiving metformin, the addition of insulin vs. a sulfonylurea was associated with an increased risk of a composite of nonfatal cardiovascular outcomes and all-cause mortality. These findings require further investigation to understand risks associated with insulin use in these patients." Propensity score matching yielded 2,436 metformin +** insulin and 1 2 1 80 metformin + sulfonylurea. Patient median follow-up was 1 4 months. There were 172 vs. 634 events for the primary outcome among patients who added insulin vs. sulfonylureas, $P = 0.009$). Acute MI **and stroke rates were 41 vs. 229 events (10.2 and 11.9 events per 1,000 person-years; $P = 0.52$), whereas all-cause death rates were 1 37 vs. 444 events, respectively (33.7 and 22.7 events per 1,000 person-years; aHR, 1.44; 95 % CI, 1.15-1.79; $P = 0.001$) (Roumie et al** 2014).

In addition overtreatment is common in the many elderly.

- Patients with risk factors for serious hypoglycemia represent a large subset of individuals receiving hypoglycemic agents. In a recent study approximately one-half had evidence of intensive treatment (Andrews and O'Malley 2014).

Sulfonylurea

Sulfonylureas such as tolbutamide glipizide, gliclazide, glimepiride, and glibenclamide have a role if needed to achieve goal and are preferred to thiazolidinediones.

- **Sulfonylureas were used successfully in addition to metformin in a recent study** (Roumie et al. 2014); the combination prevented more cardiac events compared with addition of insulin.

Thiazolidinediones

Caution: have been shown to have a mild effect on the lowering of blood glucose levels, but many have been withdrawn from the market because of adverse effects. Their use must be justified particularly in patients who are already using insulin plus metformin. Troglitazone was voluntarily withdrawn from the market because of severe hepatotoxicity. Pioglitazone (Actos) use is restricted in patients with a history of heart failure or EF < 40 %. This restriction is in place because they increase retention of sodium and water, which can precipitate or worsen heart failure.

- The European Medicines Agency has advised that there is a small increased risk of bladder cancer associated with pioglitazone use. The drug reduces peripheral insulin resistance.

These agents produce significant weight gain and they should not be prescribed to persons with familial polyposis. In addition they cause fractures. Consistent with previous trials, rosiglitazone caused an increase in heart failure and fractures (Home et al. for RECORD 2009).

Acarbose (Glucobay)

This drug is an inhibitor of intestinal alpha glucosidases and delays the digestion and absorption of starch and sucrose; it has a small but significant effect in lowering blood glucose. Flatulence can be bothersome.

- Nateglinide and repaglinide stimulate insulin release.

Exenatide (Byetta) and Nateglinide (Starlix) are licensed only for use with metformin. Exenatide and liraglutide both bind to, and activate, the GLP-1 (glucagon-like peptide-1) receptor to increase insulin secretion, suppress glucagon secretion, and slow gastric emptying. Treatment with exenatide and liraglutide is associated with the prevention of weight gain and possible promotion of weight loss which can be beneficial in overweight patients. They are both given by subcutaneous injection for the treatment of type 2 diabetes mellitus.

Dipeptidyl Peptidase-4 (DPP-4) Inhibitors (Gliptins)

- Saxagliptin, sitagliptin, and vildagliptin inhibit dipeptidyl-peptidase-4 to increase insulin secretion and lower glucagon secretion. They are approved for use in type 2 diabetes in combination with metformin or a sulfonylurea (if metformin inappropriate). **Sitagliptin (Januvia) should be avoided if eGFR less than 55 ml/min.**
- **Therapy with Gliptins appears to protect the heart**.
    The interesting investigational drug ipragliflozin improves glycemic control and decreases body weight and blood pressure.
- The FDA has approved a fixed-dose combination tablet that combines the diabetes drug sitagliptin with simvastatin, under the brand name Juvisync. The combination product comes in three strengths, all with 100 mg of sitagliptin and 10, 20, or 40 mg of simvstatin.

HbA1c values were previously aligned to the assay used in the Diabetes Control and Complications Trial (DCCT) and expressed as a percentage. A new standard, specific for HbA1c, has been created by the International Federation of Clinical Chemistry and Laboratory Medicine (IFCC), which expresses HbA1c values in mmol of glycosylated hemoglobin per mol of hemoglobin.

IFCC-HbA1c (mmol/mol)/DCCT-HbA1c (%)

42 mmol/mol = 6.0 %; 48 = 6.5; 53 = 7.0; 59 = 7.5; 64 = 8.0; 75 = 9.0 %

HbA1c estimation is not a screening test for the diagnosis of diabetes.

HYPERALDOSTERONISM

Hyperaldosteronism is usually caused by an aldosterone-producing adenoma and rarely by bilateral adrenocortical hyperplasia. Potassium depletion occurs that may produce muscular weakness. Sodium retention causes an increase in blood pressure, but hypertension is usually mild to moderate in intensity. It may be resistant to the usual antihypertensive medications. Aldosterone has a direct effect on collagen metabolism in cardiac fibroblasts and reactive perivascular and interstitial cardiac fibrosis occurs. The weak diuretics (aldosterone antagonist), spironolactone, amiloride, or eplerenone, are advisable for management of hypertension.

PHEOCHROMOCYTOMA

The lesion is usually a tumor of the adrenal medulla (~10 % are bilateral), 10 % of the time it is malignant, and 10 % of the time it is outside the adrenal medulla, where 10 % of those are familial.

Cardiovascular Features: These include severe headaches and profuse sweating, palpitations, severe labile hypertension, or sustained severe hypertension, postural hypotension, palpitations due to sinus tachycardia, and cardiac arrhythmias.

- A life-threatening myocarditis may occur, and in some, cardiomyopathy and heart failure may develop that may be reversed when the offending tumor is removed.
- Adler et al. (2008), in a review, discuss the presentation, diagnosis, management, and future directions in the management of pheochromocytoma. Figure 18-1 shows the catecholamine metabolic pathway.

Diagnosis: Plasma-free metanephrine and normetanephrine, measured by enzyme immunoassay (EIA), had a sensitivity of 66.7 % and a specificity of 100 %, but when combined (either positive), they demonstrated a 91.7 %

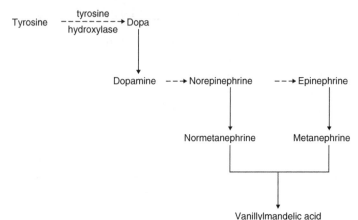

Fig. 18-1. Catecholamine metabolic pathway. Reproduced with permission from Khan M Gabriel, Hypertension. In: *Heart Disease Diagnosis and Therapy*, 2nd edition, p 340. New York: Humana Press/Springer Science + Business Media; 2005. With kind permission from Springer Science + Business Media.

sensitivity with a preserved specificity of 100 %. The EIA offers a simple and effective measurement of plasma-free metanephrines (Procopiou et al. 2009).

Plasma catecholamines may be mildly elevated with stress and essential hypertension, diuretics, prazosin, and other alpha-blockers, hydralazine, labetalol, and calcium antagonists. Elevated dopamine serum levels are estimated on the same blood samples taken for epinephrine or metanephrines, because dopamine may be the only chemical produced by some malignant pheochromocytomas.

Computer tomography (CT) or magnetic resonance imaging (MRI) may reveal a tumor. I131 meta-iodo-benzylguanidine (MIBG) enters chromaffin tissue and an MIBG scan helps identify extra-adrenal tumors.

Fiebrich and colleagues indicated that 6-[F-18]fluoro-l-dihydroxyphenylalanine positron emission tomography is superior to conventional imaging with 123I-metaiodobenzylguanidine scintigraphy, computer tomography, and magnetic resonance imaging in localizing tumors causing catecholamine excess (Fiebrich et al. 2009). Nonetheless studies are small and many of these agents are not yet in widespread clinical use.

Management: Phenoxybenzamine is a nonselective, noncompetitive alpha-adrenergic antagonist with a plasma half-life of 24 h. Oral therapy with this nonselective alpha-blocker is commenced once the blood pressure (BP) is under control or if the BP is not severely elevated after control with phentolamine or other agent. Starting dosages of 20–40 mg daily are titrated depending on the patient response; or 1–2 mg/kg daily in two or three divided doses, usually 10 mg every 8–12 h is given. Increase every 3 or 4 days by 10 mg to a maximum of 50 mg three times daily.

- Phenoxybenzamine therapy is usually required for control of BP over a period of 1–2 weeks before surgery. The drug is contraindicated in HF. Patients with pheochromocytoma are hypovolemic and alpha-blockade causes vasodilation. Thus, a marked fall in BP may occur, causing severe postural hypotension. Increase in salt intake and vigorous saline infusion are usually required during 1–2 weeks before surgery to prevent severe postural hypotension, but careful monitoring is required to prevent the precipitation of HF.

Postoperative hypotension may be avoided by discontinuing phenoxybenzamine several days before surgery. Because the presynaptic alpha 2-receptor is blocked by this agent, the release of norepinephrine from adrenergic neurons increases, causing tachycardia that may require control with a beta-blocker.

Phentolamine: Hypertensive crisis may require use of phentolamine before the administration of phenoxybenzamine; phentolamine dosage: 2–5 mg IV bolus given over 5 min, every 5 min, or an infusion of 10–20 µg/kg/min or 5–60 mg over 10–30 min at a rate of 0.1–2 mg/min. The drug has a rapid onset of action and lasts only 10–20 min.

Nitroprusside has a role and can be used to lower blood pressure during a crisis, but complicating tachyarrhythmias may occur and beta-blockers should not be used to manage arrhythmias without adequate alpha-blockade.

Calcium Antagonists: Nfedipine or other dihydropyridine calcium antagonists are useful for emergency blood pressure control. They are useful in patients who are normotensive but have paroxysmal episodes of hypertension, because they are less likely to cause significant orthostatic hypotension or overshoot hypotension. Reduction in arterial blood pressure results from inhibition of norepinephrine-mediated trans-membrane calcium influx in vascular smooth muscle (Lehmann et al. 1983). Nicardipine infusion has also been used effectively for the rapid control of hemodynamic changes intraoperatively (Proye et al. 1989; Bravo 1997).

Beta-adrenergic blockers should be commenced only after adequate pretreatment with alpha-adrenergic block-ade, because unopposed alpha-adrenergic receptor stimu-lation can precipitate a catastrophic hypertensive crisis. But labetalol has both α- and β-receptor antagonist activ-ity, is available in oral and IV preparations, and has been successfully used for the perioperative control of blood pressure in pheochromocytoma patients and in patients with metastatic disease; however, patient response may be variable (Kanto 1985).

Metyrosine (Metirosine): This agent is an inhibitor of tyrosine hydroxylase and, hence, the synthesis of cate-cholamines. The drug reduces catecholamine production by about 70 % and has a role in the preoperative manage-ment of pheochromocytomas as an alternative to phenoxybenzamine.

The drug is particularly useful for the management of inoperable tumors in combination with an alpha-blocker. A dosage of 250 mg four times daily is used and increased daily by 250 mg to reach a maximum of 4 g daily. The maximum biochemical effect is observed within 2–3 days. Adverse effects, such as severe diarrhea, sedation, extrapyramidal symptoms, and hypersensitive reactions, may occur.

Surgery: Pharmacologic agents that can be used to control blood pressure intraoperatively include phentolamine, sodium nitroprusside, nitroglycerin, magnesium sulfate, and urapidil. Tachyarrhythmias can be treated with short-acting beta-blockers and IV labetalol (Kinney et al. 2002; Mannelli 2006). Also, esmolol IV is short acting and can be used if adequate alpha-blockade is achieved. Whenever possible, pheochromocytomas should be removed using a laparoscopic approach, because this technique results in less postoperative pain, a shorter hospital stay, quicker recovery, and better cosmesis when compared with an open surgical approach.

Open procedures are reserved for very large tumors or extra-adrenal tumors in locations difficult to remove laparoscopically (Adler et al. 2008). A transabdominal incision is advisable to allow a search of all abdominal chromaffin tissue. The anesthetic agent enflurane does not stimulate catecholamine release or sensitize the myocardium to catecholamines.

Management of fluid blood volumes necessitates the use of a Swan–Ganz catheter. If the shrunken blood volume caused by excess catecholamine and blood loss is replenished, marked fluctuations in BP can be prevented. Elevated BP is controlled with nitroprusside or nitroglycerin, especially in patients where the occurrence of HF is predictable. Postoperative hypotension and HF present a greater hazard with the use of alpha-blockers and beta-blockade than with the use of nitroprusside or nitroglycerin.

Removal of the tumor may cause a precipitous fall in BP because of a shrunken blood volume and the release of the intense vasoconstriction that was produced by the pheo. A surgical cure is expected in 80 % of patients. Approximately

10 % of patients have a recurrence, and patients should be screened annually for 5 years. The 5-year survival is about 95 % for patients with benign tumors and 45 % for patients with malignant tumors.

HYPERTHYROIDISM

Cardiac Disturbances

Hyperthyroidism causes increased cardiac work, which leads to cardiac hypertrophy (Dorr et al. 2005). Cardiac output may be increased by 50–300 % over that of normal subjects; there is a combined effect of increases in resting heart rate, myocardial contractility, and ejection fraction (Biondi et al. 2002; Klein and Ojamaa 2001). Rarely, hyperthyroidism can cause chest pain, coronary artery spasm, and ECG changes suggestive of myocardial ischemia (Choi et al. 2005). Pulmonary hypertension may occur and normalize after therapy.

Shortness of breath, palpitations, tachycardia, and systolic hypertension are often observed. Sinus tachycardia is present in virtually all patients: the heart rate ranges between 110 and 150 beats/min at rest. Thus, an elevated sleeping heart rate is an important sign. From 2 to 15 % develop atrial fibrillation, with the prevalence peaking at 15 % in patients older than 70 years of age.

MANAGEMENT

A beta-blocking agent, preferably one that has membrane-stabilizing activity (propranolol), is virtually always successful in controlling the rapid heart rate caused by sinus tachycardia and is beneficial in most cases of atrial fibrillation. Propranolol is more effective than nadolol; timolol has no MSA.

In younger patients with atrial fibrillation, in the absence of structural heart disease, or other independent risk factors for embolization, the benefits of anticoagulation may be outweighed by the risk, and aspirin appears to offer a safe alternative (Klein and Danzi 2007). Tachycardia control with a beta-blocker is maintained until treatment with radioactive iodine causes destruction of the gland and symptoms and signs are completely resolved.

- An assessment of **radioiodine therapy and some insights into guidelines for adequate therapy was presented with a case vignette** (Ross 2011). Surgery should be strongly considered because of adverse effects of antithyroid drugs followed by **radioiodine therapy**. The complications of **ophthalmopathy, hypothyroidism, and relapse are more than twice as common with radioiodine therapy compared with surgery. In addition pretreatment with antithyroid drugs produces a fair amount of adverse effects**.

  - **Cardiac failure in thyroid storm. Severe life-threatening hyperthyroidism usually develops in an undiagnosed hyperthyroid patient who has another major stress or illness (infection, surgery, or traumatic injury). Clinical manifestations include fever, tachycardia, nausea, vomiting, abdominal pain, and shortness of breath culminating in cardiac failure.**

    Free T4 and T3 are elevated but no more so than in ordinary hyperthyroidism.

    Management includes
  - **IV fluids, glucose for hypoglycemia, acetaminophen, and cooling blanket for fever.**
  - **Aspirin is better than acetaminophen for reducing fever but must be avoided here as it displaces thyroid hormones from their binding** proteins.
  - Judicious use of propylthiouracil, and propranolol is required.
  - Administration of iodide (sodium ipodate) lowers serum T4 acutely.
  - Dexamethasone 2 mg IV every 6 h for 24–48 h is useful to block the peripheral conversion of T4–T3.

HYPOTHYROIDISM

Cardiac Involvement

Hypothyroidism or myxedema causes bradycardia. The pathologic heart in severe myxedema appears pale, flabby, and grossly dilated. A pericardial effusion may be present and microscopic examination shows myofibrillar swelling, interstitial fibrosis, and cardiac enlargement. Because of lack of T4 feedback to the pituitary, the sensitive TSH rapidly and accurately identifies patients who have hypo- and hyperthyroidism.

In patients with well-established hypothyroidism, TSH level is greater than 20 mIU/L. In milder or subclinical hypothyroidism, the TSH levels range from 3 to 20 mIU/L with normal T4 and T3 levels (Demers and Spencer 2003; Surks et al. 2004).

The ECG shows sinus bradycardia, low voltage, occasionally atrial arrhythmias, and prolonged QT. Rarely, torsades de pointes is precipitated particularly by medications that further prolong the QT interval. Hypercholesterolemia and hypertriglyceridemia are often found in patients with hypothyroidism and is associated with development of premature CHD. Myocardial infarction risk is increased in women with subclinical hypothyroidism (Rodondi et al. 2006). Treatment of the hypothyroid condition corrects the lipid abnormalities.

Treatment: Patients with hypothyroidism require replacement therapy with L-thyroxine, usually a dosage of 0.05–0.15 mg daily (50–150 μg/mg).

REFERENCES

ACCORD Risk-Factor Control in Type 2 Diabetes the ADVANCE Collaborative Group. Intensive blood glucose control and vascular outcomes in patients with type 2 diabetes. N Engl J Med. 2008; 358:2560–72.

ACCORD Study Group. Effects of combination lipid therapy in type 2 diabetes mellitus. N Engl J Med. 2010;362:1563–74.

ACCORD Study Group The Action to Control Cardiovascular Risk in Diabetes Study Group. Effects of intensive glucose lowering in type 2 diabetes. N Engl J Med. 2008;358:2545–59.

Adler JT, Meyer-Rochow GY, Chen H, et al. Pheochromocytoma: current approaches and future directions. Oncologist. 2008;13:779–93.

Andrews MA, O'Malley PG. Diabetes overtreatment in elderly individuals: risky business in need of better management. JAMA. 2014; 311(22):2326–7.

Biondi B, Palmieri EA, Lombardi G, et al. Effects of thyroid hormone on cardiac function: the relative importance of heart rate, loading conditions, and myocardial contractility in the regulation of cardiac performance in human hyperthyroidism. J Clin Endocrinol Metab. 2002;87:968–74.

Bravo EL. Pheochromocytoma. Curr Ther Endocrinol Metab. 1997; 6:195–7.

Castillo JG, Filsoufi F, Rahmanian PB, et al. Early and late results of valvular surgery for carcinoid heart disease. J Am Coll Cardiol. 2008;51:1507–9.

Choi YH, Chung JH, Bae SW, et al. Severe coronary artery spasm can be associated with hyperthyroidism. Coronary Artery Dis. 2005;16:135–9.

Connolly HM, Nishimura RA, Smith HC, et al. Outcome of cardiac surgery for carcinoid heart disease. J Am Coll Cardiol. 1995;25:410–6.

Connolly HM, Schaff HV, Mullany CJ, et al. Surgical management of left-sided carcinoid heart disease. Circulation. 2001;104:I36–40.

Demers LM, Spencer CA. Laboratory medicine practice guidelines: laboratory support for the diagnosis and monitoring of thyroid disease. Thyroid. 2003;13:3–126.

Dorr M, Wolff B, Robinson DM, et al. The association of thyroid function with cardiac mass and left ventricular hypertrophy. J Clin Endocrinol Metab. 2005;90:673–7.

DREAM Trial Investigators. Effect of ramipril on the incidence of diabetes. N Engl J Med. 2006;355:1551–62. DREAM.

Fiebrich H-B, Brouwers AH, Kerstens MN. 6-[F-18]Fluoro-L-Dihydroxyphenylalanine positron emission tomography is superior to conventional imaging with 123I-metaiodobenzylguanidine scintigraphy, computer tomography, and magnetic resonance imaging in localizing tumors causing catecholamine excess. J Clin Endocrinol Metab. 2009;94:3922–30.

Grosser T, Fries S, Lawson JA, et al. Drug resistance and pseudoresistance an unintended consequence of enteric coating aspirin. Circulation. 2013;127:377–85.

Haffner SM, Lehto S, Ronnemaa T, et al. Mortality from coronary heart disease in subjects with type 2 diabetes and in nondiabetic subjects with and without prior myocardial infarction. N Engl J Med. 1998;339:229–34.

Hanley AJ, Zinman B, Sheridan P, et al. Effect of rosiglitazone and ramipril on b-cell function in people with impaired glucose tolerance or impaired fasting glucose. Diab Care. 2010;33:608–13.

Kanto JH. Current status of labetalol, the first alpha- and beta-blocking agent. Int J Clin Pharmacol Ther Toxicol. 1985;23:617–28.

Khan MG. Clinical trials. In: Cardiac drug therapy. Philadelphia, PA: WB Saunders/Elsevier; 2003. p. 502.

Khan MG. Hypertension. In: Heart disease diagnosis and therapy, 2nd ed. New York: Humana Press/Springer; 2005. p. 340.

Khan MG. Hypertension. In: Encyclopedia of heart diseases. New York: Springer; 2011. p. 556.

Kinney MA, Narr BJ, Warner MA. Perioperative management of pheochromocytoma. J Cardiothorac Vasc Anesth. 2002;16:359–69.

Klein I, Danzi S. Thyroid disease and the heart. Circulation. 2007; 116:1725–35.

Klein I, Ojamaa K. Thyroid hormone and the cardiovascular system. N Engl J Med. 2001;344:501–9.

Lehmann HU, Hochrein H, Witt E, et al. Hemodynamic effects of calcium antagonists: review. Hypertension. 1983;5:II66–73.

Mannelli M. Management and treatment of pheochromocytomas and paragangliomas. Ann N Y Acad Sci. 2006;1073:405–16.

Murphy MB, Lewis PJ, Kohner E, et al. Glucose intolerance in hypertensive patients treated with diuretics: a fourteen-year follow up. Lancet. 1982;2:1293–5.

Nathan DM. Navigating the choices for diabetes prevention. NEJM. 2010;362:1533–5.

Procopiou M, Finney H, Akker SA, et al. Evaluation of an enzyme immunoassay for plasma-free metanephrines in the diagnosis of catecholamine-secreting tumors. Eur J Endocrinol. 2009;161: 131–40.

Proye C, Thevenin D, Cecat P, et al. Exclusive use of calcium channel blockers in preoperative and intraoperative control of pheochromocytomas: hemodynamics and free catecholamine assays in ten consecutive patients. Surgery. 1989;106:1149–54.

RECORD Study Team, Home PD, Pocock SJ, Beck-Nielsen H, et al. Rosiglitazone evaluated for cardiovascular outcomes in oral agent combination therapy for type 2 diabetes a multicentre, randomised, open-label trial. Lancet. 2009;373:2125–35.

Rodondi N, Aujesky D, Vittinghoff E, et al. Subclinical hypothyroidism and the risk of coronary heart disease: a meta-analysis. Am J Med. 2006;119:541–51.

Ross DS. Radioiodine therapy for hyperthyroidism. N Engl J Med. 2011;364:542–50.

Roumie CL, Greevy RA, Carlos G, Grijalva CG, et al. Association between intensification of metformin treatment with insulin vs sulfonylureas and cardiovascular events and all-cause mortality among patients with diabetes. JAMA. 2014;311(22):2288–96.

Surks MI, Ortiz E, Daniels GH, et al. Subclinical thyroid disease: scientific review and guidelines for diagnosis and management. JAMA. 2004;291:228–38.

The ACCORD Study Group. Effects of intensive blood-pressure control in type 2 diabetes mellitus. N Engl J Med. 2010;362:1575–85.

UK Prospective Diabetes Study Group. Efficacy of atenolol and captopril in reducing risk of macrovascular and microvascular complications in type 2 diabetes. BMJ. 1998;317:713–20.

19 Antiplatelet Agents, Anticoagulants, Factor Xa Inhibitors, and Thrombin Inhibitors

ANTIPLATELET AGENTS

Antiplatelet agents are used in virtually all patients with coronary heart disease (CHD). Aspirin, the pioneer hallmark agent, is of proven value for the management of:

- Acute myocardial infarction (MI).
- Post-MI prophylaxis.
- Unstable angina.
- Stable angina.
- Following coronary artery bypass graft (CABG).
- Coronary angioplasty and coronary stents when combined with clopidogrel.
- Lone atrial fibrillation in individuals aged <65 years. Here apixaban or rivaroxaban may have a role.
- Transient ischemic attacks (TIAs) or following nonhemorrhagic stroke.

Available antiplatelet agents include:

- Aspirin
- Clopidogrel
- Dipyridamole + aspirin
- Prasugrel

© Springer Science+Business Media New York 2015
M. Gabriel Khan, *Cardiac Drug Therapy*, Contemporary Cardiology,
DOI 10.1007/978-1-61779-962-4_19

- Ticagrelor
- Platelet glycoprotein IIb/IIIa receptor blockers

The patient with CHD may have to face unstable angina, MI, and early cardiac death. There is now convincing evidence that antiplatelet agents and heparin (both unfractionated [UF] and low molecular weight [LMWH]), bivalirudin, and fondaparinux improve morbidity and mortality rates in patients with CHD.

Coronary thrombosis is known to be the major cause of coronary artery occlusion resulting in acute MI. In a hallmark study by DeWood et al. (1980), coronary thrombus was present in 87 % of 126 patients who had coronary arteriography performed within 4 h of the onset of symptoms and in 65 % of those studied 12 h or more after the onset of symptoms.

Davies and Thomas (1984) observed that, of patients with sudden cardiac ischemic death, 74 of 100 had coronary thrombi; 48 (65 %) of the 74 thrombi were found at sites of preexisting high-grade stenosis. In patients with thrombi, the most common finding is an underlying fissured plaque. The contents of the plaque and denuded endothelium are highly thrombogenic and initiate thrombosis, resulting in coronary occlusion. Thus, the prevention of the atherosclerotic process, plaque rupture, and thrombosis and dissolution of thrombi with dilation of the stenotic lesions are important therapeutic goals.

Antiplatelet agents (so called because they inhibit platelet aggregation) have a role in the prevention of coronary thrombosis, MI, and cardiac death. Platelets clump onto atherosclerotic plaques, causing occlusion of the artery, and/ or embolize downstream, occluding coronary arterioles. This effect may induce fatal arrhythmias and precipitate death. Angioscopic studies (Sherman et al. 1986) have confirmed the presence of platelet clumps on eccentric atheromatous plaques in patients with unstable angina and no such platelet aggregation in patients with stable angina. It is not surprising, therefore, that aspirin, a potent antiplatelet agent, has proved effective in preventing acute MI in patients with unstable angina. A small, but timely, trial by Lewis et al. (1983) showed that aspirin 325 mg reduced nonfatal and fatal infarction rates by about 50 % in patients with unstable angina. In the second International Study of Infarct Survival (ISIS-2), patients with acute MI administered aspirin 160 mg achieved a 25 % reduction in the 35-day vascular mortality rate and a 50 % decrease in the incidence of reinfarction. The addition of aspirin to streptokinase enhanced thrombolytic efficacy, resulting in a 48 % decrease in the 35-day vascular mortality rate over the period (ISIS-2 1988a).

- Antiplatelet agents are not expected to prevent all forms of thrombotic events.
- Thrombi occurring in arteries are rich in platelets, so antiplatelet agents are effective.
- In obstructed arteries, with low flow, the thrombus consists mainly of red cells within a fibrin mesh and very few platelets. This situation is similar to venous thrombosis, in which platelets are not predominant. The contents of a ruptured plaque are highly thrombogenic. Aspirin is only partially effective in preventing coronary thrombosis following plaque rupture, the usual cause of acute MI (Clarke et al. 1991, see Chap. 11). Thus, antiplatelet agents may not help sufficiently in this situation and direct thrombin inhibitors, such as bivalirudin, hirudin, hirulog, and fondaparinux, and newer types of oral anticoagulants specific for thrombin and derivatives of atheromatous plaque contents are receiving intensive study and clinical testing.

Drug name:	**Aspirin** (acetylsalicylic acid)
Dosage:	75–81 mg [non-enteric-coated] daily for ischemic heart disease (IHD) prophylaxis or for others with atherosclerotic disease

240–324 mg [3–4 tabs, 75–81 mg] chewed and swallowed at onset of pain caused by a probable heart attack.

Table 19-1
Indications for aspirin

	Cardiovascular	*Comment*
1.	Unstable angina	Proven
2.	Stable angina	Proven
3.	Acute-onset myocardial infarction	Proven, also enhances effect of thrombolytic agents
4.	Post MI	Proven effective
5.	Silent ischemia	Strongly advisable
6.	Coronary artery bypass surgery	May prevent graft occlusion
7.	Post-coronary angioplasty	Modest decrease in reocclusion
8.	Lone atrial fibrillation	In selected patients
9.	Bioprosthetic valves	In combination with dipyridamole
10.	Transient cerebral ischemic attacks	Proven in both men and women
11.	Post-nonhemorrhagic strokes	
12.	Patients over age 45 years at high risk	Strong family history of MI and significant dyslipidemia
13.	Diabetics at high risk for CHD	Advisable

CHD coronary heart disease, *MI* myocardial infarction

UK advice: Aspirin 300 mg (chewed or dispersed in water) is recommended.

Aspirin [acetylsalicylic acid (ASA)] has rightly gained widespread use in the management of unstable angina (Lewis et al. 1983; Cairns et al. 1986) and acute MI and in the prevention of nonfatal and fatal MI during the years following infarction. Also, salutary effects have been demonstrated in patients with stable angina and TIAs and in the prevention of occlusion of CABGs (see indications, Table 19-1).

Historical Review

Although this text has not given historical reviews of pharmacologic agents, it would appear timely to document briefly a few of the historical details that led to the widespread acceptance of aspirin, a drug that can prolong life.

- Hippocrates approximately (400 BC) treated his patients for pain with willow bark, which contains salicylic acid.
- 1763: Reverend Stone of Chipping Norton described the benefit of willow bark for ague.
- 1853: Von Gerhardt of Bayer developed aspirin.
- 1899: Felix Hoffman, a Bayer chemist, treated his father for rheumatism with aspirin.
- 1948–1953: Lawrence Craven treated ~1,500 relatively healthy, overweight, sedentary men aged 40–65 years to obviate coronary thrombosis and reported his findings in the Mississippi Valley Medical Journal "In Those with Risk Factors for Coronary Artery Disease" (Craven 1953). Craven apparently started treating his patients with high doses of aspirin and finally concluded that one aspirin a day was sufficient because none of his 1,500 or more patients given this low dose for ~5 years experienced a cardiac event (Craven 1953).
- 1971: John Vane discovered that aspirin blocks the production of prostaglandins.
- 1974: Elwood et al. (1974) reported negative results of a randomized trial of aspirin in the secondary prevention of mortality from MI. Aspirin was once more forgotten until it became clear that the clinical trial had studied patients who were given the drug 2, 3, and even 12 months after infarction.
- 1972–1977: The Stroke Trial of Fields and associates (Fields et al. 1977) showed a favorable trend.
- 1978: Barnet and colleagues reported that male patients with TIAs treated with aspirin showed a significant reduction in stroke rate. These investigators emphasized that aspirin did not have beneficial effects in women in their study, and this notion was perpetuated by others for several years. The trial had enrolled ~90 % men; there were not a sufficient number of women to test the hypothesis.

- 1983: The timely randomized trial of Lewis et al. showed conclusively that one Alka-Seltzer (ASA, 325 mg) produced a 49 % reduction in nonfatal MI. Cairns et al. (1986), in a larger study, confirmed the observation using 1,300 mg aspirin daily.
- 1988: ISIS-2 confirmed an increase in survival in patients given aspirin within 6 h of the onset of infarction. Aspirin enhanced the salutary effects of streptokinase and further improved survival rates (see Chap. 11).
- 1988: **Primary prevention in 22,071 male physicians, aged 40–80 years, randomly assigned to 325 mg aspirin on alternate days, resulted in a 44 % reduction in fatal and nonfatal MI** ($p < 0.0001$).
- 1989: The American College of Chest Physicians recommended (Resnekov et al. 1989) that aspirin, 325 mg daily, be considered for virtually all individuals with evidence of CHD and selected patients with risk factors for CHD.

The Swedish Angina Pectoris Aspirin Trial studied 2,035 patients with chronic stable angina without infarction. Aspirin 75 mg reduced the occurrence of infarction and sudden death by 34 % in the treated patients versus placebo (Juul-Moller et al. 1992).

Table 19-1 gives the clinical indications for aspirin, and Table 19-2 defines patients at risk in whom aspirin is advisable.

The results of five randomized trials in patients with atrial fibrillation led to the following conclusions:

- Patients aged under 60 years with lone atrial fibrillation (no risk factors and no structural heart disease) can be treated with aspirin 60–162 mg daily. They usually do not require oral anticoagulants for stroke prevention because the risk of stroke is low (<0.5 % per year).
- In patients aged 65–75 years with lone atrial fibrillation, the stroke rate is also low (<2 % per year) and aspirin therapy is recommended by some, but anticoagulant therapy should be individualized because there are no clear answers.

Table 19-2
Patients at risk, aspirin advisable

1. Hyperlipidemia: total cholesterol level >240 mg/
   dL (5.2 mmol/L) especially if HDL-C <35 mg/dL
   (0.9 mmol/L)
2. Mild hypertension[a]
3. Diabetes, except hemorrhagic retinopathy
4. Strong family history of vascular thrombosis:
   Myocardial infarction at age <60 years, stroke at <70 years
5. Refractory smokers with any one of the above factors
   strengthens indication
6. Following hip or knee surgery for 3 weeks if oral
   anticoagulants not used

Dosage: use aspirin noncoated 75–162 mg daily with food; or
enteric coated, 81–325 mg daily

[a]Not in severe hypertension, increased risk of hemorrhagic stroke

- In patients over age 75 years, warfarin has proved more effective than aspirin, but most of this benefit was lost because of a high rate of intracranial hemorrhage caused by warfarin. In addition, the mean age of patients in these trials was 69 years, and only about 25 % were over age 75 years (Atrial Fibrillation Investigators 1994). Thus, until further trial results are available in patients older than 70 with lone atrial fibrillation, treatment should be individualized.

ACTIONS

- Acetylsalicylic acid irreversibly acetylates the enzyme cyclooxygenase. This enzyme is necessary for the conversion of platelet arachidonic acid to thromboxane A_2. The latter is a powerful platelet-aggregating agent and vasoconstrictor.
- The conversion to thromboxane A_2 and platelet aggregation can be initiated by several substances, especially those released following the interaction of catecholamine or platelets with subendothelial collagen. Endothelial and smooth

muscle cells, when stimulated by physical or chemical injury, cause cyclooxygenase to convert membrane arachidonic acid to prostacyclin (prostaglandin I2 [PGI2]), which is then released. Prostacyclin is a powerful inhibitor of platelet aggregation as well as a potent vasodilator. Prostacyclin, therefore, may help keep the vessel wall clean.

• Prostacyclin production is greatly reduced in diseased arteries. Aspirin further reduces the formation of prostacyclin in the vessel wall, and this is an undesirable effect. Low-dose aspirin inhibits thromboxane A_2 synthesis and platelet aggregation and does not inhibit PGI2 production significantly.

Dosage: The author recommends soft chewable aspirin [noncoated] 80–81 mg daily after a meal, preferably the evening meal.

General recommendation is enteric-coated aspirin 75–325 mg daily. An 80- and 81-mg enteric-coated tablet is available in North America; 60–75 mg is often used in Europe. Chewable 80–81 mg is useful, for daily use, and if chest pain occurs, the chew tablet is readily available: take 160–240 mg at the onset of symptoms of chest pain suggestive of MI.

Aspirin, 20–60 mg daily, inhibits serum thromboxane A_2 generation without affecting prostacyclin synthesis and completely suppresses platelet aggregation (Patrono and Wood 1994). It is advisable not to exceed 325 mg daily; 60–81 mg appears to be optimal. In the Aspirin Reinfarction Study, although infarction rates decreased, sudden deaths were increased (Aspirin Myocardial Infarction Study Research Group 1980). In addition, prostacyclin infusion has been shown to prevent ventricular fibrillation (VF) after circumflex artery occlusion in dogs. The importance of inhibition of prostacyclin by doses higher than 325 mg cannot be dismissed. The inhibition of prostacyclin synthesis by aspirin 1 g daily may increase the risk of sudden death during acute infarction.

The cardiovascular indications for aspirin are listed in Table 19-1.

Aspirin Resistance

The exact prevalence of aspirin resistance is unknown; estimates suggest that between 5.5 and 60 % of patients using this drug may exhibit a degree of "aspirin resistance," depending upon the definition used and parameters measured; aspirin resistance may be related to the use of nonsteroidal anti-inflammatory agents and proton pump inhibitors (Gasparyan et al. 2008). These investigators failed to consider the effect of enteric coating; however Kapoor (2008), in a letter, stated that it is important to take note of recent reports of incomplete suppression of platelet aggregation with enteric-coated aspirin as shown by Cox et al. (2006) and Maree et al. (2005). In a randomized, open-label, crossover study of healthy volunteers, incomplete thromboxane (TX) B2 inhibition was found to occur in 8 % of the aspirin group and 54.3 % of the enteric-coated aspirin group ($p = 0.0004$) (Cox et al. 2006). In another study of 131 stable cardiovascular patients treated with enteric-coated aspirin (75 mg/day), 44 % of patients failed to attain optimal inhibition of serum TX, indicating a suboptimal inhibition of platelet COX-1 activity, and those with an incomplete aspirin response were more likely to demonstrate platelet aggregation to arachidonic acid (21 % vs. 3 %; $p = 0.004$) (Maree et al. 2005).

- **It is advisable to administer 75–81 mg soft chewable aspirin daily instead of enteric-coated aspirin for the** prevention of CAD and stroke. Importantly, individuals who use soft chewable aspirin daily would have the product on hand and would be able to take 3–4 soft aspirins for chest pain that is unrelieved by nitroglycerin.
- It is important for physicians to advise patients who have symptoms suggestive of a heart attack that the immediate use of 3–4 soft aspirins could prevent a fatal or nonfatal MI, and in this setting, aspirin intake is more important than the use of nitroglycerin which does not prevent heart attacks.

- Sound advice on the use of aspirin therapy for cardiovascular disease prevention is given by the European Society of Cardiology (Halverson et al. 2014).

  <Set up as in 7 e p 335>

Drug name:	**Dipyridamole**
Trade names:	Persantine, Persantin, Persantin Retard
Supplied:	25, 50, and 75 mg; Retard 200 mg
Dosage:	50–75 mg three times; Retard 200 mg twice daily

The drug is useful only when combined with aspirin. It inhibits platelet adhesion to vessel walls and surfaces but has a low effect on platelet aggregation.

Caution: The drug may increase ischemia and angina owing to coronary steal and is contraindicated in unstable angina and immediately after MI.

The combination of dipyridamole and aspirin for the management of stroke and TIA is not advisable in patients with CHD because angina or ischemia may be precipitated.

Interaction: The drug causes an accumulation of adenosine; thus, severe hypotension may occur if IV adenosine is given for supraventricular tachycardia; the dose of adenosine should be halved.

Indications

1. Prosthetic heart valves. The combination of dipyridamole and warfarin has been shown to be more effective than oral anticoagulants alone in preventing embolization in patients at risk (i.e., those with previous embolism).
2. Patients with tissue valves who show evidence of embolization.

3. Dipyridamole combined with aspirin (Aggrenox) appears to provide beneficial effects for secondary prevention after stroke (EPS Group 1987). Dipyridamole should be added to aspirin if TIAs are recurrent.

A randomized controlled trial (RCT) indicated that dipyridamole (slow-release formulation, 200 mg plus aspirin 50 mg twice daily) resulted in a highly significant reduction in the occurrence of stroke ($p < 0.001$). The risk reduction for aspirin and dipyridamole for stroke was 37 % vs. 15 % for dipyridamole alone and 18 % for aspirin alone. At present, the combination of aspirin and dipyridamole or clopidogrel appears to be the most effective and safest therapy for secondary prevention of stroke, but see caution given above.

Drug name:	**Clopidogrel**
Trade name:	Plavix
Supplied:	75 mg
Dosage:	75 mg daily with or without food

This thienopyridine is established therapy prior to PCI for STEMI and NSTEMI. A loading dose of 600 mg is recommended prior to planned PCI. A 75 mg daily dose is continued for 1–2 years or longer in selected cases.

Studies have suggested that adverse cardiovascular outcomes with the combination of clopidogrel and a proton pump inhibitor [PPI] are explained by the individual PPI. The use of a PPI that inhibits CYP450 2C19, including lansoprazole, or rabeprazole and notably, omeprazole has been reported to significantly decrease the inhibitory effect of clopidogrel on platelet aggregation.

One study reported that the PPI pantoprazole was not associated with recurrent MI among patients receiving clopidogrel, possibly due to pantoprazole's lack of inhibition of CYP450 2C19 (Juurlink et al. 2009).

Morphine has been shown to decrease clopidogrel absorption, decrease concentrations of clopidogrel active metabolite, and diminish its salutary effects. This can cause treatment failure in susceptible patients (Hobl et al. 2014).

In the Clopidogrel and Metoprolol in Myocardial Infarction Trial/Second Chinese Cardiac Study (COMMIT/-2 2005), patients with acute MI received aspirin and were randomized to receive clopidogrel 75 mg/day or placebo. Clopidogrel caused a significant reduction in death, reinfarction, or stroke (9.2 % vs. 10.1 %; relative risk reduction, 9 %; $p = 0.002$).

The Clopidogrel for High Atherothrombotic Risk and Ischemic Stabilization, Management, and Avoidance (CHARISMA) trial (Bhat et al. 2006) showed that **clopidogrel plus aspirin administered to patients with stable CHD was not significantly more effective than aspirin alone in reducing the rate of MI, stroke, or death from cardiovascular causes.**

• Gebel points out that clinical studies provide little evidence that clopidogrel, with or without aspirin, is more efficacious for the prevention of strokes than aspirin alone (Gebel 2005). The increased risk of bleeding episodes with clopidogrel and aspirin in combination probably outweighs any small reductions in secondary event risk. In contrast, extended-release dipyridamole (ER-DP) plus aspirin reduces secondary stroke risk to a significantly greater extent (23 % relative risk reduction) than aspirin alone.

PRASUGREL

Prasugrel is a third-generation thienopyridine and a more potent blocker of the platelet P2Y12 receptor than clopidogrel, producing consistent platelet inhibition (Wiviott et al. 2007). Clopidogrel and prasugrel bind irreversibly to the platelet surface-membrane (P2Y12) receptor. Ticagrelor is a reversible

P2Y12 receptor blocker, with platelet function returning to normal, 2–3 days after discontinuation (Gurbel et al. 2009).

TRITON-TIMI 38, a double-blind, randomized controlled trial compared prasugrel with clopidogrel in patients undergoing PCI for STEMI (Montalescot et al. 2009). Patients with STEMI (3,534) were randomly assigned either prasugrel (60-mg loading, 10-mg maintenance [n = 1,769]) or clopidogrel (300-mg loading, 75-mg maintenance [n = 1,765]). The primary end point was cardiovascular death, nonfatal MI, or nonfatal stroke.

Assessment using intention to treat: at 30 days, 115 (6.5 %) individuals assigned prasugrel had met the primary end point compared with 166 (9.5 %) allocated clopidogrel (hazard ratio 0.68; p = 0.0017). This effect continued to 15 months (174 [10 %] vs. 216 [12.4 %]; 0.79; p = 0.0221). The secondary end point of cardiovascular death, MI, or urgent target vessel revascularization was significantly reduced with prasugrel at 30 days (0.75; p = 0.0205) and 15 months (0.79; p = 0.0250), as was stent thrombosis.

Life-threatening bleeding and TIMI major or minor bleeding were similar with the two treatments, and only TIMI major bleeding after CABG surgery was significantly increased with prasugrel (p = 0.0033).

In patients with STEMI undergoing PCI, prasugrel is more effective than clopidogrel for the prevention of ischemic events, without an apparent excess in bleeding (Montalescot et al. 2009).

Prasugrel showed a consistent benefit over clopidogrel for reducing cardiovascular death, MI, stroke, urgent revascularization, and stent thrombosis in patients who did (hazard ratio: 0.76) or did not receive a GP IIb/IIIa blocker (hazard ratio: 0.78). The use of a GP IIb/IIIa blocker does not accentuate the relative risk of bleeding with prasugrel as compared with clopidogrel (O'Donoghue et al. 2009). "A loading dose of 60 mg prasugrel achieves faster, more consistent, and greater inhibition of ADP-induced platelet aggregation than does 600 mg of clopidogrel, with a significant effect seen 30 min after administration of prasugrel when no effect is detectable with clopidogrel" (Wiviott et al. 2007; Wallentin et al. 2008).

• The pharmacokinetic and pharmacodynamic advantages of prasugrel over clopidogrel are clinically important when pretreatment is not possible, and fast inhibition of platelet aggregation is desirable for primary PCI for STEMI (Montalescot et al. 2009).

Prasugrel must not be administered to patients with active bleeding or a history of TIA or stroke. Patients <60 kg have an increased exposure to the active metabolite and an increased risk of bleeding on a 10-mg once-daily dose. It is advisable to lower the maintenance dose to 5 mg in patients who weigh <60 kg, although the effectiveness and safety of the 5-mg dose have not been studied prospectively.

Ticagrelor [BRILINTA: Brilique in UK]

Ticagrelor is an oral non-thienopyridine cyclopentyltriazolo-pyrimidine ADP–receptor (P2Y12) antagonist, which like prasugrel is more potent and rapid acting than clopidogrel.

Cannon and colleagues for the Platelet Inhibition and Patient Outcomes (PLATO) investigators compared ticagrelor with clopidogrel. Subjects were 13,408 (72 %) of 18,624 patients hospitalized for STEMI and NSTEMI. At 1 year, the primary composite end point occurred in fewer patients in the 6,732 ticagrelor-treated group than in the 6,676 clopidogrel group: $p = 0.0025$. Ticagrelor compared with clopidogrel significantly *reduced all-cause mortality* at 12 months in all patients (4.5 % vs. 5.9 %, hazard ratio 0.78, $p < 0.001$).

- Unlike clopidogrel and prasugrel, which bind irreversibly to the platelet surface-membrane (P2Y12) receptor, ticagrelor is a reversible P2Y12 receptor blocker, with platelet function returning to normal 2–3 days after discontinuation (Gurbel et al. 2009) compared with 5–10 days after discontinuation of clopidogrel and prasugrel. Within 30 min, a ticagrelor loading dose of 180 mg results in roughly the same level of inhibition of platelet aggregation as that achieved 8 h after a clopidogrel loading dose of 600 mg (Gurbel et al. 2009).

- Ticagrelor, compared with clopidogrel, reduced the composite of cardiovascular death, MI, and stroke in patients with extensive coronary heart disease (14.9 % vs. 17.6 %) similar to its reduction in those without extensive CAD (6.8 % vs. 8.0 %) (Kotsia et al. 2014).

In UK: Indicated in combination with aspirin for the prevention of atherothrombotic events in patients with acute coronary syndrome (with aspirin—initially 180 mg as a single dose, then 90 mg twice daily).

Caution: bradycardia, sick sinus syndrome, or second- or third-degree AV block (unless pacemaker fitted); asthma or chronic obstructive pulmonary disease; history of hyperuricemia; may elevate serum creatinine; monitor renal function 1 month after initiation.

Interactions: increases plasma concentration of simvastatin (increased risk of toxicity); interaction with digoxin, clarithromycin, erythromycin, diltiazem, paroxetine, and citalopram.

Cangrelor

Cangrelor is an IV ADP–P2Y12 receptor antagonist with a quick onset and quick offset. It has a plasma half-life of 3–6 min; platelet function returns to normal in 60 min. This rapid-acting IV antiplatelet drug, cangrelor, provided an effective bridge for patients on thienopyridine therapy, including clopidogrel, who required bypass surgery, as shown in the BRIDGE trial.

Platelet Glycoprotein IIb/IIIa Receptor Blockers

There are ~75,000 glycoprotein IIb/IIIa receptors on the surface of each platelet. Antagonism of these receptors blocks the final common pathway for platelet aggregation—the binding of fibrinogen to the platelet glycoprotein receptors. Blockade of these receptors prevents the platelet aggregation caused by thrombin, thromboxane A_2, ADP, collagen, and catecholamines, as well as shear-induced platelet aggregation.

Platelets may be activated by a myriad of agonists (thrombin, epinephrine, collagen, thromboxane, serotonin, adenosine-5′-diphosphate, von Willebrand factor, and so on) through various receptors involving complex signaling pathways. Platelet aggregation, the occurrence of cross-linking between platelets to form a "white thrombus," requires the activation of a common final pathway, the glycoprotein (GP) IIb/IIIa receptor-mediated linking of one platelet to another by binding to fibrinogen and in high-shear-stress conditions to von Willebrand factor. Given that platelets may be activated by multiple pathways but aggregate through a single pathway, the GP IIb/IIIa receptor emerged (Coller 1995).

The increasing use of clopidogrel, ticagrelor, and prasugrel, as proven alternative antiplatelet agents, and the development of direct thrombin inhibitors such as bivalirudin and fondaparinux, which cause less major bleeding, will further retard the use of platelet GP receptor blockers.

Drug name:	**Abciximab**
Trade name:	ReoPro
Dosage:	When PCI is planned within 24 h, give 0.25 mg/ kg IV bolus over at least 1 min, immediately followed by IV infusion: 0.125 µg/kg/min for 18–24 h (max. 10 µg/min), concluding 1 h after PCI. The half-life is 10–30 min

Drug name:	**Eptifibatide**
Trade name:	Integrilin
Supplied:	IV bolus prior to PCI
Dosage for ACS:	• Intravenous bolus of 180 µg/kg as soon as possible after diagnosis • Follow by continuous infusion of 2 µg/kg/min for a further 20–24 h after PCI • If the patient is to undergo CABG, eptifibatide should be discontinued • Before surgery Eptifibatide was shown in the Enhanced Suppression of the Platelet IIb/IIIa Receptor

Drug name:	**Tirofiban**
Trade name:	Aggrastat
Dosage:	Two-stage infusion: 0.40 µg/kg/min for 30 min; then 0.1 µg/kg/min for up to 48–108 h (*see* product monograph); half-life 2 h

TACTICS-TIMI 18: The Treat Angina with Aggrastat and Determine Cost of Therapy with an Invasive or Conservative Strategy (TACTICS)-TIMI 18 trial (Cannon et al. 2001) compared early invasive and conservative strategies in patients with unstable coronary syndromes treated with the GP IIb/IIIa inhibitor tirofiban and showed superiority of an invasive strategy in patients with non-ST-elevation ACS. Patients with acute NSTEMI as defined by positive troponin levels benefited the most; the drug was beneficial only in patients with ACS treated with an early invasive strategy.

TIMACS randomized 3,031 patients, 1,593 to an early invasive strategy (coronary angiography, PCI, or surgery) within 24 h of presentation and 1,438 to a delayed invasive strategy (>36 h following presentation). The relative use of various agents is notable: aspirin (98 %); clopidogrel (87 %); glycoprotein IIb/IIIa inhibitor (in only 23 %); fondaparinux

(41.5 %); heparin and low-molecular-weight heparin in 64.3 and 24.6 %, respectively; beta-blockers (86.9 %); and statins (85 %). A prior MI or significant ECG changes of ischemia were observed in 20 and 80 %, respectively, and about 77 % of the patients had elevated biomarkers indicating NSTEMI. There was no difference in the incidence of the primary outcome of death, MI, and stroke between the early invasive and delayed invasive arms (9.7 % vs. 11.4 %, hazard ratio [HR] 0.85, 95 % confidence interval [CI] 0.68–1.06, $p = 0.15$).

- There was a significant reduction in the incidence of the primary end point in the early invasive arm compared with the delayed invasive arm (14.1 % vs. 21.6 %, $p = 0.005$) in patients with a GRACE score of >140 (Mehta et al. 2009).

ANTICOAGULANTS

Drug name:	**Warfarin**
Trade names:	Coumadin
Supplied:	1, 2, 2½, 4, 5, 7½, 10 mg
Dosage:	10 mg on day 1, and 5 mg on day 2 (*preferably at bedtime*), with adjustment of dosage on the third day to about 3–7.5 mg depending on the INR; *see* text for further advice

For less urgent anticoagulation, give 5 mg daily for 4 days, and then go to international normalized ratio (INR) 2–3 (note that the 10 mg for 2 days starting dose used commonly in the 1980s can cause gangrene of the limbs, albeit rarely). Warfarin is the most commonly used coumarin oral anticoagulant. Bleeding owing to oral anticoagulant is reversed by vitamin K1 2–5 mg or fresh frozen plasma 15 mL/kg. For interactions see Table 19-3. A decrease in oral anticoagulant response has been reported with dietary sources of vitamin K1 including Ensure Plus and broccoli

Table 19-3
Oral anticoagulant drug interactions

1. *Drugs that may enhance anticoagulant response*

Alcohol
Allopurinol
Aminoglycosides
Amiodarone
Ampicillin
Anabolic steroids
Aspirin
Cephalosporins
Chloral hydrate
Chloramphenicol
Chlorpromazine
Chlorpropamide
Chlortetracycline
Cimetidine
Clofibrate (fibrates)
Co-trimoxazole
Danazol
Dextrothyroxine
Diazoxide
Dipyridamole
Disulfiram
Ethacrynic acid
Erythromycin
Fenclofenac
Fenoprofen
Flufenamic acid
Fluconazole
Isoniazid
Ketoconazole
Ketoprofen
Liquid paraffin
Mefenamic acid
Methotrexate
Metronidazole
Monoamine oxidase inhibitors
Nalidixic acid
Naproxen
Neomycin
Omeprazole
Penicillin (large doses IV)
Phenformin
Phenylbutazone
Propylthiouracil
Quinidine
Rosuvastatin
Sulfinpyrazone
Sulfonamides
Tamoxifen
Tetracyclines
Tolbutamide
Thyroxine
Tricyclic antidepressants
Trimethoprim–sulfamethoxazole
Verapamil

2. *Drugs that may decrease anticoagulant response*

Antacids
Antihistamines
Barbiturates
Carbamazepine
Cholestyramine
Colestipol
Corticosteroids
Cyclophosphamide
Dichloralphenazone
Disopyramide
Glutethimide
Griseofulvin
Mercaptopurine
Oral contraceptives
Pheneturide
Phenytoin
Primidone
Rifampicin
Vitamins K_1 and K_2

(Kempin 1983). Other foods with high vitamin K content include turnip greens, lettuce, and cabbage.

Drug name:	**Heparin**
Dosage:	60-U/kg bolus (max. 4,000 U) as an immediate bolus and then a continuous infusion of 12 U/kg (1,000 U/h) to maintain the activated partial thromboplastin time [aPTT] at 1.5–1.2 times baseline. The aPPT is assessed Q 6 h until in the target range, then every12 h

Action: Anticoagulant activity requires a cofactor, antithrombin III. Heparin binds to lysine sites on antithrombin III and converts the cofactor from a slow inhibitor to a very rapid inhibitor of thrombin. The heparin–antithrombin complex inactivates thrombin and thus prevents thrombin-induced activation of factors V and VIII. The reaction also inactivates factor X, other coagulation enzymes, and thrombin-induced platelet aggregation. The half-life is 30–60 min after a 75-U/kg IV bolus.

Low-Molecular-Weight Heparin

Drug name:	**Enoxaparin**
Trade name:	Lovenox
Supplied:	Prefilled syringes: 30, 40 mg Graduated prefilled syringes: 60, 80, 100 mg Ampules: 30 mg
Dosage:	1 mg/kg every 12 h SC; plus aspirin 100–325 mg daily for a minimum of 2 days (*see* Chaps. 11 and 22)

- The dose of LMWH should be reduced in patients over age 70 and given once daily in those with creatinine clearance (estimated GFR) 30–50 mL/min and avoided in those with estimated GFR <30 mL/min.

- The adjustment of dosage based on weight, age, and renal function is vital to reduce the increased risk of bleeding caused by LMWH.

Specific Thrombin Inhibitors

The composition of the material that causes coronary occlusion and, thus, acute MI is complex. The thrombogenic properties of ruptured atheromatous plaques cannot all be nullified by aspirin, platelet IIb/IIIa receptor blockers, and standard thrombolytic agents (t-Pa, streptokinase). Novel specific thrombin inhibitors are being sought. Direct thrombin inhibitors such as bivalirudin, fondaparinux, and hirudin do not need a cofactor to inhibit thrombin.

BIVALIRUDIN

Bivalirudin binds reversibly to thrombin. The drug cleaves to thrombin then drops off, which may explain the short half-life of 25 min and the lower adverse effects compared with hirudin and heparin.

HORIZONS-AMI (2011) was a prospective, open-label, randomized trial in patients with acute STEMI, within 12 h after onset of symptoms, undergoing PCI. Patients were randomly allocated patients 1:1 to receive bivalirudin or heparin plus a glycoprotein IIb/IIIa inhibitor [GPI].

Results at 3 years: Compared with 1,802 patients allocated to receive heparin plus a GPI, 1,800 patients allocated to bivalirudin monotherapy had lower rates of all-cause mortality (5.9 % vs. 7.7 %,), cardiac mortality (2.9 % vs. 5.1 %, $p = 0.001$), and reinfarction (6.2 % vs. 8.2 %, $p = 0.04$). Major bleeding not related to bypass graft surgery was significantly reduced (6.9 % vs. 10.5 %, $p = 0.0001$).

ISAR-REACT 4 trial (Abciximab and Heparin versus Bivalirudin for Non-ST-Elevation Myocardial Infarction): Subjects were all treated with ASA and clopidogrel 600 mg. Bivalirudin was administered to 860 and abciximab to 861 patients. There were no significant differences in deaths, or recurrent MI, but major bleeding was ~84 % increased by abciximab [4.6 %] compared with bivalirudin [2.6 %] Kastrati et al. (2011). In addition advantages include a much shorter duration of IV infusion and cost compared to the use of antiplatelet inhibitors (Kastrati et al. 2011). Bivalirudin is the preferred anticoagulant agent for PCIs:

• Avoid if eGFR less than 40 mL/min. Reduce dose if eGFR 45–60 mL/min and in elderly over age 70 because renal function is usually impaired.

UK advice: Indicated for patients undergoing PCI (in addition to aspirin and clopidogrel), IV, 750 µg/kg then by IV 1.75 mg/kg/h for up to 4 h after procedure; a reduced infusion rate of 250 µg/kg/h may be continued for a further 4–12 h if necessary. Caution renal impairment: for PCI, reduce rate of infusion to 1.4 mg/kg/h if eGFR 30–60 mL/min/1.73 m^2 and monitor blood clotting parameters; avoid if eGFR less than 30 mL/min.

Fondaparinux

Fondaparinux is a synthetic pentasaccharide that selectively inhibits factor Xa. Fondaparinux can be administered once daily without laboratory monitoring:

• In OASIS-6 [2006] which involved patients with STEMI, particularly those not undergoing primary PCI, fondaparinux significantly reduced mortality and reinfarction without increasing bleeding and strokes.
• UK advice: ST-segment elevation MI, initially IV or infusion, 2.5 mg for first day, then 2.5 mg subcutaneously once daily for up to 8 days (or until hospital discharge if sooner); treatment should be stopped 24 h before coronary artery bypass graft surgery.

Caution: Reduce dose if eGFR 40–50 mL/min or over age 75 as renal dysfunction is common. Avoid if eGFR

<40 mL/min. Unstable angina and NSTEMI, SC injection, 2.5 mg once daily for up to 8 days (or until hospital discharge if sooner).

Factor Xa Inhibitors

RIVAROXABAN [XARELTO]

Rivaroxaban has been characterized as a potent and highly selective oral direct factor Xa inhibitor. Activation of factor X to factor Xa [via the intrinsic and extrinsic pathways] plays a central role in the cascade of blood coagulation. Factor Xa initiates the final step by converting prothrombin to thrombin which converts fibrinogen to a fibrin clot. Thrombin also enhances platelet membrane activation which promotes platelet aggregation. Endothelial injury releases a cell surface glycoprotein, tissue factor, that activates Factor V11. Factor V11a activates 1X to 1Xa which activates factor X to Xa. Inhibition of factor Xa by rivaroxaban reduces thrombin generation and inhibits clot formation (Mega et al. 2012).

Acute MI Study: The ATLAS ACS–TIMI 46 RCT showed the drug effective when commenced within 7-day post-acute MI in patients stabilized following PCI or thrombolytic therapy. Patients received the first dose of rivaroxaban no sooner than 4 h after the final dose of intravenous unfractionated heparin, 2 h after the final dose of bivalirudin, and 12 h after the final dose of other intravenous or subcutaneous anticoagulants (e.g., enoxaparin or fondaparinux). Patients were randomly assigned to twice-daily administration of either 2.5 or 5.0 mg of rivaroxaban or placebo, with a maximum follow-up of 31 months.

Rivaroxaban significantly reduced the primary efficacy end point of death from cardiovascular causes, MI, or stroke, as compared with placebo. The 2.5 mg twice daily achieved efficacy without increased life-threatening bleeding (Mega et al. 2012).

Atrial Fibrillation Study (Rivaroxaban versus Warfarin in Nonvalvular Atrial Fibrillation): Patel et al., the ROCKET AF investigators (2011), randomly assigned 14,264 patients with nonvalvular atrial fibrillation who were at increased risk for stroke to receive either rivaroxaban (at a **daily dose of 20 mg**) or dose-adjusted warfarin.

The primary end point occurred in 269 patients in the rivaroxaban group (2.1 % per year) and in 306 patients in the warfarin group (2.4 % per year) $P < 0.001$ for noninferiority. Major and nonmajor clinically relevant bleeding occurred in 1,475 patients in the rivaroxaban group (14.9 % per year) and in 1,449 in the warfarin group (14.5 % per year), with significant reductions in intracranial hemorrhage (0.5 % vs. 0.7 %, $P = 0.02$) and fatal bleeding (0.2 % vs. 0.5 %, $P = 0.003$) in the rivaroxaban group.

Elderly patients had higher stroke and major bleeding rates than younger patients, but the efficacy and safety of rivaroxaban relative to warfarin did not differ with age, supporting rivaroxaban as an alternative for the elderly (Halperin et al. 2014).

Dosage: Following acute MI **2.5 mg twice daily** when patients are stabilized following PCI or thrombolytic therapy. Atrial fibrillation [approved], 20 mg daily:

- Prophylaxis of venous thromboembolism following knee replacement surgery, adult over 18 years, **10 mg once daily** for 2 weeks starting 6–10 h after surgery

Adverse effects: nausea, hemorrhage, less commonly dyspepsia, vomiting, tachycardia, dizziness, headache, renal impairment, rash; jaundice also reported.

The drug is rapidly absorbed with the maximum concentration appearing 2–4 h after tablet intake. A 10 mg or lower dose can be taken with or without food. Rivaroxaban is eliminated by both renal and metabolic routes. Approximately 66 % of a rivaroxaban dose is eliminated via the kidneys, of which 30–40 % is excreted as unchanged active drug in the urine. Metabolism occurs via cytochrome P450 (CYP) 3A4, CYP 2J2, and CYP-independent mechanisms.

The concomitant use of rivaroxaban with other strong CYP 3A4 inducers (e.g., phenytoin, carbamazepine, phenobarbitone, or St. John's wort) may also lead to a decreased rivaroxaban plasma concentration.

There is no pharmacokinetic interaction between rivaroxaban and clopidogrel, but as expected bleeding is enhanced.

DABIGATRAN [PRADAXA; PRADAX]

In patients with atrial fibrillation, the 150-mg twice-daily dose, as compared with warfarin, was associated with lower rates of stroke and systemic embolism but similar rates of major hemorrhage. There was a significantly higher rate of major gastrointestinal bleeding with dabigatran at the 150-mg dose than with warfarin (Connolly et al. 2009). Gage in an editorial emphasized that MI and gastrointestinal side effects were significantly more common with dabigatran than with warfarin. Rates of MI were 0.72 and 0.74 % with 110 and 150 mg twice daily of dabigatran, respectively, and 0.53 % with warfarin.

- Patients already taking warfarin with excellent INR control have little to gain by switching to dabigatran because of dabigatran's twice-daily dosing, the greater risk of MI, non-hemorrhagic side effects, and similar major hemorrhagic events compared with warfarin (Gage 2009).

APIXABAN [ELIQUIS]

In patients with atrial fibrillation, apixaban was superior to warfarin in preventing stroke or systemic embolism, caused less bleeding, and resulted in lower mortality (ARISTOTLE: Granger et al. 2011).

Dosage: 5 mg twice daily.

Among patients with nonvalvular atrial fibrillation who are at high risk for stroke and for whom vitamin K antagonist therapy is unsuitable, apixaban, as compared with aspirin, substantially reduced the risk of stroke, with no significant increase in the risk of major bleeding or intracranial bleeding. Apixaban, compared with warfarin, was associated with fewer intracranial hemorrhages, less adverse events following extracranial hemorrhage, and a 50 % reduction in fatal consequences at 30 days in cases of major hemorrhage (Hylek et al. 2014).

See Chap. 24

REFERENCES

ARISTOTLE, Granger CB, Alexander JH, McMurray JJV, et al. Apixaban versus warfarin in patients with atrial fibrillation. N Engl J Med. 2011;365:981–92.

Aspirin Myocardial Infarction Study Research Group. A randomized, controlled trial of aspirin in persons recovered from myocardial infarction. JAMA. 1980;243:661.

Atrial Fibrillation Investigators. Risk factor for stroke and efficacy of antithrombotic therapy in atrial fibrillation: Analysis of pooled data from 5 randomized controlled trials. Arch Intern Med. 1994;154:1449.

Cairns JA, Gent M, Singer J, et al. Aspirin, sulfinpyrazone or both in unstable angina. N Engl J Med. 1986;313:1369.

CHARISMA Investigators: Bhat DL, Keith AA, Fox KAA, Hacke W, for the CHARISMA Investigators. Prevention of atherothrombotic events. N Engl J Med. 2006;354:1706–17.

Clarke RJ, Mago G, Fitzgerald G, et al. Combined administration of aspirin and a specific thrombin inhibitor in man. Circulation. 1991;83:1510.

Coller BS. Blockade of platelet GP IIb/IIIa receptors as an antithrombotic strategy. Circulation. 1995;92:2373–80.

COMMIT-2 (Clopidogrel and Metoprolol in Myocardial Infarction Trial) Collaborative Group. Addition of clopidogrel to aspirin in 45,852 patients with acute myocardial infarction: randomised placebo-controlled trial. Lancet. 2005;366:1607–21.

Connolly SJ, Ezekowitz MD, Yusuf S, et al. Dabigatran versus warfarin in patients with atrial fibrillation. N Engl J Med. 2009;361:1139–51 [Erratum, N Engl J Med 2010;363:1877.].

Cox D, Maree AO, Dooley M, et al. Effect of enteric coating on antiplatelet activity of low-dose aspirin in healthy volunteers. Stroke. 2006;37:2153–8.

Craven LL. Experiences with aspirin (acetylsalicylic acid) in the nonspecific prophylaxis of coronary thrombosis. Miss Valley Med J. 1953;75:38.

Davies MJ, Thomas A. Thrombosis and acute coronary artery lesions in sudden cardiac ischemic death. N Engl J Med. 1984;310:1137.

DeWood MA, Spores J, Notske R, et al. Prevalence of total coronary occlusion during the early hours of transmural myocardial infarction. N Engl J Med. 1980;303:897.

Elwood PC, Cochrane AL, Burr ML, et al. A randomized controlled trial of acetylsalicylic acid in the secondary prevention of mortality from myocardial infarction. BMJ. 1974;1:436.

Fields WS, Lemak NA, Frankowski RF, et al. Controlled trial of aspirin in cerebral ischemia. Stroke. 1977;8:301.

Gage BF Can we rely on RE-LY? NEJM 2009;361:1200–1202.

Gasparyan AY, Watson T, Lip GY. The role of aspirin in cardiovascular prevention: implications of aspirin resistance. J Am Coll Cardiol. 2008;51:1829–43.

Gebel Jr JM. Secondary stroke prevention with antiplatelet therapy with emphasis on the cardiac patient. A neurologist's view. J Am Coll Cardiol. 2005;37:2059–65.

Gurbel PA, Bliden KP, Butler K, et al. Randomized double-blind assessment of the ONSET and OFFSET of the antiplatelet effects of ticagrelor versus clopidogrel in patients with stable coronary artery disease: the ONSET/OFFSET study. Circulation. 2009;120:2577–85.

Halperin JL, Hankey GJ, Wojdyla et al., on behalf of the ROCKET AF Steering Committee and Investigators. Efficacy and safety of rivaroxaban compared with warfarin among elderly patients with nonvalvular atrial fibrillation in the Rivaroxaban Once Daily, Oral, Direct Factor Xa Inhibition Compared With Vitamin K Antagonism for Prevention of Stroke and Embolism Trial in Atrial Fibrillation. Circulation. 2014;130:138–146

Halverson S, Andreotti F, ten Berg HM, et al. Aspirin therapy in primary cardiovascular disease prevention: a position paper of the European society of cardiology working group on thrombosis. J Am Coll Cardiol. 2014;64(3):319–27.

Hobl E, Stimlfl T, Ebner J, et al. morphine decreases clopidogrel concentrations and effects. A randomized double—blind placebo-controlled trial. J Am Coll Cardiol. 2014;63(7):630–5.

HORIZONS-AMI, Stone GW, Witzenbichler B, Guagliumi G, et al. Heparin plus a glycoprotein IIb/IIIa inhibitor versus bivalirudin monotherapy and paclitaxel-eluting stents versus bare-metal stents in acute myocardial infarction (final 3-year results from a multicentre, randomised controlled trial. Lancet. 2011;377(9784):2193–204.

Hylek EM, Held C, Alexander JH, et al. Major bleeding in patients with atrial fibrillation receiving apixaban or warfarin. The ARISTOTLE Trial (Apixaban for reduction in stroke and other thromboembolic events in atrial fibrillation) Predictors, characteristics, and clinical outcomes. J Am Coll Cardiol. 2014;63(20):2141–7.

ISIS-2 (Second International Study of Infarct Survival) Collaborative Group. Randomized trial of intravenous streptokinase, oral aspirin, both, or neither among 17,187 cases of suspected acute myocardial infarction: ISIS-2. Lancet. 1988a;2:349–50.

Juul-Moller S, Edvardsson N, Jhnmatz B, et al. Double-blind trial of aspirin in primary prevention of myocardial infarction in patients with stable chronic angina pectoris. Lancet. 1992;40:1421.

Juurlink DN, Gomes T, Ko DT, et al. A population-based study of the drug interaction between proton pump inhibitors and clopidogrel. CMAJ. 2009;180:713–8.

Kapoor JR. Enteric coating is a possible cause of aspirin resistance. J Am Coll Cardiol. 2008;52:1276–7.

Kastrati A, Neumann F-J, Schulz S, for the ISAR-REACT 4 Trial Investigators, et al. Abciximab and heparin versus bivalirudin for non–ST-elevation myocardial infarction. N Engl J Med. 2011;365:1980–9.

Kempin SJ. Warfarin resistance caused by broccoli. N Engl J Med. 1983;308:1229.

Kotsia A, Brilakis ES, Held C, et al. Extent of coronary artery disease and outcomes after ticagrelor administration in patients with an acute coronary syndrome: insights from the PLATelet inhibition and patient Outcomes (PLATO) trial. Am Heart J. 2014;168(1):68–75.e2.

Lev EI, Patel RT, Maresh KJ. The role of dual drug resistance. J Am Coll Cardiol. 2006;47:27–33.

Lewis HD, Davis JW, Archibald DG, et al. Protective effects of aspirin against acute myocardial infarction and death in men with unstable angina: results of a veterans administration cooperative study. N Engl J Med. 1983;309:396.

Maree AO, Curtin RJ, Dooley M, et al. Platelet response to low-dose enteric-coated aspirin in patients with stable cardiovascular disease. J Am Coll Cardiol. 2005;46:1258–63.

Mega JL, Braunwald E, Wiviott SD, et al. Rivaroxaban in patients with a recent acute coronary syndrome. N Engl J Med. 2012;366:9–19.

Mehta SR, Granger CB, Boden WE, TIMACS, et al. Early versus delayed invasive intervention in acute coronary syndromes. N Engl J Med. 2009;360:2165–75.

O'Donoghue M, Antman EM, Braunwald E, et al. The efficacy and safety of prasugrel with and without a glycoprotein IIb/IIIa inhibitor in patients with acute coronary syndromes undergoing percutaneous intervention: a TRITON–TIMI 38 (Trial to Assess Improvement in Therapeutic Outcomes by Optimizing Platelet Inhibition with Prasugrel-Thrombolysis in Myocardial Infarction 38) analysis. J Am Coll Cardiol. 2009;54:678–85. (TRITON–TIMI 38).

Patrono C, Wood AJJ. Aspirin as an anti-platelet drug. N Engl J Med. 1994;330:1287.

PLATO, Cannon CP, Harrington RA, James S, et al. for the platelet inhibition and patient Outcomes investigators. Comparison of ticagrelor with clopidogrel in patients with a planned invasive strategy for acute coronary syndromes: a randomised double-blind study. Lancet. 2010;375(9711):283–93.

Resnekov L, Chekiak J, Hirsh J, et al. Antithrombotic agents in coronary artery disease. Chest. 1989;95:528.

ROCKET AF, Patel MR, Mahaffey KW, Garg J, et al. Rivaroxaban versus warfarin in nonvalvular atrial fibrillation. N Engl J Med. 2011;365: 883–891.

Sherman CT, Litrack F, Grundfest W, et al. Coronary angioscopy in patients with unstable angina pectoris. N Engl J Med. 1986;315:913.

The ESPS Group. The European Stroke Prevention Study. Principal end points. Lancet. 1987;2:1352.

TRITON-TIMI 38 Investigators, Montalescot G, Wiviott SD, Braunwald E, et al. Prasugrel compared with clopidogrel in patients undergoing percutaneous coronary intervention for ST-elevation myocardial infarction double-blind, randomised controlled trial. Lancet. 2009;373(9665):723–31.

Wallentin L, Varenhorst C, James S, et al. Prasugrel achieves greater and faster P2Y12receptor-mediated platelet inhibition than clopidogrel due to more efficient generation of its active metabolite in aspirin-treated patients with coronary artery disease. Eur Heart J. 2008; 29:21–30.

Wiviott SD, Trenk D, Frelinger AL, et al. Prasugrel compared with high loading- and maintenance-dose clopidogrel in patients with planned percutaneous coronary intervention: the Prasugrel in comparison to clopidogrel for inhibition of platelet activation and aggregation-thrombolysis in myocardial infarction 44 trial. Circulation. 2007;116:2923–32.

20 Cardiac Drugs During Pregnancy and Lactation

Most cardiovascular agents (like all other drugs) must be avoided in the first trimester of pregnancy because they may produce congenital malformations, especially from the 3rd to the 11th week of pregnancy. When used during the second and third trimesters, several cardiac drugs may affect growth and functional development of the fetus or cause toxic effects on fetal tissues. Also, some agents must be avoided just before parturition as they may have adverse effects on labor or in the newborn.

Cardiovascular drugs are discussed mainly with an emphasis on their safety for the fetus or newborn.

The physician is commonly called to manage the following hazardous heart conditions in pregnancy:

- Acute severe hypertension caused by preeclampsia.
- Mitral stenosis and pulmonary edema that can be fatal.
- Arrhythmias that may be bothersome.
- Pulmonary hypertension that may cause sudden death.
- Peripartum cardiomyopathy causing heart failure.

ANTIHYPERTENSIVE AGENTS IN PREGNANCY

Fortunately, because of the vasodilating properties of early pregnancy, patients with mild hypertension often do not need drug therapy until after week 20 of pregnancy. In uncomplicated chronic hypertension, a target

© Springer Science+Business Media New York 2015
M. Gabriel Khan, *Cardiac Drug Therapy*, Contemporary Cardiology,
DOI 10.1007/978-1-61779-962-4_20

blood pressure of <150/100 mmHg is recommended; in women with target-organ damage as a result of chronic hypertension, and in women with chronic hypertension who have given birth, a target blood pressure of <140/90 mmHg is advised. Methyl dopa, and labetalol are antihypertensive agents commonly used in pregnancy (Seely and Ecker 2014).

The relatively safe agents commonly used from week 16 include:

- Methyldopa; discontinue 2 days prior to delivery
- Beta-adrenergic blockers with caution
- Labetalol: short term and emergencies
- Hydralazine: short term, emergencies, mainly IV use

    Caution is necessary with the following agents:

- Thiazide diuretics: short term only
- Nifedipine: short-term hypertensive crisis: fulminating preeclampsia

Angiotensin-converting enzyme (ACE) inhibitors and angiotensin receptor blockers [ARBs] nitroprusside, reserpine, diltiazem, and verapamil are contraindicated.

Achievement of blood pressure control does not eliminate a risk for the patient or baby. Intensive maternal and fetal monitoring is mandatory irrespective of successful control of blood pressure, as a risk of abruption, seizures, and disseminated intravascular coagulopathy still prevails.

Women with preeclampsia or gestational hypertension who present with a blood pressure over 150/100 mmHg should receive treatment with labetalol to achieve a target blood pressure of <150 mmHg systolic and diastolic 80–100 mmHg. If labetalol is contraindicated or intolerance develops, methyldopa is advisable and if very necessary modified-release nifedipine can be tried.

Methyldopa

Drug name:	**Methyldopa**
Trade name:	Aldomet
Supplied:	125, 250, 500 mg
Dosage:	250 mg twice daily, increasing if needed to max. 1.5 g daily

Methyldopa was the most widely used agent for the long-term management of hypertension in pregnancy for over 30 years until about 1990; since then, beta-blockers have often replaced methyldopa because depression (~22 %), sedation, and postural hypotension cause problems with compliance and lead to ~15 % of patients stopping treatment. Also, the drug causes a positive direct Coombs test, and problems may occur with cross-matching the patient's blood. The long track record of efficacy and the preservation of fetal well-being, especially the absence of neurologic effects, have established a proven role for this old drug. Several newer agents have been tried for the chronic management of hypertension, and all but a few selective beta-blocking agents have fallen aside because of various adverse effects on the fetus. Notably, most studies of antihypertensive agents in pregnancy have been used in only a few patients and with age at entry later than week 24 of gestation. Caution is therefore necessary even with relatively safe agents used early in pregnancy.

In one study, only one (0.9 %) fetal death occurred in 117 methyldopa-treated patients, and 9 (7.2 %) fetal deaths occurred in the control group of 125 women (Redman et al. 1976). Methyldopa does not cause a decrease in uteroplacental blood flow. A 7-year follow-up of children born to mothers treated with methyldopa showed no significant differences (Cockburn et al. 1982). Other randomized trials, however, have failed to show any benefit from treatment compared with beta-blockers or no treatment (Gallery et al. 1997).

Methyldopa is the recommended agent for the treatment of severe hypertension (diastolic pressure >105 mmHg) associated with severe preeclampsia, remote from delivery. Occasionally, intravenous therapy is required, 250 mg diluted in 100 mL 5 % dextrose in water, given over 30–60 min, repeated every 6 h.

Adverse effects include orthostatic hypotension, sedation, dizziness, fatigue, Coombs positivity; depression occurs in ~22 %.

Caution: *Avoid methyldopa after parturition because the drug may precipitate or worsen depression* (*see* Chap. 8).

The combination of methyldopa and beta-blockers is not advisable because both agents act centrally.

Beta-Adrenergic Blockers

Beta-blockers are relatively effective agents in controlling hypertension during pregnancy from the 16th week to about 1 week prior to labor. Although they have been used effectively in patients within 72 h before labor and during delivery, other agents are preferred during this period. Blood pressure control, if required, just prior to delivery is best achieved with the use of IV hydralazine.

Beta-blockers have advantages over methyldopa for prolonged treatment of chronic hypertension during the last trimester. These agents do not usually cause orthostatic hypotension, somnolence, or significant depression. Also, methyldopa must be taken two or three times daily as opposed to beta-blockers, which are given once daily. The most common beta-blockers used during pregnancy are *labetalol, atenolol,* and *pindolol.* Atenolol caused no fetal adverse effects in 120 pregnant women; neonates showed a minor incidence of transient bradycardia not requiring therapy, and a 1-year follow-up gave results similar to those observed with methyldopa, with no differences in development or growth indices (Reynolds et al. 1984). In another study, 4 years follow-up revealed all normal infants (Olofsson et al. 1986). Chronic atenolol therapy does not increase the incidence of neonatal respiratory distress syndrome. In one study, no child in the actively treated group required ventilation, as opposed to seven infants in the control group requiring ventilation for the respiratory distress syndrome (Rubin et al. 1983).

Other studies with atenolol have found significantly lower infant birth and placental weights compared with the nontreatment arm (Churchill and Beevers 1999), and the concern appears to be unique to atenolol used for long-term but not for short-term treatment.

Adverse effects of beta-blockers used during pregnancy include: fetal or neonatal bradycardia; premature or prolonged labor; delayed spontaneous breathing in the newborn, mainly observed with IV use; and rarely neonatal hypoglycemia. Intrauterine growth retardation is often mentioned with the use of atenolol, and low infant birth weight may occur with long-term treatment.

Drug name:	**Metoprolol**
Trade names:	Betaloc, Lopressor, Toprol XL
Supplied:	50, 100 mg
Dosage:	50 mg twice daily, max. 200 mg

The dosages of metoprolol and pindolol are much lower than those advised by the respective manufacturers.

Drug name:	**Labetalol**
Trade names:	Normodyne, Trandate
Supplied:	50, 100, 200 mg

Dosage:	Oral: 100 mg twice daily with food, increasing over 2–4 weeks to 200 mg twice daily; max. 600 mg
	For hypertensive crises in pregnancy: IV slow bolus 20–50 mg or infusion 20 mg/h titrated slowly with continuous BP monitoring to 30–160 mg/min
	The combination with hydralazine allows lower doses of both agents with fewer side effects

Hypertensive crises in pregnancy: labetalol IV infusion: 20 mg/h titrated slowly with continuous BP monitoring; the dose is doubled every 30 min if needed to 40 mg, maximum 160 mg/h . The combination with IV hydralazine allows lower doses of both agents with fewer side effects.

Labetalol is a beta-adrenergic blocking agent with $alpha_1$-blocking properties, and thus it causes vasodilation. The latter effect may result in orthostatic hypotension. **The drug may also cause fatal or life-threatening hepatic necrosis.** Labetalol is as effective as methyldopa in controlling hypertension during pregnancy. The drug is extremely useful in the acute short-term management of severe resistant hypertension just before labor or during delivery. Avoid in asthmatics. Some state that labetalol is generally safer and preferable to atenolol (Churchill and Beevers 1999).

Adverse effects include about a 27 % incidence of intrauterine growth retardation. The pregnant woman may experience perioral numbness, tingling, and itching of the scalp, and rarely a lupus-like illness, a lichenoid rash; a rare association is retroplacental hemorrhage (Lindheimer and Katz 1985). *Also, a rare but life-threatening complication is acute hepatic necrosis* (Clarke et al. 1990). **These serious side effects are not caused by other beta-adrenergic blockers.**

Labetalol use should be confined to hypertensive emergencies. The drug has a role given intravenously in the management of severe resistant hypertension (diastolic blood pressure >110 mmHg) associated with preeclampsia occurring just before or during delivery. Labetalol given intravenously appears to be more effective than IV hydralazine or methyldopa. The blood pressure-lowering effect is more predictable, and the drug causes less tachycardia and appears to cause less fetal distress than hydralazine.

Drug name:	**Hydralazine**
Trade name:	Apresoline
Supplied:	25 mg
Dosage:	25 mg twice daily, increasing to three times daily; max. 100 mg daily before the addition of a beta-blocking drug

For hypertensive crisis: IV bolus 5–10 mg.

Hydralazine is a pure arteriolar vasodilator and has been used extensively for acute control of severe hypertension in the third trimester of pregnancy.

The drug is teratogenic in animals. Safety for chronic use is not as secure as that observed with methyldopa or beta-blockers.

The drug causes reflex tachycardia and sodium and water retention, which may necessitate the use of a diuretic or a beta-blocker to blunt tachycardia as well as to enhance the antihypertensive effect.

The drug has a role in the short-term management of severe hypertension during late pregnancy unresponsive to methyldopa or beta-blockers. Acute lowering of blood pressure is necessary in severe preeclampsia to prevent cerebral hemorrhage, the main cause of the increase in maternal mortality seen in preeclampsia. The drug is very useful when a modest dose is combined with a low dose of a beta-blocking drug, such as atenolol 50 mg daily, or as an adjunct to methyldopa; combination therapy prevents tachycardia and headaches caused by hydralazine.

The chronic use of the drug is limited by adverse effects that include fetal thrombocytopenia, although this occurrence is rare. The mother may experience dizziness, postural hypotension, a lupus syndrome, palpitations, and edema.

Hydralazine is the mainstay of therapy for the treatment of acute severe hypertension (blood pressure >170/110 mmHg) occurring just before labor, during labor, or at delivery. Hydralazine remains the agent of choice, given as boluses (Patterson-Brown et al. 1994). The drug acts quickly and reduces blood pressure in a fairly well-controlled manner, although labetalol IV appears to be a reasonable alternative to hydralazine, producing a more predictable and controlled decrease in blood pressure. Also, nitroprusside is more effective but is contraindicated because of serious potential risks to the neonate. The drug does not decrease cardiac output and preserves uteroplacental blood flow.

Dosage: slow IV injection 5–10-mg bolus diluted with 10 mL 0.9 % sodium chloride given over 1–2 min, repeated in 20–30 min and then as often as necessary over several hours. The maximal effect of hydralazine is observed in 20 min. Duration of action is 6–8 h.

Hypertensive emergencies: Dosage: initially 200–300 micrograms/min; maintenance usually 50–150 micrograms/min, with continuous evaluation of heart rate and blood pressure and fetal monitoring. If hydralazine fails to control blood pressure adequately, the addition of methyldopa or labetalol is advisable. As indicated earlier, labetalol IV bolus or infusion appears to be a reasonable alternative for hydralazine-resistant hypertension. If nifedipine is chosen, caution is necessary not to give magnesium sulfate concomitantly because severe hypotension may ensue.

THIAZIDE DIURETICS

Because hypertension of pregnancy and preeclampsia are associated with reduced plasma volume, diuretics are not indicated. Fetal outcome is usually worse in women with preeclampsia who fail to expand plasma volume. Thiazides may cause neonatal thrombocytopenia, albeit rarely. Also, diuretics may exacerbate maternal carbohydrate intolerance. A meta-analysis of randomized trials involving more than 7,000 pregnant women indicated no increased incidence of adverse fetal effects (Collins et al. 1985). Other studies have shown fetal and neonatal jaundice as well as thrombocytopenia. (Furosemide is usually contraindicated during pregnancy; see later discussion of heart failure).

Calcium Antagonists

Calcium antagonists are teratogenic in animals. These agents have not been adequately tested except in a few small studies in late pregnancy for severe or accelerated hypertension in which nifedipine 5–10 mg orally has proved effective without adverse consequences (Walters and Redman 1984).

Nifedipine [unlicensed] is useful in severe hypertension or preeclampsia and has been used over a 4–6 weeks period. Nifedipine given in late pregnancy to women with accelerated severe hypertension resulted in an average fall in blood pressure of 26/20 mmHg within 20 min of oral dosing (Walters and Redman 1984).

An increase in diastolic blood pressure >110 mmHg uncontrolled by methyldopa and a beta-blocker should prompt cessation of methyldopa and commencement of the short-term use of nifedipine 20–30 mg/day.

Dosage: Modified release/long acting 20–30 mg once daily. The drug is best combined with short-term use of atenolol 25–50 mg daily or pindolol 5 mg daily. The combination used for 1–2 weeks during the last trimester of pregnancy should suffice to smother the peaking of blood pressure, and maintenance therapy with a beta-adrenergic blocking agent, with or without combination of hydralazine, may be necessary.

Nifedipine has a role to play in the management of fulminating preeclampsia and severe hypertension resistant to
therapy occurring in the last few weeks of pregnancy and for
acute hypertensive emergencies, for which controlled clinical trials are necessary to establish indications and overall
safety. Clinicians should check whether the drug is approved
for these indications.

Caution: Do not use nifedipine or calcium antagonists
concomitantly with magnesium sulfate because catastrophic
lowering of blood pressure may occur. Magnesium sulfate is
commonly used to prevent seizures in patients with severe
preeclampsia in association with resistant hypertension.

The drug may inhibit labor; manufacturer advises to
avoid before week 20; risk to fetus should be balanced
against risk of uncontrolled maternal hypertension; use only
if other treatment options are not indicated or have failed.

ACE Inhibitors

ACE inhibitors are contraindicated during pregnancy.
They may adversely affect fetal and neonatal blood pressure
control and renal function. They may cause skull defects
and oligohydramnios. These agents are teratogenic in animals and are associated with a high incidence of intrauterine
death. Acute renal failure with catastrophic consequences
has been noted in neonates of mothers given ACE inhibitors
in the third trimester.

Magnesium Sulfate

Magnesium sulfate causes only a mild and transient lowering of blood pressure. The drug remains the most useful
agent for the prevention of seizures associated with severe
preeclampsia (Saunders and Hammersley 1995). Magnesium
sulfate is a neuromuscular blocker and appears to prevent
the end-organ consequences of prolonged hypoxemia that
may occur with concomitant seizure activity. The drug is not

known to be harmful for short-term IV intravenous administration in eclampsia, but excessive doses in third trimester cause neonatal respiratory depression.

For preeclampsia prevention of seizures: IV injection over 5–20 min, 4 g followed by IV infusion, 1 g/h for 24 h; if seizure occurs, additional dose by IV injection, 2 g.

For eclampsia: treatment of seizures and prevention of seizure recurrence: IV injection over 5–20 min, 4 g, followed by IV infusion, 1 g/h for 24 h after seizure or delivery, whichever is later; if seizure recurs, increase the infusion rate to 1.5–2 g/h or give an additional dose 2 g by IV injection.

Concentration of magnesium sulfate should not exceed 20 % (dilute 1 part of magnesium sulphate injection 50 % with at least 1.5 parts of water for injections).

Caution: Magnesium sulfate is contraindicated in renal failure and hepatic dysfunction and should not be used concomitantly with calcium antagonists because severe hypotension may occur. The drug should not be used primarily for its antihypertensive effect.

Aspirin

Patients with chronic kidney disease, diabetes mellitus, autoimmune disease, or chronic hypertension are at high risk of developing preeclampsia and aspirin is advisable. Dosage 75–81 mg once daily from 12th week until the baby is born.

Patients with more than one moderate risk factor (first pregnancy, aged ≥40 years, pregnancy interval >10 years, BMI ≥35 kg/m^2 at first visit, multiple pregnancy, or family history of preeclampsia) are at risk for developing preeclampsia and aspirin 75–81 mg once daily is advised.

Mitral stenosis: In a cohort of pregnant patients with severe mitral stenosis, 67 % developed a maternal cardiac event, and 44 % of infants were born prematurely or died (Silversides et al. 2003). Women with mitral stenosis often become symptomatic during pregnancy because of significant increases in plasma volume ($\approx$50 %) and heart rate ($\approx$20–30 %). Common complications in pregnant patients include the development of pulmonary edema or atrial tachyarrhythmias/atrial fibrillation/flutter (Norrad and Salehian 2011).

Patients with significant mitral stenosis must decrease their activity and commenced on a beta-blocker [metoprolol is acceptable, except in asthmatics]. Furosemide may be needed. About 75 % of pregnant women respond to this therapy (Norrad and Salehian 2011). Medical treatment may lead to a reduction in New York Heart Association functional class III/IV to I/II (Silversides et al. 2003). Interventional and surgical options are reserved for those who deteriorate despite aggressive medical therapy. Interventional procedures should be delayed until 12–14 weeks to prevent radiation exposure during the period of organogenesis (Hameed et al. 2009). If intervention becomes necessary after 20 weeks, it is best deferred to between 26 and 30 weeks gestation to prevent complications associated with births in the extremes of prematurity (Hameed et al. 2009). Percutaneous mitral valvuloplasty is now the procedure of choice.

DRUG THERAPY FOR HEART FAILURE

Drugs are used to provide hemodynamic stability and reduce symptoms prior to prompt correction and treatment of the cause of heart failure or pulmonary edema. The common causes of heart failure or pulmonary edema in pregnancy are:

- Mitral stenosis and rarely other valvular heart disease. Mitral stenosis is the most common cause of pulmonary edema in pregnancy. Heart failure develops in more than 70 % of patients during the third trimester and early puerperium
- Systemic hypertension associated with preeclampsia
- Pulmonary hypertension
- Very rarely, peripartum cardiomyopathy

Beta-blockers are the cornerstone of treatment for the medical management of mitral stenosis during pregnancy (Al-Kasab et al. 1990), particularly for prevention of pulmonary edema in pregnant patients with mitral stenosis. Left atrial pressure rises as diastolic blood flow through the tight mitral valve is slowed. In addition, cardiac output and intravascular volume reach a peak by week 20–24. The heart rate increases an average of 10 beats/min. Increase in heart rate causes a shortened ventricular filling period and a marked increase in left atrial pressure. Sinus tachycardia, thus, may precipitate pulmonary edema, which may be fatal. Reduction in the resting heart rate from a mean of 86–78 beats/min is associated with marked clinical improvement. The dose of beta-blockers is titrated according to the patient's symptoms and heart rate. Also, with atrial fibrillation, beta-blockers are most useful to achieve a ventricular rate <80/min. Digoxin does not slow the heart rate sufficiently. If pulmonary edema develops, diuretics are added to beta-blocker therapy.

Digoxin is of no value in the management of pulmonary edema caused by pure mitral stenosis but has a small role in hypertensive heart failure and in patients with dilated cardiomyopathy or other conditions associated with poor left ventricular systolic function. The drug is not advisable except when poor left ventricular function is proved, preferably by echocardiographic evaluation. No teratogenic or untoward adverse fetal effects, except for digitalis toxicity, have been reported with the chronic use of digoxin (Rotmensch et al. 1983). Serum digoxin levels are similar in the mother and neonate (Rogers et al. 1972), but there is about a 50 % reduction in digoxin serum levels in the pregnant, as opposed to the nonpregnant, state. **Digoxin levels must be maintained 0.5 to maximum 0.9 ng/mL [0.6–1.0 nmol/l]. Toxicity can be avoided by the watchful physician;** *see* **Chap. 12.**

Diuretics

Diuretics have been discussed earlier in this chapter under antihypertensive agents. For the management of heart failure, especially in the crisis of pulmonary edema related to mitral stenosis, short-term thiazide diuretic therapy over a few days is indicated for symptomatic relief along with oxygen and morphine until mitral stenosis can be corrected by balloon valvuloplasty or by surgery. Thiazides rarely cause fetal or neonatal jaundice or thrombocytopenia, but their use is justifiable for the treatment of pulmonary edema and hypertension associated with preeclampsia. The antici-pated benefit must be weighed against the possible hazards to the fetus or neonate exposed to short-term therapy.

Caution: Furosemide is contraindicated because it causes fetal abnormalities, but it can be used for pulmonary edema in the last weeks of pregnancy and in the puerperium to manage life-threatening pulmonary edema.

Vasodilators: ACE inhibitors are contraindicated at all stages of pregnancy. If afterload reduction is deemed neces-sary for the management of heart failure, hydralazine may be used in the third trimester of pregnancy. The manufac-turer indicates hydralazine toxicity and teratogenic effects in animal studies, and this agent must be avoided during the first trimester.

ANTIARRHYTHMICS IN PREGNANCY

Adenosine

Adenosine is the drug of choice for the management of atrioventricular nodal reentrant tachycardia (AVNRT; *see* Chap. 14) (Harrison et al. 1992). The drug causes no signifi-cant change in fetal heart rate because it has a half-life of only a few seconds. A bolus of 6 mg over 2 s with cardiac monitoring followed by 12 mg after 1–2 min is usually effective; increments should not be given if high level AV block develops. Large doses may produce fetal toxicity; manufacturer advises use only if essential.

Beta-Adrenergic Blockers

Beta-blocking agents are of proven value in the management of bothersome arrhythmias during pregnancy, mainly because other antiarrhythmic agents may pose hazards for the fetus or neonate.

Acute termination of paroxysmal supraventricular tachycardia (PSVT) is achieved with the use of intravenous esmolol or atenolol and provokes few or no adverse effects in the fetus. IV beta-blockers should be avoided if possible during labor and delivery because respiratory depression may occur in the neonate, albeit rarely. See earlier discussion of beta-blockers for hypertension.

Beta-blockers are the safest antiarrhythmic agents available for the management of bothersome recurrent PSVT (chronic management; in these patients the beta-blocking agent may be used in combination with digoxin if needed) as well as for bothersome ventricular premature contractions.

- For ventricular tachycardia: beta-blockers should be tried before the use of other antiarrhythmic agents.

Disopyramide

The drug crosses the placenta and may induce labor. Sufficient data are not available to allow a firm conclusion to be made.

Lidocaine

Lidocaine crosses the placenta and does not appear to be teratogenic. Sufficient data covering use in the first trimester are not available. There is evidence of its safety during the second and third trimesters. Minimize the dose close to delivery to decrease the potential for fetal respiratory depression. The drug is indicated for life-threatening ventricular arrhythmias. Adverse effects include fetal acidosis, respiratory depression, apnea, and bradycardia in infants.

CARDIAC DRUGS DURING LACTATION

Virtually all maternally ingested drugs are excreted into breast milk, usually in amounts less than 2 % of the maternal dose. The concentration in the milk is occasionally sufficient to cause adverse pharmacologic effects in the infant. Caution is necessary because there is insufficient evidence to provide guidance on all cardiac drugs and it is advisable to administer these agents to the lactating mother only if deemed absolutely necessary.

The best time to take the drug, if administered, is immediately after a feeding. The mother is advised to express and discard the morning breast milk, which usually contains the highest concentration of the drug, and to feed the infant at least 1–2 h after the drug is given.

Factors affecting drug excretion into breast milk include:

1. **Protein binding:** Drugs that are poorly protein bound are excreted into breast milk, for example, atenolol (only 5 % bound) achieves sufficient concentration in breast milk to cause adverse effects in the infant, albeit rarely. *Atenolol, acebutolol, nadolol, and sotalol are contraindicated with breastfeeding.*
2. **Lipid solubility**: Because breast milk is an excretory pathway for lipophilic substances, which are not effectively metabolized by the body, cardiac agents that are lipophilic should be expected in higher concentration, and their use should be avoided unless alternatives are not available. Propranolol is lipophilic but is protein bound and *achieves low concentration in milk.*
3. **Molecular weight** is not an impediment to excretion into milk except for very large molecular weight agents, such as heparin and insulin, that are unable to gain passage to milk.
4. **Volume of breast milk**: Because the quantity of breast milk is greatest in the morning, transfer of the drug is maximal at this time. Consequently, this feed should be avoided if a drug that is excreted is indicated in therapy.

5. **pH of the milk**: Milk is usually acidic, with a pH of 6.35–7.65. Drugs that are weak bases, such as beta-adrenergic blockers, are trapped in the milk, but their concentration is fortunately low.

A high milk-to-plasma (MP) ratio implies an increased intake of a drug by the infant. The MP ratio may be altered by several factors, however, and is insufficiently accurate to serve as a reliable guide for prescribing most cardiac drugs. For example, a 240-mg daily dose of diltiazem achieves a concentration of about 200 ng/mL in breast milk with an MP ratio of only 1.0. Diltiazem is contraindicated with breastfeeding. Atenolol, 100 mg daily, achieves a milk concentration of about 0.6 µg/mL, MP ratio 3, and is also contraindicated. However, several agents with MP ratios of up to 3 have not indicated evidence of toxicity in infants.

The concentration of a drug in breast milk can be estimated and, when possible, agents with minimal concentrations should be prescribed. Specific drug concentrations in milk and their relation to toxicity in infants have not yet been established, and caution is required.

Drugs in breast milk may, at least theoretically, result in hypersensitivity in the infant even when drug concentration in the infant is too low to initiate a pharmacologic or toxic effect.

In addition, drugs to the mother must be avoided if the infant is premature or if either mother or infant is suspected of having hepatic or renal impairment because most drugs are metabolized or eliminated by the kidney.

Advice is given only for commonly used cardiac drugs.

ACE Inhibitors: The average concentration of captopril in breast milk is 5 µg/mL with an MP ratio of 0.1. The effect on a nursing infant has not been studied adequately, although a few reports have indicated no adverse effects. Until further information is available, ACE inhibitors should not be used during lactation except for the management of severe heart failure with poor systolic function, and breastfeeding should then be discontinued.

Adenosine: Because it has a half-life of less than 5 s, adenosine is safe during breastfeeding.

Anticoagulants: Warfarin is the most commonly used oral anticoagulant, has minimal transfer into breast milk, and rarely causes bleeding in the infant. Caution is necessary with dosing. Breastfeeding should be discontinued if the infant is premature and warfarin is deemed necessary. Ethyl biscoumacetate and phenindione are contraindicated because they are associated with a high incidence of bleeding. Low molecular weight heparins (e.g., dalteparin) are used judiciously.

Aspirin: Acetylsalicylic acid appears in breast milk. Although the concentration is low, aspirin should be avoided because interference with platelet function and metabolic acidosis may rarely occur. Also, it is necessary to avoid the rare risk of Reye's syndrome.

Beta-Blockers: Because beta-blockers are weak bases, these agents become trapped in breast milk. In addition, hydrophilic beta-blockers, atenolol, acebutolol, nadolol, and sotalol, are weakly protein bound and their concentration in the milk is much greater than that of propranolol, metoprolol, and timolol. Levels of the lipophilic agents are about 30 % lower than those of hydrophilic, loosely bound, agents (White 1984; Riant et al. 1986).

A case of atenolol toxicity in a full-term newborn infant has been reported. The mother was treated with atenolol for hypertension. Bradycardia, poor peripheral perfusion, and cyanosis were observed in the infant. Atenolol serum levels taken 48 h after cessation of breastfeeding were in the potentially toxic range for an adult (Schmimmel et al. 1989).

Caution is necessary in the use of hydrophilic beta-blockers, especially if renal dysfunction is present, as these agents are eliminated by the kidney. **If a beta-blocker is deemed necessary, it is advisable to administer propranolol**

during lactation because this drug attains an average concentration of 50 ng/mL in milk, MP ratio of 0.6. Metoprolol attains an average concentration of 1.7 μg/mL plus an MP ratio of 3, but sufficient information is not available. Pindolol and timolol attain low concentrations, but these drugs are partially excreted by the kidney and are partially lipophilic and hydrophilic; although they are not expected to be harmful; **propranolol has been well tested**. The American Academy of Pediatrics (1994) considers beta-blocker treatment to be compatible with breastfeeding.

Calcium Antagonists: Diltiazem is contraindicated because the average concentration is 200 ng/mL, MP ratio 1. Dihydropyridines have not been studied sufficiently during lactation, but nitrendipine attains a milk concentration of 5 ng/mL, MP ratio 2.5, and the concentration is believed to be too low to be harmful to the infant.

Verapamil attains an average milk concentration of about 20 μg/mL, MP ratio 0.4. The level in healthy infants has not caused adverse effects and is believed to be too low to be harmful. Accumulation and toxicity may occur, however, in the premature infant or in mothers with liver dysfunction.

Digoxin is excreted in breast milk; infant toxicity does not occur if care is taken in dosing relative to renal function. Average concentration in milk is 1.5 ng/mL, MP ratio 1.5. Digoxin is administered only if essential, with the usual precautions to avoid toxicity, and is compatible with breastfeeding.

Lidocaine (Lignocaine) is excreted in breast milk in high concentrations: up to 40 % of the maternal level (Zeisler et al. 1986). If IV lidocaine is required for the management of ventricular tachycardia, breastfeeding should cease at least 12 h after use of the drug, with the breast milk during that period being discarded. Harm to the infant is not expected. The American Academy of Pediatrics considers lidocaine treatment to be compatible with continued breastfeeding.

Methyldopa is frequently used during pregnancy to control hypertension and may be required up to delivery. Concentration in breast milk averages 1 µg/mL, MP ratio 0.3. The amount in breast milk does not appear to cause adverse effects in infants and is believed to be too small to be harmful. **Other agents, beta-blockers, are preferred after delivery because methyldopa may cause depression.**

Diuretics: Thiazides appear in breast milk. The concentration is low and usually not harmful to the infant. If large doses of thiazides beyond 25 mg daily are required, suppression of lactation may occur. The concentration of hydrochlorothiazide in breast milk is approximately 100 ng/mL, MP ratio 0.4. Because transfer to the infant is extremely small, thiazides are not contraindicated for the management of heart failure with pulmonary edema. In such a serious setting, however, breastfeeding is usually discontinued. Furosemide is more effective than thiazides for pulmonary edema.

REFERENCES

Al-Kasab S, Sabag T, Al-Zaibag M, et al. Beta-adrenergic receptor blockage in the management of pregnant women with mitral stenosis. Am J Obstet Gynecol. 1990;163:37.

Churchill D, Beevers DG. Hypertension in pregnancy. London: BMJ Books; 1999. p. 70–7.

Clarke JA, Zimmerman HF, Tanner LA. Labetalol hepatoxicity. Ann Intern Med. 1990;113:210.

Cockburn J, Moar VA, Ounsted M, et al. Final report of the study on hypertension during pregnancy: the effects of specific treatment on the growth and development of the children. Lancet. 1982;1:647.

Collins R, Yusuf S, Peto R. Overview of randomized trials of diuretics in pregnancy. BMJ. 1985;290:17.

Committee on Drugs, American Academy of Pediatrics. The transfer of drugs and other chemicals into human milk. Pediatrics. 1994;93:137.

Gallery EDM, Saunders DM, Hunyor SN, et al. Randomized comparison of methyldopa and oxprenolol for the treatment of hypertension in pregnancy. BMJ. 1997;1:1591.

Hameed A, Mehra A, Rahimtoola S. The role of catheter balloon for severe mitral stenosis in pregnancy. Obstet Gynecol. 2009;114:1336–60 (CrossRefMedline4).

Harrison JK, Greefield RA, Warton JM. Termination of acute supraventricular tachycardia by adenosine during pregnancy. Am Heart J. 1992;123:1386.

Lindheimer MD, Katz AI. Hypertension in pregnancy. N Engl J Med. 1985;313:675.

Norrad RS, Salehian O. Management of severe mitral stenosis during pregnancy. Circulation. 2011;124:2756–60.

Olofsson P, Montan S, Sartor G, et al. Effects of beta1-adrenergic blockade in the treatment of hypertension during pregnancy in diabetic women. Acta Med Scand. 1986;220:321.

Patterson-Brown S, Robson SC, Redfern N, et al. Hydralazine boluses for the treatment of severe hypertension. Br J Obstet Gynaecol. 1994;101:409.

Redman GWG, Beillin LJ, Bonnar J, et al. Fetal outcome in trial of antihypertensive treatment in pregnancy. Lancet. 1976;2:753.

Reynolds B, Butters L, Evans J, et al. The first year of life after atenolol in pregnancy associated hypertension. Arch Dis Child. 1984;59:1061.

Riant P, Urein S, Albergres E, et al. High plasma protein binding as a parameter in the selection of beta-blockers for lactating women. Biochem Pharmacol. 1986;24:4579.

Rogers MC, Willerson JT, Goldblatt A, et al. Serum digoxin concentrate in the human fetus, neonate and infant. N Engl J Med. 1972;287:1010.

Rotmensch HH, Elkayam Y, Frishman W. Antiarrhythmic drug therapy during pregnancy. Ann Intern Med. 1983;98:47.

Rubin PC, Butters L, Clark DM, et al. Placebo-controlled trial of atenolol in treatment of pregnancy-associated hypertension. Lancet. 1983; 1:431.

Saunders K, Hammersley V. Magnesium for eclampsia. Lancet. 1995; 346:788.

Schmimmel MS, Eidelman AI, Wilschanski MA, et al. Toxic effects of atenolol consumed during breastfeeding. J Pediatr. 1989;114:476.

Seely EW, Ecker J. Chronic Hypertension in Pregnancy Circulation. 2014;129:1254–1261, http://circ.ahajournals.org/search?author1=Jeffrey+Ecker&sortspec=date&submit=Submit.

Silversides C, Colman J, Sermer M, Siu S. Cardiac risk in pregnant women with rheumatic mitral stenosis. Am J Cardiol. 2003;91:1382–5.

Walters BNJ, Redman GWG. Treatment of severe pregnancy-associated hypertension with calcium antagonist nifedipine. Br J Obstet Gynaecol. 1984;91:330.

White WB. Management of hypertension during lactation. Hypertension. 1984;6:297.

Zeisler JA, Gaarder TD, Demesquita SA. Lidocaine excretion in breast milk. Drug Intell Clin Pharm. 1986;20:691.

21 Drug Interactions

Several cardiac drugs manifest some form of interaction with each other or with noncardiac drugs. It is of paramount importance for the physician to be aware of these interactions, which may be potentially harmful to patients or may negate salutary effects. In addition, the prescribing physician must be conscious of these interactions so as to avoid errors that may provoke medicolegal action.

The number of cardiac drugs available to the clinician has increased by more than 100 % over the past 25 years. Also, the drug armamentarium for the treatment of psychiatric, rheumatic, neurologic, infectious, and gastrointestinal (GI) diseases has expanded greatly. Consequently, drug interactions have increased.

Although drug interactions may have been briefly described for drug groups in earlier chapters, this chapter gives a structured summary of interactions. **This chapter deals with**:

- The interactions that occur between cardiac drugs
- The interaction of cardiovascular drugs with agents used for treating diseases of other systems and other agents with pharmacologic properties, such as caffeine, alcohol, and tobacco
- The adverse cardiovascular effects of noncardiac drugs

Drug interactions are usually:

1. **Pharmacodynamic**: Occurring between drugs that have similar or opposite pharmacologic effects or adverse effects; for example, these effects may occur because of competition

© Springer Science+Business Media New York 2015
M. Gabriel Khan, *Cardiac Drug Therapy*, Contemporary Cardiology,
DOI 10.1007/978-1-61779-962-4_21

at receptor sites or action of the drugs on the same physiologic system. In some instances, the hemodynamic effects of one agent increase or decrease the hemodynamic effects of another agent.

2. **Pharmacokinetic**: Occurring when one drug alters the absorption, distribution, metabolism, or excretion of another, thereby increasing or reducing the amount of drug available to exert its pharmacologic actions.

INTERACTIONS OF CARDIOVASCULAR DRUGS

Each cardiac drug (or drug group) interaction is discussed under the following categories:

1. Cardiovascular effects:
   (a) Vasodilator (arterial or venous, afterload, or preload reduction), hypotension, presyncope
   (b) Inotropic: positive or negative, alteration of ejection fraction (EF), propensity to precipitate congestive heart failure (CHF).
   (c) On the sinoatrial (SA) or atrioventricular (AV) node
   (d) On the conduction system
   (e) Proarrhythmic
2. Cholinergic effects
3. Plasma levels
4. Renal clearance of the drug, effect on renal function and serum potassium (K^+) concentration
5. Hematologic, including anticoagulant activity and/or immune effects
6. Hepatic and GI

ACE Inhibitors/ARBs

Cardiovascular Effects

When angiotensin-converting enzyme (ACE) inhibitors are used in combination with vasodilators, hypotension may occur. Preload-reducing agents, such as nitrates or prazosin, may cause syncope or presyncope (Table 21-1). Diuretics

Table 21-1
Angiotensin-converting enzyme inhibitors: potential interactions

- Angiotensin receptor blockers: increased risk of hyperkalemia
- Aspirin: appears to decrease salutary effects

- Corticosteroids: hypotensive effect of ACE inhibitors antagonized
  Cyclosporine: increased risk of hyperkalemia. Plasma
  concentration of aliskiren increased by cyclosporine—avoid
  concomitant use
  Lithium: reduced excretion of lithium (increased plasma
  concentration)
  Verapamil: plasma concentration of aliskiren increased by
  verapamil—manufacturer of aliskiren advises avoiding
  concomitant use
- Potassium-sparing diuretics: amiloride, Moduretic, Moduret,
  triamterene, Dyazide, Dytide, spironolactone (Aldactone),
  Aldactazide—increased risk of hyperkalemia
- Preload-reducing agents:
  Diuretics
  Nitrates
  Prazosin, other alpha blockers: enhanced hypotensive effect
- Renally excreted cardioactive agents
  Anti-arrhythmics: beta-blockers (atenolol, sotalol, nadolol)
- Digoxin: Captopril possibly increases plasma concentration
  of digoxin
- Agents that may alter immune status:
  Allopurinol: increased risk of leucopenia
  Acebutolol
  Hydralazine
  Pindolol
  Procainamide
- Tocainide
- Furosemide
- Probenecid
- NSAIDs: increased risk of renal impairment; hypotensive
  effect antagonized
- Lithium
- Cyclosporine
- Phenothiazines
- Imipramine

NSAIDS nonsteroidal anti-inflammatory drugs

stimulate the renin angiotensin system (RAS) and enhance the antihypertensive effects, producing a salutary interaction in hypertensive individuals, but hypotension may ensue in patients with CHF. The hypotensive effects are longer lasting with long-acting ACE inhibitors.

Renal Effects: ACE inhibitors and ARBs may decrease glomerular filtration rate (GFR) in some patients with renal dysfunction and may result in decreased clearance of other cardiac drugs that are eliminated by the kidney. Interaction may occur with renally excreted beta-blockers, nadolol, atenolol, sotalol, and antiarrhythmic agents. Serum K^+ may increase to dangerous levels if potassium-sparing diuretics (amiloride, eplerenone, triamterene, spironolactone, Moduretic, Moduret, Dyazide) are used concurrently. This occurrence is enhanced in patients with renal dysfunction. A normal serum creatinine level in patients with a lean body mass may not reflect underlying renal dysfunction, and **caution** is necessary, particularly in the elderly:

- **Probenecid** inhibits the tubular excretion of ACE inhibitors and increases the blood levels of these agents.
- ACE inhibitors may cause a 20–30 % decrease in digoxin clearance and an increase in digoxin levels.
- Interaction with cyclosporine may cause hyperkalemia.

Hematologic/Immune: The risk of immune adverse effects may increase with concurrent use of agents that alter the immune status: Assess antinuclear antibody levels and also assess for neutropenia with concurrent use of acebutolol, allopurinol, hydralazine, pindolol, procainamide, and tocainide.

Gastrointestinal: The absorption of fosinopril is reduced by antacids.

Interactions of Spironolactone

- Aspirin antagonizes the diuretic effect of spironolactone.
- ACE inhibitors and spironolactone both cause hyperkalemia.
- Digoxin levels are increased (laboratory reaction).
- Nonsteroidal anti-inflammatory drugs (NSAIDs) combined with spironolactone may precipitate acute renal failure.

ANTIARRHYTHMIC AGENTS

Adenosine

The electrophysiologic effects of adenosine are competitively antagonized by methylxanthines (theophylline) and are potentiated by dipyridamole, which inhibits its cellular uptake, and **severe hypotension may occur** (Table 21-2).

Amiodarone

Cardiovascular Effects

- Amiodarone has a mild vasodilator effect, and interaction may occur with antihypertensive agents, causing hypotension. This interaction is more prominent with intravenous amiodarone.
- Because of a mild inotropic effect, CHF may be precipitated, especially when amiodarone is combined with agents that possess negative inotropism (e.g., beta-blocking agents, verapamil, or diltiazem).
- Combination with verapamil or diltiazem may cause sinus arrest or AV block (Table 21-3).
- The proarrhythmic effect of amiodarone is low, but interaction may occur and may increase the risk of torsades de pointes when amiodarone is used concurrently with the following agents: diuretics, which cause hypokalemia, class IA agents (quinidine, disopyramide, procainamide), sotalol, tricyclics, phenothiazines, and erythromycin.

Oral Anticoagulants: Their activity is increased.

Table 21-2
Adenosine: potential interactions

- Carbamazepine
- Dipyridamole: **Caution**
- Methylxanthines (theophylline)
- Caffeine

Table 21-3
Amiodarone: potential interactions

- Antihypertensive agents
- Drugs that are negatively inotropic: verapamil, diltiazem, beta-blockers—**increased risk of bradycardia, AV block, and myocardial depression. Avoid concomitant use**
- Agents that inhibit SA and AV node conduction: diltiazem, verapamil—**avoid concomitant use**
- Agents that ↑ the QT interval
  Class 1A agents: quinidine, disopyramide, procainamide
  Sotalol
  Tricyclic antidepressants: **increased risk of ventricular arrhythmias—avoid concomitant use**
  Phenothiazines
  Erythromycin (other macrolides)
  Pentamidine
  Zidovudine
- Agents that decrease serum K^+ concentration (diuretics): increased cardiac toxicity with amiodarone if hypokalemia occurs with loop or thiazide diuretics
- Agents that are renally eliminated: digoxin, flecainide, procainamide—**amiodarone increases plasma concentration of digoxin (half dose of digoxin)**
- Anticoagulants: **amiodarone inhibits metabolism of coumarins (enhanced anticoagulant effect)**
- Dabigatran etexilate: amiodarone increases plasma concentration of dabigatran etexilate (reduce dose of dabigatran etexilate)
- Cimetidine: plasma concentration of amiodarone increased by cimetidine
- Cyclosporine: amiodarone possibly increases plasma concentration of cyclosporine
- Eplerenone: amiodarone increases plasma concentration of eplerenone (reduce dose of eplerenone)
- Grapefruit juice: plasma concentration of amiodarone increased by grapefruit juice
- Lithium: avoid concomitant use with lithium risk (risk of ventricular arrhythmias)
- Simvastatin: increased risk of myopathy when amiodarone given with simvastatin

AV atrioventricular, *SA* sinoatrial

Plasma Levels: Digoxin levels may double because amiodarone decreases renal clearance of digoxin. Flecainide and procainamide levels increase.

Disopyramide

Cardiovascular Effects: The negative inotropic effect of disopyramide is increased by beta-blocking agents, **verapamil, diltiazem, and flecainide**. Proarrhythmic effects, in particular torsades de pointes, are increased with agents that prolong the QT interval or cause hypokalemia. Sinus and AV node effects may occur when disopyramide is used concurrently with drugs that depress the sinus node (verapamil, diltiazem, digitalis).

Cholinergic Effects: Because disopyramide inhibits muscarinic receptors, the anticholinergic activity may cause constipation. Thus, the drug should not be combined with verapamil. Disopyramide may precipitate glaucoma, and this effect may be counteracted by timolol or betaxolol.

Flecainide

Cardiovascular Effects: The powerful, negative, inotropic effect of flecainide is worsened by negative inotropic agents; interaction occurs with **verapamil, diltiazem, beta-blockers, and disopyramide**; intraventricular conduction defects may occur when the drug is combined with class IA agents.

Plasma levels increase with concomitant **amiodarone** administration; thus, the flecainide dose should be decreased. Flecainide causes an increase in **digoxin** levels.

Lidocaine or Lignocaine

Plasma Levels: Lidocaine is metabolized in the liver. An increase in plasma levels may occur with decreased hepatic blood flow caused by **beta-blocking agents** (Ochs et al. 1980): Caution is necessary to avoid lidocaine toxicity, which may occur when lidocaine and beta-blockers are administered to patients with acute myocardial infarction. Lidocaine plasma levels decrease with **phenytoin**, which stimulates the hepatic oxidase system, resulting in accelerated breakdown of hepatically metabolized cardiovascular agents.

Mexiletine

Cardiovascular Effects: Hypotension may occur when mexiletine is combined with vasoactive agents that reduce blood pressure. AV block may worsen with the concomitant use of **amiodarone, verapamil, diltiazem, or beta-blocking drugs**.

Plasma Levels: Because the drug is partly metabolized in the liver, **phenytoin** decreases plasma levels.

Phenytoin

Phenytoin activates the hepatic oxidase system and thus accelerates the breakdown of hepatically metabolized cardiac agents, resulting in a decrease in their plasma levels: **lidocaine, hepatically metabolized beta-blockers (propranolol, metoprolol, labetalol), diltiazem, verapamil, nifedipine** (and other **dihydropyridine calcium antagonists**), **mexiletine**, and **quinidine**. Aspirin metabolism is increased; thus, phenytoin decreases the effects of aspirin.

Propafenone

Cardiovascular Effects: Hypotension may be precipitated by drugs that lower blood pressure. A prominent negative inotropic effect may be increased by other negative inotropic agents. Sinus node suppression may occur when the drug is combined with **verapamil** or **diltiazem**. AV block or conduction defects may increase with class IA agents. Digoxin level and warfarin are enhanced.

Plasma Levels: Digoxin levels are increased.

Hematologic: Oral anticoagulant activity is increased.

Procainamide

The **negative inotropic effects** of oral procainamide are increased by other negative inotropic agents. **Torsades de pointes** may be precipitated when procainamide is combined with agents that increase the QT interval. **ACE inhibitors** may enhance immune effects; both agents may cause neutropenia or agranulocytosis.

Quinidine

Hypotension: Because alpha-receptors are inhibited by quinidine, other vasoactive agents that decrease blood pressure may precipitate hypotension (e.g., **prazosin**, **verapamil**).

Intraventricular Conduction Defects: These increase when quinidine is combined with class IC agents (**flecainide, encainide, propafenone, lorcainide**).

Proarrhythmic Effects: Drugs that prolong the QT interval and diuretics that cause hypokalemia may precipitate torsades de pointes.

Hematologic: **Oral anticoagulant** activity may increase.

Plasma Levels: **Quinidine** levels decrease with phenytoin or nifedipine and increase with verapamil (Trohman et al. 1986) or **diltiazem** administration.

ANTIPLATELET AGENTS/ANTICOAGULANTS

Anticoagulants have several interactions with cardiac and noncardiac drugs (*see* Table 19-3).

Aspirin. The metabolism of aspirin is increased by agents such as **phenytoin**, **barbiturates**, and **rifampin** that induce the hepatic oxidase system. Phenytoin, therefore, decreases the effects of aspirin. The risk of bleeding is increased with concurrent administration of anticoagulants. Aspirin and thiazide **diuretics** inhibit urate excretion, whereas ACE inhibitors and sulfinpyrazone increase renal urate excretion.

Clopidogrel interacts unfavorably with atorvastatin and simvastatin. Clopidogrel and proton pump inhibitors caution: Both use the hepatic cytochrome pathway, and beneficial effect on intracoronary stent occlusion is probably reduced. See Chap. 19.

- **Morphine has been shown to decrease clopidogrel absorption, decreases concentrations of clopidogrel active metabolite, and diminishes its salutary effects. This can cause treatment failure in susceptible patients (Hobl et al.** 2014).

BETA-BLOCKERS

Cardiovascular Effects: Hypotension may be precipitated when beta-blockers are combined with calcium antagonists and other antihypertensive agents. Hypertension may ensue with concurrent use of vasoactive agents that are sympathomimetic (e.g., phenylpropanolamine).

- Effects on the SA and AV nodes: Electrophysiologic interaction occurs with **verapamil**, **diltiazem**, and **amiodarone**; severe bradycardia, complete heart block, or asystole may be precipitated (Table 21-4).

Table 21-4
Beta-adrenergic blockers: potential interactions

- Anti-arrhythmics: amiodarone, disopyramide, flecainide, lidocaine, procainamide, propafenone
- Calcium antagonists: diltiazem, verapamil, nifedipine
- Sympathomimetics (phenylpropanolamine)
- Phenytoin
- K^+-losing diuretics (sotalol only)
- Cimetidine-like agents (hepatically metabolized; metoprolol, propranolol; *see* Chap. 1)
- NSAIDs
- Fluvoxamine
- Tobacco smoking (propranolol)

- Inotropic effects: Other negative inotropic agents (**verapamil, diltiazem, flecainide, disopyramide, procainamide, propafenone**) increase the risk of CHF.
- Proarrhythmic effects: Sotalol, because of its unique class III activity, is the only beta-blocking agent with proarrhythmic effects, and it can induce torsades de pointes, especially if the serum K^+ level is low. Avoid K^+-losing diuretics. Do not combine sotalol with agents that prolong the QT interval.
- Beta-blockers must not be combined with valsartan. In **Val-HeFT**, valsartan administered in a heart failure RCT combined with a beta-blocker caused significantly more cardiac events. Often in patients with HF, a beta-blocker is needed as proven therapy. Thus an ACE inhibitor must be used.
- Caution: Valsartan must not be combined with a beta-blocker.

Plasma Levels: Metoprolol and propranolol plasma levels are increased by verapamil. Atenolol, sotalol, and nadolol plasma levels are not increased because they are not hepatically metabolized beta-blockers. Nifedipine plasma levels increase.

Immune Effects: Acebutolol and pindolol may alter immune status. The risk is additive when these agents are used concomitantly with hydralazine, procainamide, or ACE inhibitors.

CALCIUM ANTAGONISTS

Other antihypertensive agents interact favorably to lower blood pressure, but hypotension may occur. The combination of magnesium sulfate may cause severe hypotension. Verapamil decreases the hepatic metabolism of prazosin and other alpha blockers: concurrent use may cause hypotension. The combination of verapamil and quinidine may cause hypotension because of combined inhibition of peripheral alpha-receptors:

Amiodarone: increased risk of bradycardia, AV block, and myocardial depression when verapamil or diltiazem is given.

Aliskiren: Verapamil increases plasma concentration of aliskiren—manufacturer of aliskiren advises to avoid concomitant use.

Corticosteroids: The hypotensive effect of calcium-channel blockers are antagonized.

Levodopa: Enhanced hypotensive effect when calcium-channel blockers are given with statins: diltiazem increases plasma concentration of atorvastatin—possible increased risk of myopathy and increased risk of myopathy when verapamil or diltiazem is given with simvastatin. Diltiazem and verapamil increase plasma concentration of simvastatin.

Colchicine: Diltiazem, and verapamil, possibly increases risk of colchicine toxicity—suspend or reduce dose of colchicine (avoid concomitant use in hepatic or renal impairment).

Dabigatran: Verapamil possibly increases plasma concentration of dabigatran etexilate (reduce dose of dabigatran).

Digoxin: Diltiazem, verapamil, and dihydropyridines increase plasma levels.

Eplerenone: Diltiazem increases plasma concentration of eplerenone.

Lithium: Neurotoxicity may occur when diltiazem or verapamil is given ranolazine interacts with lithium.

Ticagrelor: Diltiazem increases plasma concentration.

Grapefruit juice: Concentration of amlodipine, other dihydropyridines, diltiazem, and verapamil possibly increased.

NSAIDs: Hypotensive effect of calcium-channel blockers antagonized.

St. John's Wort: Plasma concentration of verapamil significantly reduced.

Negative Inotropic Agents: Added to verapamil or diltiazem. These agents may precipitate CHF (Table 21-5).

Table 21-5
Calcium antagonists: potential interactions

- Amiodarone
- Beta-blockers
- Cyclosporine
- Digoxin
- Phenytoin
- Quinidine
- t-PA (diltiazem[a])
- Magnesium IV
- Cimetidine
- Lithium
- Carbamazepine
- Quinine, chloroquine
- Grapefruit juice
- Tobacco (smoking): hepatically metabolized agents

t-PA tissue plasminogen activator

[a]Gore et al. (1991), Becker et al. (1993)

Sinoatrial and AV Nodal Effects: Verapamil and diltiazem have electrophysiologic actions on the SA and AV nodes that are increased by beta-blocking drugs, digoxin, amiodarone, and quinidine.

Plasma Levels: Nifedipine plasma levels are increased by agents that decrease hepatic blood flow (beta-blockers). Verapamil increases metoprolol plasma levels but does not increase the levels of atenolol, sotalol, and nadolol because these agents are not metabolized in the liver. Verapamil and diltiazem interaction with digoxin results in a substantial increase in digoxin levels. Verapamil and diltiazem increase quinidine levels. Verapamil, diltiazem, and nicardipine increase cyclosporine levels. Phenytoin stimulates the hepatic oxidase system and decreases plasma levels and the activity of calcium antagonists. **Mibefradil (Posicor)**, a calcium antagonist, has been withdrawn because of serious and potential interactions with a host of cardiac drugs that are influenced by the action of cytochrome P-450 3A4. **Clinicians should be cautious with combinations of agents that interfere with cytochrome P-450**.

Hematologic: An important interaction between diltiazem and tissue plasminogen activator (t-PA) has been observed. Experimentally, the combination of t-PA and diltiazem (3d) resulted in significantly more blood loss than when t-PA was used alone (Becker et al. 1993). In the Thrombolysis in Myocardial Infarction (TIMI) phase II study, an increased risk of intracerebral hemorrhage was observed in patients who were administered calcium antagonists at study entry (Gore et al. 1991).

DIGOXIN

Digoxin interacts with several cardiac and noncardiac drugs, resulting in either an increase or decrease in digoxin levels (Table 21-6). Digoxin interacts with several cardiac drugs that have electrophysiologic effects on the SA and AV nodes. Diuretics interact by causing hypokalemia and increased sensitivity to digoxin. Cardioactive agents that decrease renal clearance of digoxin and increase digoxin plasma levels include amiodarone, flecainide, propafenone, quinidine, diltiazem, verapamil, and some dihydropyridine calcium antagonists, and ACE inhibitors. Prazosin displaces digoxin at binding sites and increases digoxin levels.

DIURETICS

Diuretics that cause hypokalemia interact with sotalol, amiodarone, and class IA agents and may precipitate torsades de pointes. Digoxin toxicity is enhanced. K^+-sparing diuretics administered with ACE inhibitors may cause an increase in serum K^+ levels. Ethacrynic acid increases the anticoagulant effect of warfarin. Both diuretics and dobutamine

Table 21-6
Digoxin: potential interactions

Agents that increase serum levels
    Atorvastatin >10 %
    Ranolazine increases levels
    Quinidine displaces digoxin at binding sites and decreases
    renal elimination (quinine, chloroquine)
    Decrease renal elimination: digoxin levels are increased by
    verapamil, diltiazem, nicardipine, felodipine, lercanidipine,
    amiodarone, flecainide, propafenone, prazosin, and ACE
    inhibitors
    Ticagrelor: plasma concentration of digoxin increased
    NSAIDs decrease renal elimination
    Lomotil and Pro-Banthine decrease intestinal motility
    Erythromycin and other macrolides: plasma concentration of
    digoxin increased (increased risk of toxicity)
    Spironolactone: Digoxin assay falsely?
Agents that decrease serum levels or bioavailability
    St John's Wort: avoid concomitant use
    Antacids, metoclopramide, cholestyramine, colestipol,
    Metamucil, neomycin, phenytoin, phenobarbital,
    salicylazosulfapyridine

ACE angiotensin-converting enzyme, *NSAIDs* nonsteroidal anti-inflammatory drugs

cause hypokalemia. Thus, caution is required when IV furosemide is administered concurrently with an infusion of dobutamine.

NITRATES

Nitroglycerin and other nitrates are preload-reducing agents and may increase the preload effect of ACE inhibitors and prazosin, resulting in syncope. High-dose IV nitroglycerin interacts with heparin, and this interaction may be important in patients with unstable angina who are treated with both agents; nitroglycerin presumably alters the antithrombin-3 molecule. Thus, a higher dose of heparin may be required. Also, excretion of heparin is increased by IV nitrates.

LIPID-LOWERING AGENTS

Statins

Fluvastatin and rosuvastatin interact with anticoagulants and cause a modest rise in INR. Administration of statins with nicotinic acid, gemfibrozil, other fibrates, cyclosporine, or erythromycin like antibiotics may cause myalgia and increase in creatinine kinase levels, myopathy, rhabdomyolysis, and possible renal failure. Fluvastatin does not alter digoxin pharmacokinetics (Blum 1994), but atorvastatin and simvastatin increase digoxin levels approx 20 % and <10 %, respectively. Among the statins simvastatin has the most interactions (*see* Table 21-7).

Bile Acid Sequestrants: Cholestyramine and colestipol decrease the absorption of digoxin, coumarin anticoagulants, diuretics, beta-blockers, HMG-CoA reductase inhibitors, L-thyroxine, and other vasoactive agents. These agents must be given 1 h before or 4 h after resin administration.

INTERACTIONS OF CARDIAC AND NONCARDIAC DRUGS

Antibiotics

Erythromycin and other macrolides may increase the QT interval and interact with cardiac agents that cause QT prolongation with the precipitation of torsades de pointes. Erythromycin may enhance the effects of digoxin (*see* Table 21-6).

Rifampin can induce the hepatic oxidase system, accelerating the metabolism of several cardiovascular drugs and thus resulting in decreased drug levels of these agents.

Table 21-7

Statins: pharmacokinetics and drug interactions

	Atorvastatin	Fluvastatin	Pravastatin	Rosuvastatin[a]	Simvastatin
Pharmacokinetics					
Lipophilic (L)	L	Both	H	Both	L or hydrophilic
Renal excretion	No	~10 % renal, ~90 % fecal	~60 %	~10 % renal, ~90 % fecal	No
Renal excretion, patient in a renal failure or elderly patient	No	Yes, if GFR <30 mL/min	Yes; caution if GFR <50 mL/min	Yes, if GFR <30 mL/min: Use cautiously if GFR is 31–50 mL/min	No
Cytochrome P-450	3A4	2C9	Not known (multiple pathways)	2C9	3A4
Drug interactions					
Warfarin—INR increased	No	Yes	No	Yes	Yes
Digoxin level increased	Yes (20 %)	<10 %		No	<10 %
Macrolide[b] Antibiotics	Yes	No	Yes	No	Yes
Antifungal agents	Yes	Yes	No	No	Yes
Antiviral agents	Yes	No	No	No	Yes
Cyclosporine	Yes	Yes	Yes	Yes[c]	Yes

(continued)

Table 21-7 (continued)

	Atorvastatin	Fluvastatin	Pravastatin	Rosuvastatin[a]	Simvastatin
Fluoxetine and similar agents	Yes	No	No	No	Yes
Fibrates[d] or niacin[d]	Yes	Yes	Yes	Yes	Yes
Grapefruit juice	Yes	No	No	No	Yes
Phenytoin	No	Yes	No	Yes	No
Verapamil, diltiazem	Yes	No	No	No	Yes
Amiodarone		No	No	No	Yes[e]

Antacids may lower levels of rosuvastatin

Ranolazine: plasma concentration of simvastatin increased by ranolazine

Ticagrelor: plasma concentration of simvastatin increased

Colchicine combination with statin to be avoided since the combination it can cause severe myopathy and rhabdomyolysis

H hydrophilic, *INR* international normalized ratio, *L* lipophilic

[a]Contraindicated if severe renal failure, GFR<30 mL/min. caution in—the elderly (age>75) often have diminished renal function yet a normal serum creatinine and estimated GFR ~50 mL/min

[b]Erythromycin, clarithromycin, troleandomycin, azithromycin

[c]Avoid concomitant use

[d]Caution: myopathy and rare rhabdomyolysis (combination of statin and fibrate or nicotinic acid is not recommended by the author)

[e]Warning: serious myopathy

Cephalosporins or aminoglycoside antibiotics interact with furosemide and may increase nephrotoxicity; the effects of oral anticoagulants are increased.

The antifungal agent pentamidine and the antiviral **zidovudine** may prolong the QT interval, may interact with cardiac drugs that increase the QT interval, and may precipitate torsades de pointes. **Amphotericin** with diuretics causes an increase in hypokalemia.

Antimalarials

Halofantrine increases the QT interval; cardioactive agents that cause QT prolongation may precipitate torsades de pointes.

Mefloquine and calcium-channel blockers may interact to cause bradycardia. Bradycardia may be increased with digoxin.

Quinine, chloroquine, and hydroxychloroquine raise plasma concentrations of digoxin. Bradycardia may occur with diltiazem and verapamil.

Anticonvulsants

The effects of carbamazepine are enhanced by verapamil and diltiazem. The effects of nifedipine and isradipine are reduced by carbamazepine, phenobarbitone, primidone, and phenytoin. Carbamazepine may increase the degree of heart block caused by adenosine.

Drugs that Affect Urate Excretion: Urate excretion is increased by ACE inhibitors, sulfinpyrazone, and probenecid. Urate excretion is decreased by diuretics and aspirin. Therefore, favorable or untoward interactions may occur. Also, probenecid decreases renal tubular secretion of captopril and may increase blood levels of ACE inhibitors.

Cyclosporine

Hyperkalemia may occur with concurrent use of ACE inhibitors or K$^+$-sparing diuretics. Plasma cyclosporine

concentrations are reduced by concurrent rifampin administration and increased by nicardipine, diltiazem, and verapamil. Cyclosporine appears to increase plasma levels of
nifedipine. Hyperkalemia may occur with the use of K^+-
sparing diuretics. Myopathy or rhabdomyolysis may occur
with coadministration of rosuvastatin.

Lithium

Both loop diuretics and thiazides decrease sodium reabsorption in the proximal tubules and may cause an increased
resorption of lithium, which may result in lithium toxicity.
ACE inhibitors reduce excretion of lithium, resulting in
increased plasma lithium concentration. Diltiazem and verapamil interact with lithium, and neurotoxicity may occur
without an increase in plasma lithium levels, ranolazine,
amiloride, eplerenone caution.

Nonsteroidal Anti-inflammatory Drugs

These agents block the production of vasodilator prostaglandins and reduce the antihypertensive effectiveness of
ACE inhibitors, diuretics, and perhaps beta-blockers.
NSAIDs decrease the diuretic effect of furosemide. There is
an increased risk of hyperkalemia with K^+-sparing diuretics
and precipitation of renal failure when indomethacin is
administered with triamterene.

Psychotropic Agents

Phenothiazines, especially thioridazine, have quinidine-
like effects on the heart; QT prolongation and interaction
with amiodarone, sotalol, and class LA agents may induce
torsades de pointes. Phenothiazines may interact with ACE
inhibitors to cause severe postural hypotension.

Tricyclic antidepressants have a class I antiarrhythmic
action. The quinidine-like effect may prolong the QT interval
and induce torsades when combined with agents, such as
sotalol, amiodarone, and others, that increase the QT interval.

These agents have anticholinergic properties (atropine-like) and interact with cardioactive agents with anticholinergic effects. Tricyclics antagonize the hypotensive effects of clonidine and increase the risk of rebound hypertension on clonidine withdrawal. Imipramine and possibly other tricyclics increase plasma concentration of diltiazem and verapamil. Because tricyclics produce a dry mouth, the effect of sublingual nitrates may be reduced.

Selective Serotonin Reuptake Inhibitors (SSRIs): fluvoxamine, fluoxetine, sertraline. SSRIs are highly protein bound and may interact with cardioactive agents that are highly protein bound, causing a shift in plasma levels of these agents, particularly warfarin and digoxin. Sinus node slowing has been reported (Ellison et al. 1990; Buff et al. 1991; Feder 1991).

Sinus bradycardia and syncope have been observed. Thus, interaction may emerge with agents that inhibit sinus node function or cause bradycardia (amiodarone, diltiazem, verapamil). Fluvoxamine increases plasma concentration of propranolol; the same interaction is likely to occur with other hepatically metabolized beta-blockers and other SSRIs.

Monoamine Oxidase Inhibitors: These agents may cause hypertensive crises with tyramine (in cheese) sympathomimetics. They increase the hypotensive effects of diuretics. They inhibit the hepatic drug metabolism enzymes. Thus, blood levels and effects of hepatically metabolized cardioactive agents may be increased.

Theophylline

Theophylline interacts with several cardioactive and non-cardioactive agents (Table 21-8). Diltiazem and verapamil enhance effects of theophylline.

Thyroxine

The metabolism of propranolol and other hepatically metabolized beta-blockers is increased, causing reduced effect.

Table 21-8
Theophylline: potential interactions

Drug	Effect[a]	Response
Adenosine	↓Effects of adenosine	
Allopurinol	↓Theophylline clearance	↓Dose of theophylline
Barbiturates	↑Theophylline clearance	↓Dose of theophylline
Carbamazepine	↑Theophylline clearance	↑Dose of theophylline
Corticosteroids	Variable metabolic effects	Monitor theophylline levels
Coumarins	Interfere with assay method for serum level resulting in falsely low values	No adjustment in dose necessary
Diltiazem	Slight ↓ in theophylline clearance	Possible ↓ in theophylline dose
Erythromycin	↓Theophylline clearance	↓Dose of theophylline
Estrogens	↓Theophylline clearance	↓Dose of theophylline
H_2-blockers		
Cimetidine	↓Theophylline clearance	↓Dose of theophylline
Ranitidine	No effect	No adjustment
Famotidine	No effect	No adjustment
Influenza vaccine	↓Theophylline clearance	↓Dose of theophylline
Interferon	↓Theophylline clearance	↓Dose of theophylline
Isoniazid	↓Theophylline clearance	↓Dose of theophylline
Isoproterenol	↑Theophylline clearance	↑Dose of theophylline
Lithium	↑Lithium clearance	↑Dose of lithium
Mexiletine	↓Theophylline clearance	↓Dose of theophylline
Nicorette	No effect	No response
Oral contraceptives	↓Theophylline clearance	↓Dose of theophylline
Pancuronium	↓Pancuronium responsiveness	↑Dose of pancuronium
Phenytoin	↑Theophylline clearance	↑Dose of theophylline
Quinolones	↓Theophylline clearance	↓Dose of theophylline
Tobacco smoking	↑Theophylline clearance	↑Dose of theophylline
Troleandomycin	↓Theophylline clearance	↓Dose of theophylline
Verapamil	↓Theophylline clearance	↓Dose of theophylline
Vidarabine	↓Theophylline clearance	↓Dose of theophylline

[a]↑, ↓, decrease

CARDIAC EFFECTS OF NONCARDIAC DRUGS

The cardiac effects of selected noncardiac drugs are summarized in Table 21-9 reached here.

Antibiotics

Erythromycin blocks a K^+ current important in cardiac repolarization. This action can predispose to early afterdepolarizations and ventricular arrhythmias (Zipes 1993).

Erythromycin IV has been reported to cause QT prolongation and, along with other macrolides, may precipitate torsades de pointes, albeit rarely. In addition, erythromycin inhibits the metabolism of astemizole and terfenadine; the increased plasma levels of terfenadine may precipitate torsades de pointes.

Antimalarials

Chloroquine has caused "cardiomyopathy."

Halofantrine: High-dose therapy has been reported to cause cardiac death (Nosten et al. 1993). Also, Mobitz type I and II block, prolongation of the QT interval, and torsades de pointes may be precipitated.

Histamine H_1 Antagonists

Astemizole and terfenadine have been reported to cause torsades de pointes and sudden cardiac death, albeit rarely. Terfenadine blocks the outward rectifier K^+ current. Increased terfenadine blood levels prolong the QT interval. Concomitant administration of agents that inhibit the hepatic oxygenase cytochrome P-450 system (erythromycin, clarithromycin, and other macrolide antibiotics; imidazole antifungal medications, such as ketoconazole or itraconazole) may further prolong the QT interval and precipitate torsades

Table 21-9
Cardiac effects of noncardiac drugs

Drug	Cardiac effect
Antimicrobials	
Erythromycin (macrolides)	↑QT interval, ↑risk of torsades de points
Co-trimoxazole	↑Risk of torsades de pointes (rare)
Ketoconazole	↑Risk of torsades de pointes
Pentamidine	↑Risk of torsades de pointes
Itraconazole	↑Risk of torsades de pointes
Spiramycin	↑Risk of torsades de pointes
Histamine H_1 antagonist	↑QT interval, ↑risk of torsades de pointes
Astemizole	↑Risk of torsades de pointes
Terfenadine	↑QT interval, ↑risk of torsades de pointes
Amantadine	↑Risk of torsades de pointes
Antimalarials	
Halofantrine	↑QT interval, ↑risk of torsades de pointes
Chloroquine	SHMD
Tricyclic antidepressants	Arrhythmias: SVT, VPBs, RBBB, conduction defect, ↑QT interval, ↑risk of torsades de pointes
Cocaine	Hypertension; LVH, arrhythmias, MI
Sumatriptan	Chest pain 3–5 %, risk of MI (rare)
Agents for treatment of AIDS	
Foscarnet (trisodium phosphate)	Acute reversible cardiac dysfunction
Zidovudine	SHMD
Pentamidine	Torsades de pointes
Cancer chemotherapeutic agents (*see* Table 21-10)	

AIDS acquired immunodeficiency syndrome, *LVH* left ventricular hypertrophy, *MI* myocardial infarction, *SHMD* specific heart muscle disease

Table 21-10
Cardiac effects of cancer chemotherapeutic agents

Chemotherapeutic agent	Cardiac effect
Busulfan	Pulmonary hypertension owing to pulmonary fibrosis
Cisplatin	Coronary artery spasm: ischemia
Cyclophosphamide	Acute SHMD, pericarditis, CHF
Doxorubicin	Early: arrhythmias, ST-T changes
	Late: SHMD 2 % (Brown et al. 1993), refractory CHF
Daunorubicin	SHMD (5 %)
5-Fluorouracil	Coronary vasospasm, ischemia (angina), myocardial infarction (rare)
Interferon-alpha	Cardiomegaly, CHF, pericardial effusion
Methotrexate	ST-T changes
Vincristine	Coronary vasospasm, ischemia

CHF congestive heart failure, *SHMD* specific heart muscle disease

de pointes (Simons et al. 1994). In addition, patients with hepatic dysfunction, hypokalemia, or hypomagnesemia, including patients with diarrhea, are at increased risk for torsades de pointes when treated with H_1 antagonists. The newer agents do not appear to cause major problems but should be used judiciously.

Antidepressants

Tricyclics: These agents predispose to a number of arrhythmic complications [Glassman et al. 1993]: ventricular premature beats (VPBs), supraventricular arrhythmias, right bundle branch block (RBBB), other intraventricular conduction delays, QT prolongation, and the risk of torsades de pointes.

SSRIs: There have been rare reports of sinus bradycardia; VPBs and complete heart block have been reported with trazodone. Monoamine oxidase inhibitors may cause VPBs, ventricular tachycardia, and hypertensive crises (particularly when combined with tyramine).

Cancer Chemotherapeutic Agents

Cardiotoxicity may occur early or late during the administration of these agents (Table 21-10). Early complications include arrhythmias, left ventricular dysfunction, electrocardiographic changes, pericarditis, myocarditis, myocardial infarction, and sudden cardiac death. Late or chronic effects include sinus tachycardia, pericardial effusion, left ventricular dysfunction, CHF, and specific heart muscle disease (cardiomyopathy).

Doxorubicin: Early cardiotoxicity may manifest by the occurrence of nonspecific ST-T wave changes, arrhythmias, left ventricular dysfunction, pericarditis, or sudden cardiac death (Lipshultz et al. 1991). These changes may occur within the first week or two of drug administration. Late cardiotoxicity: Cardiomyopathy is caused by cumulative effects of the drug at high doses. CHF may be precipitated. The incidence of specific heart muscle disease with doxorubicin is about 2 %, and that with daunorubicin is 5 % (Lipshultz et al. 1991).

Cyclophosphamide: Cardiac effects usually occur during acute treatment: Low voltage in the electrocardiogram, acute pericarditis, supraventricular arrhythmias, and nonspecific ST-T wave changes.

5-Fluorouracil may cause myocardial ischemia or chest pain owing to coronary artery spasm (Baker et al. 1986).

Cisplatin, bleomycin, vincristine, and vinblastine may cause vasospasm similar to that observed with 5-fluorouracil (Baker et al. 1986: 22), myocardial ischemia, and, rarely, myocardial infarction.

Other Agents

Proton Pump Inhibitors: Studies have suggested that adverse cardiovascular outcomes with the combination of clopidogrel and a proton pump inhibitor (PPI) are explained by the individual PPI. The use of a PPI inhibits CYP450 2C19, including omeprazole, lansoprazole, or rabeprazole. Omeprazole has been reported to significantly decrease the inhibitory effect of clopidogrel on platelet aggregation. One study reported that the PPI pantoprazole was not associated with recurrent MI among patients receiving clopidogrel, possibly due to pantoprazole's lack of inhibition of CYP450 2C19 (Juurlink et al. 2009).

Corticosteroids: Palpitations have been reported in up to 47 % of patients given steroid pulse therapy (Belmonte et al. 1986). Sudden cardiac death has been reported following large doses of steroids; VPBs may be precipitated by corticosteroid administration (Martyn et al. 1993; Belmonte et al. 1986).

Organophosphates may cause prolonged episodes of enhanced parasympathetic tone, QT alterations, ST-T wave changes, conduction defects, ventricular tachycardia, and fibrillation (Martyn et al. 1993).

Sumatriptan: This agent, used for migraine and cluster headache, may cause tightness in the chest in 3–5 % of patients (Ottervanger et al. 1993). Acute myocardial infarction has been reported, including a case in a 47-year-old woman (Ottervanger et al. 1993).

Ergotamine is known to cause coronary vasospasm and an increase in angina.

Metoclopramide: Supraventricular arrhythmias may occur, albeit rarely. Two cases of bradycardia and complete heart block have been reported (Esselink et al. 1994).

Beta$_2$-Agonists: Albuterol (salbutamol), terbutaline. These agents stimulate beta-receptors (some beta$_2$-receptors are present in the heart) and cause tachycardia. They may cause transient, but important, lowering of serum K^+ levels, which may trigger life-threatening ventricular arrhythmias, including ventricular fibrillation in patients with status asthmaticus treated with high-dose beta$_2$-agonists.

Foscarnet has been reported to cause reversible cardiac dysfunction in a patient treated for cytomegalovirus infection (Brown et al. 1993).

Ondansetron (Zofran), used as an antiemetic, may increase the risk of developing prolongation of the QT interval of the electrocardiogram, which can lead to an abnormal and potentially fatal heart rhythm, including torsades de pointes. Avoid inpatients with hypokalemia or hypomagnesemia, congestive heart failure, and bradyarrhythmias and inpatients who are taking other medications that may cause QT prolongation.

Sildenafil (Viagra) coadministration with nitrates increases the risk of life-threatening hypotension, and nitrates must not be taken within 48 h of sildenafil and similar agents. Less than 15 % of all associated cardiovascular deaths reported occurred in men who were using nitrates. Caution is required with the use of antihypertensive agents. Interaction may occur with drugs that are metabolized by or that inhibit cytochrome P-450 3A4: amlodipine, amiodarone, diltiazem, disopyramide, felodipine, losartan, mibefradil, nifedipine, ranolazine or similar agents, quinidine, verapamil, clarithromycin or similar antibiotics, antifungals, and statins.

Saint John's Wort (*Hypericum perforatum*) has been reported to cause a fall in cyclosporine serum levels that has been responsible for two cases of acute heart transplant rejection. A reduced anticoagulant effect of warfarin (decreased INR) also occurs. This and other herbal remedies induce drug-metabolizing enzymes of the cytochrome P-450 system. Thus, all herbal remedies must now be screened for interaction with prescribed medications.

Grapefruit juice (naringenin) inhibits the P-450 system and should be avoided with many medicines that use the P-450 pathways.

Herbal Drugs and Digoxin: Milkweed, lily of the valley, Siberian ginseng, oleander, squill, and hawthorn berries contain digoxin-like substances. Kushen exhibits digoxin-like properties. Kyushin and chan-su, used in Japan, cross-react with digoxin assays and cause spuriously high digoxin levels (Cheng 2002). Also, ginseng may falsely elevate digoxin levels. Licorice and opium increase the risk of digoxin toxicity. Saint John's Wort may reduce digoxin levels.

REFERENCES

Baker WP, Dainer P, Lester WM, et al. Ischemic chest pain after 5-fluorouracil therapy for cancer. Am J Cardiol. 1986;57:497.

Becker RC, Caputo R, Ball S, et al. Hemorrhagic potential of combined diltiazem and recombinant tissue-type plasminogen activator administration. Am Heart J. 1993;126:11.

Belmonte MA, Cequiere A, Roig-Escofet D. Severe ventricular arrhythmia after methylprednisolone pulse therapy in rheumatoid arthritis. J Rheumatol. 1986;13:477.

Blum CB. Comparison of properties of four inhibitors of 3-hydroxy-3-methylglutaryl-coenzyme A reductase. Am J Cardiol. 1994;73:3D.

Brown DL, Sather S, Cheitlin MD. Reversible cardiac dysfunction associated with foscarnet therapy for cytomegalovirus esophagitis in an AIDS patient. Am Heart J. 1993;125:1439.

Buff DD, Brenner R, Kirtane SS, Gilboa R. Dysrhythmia associated with fluoxetine treatment in an elderly patient with cardiac disease. J Clin Psychiatry. 1991;52:174.

Cheng TO. Interaction of herbal drugs with digoxin. J Am Coll Cardiol. 2002;40:838.

Ellison JM, Milofsky JE, Ely E. Fluoxetine-induced bradycardia and syncope in two patients. J Clin Psychiatry. 1990;51:385.

Esselink RAJ, Gerding MN, Brouwers PJAM, et al. Total heart block after intravenous metoclopramide. Lancet. 1994;343:182.

Feder R. Bradycardia and syncope induced by fluoxetine. J Clin Psychiatry. 1991;52:139.

Glassman AH, Roose SP, Bigger JT. The safety of tricyclic antidepressants in cardiac patients. JAMA. 1993;269:2673.

Gore JM, Sloan M, Price TR, and the TIMI Investigators, et al. Intracerebral hemorrhage, cerebral infarction, and subdural hematoma after acute myocardial infarction and thrombolytic therapy in the Thrombolysis in Myocardial Infarction study. Circulation. 1991;83:448.

Hobl E, Stimlfl T, Ebner J, et al. Morphine decreases clopidogrel concentrations and effects. A randomized double—blind placebo-controlled trial. J Am Coll Cardiol. 2014;63(7):630–5.

Juurlink DN, Gomes T, Ko DT, et al. A population-based study of the drug interaction between proton pump inhibitors and clopidogrel. CMAJ. 2009;180:713–8.

Lipshultz SE, Colan SD, Gelber RD, et al. Late cardiac effects of doxorubicin therapy for acute lymphoblastic leukemia in childhood. N Engl J Med. 1991;324:808.

Martyn R, Somberg JC, Kerin NZ. Proarrhythmia of non-antiarrhythmic drugs. Am Heart J. 1993;126:201.

Nosten F, terKuile FO, Luxemburger C. Cardiac effects of anti-malarial treatment with halofantrine. Lancet. 1993;341:1054.

Ochs HR, Carstens G, Greenblatt DJ. Reduction in lidocaine clearance during continuous infusion and by coadministration of propranolol. N Engl J Med. 1980;303:373.

Ottervanger JP, Paalman HJA, Boxma GL, et al. Transmural myocardial infarction with sumatriptan. Lancet. 1993;341:861.

Simons FER, Simons KJ, Wood AJJ. The pharmacology and use of H1-receptor-antagonist drugs. N Engl J Med. 1994;330:1663.

Trohman RG, Estes DM, Castellanos A, et al. Increased quinidine plasma concentration during administration of verapamil: a new quinidine-verapamil interaction. Am J Cardiol. 1986;57:706.

Zipes DP. Unwitting exposure to risk. Cardiol Rev. 1993;1:1.

22 Hallmark Clinical Trials

Results that dictate a reduction in end points observed in a few hallmark and other recent randomized clinical trials (RCTs) are given. The appropriate reference source is given so that the reader can explore the details of the RCT if required. Because of the constraints of available space, only a brief comment is given in the text regarding the results and their implications.

Prior to the assessment of these RCTs, the reader may wish to review the following brief points that relate to the interpretation of clinical trials:

Questions to ask when reading and interpreting the results of a clinical trial include (Guyatt et al. 1994)

- The "gold standard" statistical test of treatment effect is the determination of the p value using the χ^2 or Fisher's exact test. Although a p value <0.05 is at the significant level, in clinical medicine it is advisable to use $p \leq 0.02$ as a level of significant treatment effect.
- Statements describing treatment effect (Antman et al. 2002): relative risk (RR), relative risk reduction, odds ratio (OR), and absolute risk difference (ARD).
- An RR, relative risk reduction, or OR < 1 indicates treatment benefit. However, an RR reduction may give the impression of a greater treatment effect if the ARD and number needed to treat, the (1/ARD), are not given: the number of lives saved per 1,000 patients treated.
- Meta-analysis: Data pooling or quantitative review provides partial answers that may receive support from some and skepticism from others. One rule must be invoked when one

© Springer Science+Business Media New York 2015
M. Gabriel Khan, *Cardiac Drug Therapy*, Contemporary Cardiology,
DOI 10.1007/978-1-61779-962-4_22

is assessing the results derived from clinical meta-analysis: do not accept information based on subgroup analysis unless the primary end point, particularly the effect on all-cause mortality or cardiovascular mortality, showed a significant treatment effect.

- Are the results of the study valid? Was the assignment of patients to treatment randomized? Were all patients who entered the trial properly accounted for at its conclusion? Was follow-up complete and patients analyzed in the groups to which they were randomized?

ACUTE CORONARY SYNDROME RCTS

ATLAS ACS 2–TIMI 51: Rivaroxaban for ACS

In this double-blind, placebo-controlled trial, the ROCKET investigators randomly assigned 15,526 patients with a recent acute coronary syndrome (~STEMI~50 %, NSTEMI 25 %, unstable angina %) to receive twice-daily doses of either 2.5 mg or 5 mg of rivaroxaban or placebo for a mean of 13 months and up to 31 months. The primary efficacy end point was a composite of death from cardiovascular causes, myocardial infarction, or stroke (Mega et al. 2012).

Enrollment occurred within 7 days after hospital admission for an ACS. Subjects received the first dose of study drug no sooner than 4 h after the final dose of IV heparin, 2 h after the final dose of bivalirudin, and 12 h after the final dose of other intravenous or subcutaneous anticoagulants (e.g., enoxaparin or fondaparinux).

- Rivaroxaban significantly reduced the primary efficacy end point of death from cardiovascular causes, myocardial infarction, or stroke, as compared with placebo, with rates of 8.9 % and 10.7 %, respectively, $p=0.008$. The twice-daily 2.5-mg dose of rivaroxaban reduced the rates of death from cardiovascular causes (2.7 % versus 4.1 %, $p=0.002$) and from any cause (2.9 % versus 4.5 %, $p=0.002$), a survival benefit that was not seen with the twice-daily 5-mg dose.

In addition, rivaroxaban reduced the risk of stent thrombosis (Mega et al. 2012).

- The reduction in the primary efficacy end point with rivaroxaban was consistent among the subgroups except for patients with a history of stroke or transient ischemic attack (TIA). Thus the agent including apixaban and other Xa inhibitors should be avoided in patients with prior stroke or TIA.
- The 5-mg dose of rivaroxaban, as compared with placebo, did not significantly reduce the risk of death from either cardiovascular causes or any cause and differed significantly from the 2.5-mg dose of rivaroxaban ($p = 0.009$ for both comparisons) (Mega et al. 2012).

There was no significant difference in the rates of fatal bleeding associated with rivaroxaban as compared with placebo. The lower dose resulted in significantly lower rates of TIMI minor bleeding [0.9 % versus 1.6 %, and fatal bleeding (0.1 % versus 0.4 %, $p = 0.04$)]. Liver abnormalities were similar among patients treated with rivaroxaban or placebo. The advantages of the addition of rivaroxaban were observed regardless of whether patients presented with a STEMI, NSTEMI, or unstable angina (Mega et al. 2012).

- **This advantage was observed regardless of PCI or non-PCI therapy**.
  A similar RCT with the Xa inhibitor apixaban (ARISTOTLE:Granger et al 2011), which was efficacious for atrial fibrillation (See section on AF trials), was shown not effective and caused excessive bleeding but doses of the drug were obviously too high.

Bivalirudin for ACS

Acuity: The Acute Catheterization and Urgent Intervention Triage Strategy RCT evaluated the use of bivalirudin as a replacement for UF heparin and LMWH administered in the emergency department and continuing through the catheterization laboratory. The control arm of

ACUITY comprised patients treated with the heparins combined with platelet glycoprotein (GP) IIb/IIIa receptor blockers. A second arm studied bivalirudin with added GP IIb/IIIa receptor blockers; the third arm studied bivalirudin alone as monotherapy. (In the third arm, approx. 7 % of study patients received GP receptor blockers.)

- Patients who received the combination of bivalirudin with GP IIb/IIIa blockers (compared with a heparin-based regimen) had equivalent rates of bleeding and ischemia; overall patient outcomes were also equivalent.
- Bivalirudin monotherapy suppressed ischemic complications just as effectively as heparins plus GP IIb/IIIa blockers but was associated with half of the major bleeding, resulting in a significant improvement in overall patient outcomes. The trial was open labeled and had many flaws but provided important information for further trials with this hallmark thrombin inhibitor.

HORIZONS-AMI (2011) was a prospective, open-label, randomized trial in patients with acute STEMI, within 12 h after the onset of symptoms, and who were undergoing PCI. Patients were randomly allocated 1:1 to receive bivalirudin or heparin plus a glycoprotein IIb/IIIa inhibitor (GPI).

Results at 3 years: Compared with 1,802 patients allocated to receive heparin plus a GPI, 1,800 patients allocated to bivalirudin monotherapy had lower rates of all-cause mortality (5.9 % versus 7.7 %, difference -1.9 % $p=0.03$), cardiac mortality (2.9 % versus 5.1 %, $p=0.001$), and reinfarction (6.2 % versus 8.2 %, $p=0.04$).

Major bleeding not related to bypass graft surgery was significantly reduced (6.9 % versus 10.5 %, $p=0.0001$). There were no significant differences in ischemia-driven target vessel revascularization, stent thrombosis, or composite adverse events (Stone et al. 2011). Compared with 749 patients who received a bare-metal stent, 2,257 patients who received a paclitaxel-eluting stent had lower rates of ischemia-driven target lesion revascularization (9.4 % versus 15.1 %, $p < 0.0001$) after 3 years, with no significant differences in the rates of death, reinfarction, stroke, or stent thrombosis. Stent thrombosis was high (≥ 4.5 %) in both groups (Stone et al. 2011).

ISAR-REACT 4 Trial: Abciximab and Heparin versus Bivalirudin for non-ST-Elevation Myocardial Infarction: Subjects were all treated with ASA and clopidogrel 600 mg. Bivalirudin was administered to 860 and abciximab to 861 patients. A strategy of early invasive intervention (within 24 h after admission) was the standard of care at all centers for patients presenting with an ACS and elevated biomarker levels. All the patients in the trial were given 325–500 mg of aspirin and 600 mg of clopidogrel before they received a study drug. Before the guide wire had crossed the lesion, patients who were assigned to the abciximab group received a bolus dose of 0.25 mg of abciximab per kilogram of body weight, followed by an infusion of 0.125 μg of abciximab per kilogram per minute (maximum of 10 μg/min) for 12 h, and a bolus dose of 70 U of heparin per kilogram. Patients in the bivalirudin group received a bolus dose of 0.75 mg of bivalirudin per kilogram, followed by an infusion of 1.75 mg/kg/h for the duration of the procedure (Kastrati et al. 2011).

The primary end point occurred in 94 patients (10.9 %) in the abciximab group and 95 patients (11.0 %) in the bivalirudin group ($p = 0.94$).

- Cumulative incidence of primary and secondary end points in the two study groups. The secondary efficacy end point occurred in 110 patients (12.8 %) in the abciximab group and 115 patients (13.4 %) in the bivalirudin group ($p = 0.76$). Major bleeding occurred in 40 patients (4.6 %) in the abciximab group and 22 patients (2.6 %) in the bivalirudin group (relative risk, 1.84; 95 % CI, 1.10–3.07; $p = 0.02$). Profound thrombocytopenia developed in 10 patients (1.2 %) in the abciximab group and in none of the patients in the bivalirudin group ($p = 0.002$) conclusion:

- There were no significant differences in deaths, or recurrent MI, but major bleeding was ~84 % increased by abciximab (4.6 %) compared with 2.6 % for bivalirudin (Kastrati et al. 2011).
- In addition advantages include a much shorter duration of IV infusion, and cost compared to the use of antiplatelet inhibitors.
- Bivalirudin Alone Bests Heparin plus a GPI. In this rigorously performed double-blind RCT efficacy was similar and bleeding rates were remarkably lower with bivalirudin in patients undergoing PCI for NSTEMI (Kastrati et al. 2011).
- Bivalirudin is the preferred anticoagulant agent for all PCIs.

ENOXAPARIN VERSUS HEPARIN

ExTRACT-TIMI 25: Enoxaparin Versus Heparin in Acute MI

Enoxaparin and Thrombolysis Reperfusion for Acute Myocardial Infarction Treatment-Thrombolysis in Myocardial Infarction (EXTRACT-TIMI) 25 RCT (Antman et al. 2006) compared enoxaparin with heparin. A total of 20,506 patients with STEMI treated with thrombolytics received enoxaparin or weight-based UF heparin for at least 48 h. The primary efficacy end point was death or nonfatal recurrent MI.

- At 30-day follow-up: The primary end point occurred in 12.0 % of patients in the UF heparin group versus 9.9 % in the enoxaparin group (17 % reduction in RR; $p < 0.001$). Nonfatal MI occurred in 4.5 % and 3.0 %, respectively (33 % reduction in RR; $p < 0.001$); there was no difference in total mortality.
- Major bleeding occurred in 1.4 % with UF heparin versus 2.1 % with enoxaparin ($p < 0.001$).
- The exclusion of men with a creatinine level >2.5 mg/dL (220 μmol/L) and women with a creatinine level >2.0 mg/dL (177 μmol/L) was an important adjustment to prevent bleeding.

LMWH and Major Bleeding Advice

In patients aged > 70 years, use 0.75 mg/kg, and in all patients with creatinine clearance 30–50 mL/min dose once daily and avoid if the estimated GFR is <30 mL/min.

- For the conversion of serum creatinine in mg/dL, multiply × 88 (=mmol/L). The serum creatinine is only a rough measure of renal function and must not be relied on, particularly in patients older than age 70.
- Use the creatinine clearance estimated GFR rather than serum creatinine levels, but note that some electronic formulas are inaccurate in patients older than age 70 and must be adjusted in blacks (for African Americans, the laboratory-reported estimated GFR should be multiplied by a factor of 1.21 and reinterpreted accordingly).
- Patients, particularly cardiac patients, older than age 70 with a serum creatinine in the upper normal range of 1–1.2 mg/dL (88–106 µmol/L) often have a lowered GFR because of the underlying normal diminution of GFR with age. A substantial number of nephrons are lost annually beyond age 70, and in many elderly patients renal disease coexists.
- For patients older than age 75, enoxaparin 0.75 mg/kg once daily is an easy dose to recall, but it might be preferable to use the lower age cutoff: >70 years of age.
- Enoxaparin and other LMWHs should be given once daily in patients with a GFR, creatinine clearance of 40–55 mL/min. Patients in this category received enoxaparin twice daily in several RCTs; unfortunately, patients with a creatinine clearance <30 mL/min were given 1 mg/kg once daily in some RCTs.
- Importantly, if major bleeding is to be minimized in patients with ACS, LMWH should be avoided if the creatinine clearance is <30 mL/min. An estimated GFR of <30 mL/min reflects poor renal function. Clinicians most often use a creatinine clearance <15 mL/min to indicate severe renal failure. This information is correct, but end-stage renal failure (GFR < 15 mL/min) should be regarded as very severe renal failure, and drugs that have a potential to cause major

bleeding must be used only with justification. Use in patients with ACS is not justifiable because alternative therapies are available.

- Do not switch from UF heparin to LMWH and vice versa in the management of a patient with ACS.

ENOXAPARIN OR UNFRACTIONATED HEPARIN FOR PCI

In a randomized open-label trial, patients presenting with STEMI were randomly assigned (1:1) to receive an intravenous bolus of 0.5 mg/kg of enoxaparin or unfractionated heparin before primary PCI. 910 patients were assigned to treatment with enoxaparin ($n=450$) or unfractionated heparin ($n=460$) (Montalescot et al. 2011).

The primary end point was 30-day incidence of death, complication of myocardial infarction, procedure failure, or major bleeding. The main secondary end point was the composite of death, recurrent acute coronary syndrome, or urgent revascularization.

Results: The primary end point (30-day incidence of death, complication of MI, procedure failure, or major bleeding) occurred in 126 (28 %) patients with enoxaparin versus 155 (34 %) patients on unfractionated heparin ($p=0.06$). The incidence of death [enoxaparin, 17 (4 %) versus heparin, 29 (6 %) patients; $p=0.08$], complication of MI $p=0.21$; and major bleeding [20 (5 %) versus 22 (5 %); $p=0.79$] did not differ between groups. Enoxaparin resulted in a significantly reduced rate of the main secondary end point [30 (7 %) versus 52 (11 %) patients; $p=0.015$]. Death, complication of MI, or major bleeding [46 (10 %) versus 69 (15 %) patients; $p=0.03$], death or complication of MI [35 (8 %) versus 57 (12 %); $p=0.02$], and death, recurrent MI, or urgent revascularization [23 (5 %) versus 39 (8 %); $p=0.04$] were all reduced with enoxaparin.

Enoxaparin provided an improvement in net clinical benefit in patients undergoing primary PCI (Montalescot et al. 2011).

FONDAPARINUX OR ENOXAPARIN

OASIS-6: Effects of Fondaparinux on Mortality and Reinfarction in Patients With Acute ST-Segment Elevation Myocardial Infarction (STEMI).

OASIS-6 (2006) was an RCT of fondaparinux versus usual care in 12,092 STEMI patients. A 7–8-day course of fondaparinux was compared with either no anticoagulation or heparin (75 % received heparin for <48 h). Streptokinase was the main fibrinolytic used (73 % of those who received lytics). The primary outcome was a composite of death or reinfarction at 30 days.

• Conclusion: In patients with STEMI, particularly those not undergoing PCI, fondaparinux significantly reduced mortality and reinfarction without increasing bleeding and strokes (OASIS-6 Trial Investigators 2006).

In areas and in countries where PCI is not readily available, the drug can be used with streptokinase without any form of heparin administration. In addition, the one dose of fondaparinux with no adjustments for weight is a great advance in developing or developed countries.

• The addition of rivaroxaban 12 h after the final dose of fondaparinux and continued for >5 years should result in improved survival and represents a major breakthrough in the therapy for ACS.

Califf (2006) points out that a reasonable conclusion from this trial is that fondaparinux is highly beneficial in patients in whom the noninterventional approach has been predetermined and will be more preferred in settings in which the use of angiographic-based reperfusion is not routine. In addition, the absence of the need for dose adjustment is remarkable. The two large RCTs have endorsed fondaparinux as a leading antithrombotic drug in the treatment of ACS. There is no evidence that fondaparinux is inferior to either UF heparin or LMWH for the management of ACS. The reduction in bleeding in the fondaparinux group compared with the group receiving no antithrombotic therapy should give clinicians some confidence that at the dose used, fondaparinux has a desirable margin of safety (Califf (2006)). Also, heparin-induced thrombocytopenia (HIT) can be avoided. Caution with dosage is needed, however, in patients with significant renal dysfunction (estimated GFR < 50 mL/min).

INVASIVE VERSUS CONSERVATIVE STRATEGY IN ACS PATIENTS

TACTICS-TIMI 18 evaluated the superiority of an invasive strategy (stenting and use of the platelet inhibitor tirofiban) in patients with unstable angina and non-ST-elevation MI (NSTEMI). Coronary angiography was completed within 4–48 h, and PCI was accomplished in the invasive arm (TACTICS-TIMI-18 Investigators 2001). The cumulative incidence of the primary end point of death, nonfatal MI, or rehospitalization for an ACS during the 6-months follow-up period was lower in the invasive-strategy group than in the conservative-strategy group (15.9 % versus 19.4 %; OR, 0.78; $p = 0.025$). Patients with positive troponin levels (i.e., NSTEMI patients) achieved the greatest benefit from an early invasive strategy (14.3 % versus 24.2 %; $p < 0.001$; see Fig. 22-1).

Unstable angina patients were not benefited by early PCI; only patients with NSTEMI (as defined by positive troponin levels) benefited significantly.

- Patients with unstable angina with or without ischemic electrocardiographic (ECG) changes and negative troponin levels showed no significant benefit with an invasive strategy.
- Patients with unstable angina and negative troponin levels should not be considered to have ACS but simply unstable angina. These patients have not sustained infarctions and are a heterogeneous group with a markedly different prognosis compared with STEMI or NSTEMI patients.

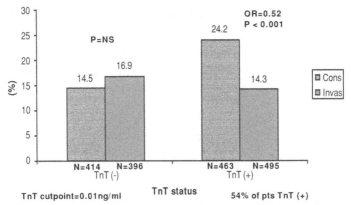

Fig. 22-1. Outcomes of invasive and conservative strategies in TACTICS-TIMI 18 according to troponin level. Reproduced with permission from Cannon CP. *Management of Acute Coronary Syndromes*, 2nd ed. Humana Press, Totowa, NJ, 2003. With kind permission from Springer Science + Business Media.

TIMACS (2009) studied the efficacy of an early invasive strategy compared with a delayed invasive strategy. Patients were randomized to either an early invasive strategy (coronary angiography as soon as possible, followed by PCI or CABG within 24 h) or a delayed strategy (coronary angiography any time >36 h followed by PCI or CABG). A total of 3,031 patients were randomized, 1,593 to an early invasive strategy, and 1,438 to a delayed invasive strategy. About 80 % had ECG changes in keeping with ischemia (ST-segment depression of 1 mm or transient ST-segment elevation or T-wave inversion of >3 mm).

About 77 % of the patients had elevated biomarkers (NSTEMI) (Mehta et al. 2009). Thus, about 77 % were NSTEMI and only 23 % were unstable angina; the presence of these 23 % lower-risk patients dilutes the treatment effects.

The median times to coronary angiography in the early and delayed arms were 14 and 50 h, respectively. PCI was conducted more often in the early invasive group (59.6 %

versus 55 %), with a median time of 16 versus 52 h; mean follow-up 6 months (Mehta et al. 2009).

- Results: An early invasive strategy was not superior to a delayed invasive strategy in patients presenting with NSTEMI and unstable angina in reducing the composite end point of death and MI.
- But there was a significant reduction in the incidence of the primary end point in the early invasive arm compared with the delayed invasive arm in **patients with a GRACE score of >140** (the third with the highest risk); the primary outcome occurred in 13.9 % of patients in the early-intervention group, as compared with 21 % in the delayed-intervention group, a reduction of 35 % in the early-intervention group (hazard ratio, 0.65; $p = 0.006$) (Mehta et al. 2009).

Patients with chest pain features of MI accompanied by ST-segment depression or transient elevation and positive troponin assays (i.e., a diagnosis of NSTEMI) should undergo an early invasive intervention if facilities are readily available.

- The TIMI or GRACE risk algorithms can be used effectively to predict the rates of death or MI for a year after hospitalization for ACS.
- In patients with elevated troponin levels if pulmonary embolism, decompensated heart failure, severe hypertension, tachycardia, anemia, and sepsis are excluded clinically, this variable along with ECG changes (two risk factors) should establish the high-risk patient.
- Fox and colleagues assessed a meta-analysis ($n = 5,467$ patients) designed to determine whether outcomes are improved despite trial differences. Conclusion: "a routine invasive strategy reduces long-term rates of cardiovascular death or MI and the largest absolute effect is seen in higher-risk patients. Even in intermediate risk populations, the benefits of an early invasive strategy are of similar magnitude as those aimed for and seen with current pharmacological interventions" (Fox et al. 2010).

TICAGRELOR VERSUS CLOPIDOGREL

PLATO: Cannon and colleagues (2010) for the platelet inhibition and patient Outcomes (PLATO) investigators compared ticagrelor with clopidogrel.

At randomization, an invasive strategy was planned for 13,408 (72 %) of 18,624 patients hospitalized for STEMI and NSTEMI. Patients were randomly assigned to ticagrelor and placebo (180 mg loading dose followed by 90 mg twice a day) or to clopidogrel and placebo (300–600 mg loading dose or continuation with maintenance dose followed by 75 mg/day) for 6–12 months. All patients were given aspirin. The primary composite end point was cardiovascular death, MI, or stroke (Cannon et al. 2010). Analyses were by intention to treat.

Results: At 1 year the primary composite end point occurred in fewer patients in the 6,732 ticagrelor-treated group than in the 6,676 clopidogrel group: 569 (event rate 9 %) versus 668 (10.7 %, hazard ratio 0.84, $p = 0.0025$).

Ticagrelor compared with clopidogrel significantly reduced all-cause mortality at 12 months in all patients (4.5 % versus 5.9 %, hazard ratio 0.78, $p < 0.001$), and in patients undergoing an early invasive strategy (3.9 % versus 5 %, $p = 0.01$).

There was no difference between clopidogrel and ticagrelor groups in the rates of total major bleeding 691 (11.6 %) versus 689 (11.5 %), or severe bleeding. These investigators concluded that ticagrelor seems to be a better option than clopidogrel for patients with STEMI OR NSTEMI, for whom an early invasive strategy is planned (Cannon et al. 2010).

During 12 months, dyspnea occurred more often in the ticagrelor group than in the clopidogrel group [924 (event rate 13.9 %) versus 527 (8 %); $p < 0.0001$]. Only 51 (0.8 %) patients in the ticagrelor group and ten (0.2 %) in the clopidogrel group permanently discontinued the study drug because of this adverse event (Cannon et al. 2010). Most episodes lasted less than a week (Wallentin et al. 2008); the levels of creatinine increased slightly more during the treatment period with ticagrelor than with clopidogrel. These minor effects can be overcome, however, by not administering the drug to patients with chronic obstructive pulmonary disease, and those with a moderate degree of renal failure or in those over age 75 because renal dysfunction may be present despite the finding of a normal serum creatinine; also, in this age group, intracranial hemorrhage is more likely to occur with potent agents that include ticagrelor and prasugrel.

Ticagrelor blocks reuptake of adenosine by red blood cells (Björkman et al. 2007), "which might explain why some patients had dyspnea and bradycardia. Inhibition of adenosine reuptake could also lead to cardiovascular benefit through reduction in blood pressure (BP), improved coronary flow, or protection against reperfusion injury".

There was a higher incidence of ventricular pauses in the first week, but not at day 30, in the ticagrelor group than in the clopidogrel group. Pauses were rarely associated with symptoms; the two treatment groups did not differ significantly with respect to the incidence of syncope or pacemaker implantation.

- Cannon and colleagues emphasized that their results show that ticagrelor might be safely initiated at first presentation and does not need to be withheld until the coronary anatomy is defined.
- The PLATO investigators estimate that "use of ticagrelor instead of clopidogrel for 1 year in 1,000 patients with acute coronary syndromes and who are planned to undergo an invasive strategy at the start of drug treatment would lead to 11 fewer deaths, 13 fewer MIs, and six fewer cases of stent thrombosis without an increase in the rates of major bleeding or transfusion" (Cannon et al. 2010).

Stone, in an editorial, emphasized that:

- Unlike clopidogrel and prasugrel, which bind irreversibly to the platelet surface-membrane (P2Y12) receptor, ticagrelor is a reversible P2Y12 receptor blocker, with platelet function returning to normal, 2–3 days after discontinuation (Gurbel et al. 2009) compared with 5–10 days after discontinuation of clopidogrel and prasugrel. The reversible action of ticagrelor is of paramount importance "in mitigating bleeding," thus allowing coronary bypass graft surgery, soon after drug discontinuation. In addition within 30 min, a ticagrelor loading dose of 180 mg results in roughly the same level of inhibition of platelet aggregation as that achieved 8 h after a clopidogrel loading dose of 600 mg (Gurbel et al. 2009). Compelling results support ticagrelor as a new standard of care in acute coronary syndromes (Stone 2010).

Ticagrelor (Brilinta) FDA approved blood-thinning drug Brilinta to treat acute coronary syndromes. *Boxed warning says daily aspirin doses above 100 mg decrease effectiveness*. In clinical trials, Brilinta was more effective than Plavix in preventing heart attacks and death, but that advantage was seen with aspirin maintenance doses of 75–100 mg once daily,

In the PLATO trial, ticagrelor compared with clopidogrel consistently reduced the primary end point and its components CV death and MI, without a difference in overall major bleeding in patients with an entry diagnosis of NSTEMI including in-hospital medically managed (Lindholm et al. 2013).

IV METOPROLOL STUDIES

- In patients with anterior Killip class < or equal to 11 ST-elevation MI undergoing PCI, early IV metoprolol before reperfusion resulted in higher long-term left ventricular ejection fraction. This administration reduced the incidence of severe left ventricular dysfunction and implantable cardioverter defibrillator indications and fewer admissions for heart failure (Pizarro et al. 2014).

COMMIT/CCS-2: *Second Chinese Cardiac Study (CCS-2) (31)*

This trial was conducted on the emergency treatment of STEMI patients. Patients received aspirin and were randomized to receive clopidogrel 75 mg/day or placebo; within these two groups, patients were then randomized to metoprolol (15 mg IV in three equal doses followed by 200 mg/day oral) or placebo. Patients were randomized within 24 h of suspected acute MI and demonstrated ST elevation or other ischemic abnormality and excluded if they were undergoing PCI. The primary end point varied between study drugs: for clopidogrel, it was death or the combination of death, reinfarction, or stroke up to 4 weeks in the hospital or prior to discharge; for metoprolol, it was death or death, reinfarction, or cardiac arrest/ventricular fibrillation (VF) up to 4 weeks in the hospital or prior to discharge.

- Metoprolol produced a significant 18 % relative risk reduction in reinfarction (2.0 % versus 2.5 %; $p=0.001$) as well as a 17 % relative risk reduction in ventricular fibrillation (2.5 % versus 3.0 %; $p=0.001$); there was no effect on mortality (7.7 % versus 7.8 %). Metoprolol significantly increased the relative risk of death from cardiogenic shock by 29 %, with the greatest risk of shock occurring primarily on day 0–1 (COMMIT/CCS-2 2005).
- Cardiogenic shock understandably was more evident in patients in Killip classes II and III; this adverse effect was largely iatrogenic because the dose of metoprolol was excessive. Oral beta-blocker therapy is preferred, and the IV use is cautioned against.
- **Importantly. metoprolol IV was administered to patients who were hemodynamically unstable, a situation that must be avoided. (See Chap. 2, Beta-Blocker Controversies.)**

The METOCARD-CNIC

Effect of Metoprolol in Cardioprotection During an Acute Myocardial Infarction trial

- The study randomized 270 patients Killip class II anterior STEMI presenting early after symptom onset (<6 h) to pre-reperfusion IV metoprolol or control group. Long-term magnetic resonance imaging (MRI) was performed on 202 patients (101 per group) 6 months after STEMI. Patients had a minimal 12-month clinical follow-up (Pizarro et al. 2014).

"Results Left ventricular ejection fraction (LVEF) at the 6 months MRI was higher after IV metoprolol (9.9 % versus 11.7 % in control subjects p ¼ 0.025). The occurrence of severely depressed LVEF (35 %) at 6 months was significantly lower in patients treated with IV metoprolol (11 % versus 27 %, p ¼ 0.006). The proportion of patients fulfilling Class I indications for an implantable cardioverter-defibrillator (ICD) was significantly lower in the IV metoprolol group (7 % versus 20 %, p ¼ 0.012). At a median follow-up of 2 years, occurrence of the pre-specified composite of death, heart failure admission, reinfarction, and malignant arrhythmias was 10.8 % in the IV metoprolol group versus 18.3 % in the control group. Heart failure admission was significantly lower in the IV metoprolol group" (Pizarro et al. 2014).

In patients with anterior Killip class II STEMI undergoing pPCI, early IV metoprolol before reperfusion resulted in higher long-term LVEF, reduced incidence of severe LV systolic dysfunction and ICD indications, and fewer heart failure admissions (Pizarro et al. 2014).

The results of the COMMIT (2005), which showed no short-term net clinical benefit of early metoprolol in STEMI patients undergoing thrombolysis, discourage some from using the drug. But in that study the high dose of metoprolol given to patients with a systolic blood pressure <110 mmHg was inappropriate (Khan 2007).

ASPIRIN FOR CARDIOVASCULAR DISEASE PREVENTION

Aspirin Pseudoresistance

Grosser et al. (2013) assessed aspirin resistance and identified a high occurrence of pseudoresistance that is clinically meaningful.

Healthy volunteers ($n = 400$) were screened for their response to a single dose of 325-mg immediate release or enteric coated aspirin. Response parameters reflected the activity of the molecular target of aspirin, cyclooxygenase-1. Absorption proved very variable and caused up to 49 % apparent resistance to a single dose of enteric coated aspirin but not to immediate release aspirin (0 %). Conclusion: pharmacologic resistance to aspirin is rare; the study failed to identify a single case of true aspirin resistance. Pseudoresistance, reflecting delayed and reduced drug absorption, complicates enteric coated but not immediate release aspirin administration.

The author abandoned the use of enteric coated aspirin in 2009 and instead prescribes soft chewable aspirin 81 mg for CVD prevention.

Sound advice on the use of aspirin therapy for cardiovascular disease prevention is given by the European society of cardiology (Halverson et al. 2014).

ANGINA RCTS

PCI Versus Optimal Medical Therapy

COURAGE: The Clinical Outcomes Utilizing Revascularization and Aggressive Drug Evaluation (trial compared an initial strategy of PCI plus optimal medical therapy with optimal medical therapy alone for patients with stable angina. This RCT studied 2,287 patients who had objective evidence of myocardial ischemia, 1,149 patients to undergo PCI with optimal medical therapy (PCI group), and 1,138 to receive optimal medical therapy alone (medical-therapy group). The primary outcome was death from any cause and nonfatal MI during a median follow-up of 4.6 years). There were 211 primary events in the PCI group and 202 events in the medical-therapy group. The 4.6-years cumulative primary-event rates were 19 % in the PCI group and 18.5 % in the medical-therapy group.

In patients with stable angina, PCI did not reduce the risk of death, MI, or other major cardiovascular events when added to optimal medical therapy (Boden et al. for the COURAGE Trial Research 2007).

During the trial period, 21 % crossed over and received PCI. There was rapidity of improvement in health status in both treatment groups; the majority of patients who received optimal medical therapy alone had improved symptoms within 3 months. This suggests that optimal antianginal medications are underused in practice.

- The "take-home" message from the COURAGE trial is to pursue optimal medical therapy initially as it is effective in 75 % and if this is ineffective in 25 %, resort to PCI.

- Pooled together the results of 17 randomized trials comparing PCI and medical treatment as strategies in patients with stable angina and no acute coronary syndromes, this meta-analysis concluded that a PCI-based invasive strategy may improve long-term survival in patients with stable coronary artery disease (CAD), and that this justifies a new clinical trial sufficiently powered to evaluate the impact of PCI on long-term mortality.

- Based on the strength of available evidence, however, O'Rourke recommends "more aggressive medical therapy for patients with moderate to severe angina, and PCI or CABG for patients whose symptoms persist. Optimal medical therapy is a proven option for chronic stable angina" (O'Rourke 2008).

Carvedilol in Postinfarct Patients

CAPRICORN: In the Carvedilol Postinfarct Survival Controlled Evaluation trial, patients with acute MI and ejection fraction (EF)<40 % (mean 32.8), 1–21 day prior to randomization, treated with an angiotensin-converting enzyme (ACE) inhibitor, were randomly assigned; the treatment arm received carvedilol 6.25 mg, which was increased progressively to 25 mg twice daily in 74 % of treated patients.

- Carvedilol caused a significant 23 % reduction in all-cause mortality in patients with acute MI observed for 2.5 years [mortality 116 (12 %) in the treated versus 151 (15 %) in the placebo arm; $p=0.031$] (CAPRICORN Investigators 2001).
- The absolute reduction in risk was 2.3 %: 43 patients need to be treated for 1 year to save one life; this reduction is somewhat better than that observed in a meta-analysis of three ACE inhibitor trials, SAVE, AIRE, and TRACE.
- Notably, the reduction by carvedilol is in addition to those of ACE inhibitors alone.

ATRIAL FIBRILLATION RCTS

Lenient Rate Control

Van Gelder and colleagues (2010) randomly assigned 614 patients with permanent atrial fibrillation to undergo a lenient rate-control strategy (resting heart rate <110/min) or a strict rate-control strategy (resting heart rate <80/min and heart rate during moderate exercise <110 beats/min). The primary outcome was a composite of death from cardiovascular causes, hospitalization for HF, and stroke, and systemic embolism.

Results: The estimated cumulative incidence of the primary outcome at 3 years was 12.9 % in the lenient-control group and 14.9 % in the strict-control group, with an absolute difference with respect to the lenient-control group of –2 % points $p<0.001$ for the prespecified noninferiority margin. The frequencies of the components of the primary outcome were similar in the two groups.

More patients in the lenient-control group met the heart-rate target or targets [304 (97.7 %), versus 203 (67 %) in the strict-control group; $p < 0.001$] with fewer total visits [75 (median, 0), versus 684, $p < 0.001$].

The frequencies of symptoms and adverse events were similar in the two groups.

In patients with permanent atrial fibrillation, lenient rate control is safe (resting heart rate 70 to <110/min), and as effective as strict rate control, and is easier to achieve with fewer total visits. **In Canada the goal rate is <100/min.**

Rate Versus Rhythm Control in Atrial Fibrillation

AFFIRM 2002: The Atrial Fibrillation Follow-up Investigation of Rhythm Management (AFFIRM) was a well-run rate versus rhythm control RCT with 2–5 years of follow-up.

Conclusions: Rate control is an acceptable primary therapy. In the rate-control arm, 51 % received digoxin and 49 % a beta-blocker. At 2 years of follow-up, the perceived benefit of restoring and maintaining sinus rhythm did not alter mortality. Patients in the rhythm control arm still required warfarin (70 %). Mortality, stroke rate, and hospitalizations were slightly increased, and bradycardiac arrest and torsades de pointes were of concern. Amiodarone was used in approx. 39 %, sotalol in approx. 33 %, and propafenone in approx. 10 % to maintain rhythm control, which required frequent changes in drug and dosing schedule.

An RCT conducted in The Netherlands in patients with persistent atrial fibrillation <1 year randomly assigned to electrical conversion and rhythm control versus rate control indicated that rate control was not inferior to rhythm control. Nonfatal end points were slighter greater in the rhythm control group; cardiovascular mortality was the same in both groups.

Newer Anticoagulants for Reduction in Stroke

ARISTOTLE Granger et al. 2011: Patients, 18,201 with atrial fibrillation and at least one additional risk factor for stroke were enrolled in the trial and were randomly assigned to receive the direct factor Xa inhibitor apixaban (at a dose of 5 mg twice daily) or warfarin [target international normalized ratio (INR), 2.0–3.0].

Results: apixaban was not only noninferior to warfarin, but actually superior, reducing the risk of stroke or systemic embolism by 21 % and the risk of major bleeding by 31 %. In predefined hierarchical testing, apixaban, as compared with warfarin, also reduced the risk of death from any cause by 11 % (Granger et al. 2011). The reduction in stroke was mainly due to a lower rate of hemorrhagic stroke (0.24 % versus 0.47 % per year; HR 0.51). The dabigatran and riva-roxaban versus warfarin clinical trials showed a similar reduction in this end point.

- 25.3 % of patients on apixaban discontinued the study drug versus 27.5 % for warfarin.
- Adverse events were similar (81.5 % versus 83.1 %) and serious adverse events (35 % versus 36.5 %) in the two groups.

RE-LY 2010: Dabigatran Versus Warfarin in Patients with Atrial Fibrillation

The RE-LY study assigned 18,113 patients who had atrial fibrillation and a risk of stroke to receive, in a blinded fashion, fixed doses of dabigatran, an oral factor Xa inhibitor—110 mg or 150 mg twice daily—or, in an unblinded fashion, adjusted-dose warfarin (Connolly et al. 2009).

Dabigatran given at a dose of 110 mg was associated with rates of stroke and systemic embolism that were similar to those associated with warfarin, as well as lower rates of major hemorrhage. Dabigatran administered at a dose of 150 mg, as compared with warfarin, was associated with lower rates of stroke and systemic embolism but similar rates of major hemorrhage (Connolly et al. 2009).

ROCKET: RIVAROXABAN VERSUS WARFARIN IN NONVALVULAR ATRIAL FIBRILLATION

This RCT assigned 14,264 patients with nonvalvular atrial fibrillation who were at increased risk for stroke to receive either rivaroxaban an oral factor Xa inhibitor (at a once daily dose of 20 mg) or dose-adjusted warfarin.

Results: The median duration of treatment exposure was 590 days; the median follow-up period was 707 days. The primary end point occurred in 188 patients in the rivaroxaban group and in 241 in the warfarin group ($p<0.001$ for noninferiority). In the intention-to-treat analysis, the primary end point occurred in 269 patients in the rivaroxaban group and in 306 patients in the warfarin group ($p<0.001$ for noninferiority; $p=0.12$ for superiority).

Major and nonmajor clinically relevant bleeding occurred in 1,475 patients in the rivaroxaban group (14.9 % per year) and in 1,449 in the warfarin group (14.5 % per year) ($p=0.44$). There were significant reductions in intracranial hemorrhage (0.5 % versus 0.7 %, $p=0.02$) and fatal bleeding (0.2 % versus 0.5 %, $p=0.003$) in the rivaroxaban group.

Conclusion: In patients with atrial fibrillation, rivaroxaban was noninferior to warfarin for the prevention of stroke or systemic embolism. There was no significant between-group difference in the risk of major bleeding, although intracranial and fatal bleeding occurred less frequently in the rivaroxaban group.

The FDA has approved rivaroxaban (Xarelto) for the prevention of stroke in patients with nonvalvular atrial fibrillation. Mega (2011) emphasized the following:

- In the RE-LY trial, the assignments to dabigatran or warfarin were not concealed. In contrast, the ROCKET AF and ARISTOTLE trials successfully achieved a double-blind design. Rivaroxaban is administered once daily and the other agents are given twice daily.

- **Switching to a newer agent may not be necessary for patients in whom the INR has been well controlled with warfarin for years**.
- Although the newer anticoagulants have a more rapid onset and termination of anticoagulant action than does warfarin, **agents to reverse the effect of the drugs are still under development**.

For Edoxaban in patients with atrial fibrillation, **see Chaps. 19 and 24.**

COLCHICINE FOR CARDIOVASCUALR DISEASE

Colchicine for Stable Coronary Artery Disease

A study to determine whether colchicine 0.5 mg/day can reduce the risk of CVD events in patients with stable coronary disease. Activated neutrophils are observed in culprit atheroma plaques of patients with acute coronary syndrome (ACS). The inhibition of neutrophil function with colchicine may reduce the risk of plaque instability and thereby improve clinical outcomes in patients with stable disease (Nidorf et al. 2013).

In a clinical trial with a prospective, randomized, observer-blinded end point design, 532 patients with stable coronary disease receiving aspirin and/or clopidogrel (93 %) and statins (95 %) were randomly assigned colchicine 0.5 mg/day or no colchicine and followed for a median of 3 years. The primary analysis was by intention to treat.

The primary outcome: the composite incidence of ACS, out-of-hospital cardiac arrest, or noncardioembolic ischemic stroke occurred in 15 of 282 patients (5.3 %) who received colchicine and 40 of 250 patients (16.0 %) assigned no colchicine (hazard ratio: 0.33; 95 % $p<0.001$; number needed to treat: 11).

Conclusions: Colchicine 0.5 mg/day appears beneficial for the prevention of CVD events in patients with stable coronary disease (Nidorf et al. 2013). Unfortunately a statin is required in virtually all patients with CVD and must not be combined with colchicine.

- **Caution: Colchicine combined with statins may cause serious myopathy and rhabdomyolysis. See Table** 21-7.

Colchicine for pericarditis

"Colchicine added to conventional anti-inflammatory treatment significantly reduced the rate of subsequent recurrences of pericarditis in patients with multiple recurrences. Taken together with results from other randomised controlled trials, these findings suggest that colchicine should be probably regarded as a first-line treatment for either acute or recurrent pericarditis in the absence of contraindications or specific indications" (Imazio et al. 2014).

- *See Colchicine for post-op atrial fibrillation under section atrial fibrillation.*

Colchicine for Post-op Atrial Fibrillation

The Colchicine for the Prevention of the Postpericardiotomy Syndrome (COPPS) POAF substudy is the first trial designed to assess the efficacy and safety of colchicine for paroxysmal atrial fibrillation (POAF) prevention. It is a substudy of the COPPS trial, in which colchicine halved the occurrence of the postpericardiotomy syndrome (PPS).

The COPPS POAF substudy included 336 patients (mean age, 65.7 ± 12.3 years; 69 % male) of the COPPS trial, a multicenter, double-blind, randomized trial. Substudy patients were in sinus rhythm before starting the intervention [placebo/colchicine 1.0 mg twice daily starting on postoperative day 3 followed by a maintenance dose of 0.5 mg twice daily for 1 month Imazio et al. (2011)].

Patients on colchicine had a reduced incidence of paroxysmal atrial fibrillation (POAF) (12.0 % versus 22.0 %, respectively; $p = 0.021$; relative risk reduction, 45 %; number needed to treat, 11). The POAF events after the start of the intervention (placebo/colchicine) numbered 35 of 167 versus 20 of 169, respectively. The duration of POAF was shorter in the colchicine group compared with the placebo group (3.0 ± 1.2 versus 7.7 ± 2.5 days, respectively; $p < 0.001$). Patients treated with colchicine had a shorter in-hospital stay (9.4 ± 3.7 versus 10.3 ± 4.3 days; $p = 0.040$), rehabilitation stay (12.1 ± 6.1 versus 13.9 ± 6.5 days; $p = 0.009$), and overall hospital stay [cardiac surgery plus rehabilitation Imazio et al. (2011)].

The rates of adverse effects and drug withdrawal were similar in the colchicine and placebo groups [9.5 % versus 4.8 %, respectively ($p = 0.137$), for side effects, and 11.8 % versus 6.6 % ($p = 0.131$) for drug withdrawal]. No severe adverse effects were noted (Imazio et al. 2011).

Gastrointestinal intolerance was the only side effect recorded during the study in colchicine-treated patients. One case of myotoxicity was recorded in the placebo group and was related to concomitant use of a statin. Statins should not be given concomitantly.

- **In the COPPS trial, colchicine halved the incidence of the postpericardiotomy syndrome**.

Interactions occur with amiodarone and statins, particularly simvastatin; these agents should be avoided during the course of colchicine.

Conclusion: Colchicine represents an inexpensive and safe option for the prevention of both postpericardiotomy syndrome (PPS) and POAF (Imazio et al. 2011).

A study to determine whether colchicine 0.5 mg/day can reduce the risk of CVD events in patients with stable coronary disease. Activated neutrophils are observed in culprit atheroma plaques of patients with acute coronary syndrome (ACS). The inhibition of neutrophil function with colchicine may reduce the risk of plaque instability and thereby improve clinical outcomes in patients with stable disease (Nidorf et al. 2013).

In a clinical trial with a prospective, randomized, observer-blinded endpoint design, 532 patients with stable coronary disease receiving aspirin and/or clopidogrel (93 %) and statins (95 %) were randomly assigned colchicine 0.5 mg/day or no colchicine and followed for a median of 3 years. The primary analysis was by intention to treat.

The primary outcome: the composite incidence of ACS, out-of-hospital cardiac arrest, or noncardioembolic ischemic stroke occurred in 15 of 282 patients (5.3 %) who received colchicine and 40 of 250 patients (16.0 %) assigned no colchicine (hazard ratio: 0.33; 95 % $p < 0.001$; number needed to treat: 11).

Conclusions Colchicine 0.5 mg/day in addition to statins and other standard prevention therapies appears beneficial for the prevention of CVD events in patients with stable coronary disease (Nidorf et al. 2013).

Caution: colchicine combined with statins may cause serious myopathy and rhabdomyolysis.

HEART FAILURE RCTS

COPERNICUS 2001: Carvedilol in Severe Chronic HF

The Carvedilol Prospective Randomized Cumulative Survival Study involved 2,289 patients with severe heart failure (HF; EF 19.8 ± 4 %). There were 190 deaths in placebo recipients and 130 in those given carvedilol, a 35 % decrease in the risk of death ($p = 0.0014$). The dose of carvedilol was 6.25 mg, with a slow increase to 25 mg twice daily. An ACE inhibitor, digoxin, and spironolactone were used in 97 %, 66 %, and 20 % of patients, respectively.

HEART FAILURE TRIALS

MERIT-HF 2000: Metoprolol CR/XL in Chronic Heart Failure

The Metoprolol CR/XL Randomized Intervention Trial in Congestive Heart Failure (MERIT-HF) trial studied metoprolol succinate (not tartrate) in patients with class II and III HF (mean EF 0.28). An ACE inhibitor or angiotensin receptor blocker (ARB) and digoxin were used in 95 % and 64 % of patients, respectively.

Metoprolol succinate caused significant reductions in the primary outcomes. Importantly, worldwide mainly the tartrate formulation is widely used; the sustained release product does not have a 24 h duration of action and is not recommended.

A-HeFT 2004: Isosorbide Dinitrate and Hydralazine in Blacks with HF In the African-American Heart Failure Trial (AHeFT), 1,050 black patients who had class III or IV HF with dilated ventricles were randomly assigned to receive 37.5 mg of hydralazine hydrochloride and 20 mg of isosorbide dinitrate three times daily. The dose was increased to two tablets three times daily, for a total daily dose of 225 mg of hydralazine hydrochloride and 120 mg of isosorbide dinitrate. (It is surprising that nitrate tolerance did not alter the results.)

- The study was terminated early (at 18 months) because of a significantly higher mortality rate in the placebo group than in the group given isosorbide dinitrate plus hydralazine (10.2 % versus 6.2 %; $p = 0.02$). There was a 43 % reduction in the rate of death from any cause (HR, 0.57; $p = 0.01$) and a 33 % relative reduction in the rate of first hospitalization for HF (16.4 % versus 22.4 %; $p = 0.001$) (14).

THE SENIORS STUDY: NEBIVOLOL FOR HEART FAILURE

These investigators studied 2,111 patients; 1,359 (64 %) had impaired (35 %) EF (mean 28.7 %) and 752 (36 %) had preserved (>35 %) EF (mean 49.2 %).

During follow-up of 21 months, the primary end point occurred in 465 patients (34.2 %) with impaired EF and in 235 patients (31.2 %) with preserved EF. The effect of nebivolol on the primary end point [hazard ratio (HR) of nebivolol versus placebo] was 0.86 (95 % confidence interval: 0.72–1.04) in patients with impaired EF and 0.81 (95 % confidence interval: 0.63–1.04) in preserved EF ($p = 0.720$ for subgroup interaction). Effects on all secondary end points were similar between groups (HR for all-cause mortality 0.84 and 0.91, respectively). Conclusions: The effect of beta-blockade with nebivolol in elderly patients with HF in this study was similar in those with preserved and impaired EF (Flather et al. 2005; van Veldhuisen et al. 2009).

- Nebivolol is a unique, highly selective beta-blocker with vasodilatory properties mediated through the nitric oxide pathway. This cardioactive agent is a highly selective b1-adrenergic receptor blocker, and is the only beta-blocker known to induce vascular production of nitric oxide, the main endothelial vasodilator. Nebivolol induces nitric oxide production via activation of b3-adrenergic receptors and stimulates the b3-adrenergic receptor-mediated production of nitric oxide in the heart; this stimulation results in a greater protection against HF (Maffei and Lembo 2009).
- Nebivolol reduces P-wave dispersion on the electrocardiogram, which would attenuate the risk of atrial fibrillation (Tuncer et al. 2008).

Aldosterone Antagonist Trials

RALES: Spironolactone in Severe HF Patients: significant results were obtained in the Randomized Aldactone Evaluation Study (RALES) trial (1999) with the use of spironolactone (Aldactone) in patients with severe HF classes III and IV (EF 25 ± 6.8). ACE inhibitors and digoxin were used in 95 % and 74 % of patients, respectively. The old drug spironolactone (Aldactone) is a major addition to our HF armamentarium.

EPHESUS: EPLERENONE IN POST-ACUTE MI

The Eplerenone Post-Acute MI and HF Efficacy and Survival Study (EPHESUS 2003) showed that eplerenone, a selective aldosterone blocker, added to optimal medical therapy in patients with acute MI and heart failure (EF < 35 %), significantly reduced mortality and morbidity. The trial randomized 6,600 patients. An eplerenone dose of 25 mg was titrated up to 50 mg daily. Gynecomastia was not observed, but significant hyperkalemia occurred in 5.5 % and 3.9 % of patients in the treated and placebo groups, respectively ($p = 0.002$).

Caution: This useful replacement for spironolactone should not be used in patients with serum creatinine > 1.5 mg/dL (133 μmol/L), particularly in patients older than age 75 or in type 2 diabetics and in all patients with GFR < 50 mL/min because hyperkalemia may be precipitated. Most important, the serum creatinine does not reflect creatinine clearance, particularly in the elderly, who are most often treated for HF.

ACE INHIBITORS AND ARB RCTS

HOPE 2000: The Heart Outcomes Prevention Evaluation (HOPE) trial studied high-risk patients [diabetes 38 %, MI 52 %, angina 80 %, peripheral vascular disease (PVD) 43 %, hypertension 47 %] without known significant left ventricular dysfunction.

- Ramipril significantly reduced the rates of death, MI, and stroke: 651 for ramipril versus 826 for placebo; the RR of the composite outcome in the ramipril group compared with the placebo group was 0.78. Treatment of 1,000 patients for 4 years prevents approx. 150 events in approx. 70 patients.

  Total mortality was only modestly reduced after 4 years of therapy: ramipril 482 versus 569 for placebo; a 15.2 % decrease in total deaths.

- **When this trial was conducted these high-risk patients were not given optimal therapy: beta-blockers, aspirin, and statins. ACE inhibitors and ARBs may be over prescribed**.

ONTARGET Granger et al. 2008: the investigators conducted an RCT in patients with vascular disease or high-risk diabetes but absence of heart failure (HF), and assigned 8,576 patients to receive 10 mg of ramipril per day, and 8,542 to receive 80 mg of the ARB telmisartan per day, and 8,502 assigned to receive both drugs (combination therapy). The primary composite outcome was death from cardiovascular causes, MI, stroke, or hospitalization for HF.

- Results: At a median follow-up of 56 months, the primary outcome was reported in 1,412 patients in the ramipril group (16.5 %), and in 1,423 patients in the telmisartan group (16.7 %).
- Telmisartan was equivalent to ramipril in this study. Without a placebo group this trial is flawed. Of course a placebo group would be unethical.

The combination of the two drugs was associated with more adverse events with no improvement in outcomes (ONTARGET Granger et al. 2008).

Because telmisartan was shown equivalent to ramipril in ONTARGET but without effect in TRANSCEND (Yusuf et al. 2008) there is some concern regarding the effectiveness of ARBs.

- **The efficacy of the ARB telmisartan raises some concern because of poor efficacy in two large RCTs: TRANSCEND and PRoFESS (2008). It is important to reassess the benefits of ramipril in the HOPE study**.

  – Weinsaft (2000) indicated that the population studied in HOPE was one in which a considerable number of high-risk patients were being treated with suboptimal medication regimens, according to current treatment guidelines. **Although 65.4 % of the treated group had documented hyperlipidemia, only 28.4 % were taking statins. In addition 51.9 % had had a documented MI and 54.8 % had a history of stable angina, only 39.2 % were taking beta-blockers**.

- **Thus, one may question whether the benefits associated with r**amipril in the HOPE study would have been maintained if patients had been treated with appropriate regimens of aspirin, beta-blockers, and lipid-lowering agents.

TRASCEND 2008: Telmisartan was tested against a placebo population that was administered near-optimal cardiovascular protective agents.

Telmisartan appeared equivalent to ramipril as indicated by ONTARGET, but each of these two agents may not show significant benefit in patients administered optimal medical therapy that includes statins to maintain LDL-C <1.8 mmol/L, a non-atenolol beta-blocker, and soft non-coated aspirin.

The TRANSCEND Investigators (Yusuf et al. 2008) studied the effects of telmisartan on cardiovascular events in 5,926 high-risk patients intolerant to ACE inhibitors.

Many patients receiving concomitant proven therapies were randomized to receive telmisartan 80 mg/day ($n = 2,954$) or placebo ($n = 2,972$). The primary outcome was the composite of cardiovascular death, MI, or hospitalization for HF.

After a median duration of follow-up of 56 months, 465 (15.7 %) patients experienced the primary outcome in the telmisartan group compared with 504 (17 %) in the placebo group, $p = 0.216$. Total **cardiovascular deaths > telmisartan 227** versus **223 for placeb**o; **the total mortality was unfortunately not given but is certainly not reduced by telmisartan**.

Telmisartan administration for 56 months in high-risk patients intolerant to ACE inhibitors surprisingly had no significant effect on the primary outcome, which included hospitalizations for HF (Yusuf et al. 2008). GFR decreased significantly more in the telmisartan group than placebo.

In addition, in the well-run RCT PRoFESS, telmisartan failed to decrease recurrent stroke (Yusuf et al. for the PRoFESS Study Group 2008). The efficacy of the ARB telmisartan raises some concern because of poor efficacy in two large RCTs.

PRoFESS *2008: Telmisartan to Prevent Recurrent Stroke*

The trialists randomly assigned 10,146 patients with recent ischemic stroke to receive telmisartan (80 mg daily) and 10,186 to receive placebo. The primary outcome was recurrent stroke. Secondary outcomes were death from cardiovascular causes, recurrent stroke, or MI. At a mean follow-up of 2.5 years, the mean blood pressure was 3.8/2 mmHg lower in the telmisartan group than in the placebo group. A total of 880 patients (8.7 %) in the telmisartan group and 934 patients (9.2 %) in the placebo group had a subsequent stroke ($p=0.23$). Secondary outcomes occurred in 1,367 patients (13.5 %) in the telmisartan group and 1,463 patients (14.4 %) in the placebo group; $p=0.11$.

- **Conclusion: Telmisartan therapy commenced soon after an ischemic stroke and continued for 2.5 years did not significantly lower the rate of recurrent stroke** (Yusuf et al. 2008).
- In addition it is a concern that telmisartan failed to prevent HF in patients intolerant to ACE inhibitors in TRANSCEND (2008); further studies are required to prove the value of this particular ARB. In addition, an increased cancer risk has been observed with some ARBs. **The FDA is reviewing the safety of the angiotensin-receptor blocker olmesartan after two ongoing trials among patients with type 2 diabetes and suggested increased risk for cardiovascular death with the drug**.

- It is now important for the physician to select an appropriate ARB with the understanding that all ARBs are not alike.

CANCER RISK WITH ARBS

Angiotensin-receptor blockers (ARBs) are associated with a modestly increased risk for cancer, according to a meta-analysis published in the Lancet Oncology. Researchers, examining data from five randomized trials comprising nearly 62,000 patients, found that those taking ARBs (*85 % were using telmisartan*) had a significantly greater risk for new cancer than did controls (7.2 % versus 6 %). When cancer type was analyzed, only lung cancer risk was significantly increased. The authors estimate that 143 patients would need to be treated for roughly 4 years for one excess cancer to occur (Sipahi et al. 2010). In an accompanying commentary, Nissen (2010) states that until we have more data, clinicians "should use ARBs, particularly telmisartan, with greater caution." He recommends reserving the drugs for patients who cannot tolerate ACE inhibitors.

ACE INHIBITORS AND CORONARY BYPASS SURGERY

Miceli and colleagues (2009) conducted a retrospective, observational, cohort study of prospectively collected data on 10,023 consecutive patients undergoing isolated CABG to May 2008. Of these, 3,052 patients receiving preoperative ACEI were matched to a control group by propensity score analysis.

Overall rate of mortality was 1 %. Preoperative ACEI therapy was associated with a doubling in the risk of death (1.3 % versus 0.7 %; $p = 0.013$). There was also a significant difference between the ACEI and control group in the risk of postoperative renal dysfunction (PRD) (7.1 % versus 5.4 %; $p = 0.006$), atrial fibrillation (25 % versus 20 %; $p < 0.0001$), and increased use of inotropic support (45.9 %

versus 41.1 %; $p < 0.0001$). In a multivariate analysis, preoperative ACEI treatment was an independent predictor of mortality ($p = 0.04$), PRD ($p = 0.0002$), use of inotropic drugs ($p < 0.0001$), and AF ($p < 0.0001$).

Conclusions: CAUTION **Preoperative treatment with ACE inhibitor is associated with an increased risk of mortality, use of inotropic support, PRD, and new onset of postoperative AF** (Miceli et al. 2009).

Bach (2009) makes the following points: suspending ACEI therapy before CABG and restarting it postoperatively might improve early surgical outcomes, while retaining the long-term cardioprotective effects of therapy.

This study, however, comes in the context of several others suggesting similar conclusions regarding long-term ACE inhibitor therapy. Bach (2009) emphasized that the EUROPA (EURopean Trial (2003) on reduction of cardiac events with perindopril in stable coronary Artery disease) study found that 50 patients would need to be treated for 4 years to prevent one major cardiac adverse event (the EUROPA study 2003).

The ACE Inhibitor Myocardial Infarction Collaborative Group found that only five lives would be saved per 1,000 patients treated with ACEI therapy and that therapy was associated with a twofold incidence of both persistent hypotension and renal dysfunction (ACE Inhibitor Myocardial Infarction Collaborative Group 1998). ARBs are less effective than ACE inhibitors; thus there salutary benefits are minimal (see Chaps. 3 and 4).

HYPERTENSION TRIALS

ALLHAT 2002

ACE Inhibitor or Calcium Channel Blocker Versus Diuretic to Prevent HF: The Antihypertensive and Lipid-Lowering Treatment to Prevent Heart Attack Trial (ALLHAT) is a hallmark clinical trial. A total of 33,357 hypertensive patients (mean age, 67) were randomized to receive chlorthalidone, 12.5–25 mg/day (n=15,255); amlodipine, 2.5–10 mg/day (n=9,048); or lisinopril, 10–40 mg/day (n=9,054), with a follow-up of 4.9 years. There was good representation for women (47 %) and blacks (35 %); 36 % were diabetics.

The primary outcome, combined fatal CHD or nonfatal MI, occurred in 2,956 participants, with no difference between treatments. All-cause mortality did not differ between groups.

- The doxazosin arm of the trial was halted because of a marked occurrence of HF (47 %) caused by doxazosin. No significant increase in cholesterol was caused by chlorthalidone.
- The primary outcomes for amlodipine versus chlorthalidone were similar except for a higher 6-year rate of HF with amlodipine.
- The 6-year rate for HF with amlodipine was 10.2 % versus 7.7 % with chlorthalidone; a 32.5 % higher risk of HF (p<0.001) with a 6-year absolute risk difference of 2.5 % and a 35 % higher risk of hospitalized/fatal HF (p<0.001). Elderly patients had a higher incidence of HF, which was even greater in black individuals. Importantly, because BP goal was achieved with chlorthalidone monotherapy in <30 % of patients, added therapy was atenolol 25–100 mg, and in some reserpine or clonidine. **It appears that a beta-blocker was used in >60 % of patients in this arm of the study and yet not now recommended by JNC8 experts**.

Nebivolol Combined with Valsartan Study

A double-blind treatment study with nebivolol and valsartan fixed-dose combination (5 and 80 mg/day, 5 and 160 mg/day, or 10 and 160 mg/day), nebivolol (5 mg/day or 20 mg/day), valsartan (80 mg/day or 160 mg/day), or placebo (Giles et al. 2014).

Doses were doubled in weeks 5–8; results are reported according to the final dose. Staff were masked to treatment allocation. The primary and key secondary end points were changes from baseline to week 8 in diastolic and systolic blood pressure, respectively. 4,161 patients were randomly assigned (277 to placebo and 554–555 to each active comparator group), 4,118 of whom were included in the primary analysis. At week 8, the fixed-dose combination nebivolol 20 and valsartan 320 mg/day group had significantly greater reductions in diastolic blood pressure from baseline than both nebivolol 40 mg/day and valsartan 320 mg/day; all other comparisons were also significant, favoring the fixed-dose combinations (all $p < 0.0001$). All systolic blood pressure comparisons were also significant (all $p < 0.01$) (Giles et al. 2014).

- At least one treatment-emergent adverse event was experienced by 30–36 % of participants in each group.
- Nebivolol and valsartan fixed-dose combination appears to be an effective and well-tolerated treatment option for patients with hypertension.

But the combination of valsartan and beta-blocker in a heart failure study showed increase in mortality. Among those who were receiving both drugs at baseline, valsartan had an adverse effect on mortality ($p = 0.009$) and was associated with a trend toward an increase in the combined end point of mortality and morbidity (Cohn and Tognoni 2001),

These investigators concluded "the post hoc observation of an adverse effect on mortality and morbidity in the subgroup receiving valsartan, an ACE inhibitor, and a beta-blocker raises concern about the potential safety of this specific combination" (Cohn and Tognoni 2001).

The Author advises a combination of nebivolol and ramipril (if cough use candesartan not diovan).

DYSLIPIDEMIA RCTS

Early and Late Benefits of High-Dose Atorvastatin

PROVE IT-TIMI 22 (2005): In this RCT 4,162 patients [hospitalized for an acute coronary syndrome—either STEMI, NSTEMI or high-risk unstable angina—in the preceding 10 days and with a total cholesterol level of 240 mg/dL (6.21 mmol/L) or less] were randomized to receive atorvastatin 80 mg (intensive statin therapy) or pravastatin 40 mg (standard therapy, moderate lipid lowering). The primary end point was a composite of death from any cause, MI, documented unstable angina requiring rehospitalization, revascularization (performed at least 30 days after randomization), and stroke (Cannon et al. 2004).

The median LDL cholesterol level achieved during treatment was 95 mg/dL (2.46 mmol/L) in the standard-dose pravastatin group and 62 mg/dL (1.60 mmol/L) in the high-dose atorvastatin group ($p < 0.001$). Results: The composite triple end point of death, MI, or rehospitalization for recurrent ACS at 30 days occurred in 3 % of patients receiving atorvastatin 80 mg versus 4.2 % of patients receiving pravastatin 40 mg ($p = 0.046$) (Cannon et al. 2004).

- There were nonsignificant reductions in the rates of death from any cause ($p = 0.07$) and of death or MI (, $p = 0.06$). The risk of the secondary end point of death due to CHD, MI, or revascularization was reduced by 14 % in the atorvastatin group ($p = 0.029$), with a 2-year event rate of 19.7 %, as compared with 22.3 % in the pravastatin group. The risk of death, MI, or urgent revascularization was reduced by 25 % in the atorvastatin group ($p < 0.001$).
  - Benefit appeared to be greater among patients with a baseline LDL-C of at least 125 mg/dl (3.5 mmol/L) a prespecified subgroup, with a 34 % reduction in the hazard ratio, as compared with only a 7 % reduction among patients with a baseline LDL cholesterol below 125 mg/dl (3.5 mmol/L) Cannon et al. (2004).

- The LDL interquartile range for pravastatin and atorvastatin was 87–127 and 89–128 mg/dL, respectively. How many subjects had an LDL level > 124 is not stated. In addition to reducing first events in patients after an ACS, Murphy and colleagues hypothesized that high-dose atorvastatin 80 mg would also reduce recurrent cardiovascular events, and therefore total events, compared with pravastatin 40 mg during a 2-year follow-up. Overall, there were 138 fewer primary efficacy events with atorvastatin 80 mg versus pravastatin 40 mg ($n = 739$ versus $n = 877$, respectively; $p = 0.001$) (Murphy et al. 2009). Based on the primary end point results, the number of patients needed to treat to prevent the first occurrence of the primary end point is 26. When considering total events, however, the needed-to-treat number to prevent 1 event is much lower, at 14 (Murphy et al. 2009).

ASTEROID (2006): high-intensity statins for atheroma regression.

A Study to Evaluate the Effect of Rosuvastatin on Intravascular Ultrasound-Derived Coronary Atheroma Burden (ASTEROID) assessed whether very intensive statin administration could regress coronary atheroma as evaluated by intravascular ultrasound (IVUS) imaging using percent atheroma volume (PAV), the most rigorous IVUS measure of disease progression and regression. A baseline IVUS examination was done on 507 patients who received rosuvastatin 40 mg daily. After 24 months, 349 patients had serial IVUS examinations. Two primary efficacy parameters were prespecified: the change in PAV and the change in nominal atheroma volume in the 10-mm subsegment with the greatest disease severity at baseline. Findings at 24 months were as follows:

The mean (SD) change in PAV for the entire vessel was −0.98 % (3.15 %), with a median of −0.79 % (97.5 % CI, −1.21 to −0.53 %; $p < 0.001$ versus baseline). The mean (SD) change in atheroma volume in the most diseased

10-mm subsegment was −6.1 (10.1) mm^3, with a median of −5.6 mm^3 (97.5 % CI, −6.8 to −4.0 mm^3; $p < 0.001$ versus baseline). Change in total atheroma volume showed a 6.8 % median reduction, with a mean (SD) reduction of −14.7 (25.7) mm^3 and a median of −12.5 mm^3 (95 % CI, −15.1 to −10.5 mm^3; $p < 0.001$ versus baseline). The mean (SD) baseline LDL-C level of 130.4 (34.3) mg/dL was reduced to 60.8 (20.0) mg/dL (53.2 %; $p < 0.001$). The mean (SD) high-density lipoprotein cholesterol (HDL-C) level at baseline was 43.1 (11.1) mg/dL; it increased to 49.0 (12.6) mg/dL (14.7 %; $p < 0.001$) (20). Adverse events were infrequent and similar to those of other statin trials.

Nissen and colleagues concluded that very high-intensity statin therapy with rosuvastatin 40 mg/d achieved an average LDL-C of 60.8 mg/dL and increased HDL-C by 14.7 %. This lipid change caused significant regression of atheroma for all three prespecified IVUS measures of disease burden (ASTEROID 2006). Blumenthal and Kapur (2006), however, stated that the trial has some concerns, including lack of a control group receiving a somewhat less intensive LDL-C-lowering regimen and the absence of paired IVUS measurements in less diseased coronary segments to demonstrate reproducibility of atheroma volume measurements. The study does not provide definitive information regarding the relationship of LDL-C lowering and extent of atheroma regression to determine whether high-intensity treatment is necessary to obtain regression. Nonetheless, it is the first clear evidence that coronary atheroma can regress significantly when LDL-C is markedly lowered.

SATURN trial: Nicholls et al. (2011) performed serial intravascular ultrasonography in 1,039 patients with coronary disease, at baseline and after 104 weeks of treatment with either atorvastatin, 80 mg daily, or rosuvastatin, 40 mg daily, and assessed the effect of these two intensive regimens on the progression of coronary atheroma.

After 104 weeks, the rosuvastatin group had lower levels of LDL cholesterol than the atorvastatin group [62.6 versus 70.2 mg per deciliter (1.62 versus 1.82 mmol/L)], and higher levels of HDL cholesterol [50.4 versus 48.6 mg/dL (1.30 versus 1.26 mmol/L)]. The primary efficacy end point, percent atheroma volume (PAV), decreased by 0.99 % with atorvastatin and by 1.22 % with rosuvastatin ($p = 0.17$). The effect on the secondary efficacy end point, normalized total atheroma volume (TAV), was more favorable with rosuvastatin than with atorvastatin: 6.39 mm^3 (95 % CI, −7.52 to −5.12), as compared with −4.42 mm^3 ($p = 0.01$). Both agents induced regression in the majority of patients: 63.2 % with atorvastatin and 68.5 % with rosuvastatin for PAV ($p = 0.07$) and 64.7 % and 71.3 %, respectively, for TAV ($p = 0.02$) Nicholls et al. (2011).

MRC/BHF Heart Protection Study (2002) Cholesterol Lowering to Reduce Event Risk. The Study indicated that in vascular high-risk patients, 40 mg simvastatin safely reduced the risk of heart attack, of stroke, and of revascularization by at least one-third. Among the 4,000 patients with a total cholesterol < 5 mmol/L (192 mg/dL), a clear reduction in major events was observed.

- All-cause mortality was significantly reduced [1,328 (12.9 %) deaths among 10,269 allocated simvastatin versus 1,507 (14.7 %) among 10,267 allocated placebo; $p = 0.0003$], owing to a highly significant 18 % proportional reduction in the coronary death rate [587 (5.7 %) versus 707 (6.9 %); $p = 0.0005$]. There were highly significant reductions of about one-fourth in the first-event rate for fatal and nonfatal MI [898 (8.7 %) versus 1,212 (11.8 %); $p < 0.0001$], for nonfatal or fatal stroke [444 (4.3 %) versus 585 (5.7 %); $p < 0.0001$], and for coronary or noncoronary revascularization [939 (9.1 %) versus 1,205 (11.7 %); $p < 0.0001$].

PROSPER: Pravastatin in the Elderly. In the Prospective Study of Pravastatin in the Elderly at Risk (PROSPECT 2002), pravastatin 40 mg was administered to 5,804 randomized elderly patients aged 70–82. At the short, 3.5-year follow-up, there was no difference in the number of strokes, but CHD death was reduced by 24 %. There were 245 new cases of cancer in the pravastatin group, versus 199 in the placebo group. Breast and gastrointestinal cancers showed the largest increases.

• New cancer diagnoses were more frequent on pravastatin than on placebo (HR, 1.25; 95 % CI, 1.04–1.51, $p = 0.020$).
• Caution is required because in the CARE study (1996) there were 12 cancers in the pravastatin-treated patients versus 1 in the control group (see Chap. 18, Statin Controversies).

LIPID (1998): Pravastatin for Prevention. This RCT compared the effects of 40 mg pravastatin with those of a placebo in 9,014 patients with past MI, hospitalization for unstable angina, and cholesterol levels of 155–271 mg/dL who were 31–75 years of age. Both groups received advice on following a cholesterol-lowering diet. The primary study outcome was mortality from coronary heart disease. At a mean follow-up of 6.1 year, overall mortality was 14.1 % in the placebo group and 11.0 % in the pravastatin group (relative reduction in risk, 22 %; $p < 0.001$). Death from CHD occurred in 8.3 % of the patients in the placebo group and 6.4 % of those in the pravastatin group, a relative reduction in risk of 24 % (95 % CI, 12–35 %; $p < 0.001$). Importantly, there were no differences in cancer deaths (128 for pravastatin versus 141 for placebo).

NIACIN study: AIM-HIGH Investigators (2011) assigned 3,414 patients to receive extended-release niacin (1,718), 1,500–2,000 mg per day, or matching placebo (1,696). All patients received simvastatin, 40–80 mg per day, plus ezetimibe, 10 mg per day, if needed, to maintain an LDL cholesterol level of 40–80 mg per deciliter (1.03–2.07 mmol/L). The primary end point was the first event of the composite of death from coronary heart disease, nonfatal MI, ischemic stroke, hospitalization for ACS, or revascularization.

- **The trial was stopped after a mean follow-up period of 3 years owing to a lack of efficacy. There was a small excess of ischemic strokes in the niacin group**.

At 2 years, niacin therapy had significantly increased the median HDL cholesterol level from 35 mg per deciliter (0.91 mmol/L) to 42 mg/dL (1.08 mmol/L), lowered the triglyceride level from 164 mg/dL (1.85 mmol/L) to 122 mg/dL (1.38 mmol/L), and lowered the LDL cholesterol level from 74 mg/dL (1.91 mmol/L) to 62 mg/dL (1.60 mmol/L). The primary end point occurred in 282 patients in the niacin group (16.4 %) and in 274 patients in the placebo group (16.2 %) $p = 0.79$.

Conclusion: Among patients with cardiovascular disease and LDL cholesterol levels of less than 70 mg per deciliter (1.81 mmol/L), there was no clinical benefit from the addition of niacin to statin therapy during a 36-month follow-up period, despite significant improvements in HDL cholesterol and triglyceride levels. Rhabdomyolysis occurred in one patient in the placebo group and four in the niacin group. The disappointing results of AIM-HIGH do not provide support for the use of niacin as an add-on therapy to statins in patients with preexisting stable cardiovascular disease who have well-controlled LDL cholesterol levels. Given the lack of efficacy, the frequent occurrence of flushing that some patients find intolerable, and the increased risk of ischemic stroke, one can hardly justify the continued expenditure of nearly $800 million per year in the United States for branded extended-release niacin (Giugliano 2011). Importantly, the drug should not be combined with statins. Niacin use is not justifiable; see Chap. 17.

ARRHYTHMIA RCTS

AFFIRM (2002): Rate Versus Rhythm Control in Atrial Fibrillation

The Atrial Fibrillation Follow-up Investigation of Rhythm Management (AFFIRM) was a well-run rate versus rhythm control RCT with 2–5 years of follow-up.

Conclusions: Rate control is an acceptable primary therapy. In the rate control arm, 51 % received digoxin and 49 % a beta-blocker. At 2 years of follow-up, the perceived benefit of restoring and maintaining sinus rhythm did not alter mortality. Patients in the rhythm control arm still required warfarin (70 %); mortality, stroke rate, and hospitalizations were slightly increased, and bradycardiac arrest and torsades de pointes were of concern. Amiodarone was used in approx. 39 %, sotalol in approx. 33 %, and propafenone in approx. 10 % to maintain rhythm control, which required frequent changes in drug and dosing schedule. An RCT conducted in The Netherlands in patients with persistent atrial fibrillation <1 year randomly assigned to electrical conversion and rhythm control versus rate control indicated that rate control was not inferior to rhythm control. Nonfatal end points were slighter greater in the rhythm control group; cardiovascular mortality was the same in both groups.

BETA-BLOCKERS AND DIABETES

GEMINI (2004): Beta-Blockers for Hypertensive Diabetics

The Glycemic Effects in Diabetes Mellitus: Carvedilol-Metoprolol Comparison in Hypertensives trial addressed concerns regarding the increased incidence of type 2 diabetes caused by beta-blockers. Carvedilol is a unique beta-blocker with properties that are subtly different from other beta-blockers. This randomized, double-blind, parallel-group trial compared the effects of carvedilol and metoprolol tartrate on glycemic control in the context of cardiovascular (CDV) risk factors in 1,235 individuals with hypertension and type 2 diabetes mellitus [glycosylated hemoglobin (HbA1c), 6.5–8.5 %] who were receiving ACE inhibitors or ARBs. Patients were randomized to receive a 6.25–25-mg dose of carvedilol or 50–200-mg dose of metoprolol tartrate each twice daily.

- At 35 weeks of follow-up, the mean (SD) HbA1c increased with metoprolol [0.15 % (0.04 %); $p < 0.001$] but not carvedilol [0.02 % (0.04 %); $p = 0.65$].
- Insulin sensitivity improved with carvedilol (−9.1 %; $p = 0.004$) but not metoprolol (−2.0 %; $p = 0.48$).
- Carvedilol treatment had no effect on HbA1c [mean (SD) change from baseline to end point [0.02 % (0.04 %); 95 % CI, −0.06–0.10 %; $p = 0.65$], whereas metoprolol increased HbA1c [0.15 % (0.04 %); 95 % CI, 0.08–0.22 %; $p < 0.001$].
- Blood pressure was similar between groups.
- Metoprolol increased triglycerides (13 %, $p < 0.001$), whereas carvedilol had no effect. Significant weight gain was observed in the metoprolol group 1.2 kg for metoprolol, $p < 0.001$ versus 0.2 kg for carvedilol, $p = 0.36$].

CLOPIDOGREL

PCI-Clarity: Clopidogrel Before PCI

PCI-Clopidogrel as Adjunctive Reperfusion Therapy (PCI-CLARITY) (29) was an RCT of the 1,863 patients undergoing PCI after mandated angiography in CLARITY-TIMI, an RCT of clopidogrel. All patients received aspirin and were randomized to receive either clopidogrel (300 mg loading dose and then 75 mg once daily) or placebo initiated with thrombolytics and given until coronary angiography was performed 2–8 days after initiation of the study drug. For patients undergoing coronary artery stenting, it was recommended that open-label clopidogrel (including a loading dose) be administered after the diagnostic angiogram. The primary outcome was the incidence of the composite of CVD death, recurrent MI, or stroke from PCI to 30 days after randomization.

- Pretreatment with clopidogrel significantly reduced the incidence of CVD death, MI, or stroke following PCI [34 (3.6 %) versus 58 (6.2 %); adjusted OR, 0.54; $p = 0.008$]. Pretreatment with clopidogrel also reduced the incidence of MI or stroke prior to PCI [37 (4.0 %) versus 58 (6.2 %); OR, 0.62; $p = 0.03$]. Overall, pretreatment with clopidogrel resulted in a highly significant reduction in cardiovascular death, MI, or stroke from randomization through 30 days [70 (7.5 %) versus 112 (12.0 %); adjusted OR, 0.59; $p = 0.001$; number needed to treat = 23]. There was no significant excess in the rates of bleeding (29).

Clopidogrel caused a significant reduction in death, reinfarction, or stroke (9.2 % versus 10.1 %; relative risk reduction, 9 %; $p = 0.002$). Clopidogrel was equally effective with or without thrombolytic therapy.

FOLIC ACID/B6, B12

HOPE-2: Homocysteine Lowering

The Heart Outcomes Prevention Evaluation (HOPE) study (2006) randomly assigned 5,522 patients 55 years of age or older who had vascular disease or diabetes to treatment either with the combination of 2.5 mg of folic acid, 50 mg of vitamin B6, and 1 mg of vitamin B12 or with placebo. At 5-year follow-up, this therapy did not reduce the risk of major CVD events in patients with vascular disease.

Mean plasma homocysteine levels decreased by 2.4 μmol/L (0.3 mg/L) in the active-treatment group and increased by 0.8 μmol/L (0.1 mg/L) in the placebo group. Primary outcome events occurred in 519 patients (18.8 %) assigned to active therapy and 547 (19.8 %) assigned to placebo (RR, 0.95; 95 % CI, 0.84–1.07; $p = 0.41$). **This extensive, well-run RCT should convince clinicians and the public that lowering homocysteine levels does not decrease risk for CVD**.

REFERENCES

ACE Inhibitor Myocardial Infarction Collaborative Group. Indications for ACE inhibitors in the early treatment of acute myocardial infarction. Systematic overview of individual data from 100,000 patients in randomized trials. Circulation. 1998;97:2202–12.

AFIRM: The Atrial Fibrillation Follow-up Investigation of Rhythm Management Investigators. A comparison of rate control and rhythm control in patients with atrial fibrillation. N Engl J Med. 2002;347:1825.

A-HeFT, Taylor AL, Ziesche S, Yancy C, et al. Combination of isosorbide dinitrate and hydralazine in blacks with heart failure. N Engl J Med. 2004;351:2049–57.

AIM-HIGH Investigators. Niacin in patients with low HDL cholesterol levels receiving intensive statin therapy. N Engl J Med. 2011; 365:2255–67.

Antman EM, Califf RM, Kupersmith J. Tools for assessment of cardiovascular tests and therapies. In: Antman EM, editor. Cardiovascular therapeutics. 2nd ed. Philadelphia, PA: WB Saunders; 2002. p. 1–19.

Antman EM, Morrow DA, McCabe CH, et al. with fibrinolysis for ST-elevation myocardial infarction for the ExTRACT-TIMI 25 Investigators. N Engl J Med. 2006; 354:1477–88.

ARISTOTLE, Granger CB, Alexander JH, McMurray JJV, et al. Apixaban versus warfarin in patients with atrial fibrillation. N Engl J Med. 2011;365:981–92.

ASTEROID, Nissen SE, Nicholls SJ, Sipahi I, et al. Effect of very high-intensity statin therapy on regression of coronary atherosclerosis: the ASTEROID trial. JAMA. 2006;295:1556–65.

Bach DS. Angiotensin-converting enzyme inhibitor therapy at the time of coronary artery bypass surgery when a friend turns meanspirited. J Am Coll Cardiol. 2009;54(19):1785–6.

Björkman J-A, Kirk I, van Giezen JJ. AZD6140 inhibits adenosine uptake into erythrocytes and enhances coronary blood flow after local ischemia or intracoronary adenosine infusion. Circulation 2007;116 Suppl II: II–28, (abstr).

Blumenthal RS, Kapur NK. Can a potent statin actually regress coronary atherosclerosis? JAMA. 2006;295:1583–4.

Califf RM. Fondaparinux in ST-segment elevation myocardial infarction. The drug, the strategy, the environment, or all of the above? JAMA. 2006;295:1579–80.

Cannon CP, Braunwald E, McCabe CH, et al. Intensive versus moderate lipid lowering with statins after acute coronary syndromes. N Engl J Med. 2004;350:1495–504.

CAPRICORN Investigators. Effect of carvedilol on outcome after MI in patients with left ventricular dysfunction; the CAPRICORN randomized trial. Lancet 2001;357:1385–90.

CARE: For the Cholesterol and Recurrent Events Trial Investigators. The effect of pravastatin on coronary events after myocardial infarction in patients with average cholesterol levels. N Engl J Med. 1996;335:1001.

COMMIT (Cl Opidogrel and Metoprolol in Myocardial Infarction Trial) Collaborative Group. Addition of clopidogrel to aspirin in 45,852 patients with acute myocardial infarction: randomised placebo-controlled trial. Lancet. 2005;366:1607–21.

COMMIT/CCS-2 (Clopidogrel and Metoprolol in Myocardial Infarction Trial) Collaborative Group. Early intravenous then oral metoprolol in 45,852 patients with acute myocardial infarction: Randomised placebo-controlled trial. Lancet 2005;366:1622–32.

Connolly SJ, Ezekowitz MD, Yusuf S, et al. Dabigatran versus warfarin in patients with atrial fibrillation. N Engl J Med. 2009;361: 1139–51,(Erratum, N Engl J Med 2010;363:1877).

COPERNICUS: Carvedilol Prospective Randomized Cumulative Survival Study Group. Effect of carvedilol on survival in severe chronic heart failure. N Engl J Med. 2001;344:1651–8.

COURAGE trial, Boden WE, O'Rourke RA, Teo KK, et al. Optimal medical therapy with or without PCI for stable coronary disease. N Engl J Med. 2007;356:1503–16.

EPHESUS: Pitt B, Remme W, Zannad F, et al. for the Eplerenone Post-Acute Myocardial Infarction Heart Failure Efficacy and Survival Study Investigators. Eplerenone, a selective aldosterone blocker, in patients with left ventricular dysfunction after myocardial infarction. N Engl J Med. 2003;348:1309–21.

EUROPA: The European Trial on Reduction of Cardiac Events with Perindopril in Stable Coronary Artery Disease Investigators. Efficacy of perindopril in reduction of cardiovascular events among patients with stable coronary artery disease: randomized, double-blind, placebo-controlled, multicenter trial. Lancet. 2003;362:782–88.

Fox KAA, Clayton TC, Damman P, et al. for the FIR Collaboration. Long-term outcome of a routine versus selective invasive strategy in patients with non-ST-segment elevation acute coronary syndrome. A meta-analysis of individual patient data. J Am Coll Cardiol. 2010;55: 2435–45.

GEMINI, Bakris GL, Fonseca V, Katholi RE, et al. Metabolic effects of carvedilol vs metoprolol in patients with type 2 diabetes mellitus and hypertension: a randomized controlled trial. JAMA. 2004;292: 2227–36.

Giles TD, Weber MA, Basile J, et al. for the NAC-MD-01 Study Investigators. Efficacy and safety of nebivolol and valsartan as fixed-dose combination in hypertension: a randomised multicentre study. Lancet 2014;383:1889–98.

Giugliano RP. Niacin at 56 years of age — time for an early retirement? N Engl J Med. 2011;365:2318–20.

Grosser T, Fries S, Lawson JA, et al. Drug resistance and pseudoresistance an unintended consequence of enteric coating aspirin. Circulation. 2013;127:377–85.

Gurbel PA, Bliden KP, Butler K, et al. Randomized double-blind assessment of the ONSET and OFFSET of the antiplatelet effects of ticagrelor versus clopidogrel in patients with stable coronary artery disease: the ONSET/OFFSET study. Circulation. 2009;120: 2577–85.

Guyatt GH, Sackett DL, Cook DJ. The medical literature: users' guide to the medical literature: II. How to use an article about therapy or prevention. B. What were the results and will they help me in caring for my patients? JAMA. 1994;271:59–63.

Halverson S, Andreotti F, ten Berg HM, et al. Aspirin therapy in primary cardiovascular disease prevention: a position paper of the European Society of Cardiology Working Group on Thrombosis. J Am Coll Cardiol. 2014;64(3):319–27.

Heart Protection Study Collaborative Group. MRC/BHF heart protection study of cholesterol lowering with simvastatin in 20,536 high-risk individuals: a randomised placebo-controlled trial. Lancet. 2002; 360:7–22.

HOPE 2: The Heart Outcomes Prevention Evaluation (HOPE) 2 Investigators. Homocysteine lowering with folic acid and B vitamins in vascular disease. N Engl J Med. 2006;354:1567–77.

HOPE: Heart Outcomes Prevention Evaluation Study Investigators. Effects of an angiotensin-converting enzyme inhibitor, ramipril, on cardiovascular events in high risk patients. N Engl J Med. 2000; 342:145–53.

HORIZONS-AMI: Stone GW, Witzenbichler B, Guagliumi G, et al. Heparin plus a glycoprotein IIb/IIIa inhibitor versus bivalirudin monotherapy and paclitaxel-eluting stents versus bare-metal stents in acute myocardial infarction: final 3-year results from a multicentre, randomised controlled trial. Lancet. 2011;377(9784):2193–204.

Imazio M, Brucato A, Ferrazzi P, et al. Colchicine reduces postoperative atrial fibrillation: results of the colchicine for the prevention of the postpericardiotomy syndrome (COPPS) atrial fibrillation substudy. Circulation. 2011;124(21):2290–5.

Imazio M, Belli R, Brucato A. Efficacy and safety of colchicine for treatment of multiple recurrences of pericarditis (CORP-2): a multicentre, double-blind, placebo-controlled, randomised trial. Lancet. 2014; 383(9936):2232–7.

Kastrati A, Neumann F-J, Schulz S, et al. for the ISAR-REACT 4 Trial Investigators. Abciximab and heparin versus bivalirudin for non-ST-elevation myocardial infarction. N Engl J Med. 2011; 365:1980–89.

Khan MG. Hallmark clinical trials. In: Cardiac drug therapy 7e. New York: Springer; 2007. p. 391.

Lindholm D, Varenhorst C, Cannon C. Ticagrelor versus clopidogrel in patients with non-ST-elevation acute coronary syndrome: results from the PLATO trial. Am Coll Cardiol. 2013;61(10 S).

LIPID Study Group. Prevention of cardiovascular events and death with pravastatin in patients with coronary heart disease and a broad range of initial cholesterol levels. N Engl J Med. 1998;339:1349–57.

Maffei A, Lembo G. Nitric oxide mechanisms of nebivolol. Ther Adv Cardiovasc Dis. 2009;3(4):317–27.

Mega JL. A new era for anticoagulation in atrial fibrillation. N Engl J Med. 2011;365:1052–4.

Mega JL, Braunwald E, Wiviott SD, et al. Rivaroxaban in patients with a recent acute coronary syndrome. N Engl J Med. 2012;366:9–19.

MERIT-HF Study Group. The metoprolol CR/XL randomized intervention trial in CHF. Effects of controlled-release metoprolol on total mortality, hospitalizations and well-being in patients with heart failure. JAMA. 2000;283:1295–302.

Miceli A, Capoun R, Fino C, et al. Effects of angiotensinconverting enzyme inhibitor therapy on clinical outcome in patients undergoing coronary artery bypass grafting. J Am Coll Cardiol. 2009;54:177–84.

Montalescot G, Zeymerc U, Silvain J, et al. for the ATOLL Investigators. Intravenous enoxaparin or unfractionated heparin in primary percutaneous coronary intervention for ST-elevation myocardial infarction: the international randomised open-label ATOLL trial. Lancet 2011; 378(9792):693–703

Murphy SA, Cannon CP, Wiviott SD, et al. Reduction in recurrent cardiovascular events with intensive lipid-lowering statin therapy compared with moderate lipid-lowering statin therapy after acute coronary syndromes: from the PROVE IT–TIMI 22 (Pravastatin or Atorvastatin Evaluation and Infection Therapy – Thrombolysis in Myocardial Infarction 22) trial. J Am Coll Cardiol. 2009;54:2358–62.

Nicholls SJ, Ballantyne CM, Barter PJ, et al. Effect of two intensive statin regimens on progression of coronary disease. N Engl J Med. 2011; 365:2078–87.

Nidorf SM, Eikelboom JW, Budgeon CA, et al. Low-dose colchicine for secondary prevention of cardiovascular disease. J Am Coll Cardiol. 2013;61(4):404–10.

Nissen SE (2010) Angiotensin-receptor blockers and cancer: urgent regulatory review needed. Lancet Oncol. doi:10.1016/S1470-2045(10)70142-XCite, Early Online Publication

OASIS-6 Trial Investigators. Effects of fondaparinux on mortality and reinfarction in patients with acute ST-segment elevation myocardial infarction. The OASIS-6 randomized trial. JAMA 2006;295: 1519–1530.

O'Rourke RA. Optimal medical therapy is a proven option for chronic stable angina. J Am Coll Cardiol. 2008b;52:905–7.

ONTARGET Investigators. Telmisartan, ramipril, or both in patients at high risk for vascular events. N Engl J Med. 2008;358:1547–59.

Pizarro G, Fernandez-Friera L, Fuster V. Long-term benefit of early pre-reperfusion metoprolol administration in patients with acute MI: results from the METOCARD-CNTC trial (effect of metoprolol in cardioprotection during an acute myocardial infarction). J Am Coll Cardiol. 2014;63(22):2356–62.

PLATO: Cannon CP, Harrington RA, James S, et al. for the PLATelet inhibition and patient Outcomes investigators. Comparison of ticagrelor with clopidogrel in patients with a planned invasive strategy for acute coronary syndromes: a randomised double-blind study. Lancet 2010;375(9711):283–93.

PRoFESS :Yusuf S, Diener H-C, Sacco RL et al Telmisartan to preventre-current stroke and cardiovascular events. N Eng J Med 2008 359(12):1225–1237.

PROSPECT :Shepherd J, Blauw GJ, Murphy MB, et al. Pravastatin in elderly individuals at risk of vascular disease: A randomised controlled trial. Lancet 2002;360:1623–1630.

PROVE IT-TIMI 22: Ray KK, Cannon CP, McCabe CH, et al. for the PROVE IT-TIMI 22 Investigators. Early and late benefits of high-dose atorvastatin in patients with acute coronary syndromes: Results from the PROVE IT-TIMI 22 trial. J Am Coll Cardiol 2005;46: 1405–1410.

RALES: The Randomized Aldactone Evaluation Study Investigators. The effect of spironolactone on morbidity and mortality in patients with severe heart failure. N Engl J Med 1999;341:709–717.

ROCKET: Patel MR, Mahaffey KW, Garg J, et al. Rivaroxaban versus warfarin in nonvalvular atrial fibrillation. N Engl J Med 2011; 365:883–891.

SENIORS: Flather MD, Shibata MC, Coats AJ, et al. Randomized trial to determine the effect of nebivolol on mortality and cardiovascular hospital admission in elderly patients with heart failure. Eur Heart J. 2005;26:215–25.

SENIORS Investigators, van Veldhuisen DJ, Cohen-Solal A, Bohm M, et al. Beta-blockade with nebivolol in elderly heart failure patients with impaired and preserved left ventricular ejection fraction: data from SENIORS (study of effects of nebivolol intervention on outcomes and rehospitalization in seniors with heart failure). J Am Coll Cardiol. 2009;53:2150–58.

Sipahi I, Debanne SM, Rowland DY (2010) Angiotensin-receptor blockade and risk of cancer: meta-analysis of randomised controlled trials. Lancet Oncol. doi:10.1016/S1470-2045(10)70106-6, Early Online Publication.

Stone GW. Ticagrelor in ACS: redefining a new standard of care? Lancet 2010;375(9711):263–5.

Stone GW, McLaurin BT, Cox DA, et al. for the ACUITY Investigators. Bivalirudin for patients with acute coronary syndromes. N Engl J Med 2006;355:2203–16.

The ALLHAT Officers and Coordinators for the ALLHAT Collaborative Research Group. Major outcomes in high-risk hypertensive patients randomized to angiotensin-converting enzyme inhibitor or calcium channel blocker vs diuretic. The Antihypertensive and Lipid-Lowering Treatment to Prevent Heart Attack Trial (ALLHAT). JAMA 2002;288:2981–2997.

TIMACS: Mehta SR, Granger CB, Boden WE et al. for the TIMACS Investigators (2009) Early versus delayed invasive intervention in acute coronary syndromes. N Engl J Med 360:2165–2175

TRANSCEND: Yusuf S, Teo K, Anderson C et al for the Effects of the angiotensin-receptor blocker telmisartan on cardiovascular events in high-risk patients intolerant to angiotensin-converting enzyme inhibitors: a randomised controlled trial. Lancet 2008, 372:1174–1183.

Tuncer M, Fettser DV, Gunes Y, et al. Comparison of effects of nebivolol and atenolol on P-wave dispersion in patients with hypertension. Kardiologiia. 2008;48:42–5 (in Russian).

Val-HeFT, Cohn JN, Tognoni G. A randomized trial of the angiotensin-receptor blocker valsartan in chronic heart failure. N Engl J Med. 2001;345:1667–75.

Van Gelder IC, Groenveld HF, Crijns HJGM et al. For the RACE II Investigators (2010) Lenient versus strict rate control in patients with atrial fibrillation. N Engl J Med 362:1363–73

Wallentin L, Varenhorst C, James S, et al. Prasugrel achieves greater and faster P2Y12 receptor-mediated platelet inhibition than clopidogrel due to more efficient generation of its active metabolite in aspirin-treated patients with coronary artery disease. Eur Heart J. 2008; 29:21–30.

Weinsaft JW. Effect of ramipril on cardiovascular events in high risk patients. N Engl J Med. 2000;343:64–6.

23 Management of Cardiomyopathies

An appropriate classification of cardiomyopathies is as follows:

1. Hypertrophic cardiomyopathy
2. Dilated cardiomyopathy
3. Restrictive cardiomyopathy
4. Arrhythmogenic right ventricular cardiomyopathy (right ventricular dysplasia)
5. Unclassified cardiomyopathy: diseases that do not have features of 1 through 4 and include fibroelastosis and mitochondrial disease
6. Specific cardiomyopathies (specific heart muscle diseases formerly called secondary cardiomyopathy)

HYPERTROPHIC CARDIOMYOPATHY

Hypertrophic cardiomyopathy (HCM) is now recognized as a genetic disorder caused by more than 1,400 mutations in 11 or more genes encoding proteins of the cardiac sarcomere (Maron and Maron 2013). HCM is often inherited in an autosomal dominant pattern, but there are many patients without any relatives who are known to have the disease (Fifer and Vlahakes 2008).

- HCM is the most common genetic cardiovascular disease. In the majority of patients the disease runs a benign course, but is the most common cause of sudden cardiac death in young individuals including athletes.

© Springer Science+Business Media New York 2015
M. Gabriel Khan, *Cardiac Drug Therapy*, Contemporary Cardiology,
DOI 10.1007/978-1-61779-962-4_23

Maron et al. (1986) indicate that HCM may cause sudden death in individuals of all ages. But sudden death occurs in asymptomatic or mildly symptomatic patients (Maron 2010).

Sudden death results primarily from ventricular arrhythmias that, in turn, are likely related to an abnormal substrate of disorganized muscle cell structure and a multitude of possible inciting events, such as ischemia, abnormal autonomic milieu, atrial arrhythmias, or bradycardia. These devastating events occur infrequently, but pose a management dilemma for clinicians (Nishimura and Ommen 2007). Approximately 70 % of patients have outflow obstruction at rest or with exercise; about 33 % will have the non-obstructive form without capacity to generate significant outflow gradients (Maron et al. 2006).

"In children with hypertrophic cardiomyopathy, the risk of death or heart transplantation was greatest for those who presented as infants or with inborn errors of metabolism or with mixed hypertrophic and dilated or restrictive cardiomyopathy" (Lipshultz et al. 2013).

Pathophysiology

Most patients show asymmetric hypertrophy of the septum and a hypertrophied non-dilated left and or right ventricle. The septum may be diffusely hypertrophied or only in its upper, mid, or apical portion. Hypertrophy extends to the free wall of the left ventricle. There is decreased compliance and incomplete relaxation of the thickened and stiff left ventricular muscle that causes impedance to filling of the ventricles during diastole (diastolic dysfunction). The rapid powerful contraction of hypertrophied left ventricle expels most of its contents during the first half of systole. This hyperdynamic systolic function is apparent in most patients with HCM.

The anterior leaflet of the mitral valve is displaced toward the hypertrophied septum. Mitral regurgitation is virtually always present in the obstructive phase of the disease. The sequence of events is eject, obstruct, and leak. A variable LV outflow pressure gradient at rest occurs in approximately 35 % of patients. A further 25 % develop a similar gradient precipitated by conditions that increase myocardial contractility or decrease ventricular volume. Thus, diuretics and other causes of hypovolemia and preload-reducing agents that reduce the volume of the small ventricular cavity may worsen outflow tract obstruction.

Clinical Diagnosis

The palpable left atrial beat preceding the LV thrust is a most important sign because it can occur in the absence of gradient or murmur.

- A murmur is heard and has typical characteristics, but the entire examination may reveal little or no abnormalities depending on the stage of the disease.

The murmur has typical features:

- Crescendo–decrescendo starts well after the first heart sound (S1) and ends well before the second heart sound (S2). It is best heard between the apex and left sternal border.
- Radiates poorly to the neck, if at all.
- Intensity increases with maneuvers or drugs that decrease preload (Valsalva, standing, amyl nitrite) and decreases in intensity with an increase in afterload (squatting, hand grip, phenylephrine).
- Easy to distinguish from aortic valvular stenosis, in which the murmur starts soon after the S1 and radiates well to the neck.
- A mitral regurgitant murmur is often heard in the last half of systole with radiation to the axilla. It is usually associated with an outflow tract gradient.

Diagnosis of HCM requires the finding of a hypertrophied non-dilated left ventricle without evidence of any other cardiac or systemic disease (e.g., systemic hypertension) that could produce the extent of hypertrophy observed (Maron et al. 2003).

ELECTROCARDIOGRAPHIC FINDINGS

The ECG is abnormal in >90 % of patients with significant symptomatic HCM and about ~85 % abnormal in asymptomatic patients.

McLeod et al. (2009) in a study concluded: almost 6 % of patients presenting with demonstrable echocardiographic evidence of HCM had a normal ECG at the time of diagnosis. This subset of **patients with normal ECG-HCM appears to exhibit a less severe phenotype with better cardiovascular outcomes.** None of these patients had a cardiac death at follow-up.

The ECG may be abnormal when the echocardiogram shows no significant abnormality.

ECG findings include:

- Deep narrow Q waves in about 30 % of subjects in leads II, III, aVF, V5, and V6, or in I, aVL, V5, and V6, and rarely V1 through V3, which at times reflect septal hypertrophy and may mimic myocardial infarction
- Intraventricular conduction delay in over 80 %.
- High QRS voltage LV hypertrophy (LVH).
    - Left atrial abnormality indicating enlargement and/or hypertrophy.

- Diffuse T-wave changes in some patients or T waves of LVH.
- Giant inverted T waves, very high precordial QRS voltage with apical HCM
    - There can be marked ST-segment elevation in V2–V4 with prominent negative waves in V2–V4 as shown in Fig. 23-1.

- ST-segment depression in some.
- PR interval occasionally short; preexcitation may be seen.

    - Over time atrial fibrillation occurs in ~20 %

- The ECG is a good screening test because <7 % of individuals with HCM are expected to have a normal electrocardiogram, and these patients probably are at low risk. Sensitivity and specificity are equal to that of echocardiography.

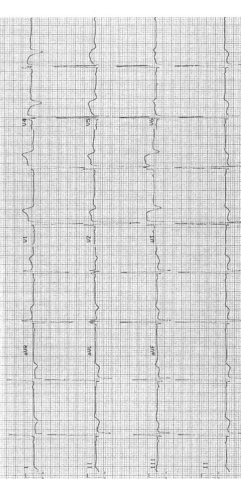

Fig. 23-1. Hypertrophic cardiomyopathy. ECG shows voltage criteria for LVH. There is marked ST-segment elevation V2–V4 with prominent negative waves in V2–V4; Q waves in leads II–III, aVF, V5, and V6 in keeping with septal hypertrophy. From an asymptomatic 20 year old, played soccer, rugby, and hockey from age 15–20. Routine physical revealed a grade II systolic murmur. Echocardiogram showed marked asymmetric septal hypertrophy, septal thickness 36 mm (normal less than 11 mm). No dynamic outflow obstruction at rest. At age 22, one episode of presyncope and one episode of syncope after exercise; ICD implanted. Reproduced with permission from Khan MG, *Encyclopedia of Heart Diseases*, 2nd edition. New York: Springer Science + Business Media; 2011. With kind permission from Springer Science + Business Media.

ECHOCARDIOGRAPHY

Two-dimensional echocardiographic observation of a LV myocardial segment of 1.5 cm or more in a normal-sized adult is considered diagnostic if there is no other evident cause. Continuous-wave Doppler echocardiography defines the degree of LV outflow-tract gradient. Asymmetric septal hypertrophy involving most of the septum is the most common variant form of hypertrophy; see Fig. 23-2.

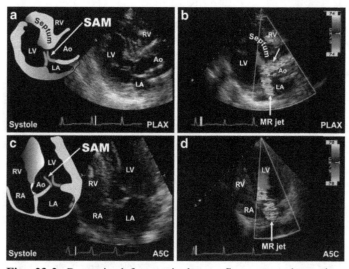

Fig. 23-2. Dynamic left ventricular outflow tract obstruction. Dynamic left ventricular outflow tract obstruction with systolic anterior motion of the mitral valve leaflets (SAM) are shown in this parasternal long-axis (PLAX) view (**a**). Suboptimal mitral leaflet coaptation accompanies SAM and is typically accompanied by a posteriorly directed mitral regurgitant jet. Note the turbulence created within the left ventricular outflow tract (*arrow*, **b**). Apical five-chamber (A5C) views of the same features above are shown (**c, d**). Reproduced with permission from Bulwer BE, Solomon SD: Cardiomyopathies. In: Solomon SD, Bulwer BE, editors. *Essential Echocardiography: A Practical Handbook.* Totowa, NJ: Humana Press, 2007; p. 175. With kind permission from Springer Science + Business Media.

Therapy

Management necessitates the accomplishment of the following:

1. Activity restriction with avoidance of volume depletion.
2. Control of symptoms.
3. Prevention of sudden death.
4. Screening of relatives.
5. Symptomatic relief (unrelated to protection from sudden death) can often be accomplished by pharmacologic therapy designed to: Block the effects of catecholamines and diminish myocardial contractility that exacerbate outflow tract obstruction. Slowing of the heart rate to 50–60 beats per minute (BPM) to enhance diastolic filling. Administration of an appropriate beta-blocking drug (timolol, carvedilol, or nebivolol, propranolol in nonsmokers) and in carefully selected cases, the calcium antagonist, verapamil.

Some patients with obstructive HCM may benefit from disopyramide, which shares a negative inotropic action with beta-blockers and verapamil, and because of its atrial antiarrhythmic properties, disopyramide may be of particular benefit in patients with atrial fibrillation.

Patients must be instructed to avoid strenuous competitive exercise because it can cause sudden death. A decrease in ventricular volume or increase in ventricular contractility increases the outflow gradient.

- **Dehydration and the use of preload-reducing agents, such as diuretics, nitrates, or angiotensin converting enzyme (ACE) inhibitors, should be avoided. Beta-agonists increase contractility and are contraindicated.**

Digoxin increases contractility and its use should be avoided, except in the management of chronic atrial fibrillation, a fast ventricular response uncontrolled by amiodarone, beta-blockers, or verapamil.

An algorithm for the management of symptomatic HCM in the absence of high risk advises the following (Fifer and Vlahakes 2008):

- Commence a beta-blocking drug (experience mainly with propranolol).
- If there is a contraindication to a beta-blocker or adverse effects, verapamil can be tried. Caution: watch for bradycardia, sinus arrest, AV block, hypotension, and heart failure.
- In the presence of significant LV outflow tract gradient and persistent symptoms, add disopyramide with caution or consider mechanical therapy.
- Refractory symptoms despite above treatment consider mechanical therapy:
  - Septal myectomy or ablation—(Fifer and Vlahakes 2008)

Beta-Adrenergic Blocking Agents

A study with propranolol was done in 22 patients with HOCM. Average propranolol dosage was 462 mg/day. Mean follow-up was 5 years. Dyspnea, angina, palpitations, dizziness, and syncope all improved (by 58–100 %) on propranolol (Frank et al. 1978).

Beneficial effects of beta-blocking agents include the following:

- Decrease in myocardial contractility causes a decrease in "venturi" effect and therefore less obstruction.
- Relief of dyspnea in about 40 % of patients.
- Significant relief of angina in 33–66 % of patients.
- The heart rate should be maintained between 52 and 60 BPM; this results in an improvement in ventricular filling during prolonged diastole; also increased coronary filling occurs because of prolongation of the diastolic interval and relaxation of the ventricular muscle.
- Improvement in diastolic dysfunction.
- Partial control of supraventricular and ventricular arrhythmias.

The therapeutic activity of beta-blockers, particularly propranolol, metabolized in the liver, and calcium antagonists are blunted by cigarette smoking. It is important for patients with HCM to desist smoking because of other adverse effects, as well as the decrease in effectiveness of the two major pharmacologic interventions.

- Only lipophilic beta-blocking agents have been shown to prevent sudden cardiac death (timolol in smokers and non-smokers, propranolol in nonsmokers). These agents are advisable.
- Atenolol is hydrophilic, poorly effective, and should not be used. Sufficient attention has not been paid by the medical profession and researchers, regarding the subtle differences that exist amongst the available beta-blocking drugs (Khan 2005).
- Nebivolol reduces P-wave dispersion on the electrocardiogram, which might attenuate the risk of atrial fibrillation (Tuncer et al. 2008).

Propranolol: Supplied as 20-, 40-, 80-, and 120-mg tablets (Inderal LA): 80, 120, and 160 mg. A dosage of 10 mg three times daily is given and increased slowly to 120–240 mg daily. A slow buildup of the dosage to 320 mg may be required. Propranolol is not effective in smokers.

CALCIUM ANTAGONISTS

Considerable experience with verapamil is now available, but the initial high expectations have not materialized, and the drug has caused deaths. Verapamil decreases dyspnea and increases exercise capacity in some patients but does not improve survival and has precipitated life-threatening pulmonary edema in a significant number of patients; these vasodilators can unpredictably increase the obstruction with resultant pulmonary edema, cardiogenic shock, and death. It is contraindicated in patients with severe obstruction or end-stage disease associated with ventricular dilation and HF. Verapamil: a dosage of 40 mg three times daily or 80 mg twice daily is used and increases slowly over weeks to 240–360 mg daily under close observation.

Implantable Cardioverter-Defibrillators

Implantable cardioverter-defibrillators (ICDs) are an effective therapy to prevent sudden death in patients with HCM. The decision to recommend an ICD is by no means a simple task and raises concerns regarding overtreatment because many individuals run a benign course.

ICD-related complications include infection in about 5 %, lead fractures, and fatal device malfunction. Also, there is a risk of severe tricuspid regurgitation after device implantation. Patients with two or more risk factors likely present a high-enough risk to warrant implantation of an ICD (Nishimura and Ommen 2007).

Maron provided an extensive review relating insights and strategies for risk stratification and prevention of sudden death in hypertrophic cardiomyopathy (Maron 2010).

> "The risk-factor algorithm used in hypertrophic cardiomyopathy is incomplete, as shown by infrequent sudden deaths in patients judged clinically not to be at high risk. A subgroup of patients with genetic mutations but without left-ventricular hypertrophy has emerged, with unresolved natural history. Now, after more than 50 years, hypertrophic cardiomyopathy has been transformed from a rare and largely untreatable disorder to a common genetic disease with management strategies that permit realistic aspirations for restored quality of life and advanced longevity" (Maron and Maron 2013).

Risk Factors for Sudden Death and Guide for ICD Include

Secondary prevention: Cardiac arrest or sustained ventricular tachycardia (there is no dispute here).

Conventional primary prevention risk markers: Family history of sudden death due to HCM; unexplained recent syncope; multiple repetitive non-sustained VT; hypotensive or attenuated blood pressure response to exercise; massive left-ventricular hypertrophy (thickness ≥ 30 mm) (Maron et al. 2007; Maron 2010).

Surgery

Surgery for HCM is considered for patients with resting or provocable LV outflow tract obstruction with gradient equal to or >30 mmHg at rest or equal to or >50 mmHg during exercise and who have substantial symptoms that are refractory to optimal medical therapy (Fifer and Vlahakes 2008).

Surgical myectomy is the preferred treatment in the USA and Canada, but discarded in much of Europe in favor of alcohol ablation (Maron et al. 2011).

Septal Ablation

In skilled hands in high volume centers, nonsurgical septal ablation with intracoronary alcohol results in a marked immediate decrease in outflow tract gradient in about 80 % of patients (Faber et al. 2007).

Alcohol septal ablation increases arrhythmogenicity and is associated with an increased risk for complications such as heart block (requiring permanent pacing), generally less efficacious relief of gradient and symptoms (Maron and Nishimura 2014).

Apical HCM shows relatively small burden of myocardial fibrosis and less severe diastolic dysfunction, and subsequently more favorable clinical manifestations in comparison with other HCMs. This may be one explanation of why most patients with apical HCM show a benign course of disease compared to non-apical HC (Kim et al.2014).

DILATED CARDIOMYOPATHY

Diagnosis

A diagnosis of dilated cardiomyopathy (DCM) should be considered in a patient with right and left HF, documented global hypokinesis and dilatation of the left and/or right ventricles, and reduced systolic function in the absence of evidence of coronary artery disease, congenital, specific valvular, hypertensive, or specific heart muscle disease, and chronic excessive alcohol consumption.

- DCM is not caused by alcohol but can be exaggerated by it. A previous viral infection has been suspected in about 33 % of cases. Although previously considered to be only rarely familial, it is now known that a genetic basis exists; the locus affected appears to be associated with immunoregulation.
- Patients usually present at age 20–50, but the disease also occurs in children and in the elderly. More than 75 % of patients present with an initial episode of heart failure, New York Heart Association class III or IV. Careful screening of relatives has shown that up to 35 % of patients with DCM had a familial disease (Mestroni et al. 1999). Routine echocardiographic evaluation in all first degree relatives is therefore recommended.

A number of distinct subtypes of familial DCM have been identified:

1. Autosomal dominant, the most frequent form (56 %).
2. Autosomal recessive (16 %), characterized by worse prognosis.
3. X-linked (10 %), with different mutations of the dystrophin (Mestroni et al. 1999).

The disorder is characterized by enlargement of cardiac chambers, thin ventricular walls with poor contractility. Myocyte loss and interstitial fibrosis are the main histologic findings. Progressive dyspnea on exertion over weeks or months, USUALLY culminates in orthopnea, paroxysmal nocturnal dyspnea, and edema.

Physical Signs

Signs of right and left heart failure are prominent in late cases.

- The apex beat is displaced downward and outward to the left due to LV dilatation.
- Left lower parasternal lift or pulsation indicates right ventricular dilatation.

- The jugular venous pressure may be elevated and may show a systolic wave of tricuspid regurgitation.
- A soft grade I–II/VI systolic mitral murmur and a soft tricuspid systolic murmur are commonly present because of mitral and tricuspid regurgitation as a result of dilatation of the ventricles and valve rings, as well as papillary muscle dysfunction.
- S4 and S3 are constantly present, as well as sinus tachycardia; thus, a summation gallop is a frequent finding.
- The loud S3 is present in virtually all cases and is often heard when heart failure is absent. This hallmark serves to differentiate dilated cardiomyopathy from a class 4 ventricle due to coronary artery disease where a soft S3 is heard during episodes of heart failure, but is frequently absent or quite soft when the individual is assessed not to have heart failure and in the absence of LV aneurysm.

Echocardiogram

Findings include:

1. 1 Severe dilatation of both ventricles; there is global hypokinesis and commonly paradoxical movement of the septum;
2. Increased end systolic and end diastolic dimensions;
3. Ejection fraction (EF) usually less than 35 %; in the presence of heart failure. EF is usually 10–30 %;
4. Atrial enlargement and ventricular thrombi are commonly seen;
5. A small pericardial effusion is frequent.

Echocardiographic diagnosis can be made before overt heart failure has developed. Figure 23-3 shows salient features of dilated cardiomyopathy.

Therapy

Optimal management for heart failure should be instituted:

- Salt restriction.
- Avoidance of alcohol is necessary in all patients with heart failure and especially in the patient with a class 3 or 4 ventricle, because alcohol decreases the EF.

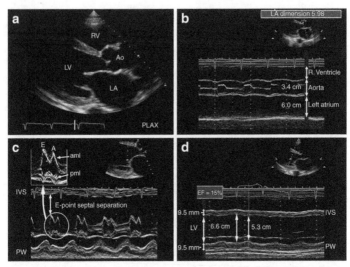

Fig. 23-3 Dilated cardiomyopathy. Left ventricular, left atrial, and right ventricular dilatation are seen in the parasternal long-axis view. (**a**) Wall thicknesses were within normal limits. Severe hypokinesis with akinetic segments and poor wall thickening are seen. Reduced systolic function leads to poor aortic valve opening, premature closure secondary to reduced stroke volume, and reduced anterior motion of aortic root during systole. (**b**) M-mode at the mitral valve level shows increased E-point septal separation. Note poor mitral valve closure, the akinetic septum, and the relatively preserved postero-basal segment. (**c**) M-mode more just distal to the mitral leaflets. (**d**) Shows dilated ventricular chambers with minimal excursion of the ventricular walls, little difference between systole and diastole, and calculated ejection fraction of 15 %. Reproduced with permission from Bulwer BE, Solomon SD: Cardiomyopathies. In: Solomon SD, Bulwer BE, editors. *Essential EchocardiographyN A Practical Handbook*. Totowa, NJ: Humana Press, 2007; p. 164. With kind permission from Springer Science+Business Media

Patients should be assessed for the presence of macroovalocytes, decreased platelet counts, and increased levels of gamma glutamyl transferase, which may indicate alcohol abuse with the patient's denial.

DIGOXIN

Digoxin provides some benefit in heart-failure patients in sinus rhythm and is indicated for atrial fibrillation with uncontrolled ventricular response. The dose should be adequate, but care is needed to avoid digitalis toxicity and to maintain a digoxin level 0.5–0.9 ng/mL (nmol/L) particularly in women. In patients with refractory heart failure, IV dobutamine may cause temporary "improvement."

DIURETICS

Diuretics play a vital role in the relief of symptoms and cannot be replaced by ACE inhibitors. The four groups of drugs, diuretics, digoxin, beta-blockers, and ACE inhibitors, are complimentary.

Furosemide at dosage of 40–80 mg daily is often necessary. The use of ACE inhibitors is often limited by hypotension. Patients with poor systolic function often have low systolic pressures (<110 mmHg), and it is sometimes necessary to discontinue diuretics for 24–48 h to permit the selected ACE inhibitors to be commenced. Caution is needed to avoid hypokalemia and magnesium depletion. The latter can be treated with magnesium glycerophosphate (3–6 g daily).

ACE INHIBITORS

These agents have made a major contribution to survival of patients with heart failure; however, diastolic dysfunction in patients with dilated cardiomyopathy tends to worsen with ACE inhibitor therapy.

BETA-BLOCKERS

Carvedilol, bisoprolol, metoprolol, and nebivolol are appropriate beta-blocking drugs; *the commonly prescribed atenolol is not advisable.*

Nebivolol: Fortunately, all beta-blockers are not alike. Nebivolol is a highly selective $beta_1$-adrenergic receptor blocker and is the only beta-blocker known to induce vascular production of nitric oxide, the main endothelial vasodilator. Nebivolol induces nitric oxide production via activation of beta$_3$-adrenergic receptors and stimulates the beta$_3$-adrenergic receptor-mediated production of nitric oxide in the heart; this stimulation results in a greater protection against heart failure (Maffei and Lembo 2009).

The SENIORS investigators studied 2,111 patients; 1,359 (64 %) had impaired (equal to or <35 %) EF (mean 28.7 %) and 752 (36 %) had preserved (>35 %) EF (mean 49.2 %). During follow-up of 21 months, the primary end point occurred in 465 patients (34.2 %) with impaired EF and in 235 patients (31.2 %) with preserved EF. The effect of nebivolol on the primary end point (hazard ratio (HR) of nebivolol versus placebo) was 0.86 (95 % confidence interval: 0.72–1.04) in patients with impaired EF and 0.81 [in preserved EF ($p=0.720$) for subgroup interaction].

The effect of beta-blockade with nebivolol in elderly patients with HF in this study was similar in those with preserved and impaired EF (van Veldhuisen et al. 2009).

Nebivolol requires further testing in large RCTs of heart failure patients including DCM.

ORAL ANTICOAGULANTS

Warfarin is advisable in most patients to prevent embolization from atrial and ventricular thrombi. The drug is necessary if there is atrial fibrillation.

RESTRICTIVE CARDIOMYOPATHY

The most common cause of RCM is endomyocardial fibrosis in tropical regions. In temperate climates, hypereosinophilic heart disease (Loffler's disease) may involve organs other than the heart. Myocardial involvement by amyloid, not associated with multiple organ involvement, is another cause of RCM in the Western world.

Cardiac disease resulting from amyloid-associated multiple organ involvement, sarcoid, hemochromatosis, eosinophilic syndromes, scleroderma, adriamycin toxicity, and infectious agents, including tuberculosis, causing restrictive physiology is considered as specific heart muscle.

Clinical Features

Clinical hallmarks of endomyocardial fibrosis include:

- Intermittent fever, shortness of breath, cough, palpitations, edema, and tiredness.
- Hypereosinophilia with abnormal eosinophil degranulationis seen in temperate climates (hypereosinophilic heart disease).
- Hypereosinophilia is less severe in tropical EMF.
- S3 and S4 gallops may be visible and audible in the absence of heart failure.
- Symptoms and signs of heart failure and of moderate to severe mitral and tricuspid regurgitation due to involvement of the papillary muscles serve to differentiate.

RCM from constrictive pericarditis, as does the greater degree of cardiac enlargement on chest X-ray in the former condition.

- During the early stages, EMF may mimic the hemodynamic and clinical features of constrictive pericarditis.

Chest X-Ray: The chest X-ray in patients with EMF may show extensive calcification of the right or left ventricular apical myocardium.

ECG findings are nonspecific. Marked ST-segment changes, deep T wave inversion, and LVH may be observed (See Fig. 23-4).

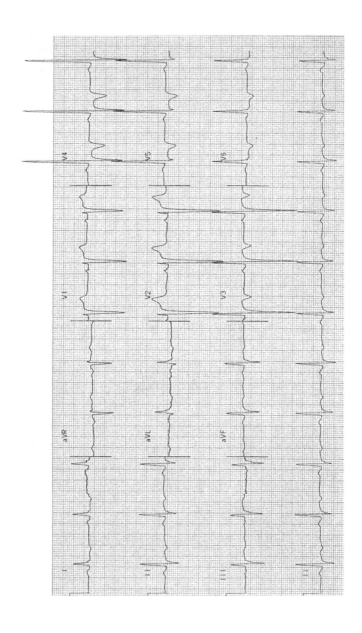

Fig. 23-4. ECG recording from a 29-year-old male with endomyocardial fibrosis, left ventricular hypertrophy, left atrial abnormality, and diffuse sinister looking ST-T-wave changes. These changes are unusual findings for individuals under age 30. Findings of deep T-wave inversion in the ECG of young individuals of African origin should suggest a diagnosis of restrictive cardiomyopathy. Echocardiogram showed extensive calcification and fibrosis of the endocardium of the LV apex and papillary muscles. Thrombus within the calcific fibrotic mass cannot be excluded. Numerous echogenic areas can be seen throughout the left ventricular endocardium. Some 20 years later, this man continues to have a normal lifestyle; walks up six flights of stairs without shortness of breath. He is relatively asymptomatic at age 50. His initial summation gallop rhythm at age 29 became subdued after about 10 years of daily enalapril 10 mg. The ECG remains as abnormal as it was 20 years ago. Reproduced with permission from Khan MG, *Encyclopedia of Heart Diseases*, 2nd edition. New York: Springer Science + Business Media; 2011. With kind permission from Springer Science + Business Media.

ECHOCARDIOGRAPHIC FINDINGS

- Obliteration of the apices of the ventricles by echogenic masses, likened to a boxing glove.
- Numerous echogenic areas are usually observed throughout the ventricular endocardium and myocardium.
- Also, myocardial calcification may be detected, and in later stages, mitral and tricuspid regurgitation may require further assessment.

Therapy

Medical therapy is unrewarding. Steroids may be helpful in the early acute inflammatory phase associated with hypereosinophilia. Hydroxyurea and vincristine have been used. Anticoagulants are necessary because thromboembolism is common. Restriction to filling does not respond to digoxin, diuretics, or vasodilators. Digoxin may be required to control the ventricular rate in patients with atrial fibrillation. If dyspnea is prominent, judicious trial of enalapril, 2.5–5 mg daily, should be tried; a salutary response has been observed in some patients. Arrhythmias may respond to small doses of beta-blockers, particularly nebivolol, which has shown salutary effects in patients with heart failure and normal EF.

- Potentially lethal arrhythmias may require amiodarone therapy.

Resection of masses of obliterating endocardial tissue with valve repair has produced apparent relief in some patients with EMF for a few years.

PERIPARTUM CARDIOMYOPATHY

Peripartum cardiomyopathy (PPCM) is a disorder in which initial left ventricular systolic dysfunction and symptoms of heart failure HF occur between the late stages of pregnancy and the early postpartum period (Sliwa et al. 2006a, b).

Criteria for diagnosis (1) the development of HF in the last month of pregnancy or within 5 months of delivery; (2) the absence of a determinable etiology for HF; and (3) the absence of demonstrable heart disease before the last month of pregnancy. (4) left ventricular systolic dysfunction with EF <45 %, fractional shortening <30 %, or both (Gersh et al. 2011 ACCF/AHA Guideline).

The cause and mechanism of pathogenesis of peripartum cardiomyopathy (PPCM) remain unknown, and many hypotheses have been proposed. Immune activation appears to contribute to the pathogenesis of PPCM (Sliwa et al. 2006a, b, 2000). There is no clear evidence to suggest viral involvement similar to that found in dilated cardiomyopathy.

Risk factors associated with PPCM have included age, gravidity, and most important African origin. An estimated incidence reveals one case per 299 live births in Haiti (Fett et al. 2005), one case per 1,000 live births in South Africa (Desai et al. 1995) to one case per 4,000 live births in the USA (Mielniczuk et al. 2006; Pearson et al. 2000).

- Gentry et al. indicated that African–American women have a higher risk for developing peripartum cardiomyopathy (Gentry et al. 2010).

Treatment

Anti-heart failure medications are used judiciously.

1. Furosemide 40–60 mg daily with maintenance of a normal serum potassium and avoidance of hypotension.
2. Beta-blockers: the use of beta-1-selective beta-blockers (bisoprolol, metoprolol) is preferred, because nonselective beta-blockade could facilitate uterine activity. These agents control tachycardia and arrhythmias and are necessary for the treatment of HF Class II–III. They can be used for compensated class IV HF. A small dose of bisoprolol 2.5 mg daily increased only after several days if needed to 5 mg

should suffice. See Chap. 20 for advice on drugs in mother's milk; propranolol is advisable.

3. Hydralazine for after-load reduction replaces ACE inhibitors that are contraindicated in pregnancy.
4. Digoxin is useful and safe when used by a watchful physician with regard for renal dysfunction and maintaining a digoxin level in the low range: 0.5–1.0 ng/mL.
5. Pentoxifylline promising results have been obtained with pentoxifylline in a non-randomized trial (Sliwa et al. 2005).
6. Data from 40 patients with longitudinal follow-up of 30±29 months showed that improvement usually occurred within the first 6 months after the diagnosis (Elkayam 2011).

Elective cesarean section is advisable. This can be done more rapidly and allows better planning of the time of delivery. Also, it assures the presence of the most experienced medical team during the delivery (Gersh et al. 2011 ACCF/AHA Guideline).

REFERENCES

Desai D, Moodley J, Naidoo D. Peripartum cardiomyopathy: experiences at King Edward VIII Hospital, Durban, South Africa and a review of the literature. Trop Doct. 1995;25:118–23.

Elkayam U. Clinical Characteristics of peripartum cardiomyopathy in the United States: diagnosis, prognosis, and management. J Am Coll Cardiol. 2011;58:659–70.

Faber L, Welge D, Fassbender D, et al. Percutaneous septal ablation for symptomatic hypertrophic obstructive cardiomyopathy: managing the risk of procedure-related AV conduction disturbances. Int J Cardiol. 2007;19:163–7.

Fett JD, Christie LG, Carraway RD, et al. Five-year prospective study of the incidence and prognosis of peripartum cardiomyopathy at a single institution. Mayo Clin Proc. 2005;80:1602–6.

Fifer MA, Vlahakes GJ. Management of symptoms in hypertrophic cardiomyopathy. Circulation. 2008;117:429–39.

Frank MJ, Abdulla AM, Canedo MI, et al. Long-term medical management of hypertrophic obstructive cardiomyopathy. Am J Cardiol. 1978;42:993–1001.

Gentry MB, Dias JK, Luis A, et al. African-American women have a higher risk for developing peripartum cardiomyopathy. J Am Coll Cardiol. 2010;55:654–9.

Gersh BJ, Maron BJ, Bonow RO, et al. ACCF/AHA Guideline for the Diagnosis and Treatment of Hypertrophic Cardiomyopathy: a report of the American College of Cardiology Foundation/American Heart Association Task Force on Practice Guidelines American Association for Thoracic Surgery, American Society of Echocardiography, American Society of Nuclear Cardiology, Heart Failure Society of America, Heart Rhythm Society, Society for Cardiovascular Angiography and Interventions, Society of Thoracic Surgeons. J Am Coll Cardiol. 2011;58:e212–60. doi:10.1016/j.jacc.2011.06.011.

Khan MG. Acute myocardial infarction. In: Heart disease diagnosis and therapy, a practical approach. Totowa, NJ: Humana Press; 2005. p. 55.

Lipshultz SE, Orav EJ, Wilkinson JD, et al. Risk stratification at diagnosis for children with hypertrophic cardiomyopathy: an analysis of data from the Pediatric Cardiomyopathy Registry. Lancet. 2013;382: 1889–97.

Maffei A, Lembo G. Nitric oxide mechanisms of nebivolol. Ther Adv Cardiovasc Dis. 2009;3(4):317–27.

Mestroni L, Rocco C, Gregori D, et al. Familial dilated cardiomyopathy: evidence for genetic and phenotypic heterogeneity. Heart Muscle Disease Study Group. J Am Coll Cardiol. 1999;34:181–90.

Maron BJ. Contemporary insights and strategies for risk stratification and prevention of sudden death in hypertrophic cardiomyopathy. Circulation. 2010;121(3):445–56.

Maron BJ, Olivotto I, Spirito P, et al. Epidemiology of hypertrophic cardiomyopathy-related death: revisited in a large non-referral-based patient population. Circulation. 2000;102:858–64.

Maron BJ, Epstein SE, Roberts WC. Causes of sudden death in competitive athletes. J Am Coll Cardiol. 1986;7(1):204–14.

Maron BJ, McKenna WJ, Danielson GK, et al. For the Task Force on Clinical Expert Consensus Documents, American College of Cardiology; Committee for Practice Guidelines, European Society of Cardiology. American College of Cardiology/European Society of Cardiology clinical expert consensus document on hypertrophic cardiomyopathy: a report of the American College of Cardiology Foundation Task Force on Clinical Expert Consensus Documents and the European Society of Cardiology Committee for Practice Guidelines. J Am Coll Cardiol. 2003;42:1687–713.

Maron BJ, Spirito P, Shen W-K, et al. Implantable cardioverter defibrillators and prevention of sudden cardiac death in hypertrophic cardiomyopathy. JAMA. 2007;298:405–12.

Maron MS, Olivotto I, Zenovich AG, et al. Hypertrophic cardiomyopathy is predominantly a disease of left ventricular outflow tract obstruction. Circulation. 2006;114:2232–9.

Maron BJ, Maron MS. Hypertrophic cardiomyopathy. Lancet. 2013;381(9862):242–55.

Maron BJ, Nishimura RA. Revisiting arrhythmic risk after alcohol septal ablation: is the pendulum finally swinging … back to myectomy?* JCHF. http://clicks.skem1.com/trkr/?c=14833&g=156879&p=3b08379 2ca737c74e545411369a4fd3f&u=006620f95d14b895ee34b24076ca14 38&q=&t=1. Accessed 22 Oct 2014. doi:10.1016/j.jchf.2014.07.008.

Maron BJ, Yacoub M, Dearani JA. Benefits of surgery in obstructive hypertrophic cardiomyopathy: bring septal myectomy back for European patients. Eur Heart J. 2011;32:1055–8.

McLeod CJ, Ackerman MJ, Nishimura RA, Tajik AJ, Gersh BJ, Ommen SR. Outcome of patients with hypertrophic cardiomyopathy and a normal electrocardiogram. J Am Coll Cardiol. 2009;54:229–33.

Mielniczuk LM, Williams K, Davis DR, et al. Frequency of peripartum cardiomyopathy. Am J Cardiol. 2006;97:1765–8.

Nishimura RA, Ommen SR. Hypertrophic cardiomyopathy, sudden death, and implantable cardiac defibrillators how low the bar? JAMA. 2007;298:452–4.

Pearson GD, Veille JC, Rahimtoola S, et al. Peripartum cardiomyopathy. National heart, lung, and blood institute and office of rare diseases (National Institutes of Health) workshop recommendations and review. JAMA. 2000;283:1183–8.

Sliwa K, Damasceno A, Mayosi B. Cardiomyopathy in Africa. Circulation. 2005;112:3577–83.

Sliwa K, Fett J, Elkayam U. Peripartum cardiomyopathy. Lancet. 2006a;368:687–93.

Sliwa K, Forster O, Libhaber E, et al. Peripartum cardiomyopathy: inflammatory markers as predictors of outcome in 100 prospectively studied patients. Eur Heart J. 2006b;27:441–6.

Sliwa K, Skudicky D, Bergemann A, et al. Peripartum cardiomyopathy: analysis of clinical outcome, left ventricular function, plasma levels of cytokines and Fas/Apo-1. J Am Coll Cardiol. 2000;35:701–5.

Sliwa K, Skukicky D, Candy G, et al. The addition of pentoxifylline to conventional therapy improves outcome in patients with peripartum cardiomyopathy. Eur J Heart Fail. 2002;4:305–9.

Tuncer M, Fettser DV, Gunes Y, et al. Comparison of effects of nebivolol and atenolol on P-wave dispersion in patients with hypertension (in Russian). Kardiologiia. 2008;48:42–5.

van Veldhuisen DJ, Cohen-Solal A, Bohm M, SENIORS Investigators, et al. Beta-blockade with nebivolol in elderly heart failure patients with impaired and preserved left ventricular ejection fraction: data from SENIORS (Study of Effects of Nebivolol Intervention on Outcomes and Rehospitalization in Seniors with Heart Failure). J Am Coll Cardiol. 2009;53:2150–58.

24 Newer Agents

APIXABAN

Patients with AF have a fivefold increased risk of stroke, particularly in patients with valvular heart disease and in the elderly. It is estimated that 15–20 % of all strokes are attributable to AF. Four new agents [apixaban, dabigatran, edoxaban, and rivaroxaban] are vying to replace or greatly reduce the use of the well-tried warfarin. There is little doubt that warfarin is underused and in many the international normalized ratio [INR] is not in the desired range 2–3.

Apixaban is an oral direct factor Xa inhibitor. Bioavailability is high. Importantly, **elimination is only 25 % renal**, and half-life ≈ 12 h. Similar to rivaroxaban, cytochrome P450 3A4 is involved in the metabolism so that strong inhibitors substantially increase drug levels (Eikelboom and Weitz 2010).

ARISTOTLE.Granger et al 2011: [Apixaban for Reduction in Stroke and Other Thromboembolic Events in Atrial Fibrillation trial] In this double-blind design trial 18,201 patients with nonvalvular atrial fibrillation and at least one additional risk factor for stroke were enrolled and randomly assigned to receive the direct factor Xa inhibitor apixaban (at a dose of 5 mg twice daily) or warfarin (target INR, 2.0–3.0).

Results: Apixaban was not only noninferior to warfarin, but actually superior, reducing the risk of stroke or systemic embolism by 21 % and the risk of major bleeding by 31 %. As compared with warfarin, apixaban significantly reduced the risk of death from any cause by 11 %. Apixaban is the

© Springer Science+Business Media New York 2015
M. Gabriel Khan, *Cardiac Drug Therapy*, Contemporary Cardiology,
DOI 10.1007/978-1-61779-962-4_24

Table 24-1
Newer anticoagulants compared with Warfarin

	Total mortality	Stroke
Apixaban	3.52 % / *3.94 %; p=0.047	1.27 %/*1.60 % P 0.01
Dabigatran#	3.75 % / *4.13 %; p=0.13	1.1 % / *1.69 P<0.001
Rivaroxaban	4.5 % / *4.9 %; p=0.15	2.12 / *2.42 P 0.12
Major bleeding		
Apixaban	2.13 % / *3.09 %; p <0.001	
Dabigatran#	3.64 % / *4.13 %; p=0.13	
Rivaroxaban	3.6 % / *3.45 %; p=0.58	

/* Warfarin column

Apixaban 5 mg twice daily renal elimination ~25 %

#Dabigatran 150 mg twice daily [110 mg twice daily stroke 1.5 vs warfarin 1.7 p 0.34; but major bleeding significantly reduced 2.7 % vs 3.36 % p 0.003] caution, ~80 % renal elimination

Rivaroxaban 20 mg daily renal elimination ~ 33 %

Caution: no antidote/agent is available if bleeding occurs with newer agents.

Modified with permission from Granger, CB, Armaganijan, LV. Should newer oral anticoagulants be used as first-line agents to prevent thromboembolism in patients with atrial fibrillation and risk factors for stroke or thromboembolism? *Circulation* January 3 2012; 125: 159–64

first of the newer anticoagulants to show a significant reduction in the risk of death from any cause as compared with warfarin (hazard ratio, 0.89; $P = 0.047$). See Table 24-1.

AVERROES compared the efficacy of apixaban 5 mg twice daily with aspirin (81–325 mg once daily) for stroke and systemic embolism prevention in 5599 AF patients considered unsuitable for vitamin K antagonist treatment. The trial was stopped early on recommendation by the Data and Safety Monitoring Board because of clear benefits in regard to stroke reduction favoring apixaban (hazard ratio, 0.46;

$P < 0.001$). Strikingly, apixaban was associated with rates of major bleeding similar to those observed with aspirin (Connolly et al 2011).

Apixaban was better tolerated than aspirin. At 2 years, the rates of permanent discontinuation of the study medication were 17.9 % per year in the apixaban group and 20.5 % per year in the aspirin group (Connolly et al 2011). Apaxiban, compared with warfarin, was associated with fewer intracranial hemorrhages, less adverse events following extracranial hemorrhage, and a 50 % reduction in fatal consequences at 30 days in cases of major hemorrhage (Hylek et al. 2014).

In an RCT Apixaban was superior to enoxaparin VTE prophylaxis after hip replacement.

- Apixaban renal elimination, 25 % is better than dabigatran 80 %, *edoxaban* 40 % rivaroxaban 33 %. Atrial fibrillation is most common in the elderly,and renal function is abnormal in more than 50 % of elderly subjects.

RIVAROXABAN

Rivaroxaban is an oral direct inhibitor of factor Xa with high bioavailability, **Elimination is 33**% **renal**; the half-life ≈ 9–12 h, peak plasma level 2.5–4 h (Abrams and Emerson 2009)

A new drug for myocardial infarction: Rivaroxaban

The ROCKET investigators (Mega et al. 2012) randomly assigned 15,526 patients with a recent acute coronary syndrome [~ STEMI ~ 50 %, NSTEMI ` 25 %, unstable angina %] to receive twice-daily doses of either 2.5 mg or 5 mg of rivaroxaban or placebo for a mean of 13 months and up to 31 months. The primary efficacy end point was a composite of death from cardiovascular causes, myocardial infarction, or stroke (Mega et al. 2012). Rivaroxaban significantly reduced the primary efficacy end point of death from cardiovascular causes, myocardial infarction [MI], or stroke, as compared with placebo, with rates of 8.9 % and 10.7 %, respectively, $P = 0.008$. The twice-daily 2.5-mg dose of rivaroxaban reduced the rates of death from cardiovascular causes (2.7 % vs. 4.1 %, $P=0.002$) and from any cause (2.9 % vs. 4.5 %, $P=0.002$). Importantly, rivaroxaban reduced the risk of stent thrombosis (Mega et al. 2012).

ROCKET AF. (Patel et al. 2011) compared *a once-daily*, fixed dose of rivaroxaban [20 mg] with adjusted-dose warfarin in patients with nonvalvular atrial fibrillation who were at moderate-to-high risk for stroke; rivaroxaban was noninferior to warfarin in the prevention of subsequent stroke or systemic embolism. There was no significant between-group difference in the risk of major bleeding, although intracranial and fatal bleeding occurred less frequently in the rivaroxaban group. In this double-blind design trial rates of intracranial hemorrhage were significantly lower in the rivaroxaban group than in the warfarin group (0.5 % vs. 0.7 % per year; hazard ratio, 0.67; $P=0.02$).

- Elderly patients had higher stroke and major bleeding rates than younger patients, but the efficacy and safety of rivaroxaban relative to warfarin did not differ with age, supporting rivaroxaban as an alternative for the elderly (Halperin et al. 2014).

The FDA has approved the oral direct factor Xa inhibitor rivaroxaban (Xarelto) for prevention of stroke in patients with **nonvalvular a**trial fibrillation. See Chap. 22 for details.

DABIGATRAN

Dabigatran etexilate is hydrolyzed to the active dabigatran, with maximum activity ≈ 1 h after administration. ***Elimination is 80 % renal***; the half-life is 12–17 h.

The RE-LY trial evaluated the direct thrombin inhibitor dabigatran 110 mg and 150 mg, administered twice daily in patients with no valvular atrial fibrillation. **The assignments to dabigatran or warfarin were, however, not**

concealed. The ROCKET AF and ARISTOTLE trials achieved a double-blind design.

In patients with *nonvalvular* atrial fibrillation, dabigatran given at a dose of 110 mg was associated with rates of stroke and systemic embolism that were similar to those associated with warfarin, as well as lower rates of major hemorrhage, but this dose is not approved by some National bodies. The 150 mg dose, approved by the FDA as compared with warfarin, was associated with lower rates of stroke, but similar rates of major hemorrhage (Connolly et al. 2009).

The rate of MI, however, was 0.53 % per year with warfarin and was higher with dabigatran: 0.72 % per year in the 110-mg group (relative risk, 1.35; 95 % CI, 0.98–1.87; $P=0.07$) and 0.74 % per year in the 150-mg group (relative risk, 1.38, $P=0.048$) (Connolly et al. 2009).

There was a significantly higher rate of major gastrointestinal bleeding with dabigatran at the 150-mg dose than with warfarin. Rates of dyspepsia and including abdominal pain were more common with dabigatran (11.8 % in the 110-mg group and 11.3 % in the 150-mg group) as compared with warfarin (5.8 %) (Connolly et al. 2009).

- Because of dabigatran's twice-daily dosing, mainly renal elimination [=higher risk in elderly], greater risk of non-hemorrhagic side effects and controversy relating to an increased MI risk patients already taking warfarin with excellent INR control have little to gain by switching to dabigatran.
- Follow-up was 2 years, so the hepatic risks of long-term use are unclear (Gage 2009). The 110 mg dose [not FDA approved] is advisable in selected patients over age 75 if renal function is not much diminished > 55 ml/min. Avoid in patients with more severe renal dysfunction.

Gastrointestinal bleeding was more common with higher-dose dabigatran than warfarin, and dyspepsia was more common with dabigatran (11.8 % of patients with 110 mg and 11.3 % of patients with 150 mg compared with 5.8 %

with warfarin; $P < 0.001$ for both) (Connolly et al. 2009). There was a small increased risk for acute MI.

Edoxaban

This oral, direct factor Xa inhibitor attains maximum plasma concentration in < 2 h; the half-life is 8–10 h. Elimination is ~ 40 % renal (Ruff et al 2010). The Effective Anticoagulation With Factor Xa Next Generation in Atrial Fibrillation (ENGAGE AF-TIMI 48) trial has randomized >20,000 patients who have AF and a CHADS2 score of ≥2. (Acronym for heart failure, hypertension, age ≥75 years, diabetes, and prior stroke or TIA).

Patients were randomized in a double-blind fashion to warfarin (target INR, 2.0–3.0) or 1 of 2 doses of edoxaban given once daily, 25 with dose adjustments both at baseline and subsequently for factors associated with higher drug exposure, including renal insufficiency (Ruff et al 2010). Both once-daily administration of edoxaban were noninferior to warfarin for the prevention of stroke or systemic embolism and were associated with significantly lower rates of bleeding and death from cardiovascular causes (Giugliano et al. 2013).

CONCLUSION

There are disadvantages of newer agents (Ansell 2012)

- Cost: the estimated cost of one of the new agents already on the market is ≈ \$3,000 per year versus ≈ \$50 per year for warfarin (Avorn 2011).
- Interactions: the serum levels of most of the new agents may be altered because these agents are metabolized, in part, by the P450 cytochrome system in the liver (particularly CYP 3A4) (Walenga and Adiguzel 2010).
- Because dabigatran is predominantly eliminated unchanged by the kidney and other agents have greater or lesser degrees of renal elimination, fluctuating renal function is another variable that must be considered carefully, particularly

decreased renal function in most elderly. **Chronic atrial fibrillation is a disease mainly of the elderly; thus dabigatran use may be is restricted**.

- Although apixaban, rivaroxaban, endoxaban, and dabigatran have a more rapid onset and termination of anticoagulant action than warfarin, agents to reverse the effect of the drugs are not available. Costs mainly will perpetuate the continued use of warfarin worldwide in most patients with atrial fibrillation.

- Apixaban presently has advantages over the three other agents: mortality benefit shown, and low renal elimination would lend to less major bleeding in the elderly with unsuspected renal dysfunction. Also less GI bleeding has been observed compared with dabigatran and rivaroxaban.

- **Most important, patients at high risk, particularly the many with valvular heart disease, require warfarin therapy until these agents are tested in RCTs**.

OMECAMTIV MECARBILA

This selective cardiac myosin activator prolongs systole. This agent has reached the phase 2 stage of clinical development for treatment of systolic heart failure. Omecamtiv mecarbil improved cardiac function in patients with heart failure caused by left ventricular dysfunction and could be the first in class of a new therapeutic agent and might provide an alternative to existing inotropic drugs. See Chap. 22 for details (Cleland et al 2011).

The first-in-man data show highly dose-dependent augmentation of left ventricular systolic function in response to omecamtiv mecarbil and support potential clinical use of the drug in patients with heart failure (Teerlink et al 2011).

CELIVARONE

This is a new benzofuran derivative with an electrophysiologic profile similar to amiodarone which showed promising results in a pilot ICD study. It can be considered a daughter of dronedarone. Implantable cardioverter defibrillators (ICDs) improve survival in patients at risk of VT/VF. Many ICD patients need adjunctive therapy with amiodarone or sotalol that have incomplete efficacy in preventing bothersome frequency of ICD shocks, VT/VF, or sudden death. A total of 486 patients with an ICD, EF≤40 %, and at least one appropriate ICD intervention or implanted during the previous month were randomized to receive celivarone 50 mg, 100 mg, 300 mg, placebo, or amiodarone 200 mg (after loading dose of 600 mg for 10 days) once daily.

The drug failed to prevent events: a negative trial. Amiodarone significantly prevented shocks but increased mortality including sudden death (Kowey for the ALPHEE Investigators AHA scientific meeting 2011).

DRONEDARONE

Dronedarone is a multichannel blocking antiarrhythmic drug with electrophysiologic properties similar to amiodarone, but it does not contain iodine. In the UK dronedarone is an option for the treatment of non-permanent atrial fibrillation only in patients who are not controlled on first-line therapy (usually including beta-blockers) and do not have unstable III or IV heart failure. Adverse effects include QT prolongation, increases in serum creatinine, and rarely liver injury, including life-threatening acute liver failure.

The international multicenter PALLAS Study enrolled patients with documented permanent AF for greater than 6 months who also had prior stroke, MI, coronary artery disease, EF≤40 %, and heart failure symptoms with hospitalization for heart failure between 1 and 12 months prior to enrolment. Patients were randomized to receive either dronedarone 400 mg BID or matching double-blind placebo.

After enrolment of 3,149 patients, the Data Monitoring Committee recommended that the study be stopped due to highly significant excesses of events in the active group for both co-primary outcomes as well as hospitalizations and heart failure events with no evidence of benefit in other secondary end points (Connolly et al. 2011 AHA scientific session). **The drug is not advisable**; **use is not justified**.

NEBIVOLOL

Licensed for stable mild-to-moderate heart failure in patients over 70 years; the drug is a useful addition to our therapeutic armamentarium. Proven for heart failure in the elderly and particularly in those with a preserved EF (Seniors 2009).

Dosage: For heart failure, mainly in patients 70 years and older: initially 1.25 mg once daily, then if tolerated increased at intervals of 1–2 weeks to 2.5 mg once daily, then to 5 mg once daily, and then to max. 10 mg once daily. Caution in patients with renal failure. See Chap. 13. Importantly nebivolol appears to be the only agent shown to have salutary effects in heart failure patients with preserved EF.

Nebivolol and valsartan fixed-dose combination proved to be an effective and well-tolerated treatment option for patients with hypertension (Giles et al. 2014).

PRASUGREL [EFIENT IN UK]

In TRITON–TIMI 38 RCT, prasugrel showed a consistent benefit over clopidogrel for reducing cardiovascular death, MI, stroke, urgent revascularization, and stent thrombosis in patients who did or did not receive a GP IIb/IIIa blocker ."A loading dose of 60 mg prasugrel achieves faster, more consistent, and greater inhibition of ADP-induced platelet aggregation than does 600 mg of clopidogrel, with a significant effect seen 30 min after administration of prasugrel when no effect is detectable with clopidogrel" (Wiviott et al. 2007, Wallentin et al. 2008). Prasugrel is more effective than clopidogrel for the prevention of ischemic events, without an apparent excess in bleeding (Montalescot et al. 2009). Caution: Renal or hepatic dysfunction. Contraindications are active bleeding and history of stroke or transient ischemic attack.

Among patients with unstable angina or non-ST segment elevation MI, prasugrel did not significantly reduce the frequency of the primary end point, as compared with clopidogrel, and similar risks of bleeding were observed (Roe et al. 2012).

TICAGRELOR [BRILINTA; BRILIQUE IN UK]

The PLATO investigators (2010) compared ticagrelor with clopidogrel. Subjects were 13,408 (72 %) of 18,624 patients hospitalized for STEMI and NSTEMI. Patients were randomly assigned to ticagrelor and placebo (180-mg loading dose followed by 90 mg twice a day) or to clopidogrel and placebo (300–600-mg loading dose or continuation with maintenance dose followed by 75 mg/day) for 6–12 months. All patients were given aspirin. At 1 year, the primary composite end point occurred in fewer patients in the 6,732 ticagrelor-treated group than in the 6,676 clopidogrel group: 569 (event rate 9 %) versus 668 (10.7 %, hazard ratio 0.84, $p=0.0025$).

- Importantly, ticagrelor compared with clopidogrel significantly reduced all-cause mortality at 12 months in all patients (4.5 % vs. 5.9 %, hazard ratio 0.78, $p<0.001$) and in patients undergoing an early invasive strategy (3.9 % vs. 5 %, hazard ratio 0.81, $p=0.01$).
- Unlike clopidogrel and prasugrel, which bind irreversibly to the platelet surface-membrane (P2Y12) receptor, ticagrelor is a reversible P2Y12 receptor blocker, with platelet function returning to normal, 2–3 days after discontinuation (Gurbel et al. 2009) compared with 5–10 days after discontinuation of clopidogrel and prasugrel. In addition within 30 min, a ticagrelor loading dose of 180 mg results in roughly the same level of inhibition of platelet aggregation as that achieved 8 h after a clopidogrel loading dose of 600 mg (Gurbel et al. 2009).

CAUTION: Asthma or chronic obstructive pulmonary disease; history of hyperuricemia; assess renal function within 1 month interactions may occur: see Chap. 22.

CANGRELOR

Cangrelor has been shown to significantly reduce the rate of ischemic events, including stent thrombosis, during PCI, with no significant increase in severe bleeding (Bhatt et al. 2013). Patients with an acute coronary syndrome may benefit from prasugrel or ticagrelor before PCI, as compared with clopidogrel, but these are oral agents. Some patients undergoing PCI may benefit from an intravenous ADP-receptor antagonist, such as cangrelor, but the routine use of this therapy for all patients undergoing PCI is not yet justified (Lange and Hillis 2013).

EVACETRAPIB

In combination with statin therapy, evacetrapib, 100 mg/day, produced increases in HDL-C of 42.1–50.5 mg/dL (78.5 % to 88.5 %; $P<0.001$ for all compared with statin monotherapy) and decreases in LDL-C of −67.1 to −75.8 mg/dL (−11.2 % to −13.9 %; $P<0.001$ for all compared with statin monotherapy). Compared with placebo or statin monotherapy, evacetrapib as monotherapy or in combination with statins increased HDL-C levels and decreased LDL-C levels and no adverse effects were observed (Nicholls et al. 2011). "165 Japanese patients with elevated LDL-C or low HDL-C levels were randomly assigned to receive placebo, evacetrapib monotherapy 30 mg, 100 mg, or 500 mg, atorvastatin 10 mg, or evacetrapib 100 mg in combination with atorvastatin 10 mg. After 12 weeks, evacetrapib monotherapy increased HDL-C levels by 74 %, 115 %, and 136 % and decreased LDL-C levels by 15 %, 23 %, and 22 % and CETP activity by 50 %, 83 %, and 95 % (for the 30-mg, 100-mg, and 500-mg dose groups, respectively) versus placebo" (Teramoto et al. 2014).

REFERENCES

Abrams PJ, Emerson CR. Rivaroxaban: a novel, oral, direct factor Xa inhibitor. Pharmacotherapy. 2009;29:167–81.

Ansell J. Should newer oral anticoagulants be used as first-line agents to prevent thromboembolism in patients with atrial fibrillation and risk factors for stroke or thromboembolism?: new oral anticoagulants should not be used as first-line agents to prevent thromboembolism in patients with atrial fibrillation. Circulation. 2012;125:165–70.

ARISTOTLE, Granger CB, Alexander JH, McMurray JJV, et al. Apixaban. GRANGER IS IN versus warfarin in patients with atrial fibrillation. N Engl J Med. 2011;365:981–92.

Avorn J. The relative cost-effectiveness of anticoagulants: obvious, except for the cost and the effectiveness. Circulation. 2011;123:2519–21.

Bhatt DL, Stone GW, Mahaffey KW, et al. Effect of platelet inhibition with cangrelor during PCI on ischemic events. N Engl J Med. 2013;368:1303–13.

Cleland JGF, Teerlink JR, Senior R, et al. The effects of the cardiac myosin activator, omecamtiv mecarbil, on cardiac function in systolic heart failure: a double-blind, placebo-controlled, crossover, dose-ranging phase 2 trial. Lancet. 2011;378:676–83.

Connolly SJ, EzekowitzMD, Yusuf S, et al. Dabigatran versus warfarin in patients with atrial fibrillation. N Engl J Med. 2009;361:1139–51. (and the RE-LY Steering Committee and Investigators).

Connolly SJ, Eikelboom J, Joyner C, et al. for the AVERROES Steering Committee and Investigators .Apixaban in patients with atrial fibrillation. N Engl J Med. 2011;364:806–17.

Eikelboom JW, Weitz JI. New anticoagulants. Circulation. 2010;121: 1523–32.

Gage BF. Can we rely on RE-LY? N Engl J Med. 2009;361:1200–2.

Giles TD, Weber MA, Basile J, for the NAC-MD-01 Study Investigators, et al. Efficacy and safety of nebivolol and valsartan as fixed-dose combination in hypertension: a randomised, multicentre study. Lancet. 2014;383:1889–98.

Giugliano RP, Ruff CT, Braunwald E, et al. Edoxaban versus warfarin in patients with atrial fibrillation. N Engl J Med. 2013;369(22):2093–104.

Gurbel PA, Bliden KP, Butler K, et al. Randomized double-blind assessment of the ONSET and OFFSET of the antiplatelet effects of ticagrelor versus clopidogrel in patients with stable coronary artery disease: the ONSET/OFFSET study. Circulation. 2009;120(2577–2585):2009.

Hylek EM, Held C, Alexander JH, et al. Major bleeding in patients with atrial fibrillation receiving apixaban or warfarin The ARISTOTLE Trial (Apixaban for reduction in stroke and other thromboembolic events in atrial fibrillation) Predictors, characteristics, and clinical outcomes. J Am Coll Cardiol. 2014;63(20):2141–7.

Lange RA, Hillis LD. The duel between dual antiplatelet therapies. N Engl J Med. 2013;368:1356–7.

Mega JL, Braunwald E, Wiviott SD, et al. Rivaroxaban in patients with a recent acute coronary syndrome. N Engl J Med. 2012;366:9–19.

Nicholls SJ, Ballantyne CM, Barter PJ, et al. Effect of two intensive statin regimens on progression of coronary disease. N Engl J Med. 2011;365:2078–87.

PLATO (for the PLATelet inhibition and patient Outcomes investigators), Cannon CP, Harrington RA, James S, et al. Comparison of ticagrelor with clopidogrel in patients with a planned invasive strategy for acute coronary syndromes: a randomised double-blind study. Lancet. 2010;375(9711):283–93.

ROCKET: AF, Patel MR, Mahaffey KW, Garg J, et al. Rivaroxaban versus warfarin in nonvalvular atrial fibrillation. N Engl J Med. 2011;365:883–91.

ROCKET AF: Halperin JL, Hankey GJ, Wojdyla DM, On behalf of the ROCKET AF Steering Committee and Investigators. Efficacy and safety of rivaroxaban compared with warfarin among elderly patients with nonvalvular atrial fibrillation in the rivaroxaban once daily, oral, direct factor Xa inhibition compared with vitamin K antagonism for prevention of stroke and embolism trial in atrial fibrillation. Circulation. 2014;130:138–46.

Roe MT, Armstrong PW, Fox KAA, et al. Prasugrel versus clopidogrel for acute coronary syndromes without revascularization. N Engl J Med. 2012;367:1297–309.

Ruff CT, Giugliano RP, Antman EM, Crugnale SE, Bocanegra T, Mercuri M, et al. Evaluation of the novel factor Xa inhibitor edoxaban compared with warfarin in patients with atrial fibrillation: design and rationale for the Effective Anticoagulation With Factor Xa Next Generation in Atrial Fibrillation-Thrombolysis in Myocardial Infarction Study 48 (ENGAGE AF-TIMI 48). Am Heart J. 2010;160:635–41.

SENIORS Investigators, van Veldhuisen DJ, Cohen-Solal A, Bohm M, et al. Beta-blockade with nebivolol in elderly heart failure patients with impaired and preserved left ventricular ejection fraction: data from SENIORS (Study of Effects of Nebivolol Intervention on Outcomes and Rehospitalization in Seniors With Heart Failure). J Am Coll Cardiol. 2009;2009(53):2150–8.

Teerlink JR, Clarke CP, Saikali KG, et al. Dose-dependent augmentation of cardiac systolic function with the selective cardiac myosin activator, omecamtiv mecarbil: a first-in-man study. Lancet. 2011;378:667–75.

Teramoto T, Takeuchi M, Morisaki Y, et al. Efficacy, safety, tolerability, and pharmacokinetic profile of *Evacetrapib* administered as monotherapy or in combination with *Atorvastatin* in Japanese patients with dyslipidemia. Am J Cardiol. 2014;113:2021–9.

TRITON-TIMI 38 Investigators, Montalescot G, Wiviott SD, Braunwald E, et al. Prasugrel compared with clopidogrel in patients undergoing percutaneous coronary intervention for ST-elevation myocardial infarction (TRITONTIMI 38): double-blind, randomised controlled trial. Lancet. 2009;373(9665):723–31. (TRITON-TIMI 38 Investigators).

Walenga JM, Adiguzel C. Drug and dietary interactions of the new and emerging oral anticoagulants. Int J Clin Pract. 2010;64:956–67.

Wallentin L, Varenhorst C, James S, et al. Prasugrel achieves greater and faster P2Y12receptor-mediated platelet inhibition than clopidogrel due to more efficient generation of its active metabolite in aspirin-treated patients with coronary artery disease. Eur Heart J. 2008;29:21–30.

Wiviott SD, Trenk D, Frelinger AL, et al. Prasugrel compared with high loading- and maintenance-dose clopidogrel in patients with planned percutaneous coronary intervention: the Prasugrel in comparison to clopidogrel for inhibition of platelet activation and aggregation-thrombolysis in myocardial infarction 44 trial. Circulation. 2007;116:2923–32.

INDEX

© Springer Science+Business Media New York 2015
M. Gabriel Khan, *Cardiac Drug Therapy*, Contemporary Cardiology,
DOI 10.1007/978-1-61779-962-4

CPSIA information can be obtained
at www.ICGtesting.com
Printed in the USA
LVHW081935231118
597991LV00001B/1/P